2015 International Conference on

Computer Science and Engineering Technology (CSET2015), Medical Science and Biological Engineering (MSBE2015)

2015 International Conference on

Computer Science and Engineering Technology (CSET2015), Medical Science and Biological Engineering (MSBE2015)

Editors

Jiamei Deng

Kingston University, United Kingdom
Guest Editor of CSET2015

Qingjun Liu

Zhejiang University, China
Guest Editor of MSBE2015

World Scientific

NEW JERSEY • LONDON • SINGAPORE • BEIJING • SHANGHAI • HONG KONG • TAIPEI • CHENNAI

Published by

World Scientific Publishing Co. Pte. Ltd.
5 Toh Tuck Link, Singapore 596224
USA office: 27 Warren Street, Suite 401-402, Hackensack, NJ 07601
UK office: 57 Shelton Street, Covent Garden, London WC2H 9HE

British Library Cataloguing-in-Publication Data
A catalogue record for this book is available from the British Library.

COMPUTER SCIENCE AND ENGINEERING TECHNOLOGY (CSET2015) &
MEDICAL SCIENCE AND BIOLOGICAL ENGINEERING (MSBE2015)
Proceedings of the 2015 International Conference on CSET & MSBE

ISBN 978-981-4651-00-4

Editorial

This proceedings published by World Scientific consists of one hundred and five selected papers presented in the joint conferences of 2015 International Conference on Computer Science and Engineering Technology (CSET2015) and 2015 International Conference on Medical Science and Biological Engineering (MSBE2015), which was successfully held in Hong Kong during May 30–31, 2015.

This proceedings covers a wide areas of research and applications in computer science, mechanical engineering, control engineering, building material and civil engineering, material science and engineering, technology for education, and medical science and biological engineering. The joint conferences of CSET2015 and MSBE2015 provided an international forum to bring together industry professionals, academics, and individuals from institutions, industrials and government agencies to exchange research results and findings, to discuss potential of new emerging technologies, and seek possible collaboration in computing and biomedical engineering.

The aims of the proceedings of CSET2015 and MSBE2015 intended to compile and put together the latest research results and applications in computing and biomedical research. All accepted papers were subjected to strict peer reviewing by two to four expert referees.

Finally, on behalf of the organizing committees of CSET2015 and MSBE2015, we would like to take this opportunity to express our sincere appreciations to all authors for their contributions to these two conferences. We would like to extend our thanks to all the referees for their constructive comments on all submitted papers; especially, we would like to thank Dr. Yan H. Ng from World Scientific for his support and dedication in the publication of this proceedings.

Dr. Jiamei Deng, Kingston University, United Kingdom
Guest Editor of CSET2015

Prof. Qingjun Liu, Zhejiang University, China
Guest Editor of MSBE2015

Contents

Chapter 3: Medical Science and Biological Engineering

Chapter 6: Material Science and Engineering

CHAPTER 1

Mechanical and Control Engineering

The Design of High Frequency Induction Heating Power Supply Based on DSP and FPGA Dual Core Processors

Liu Lina

Bao Tou Light Industry Vocational Technical College, Bao Tou, China
E-mail: Liulina_bt@126.com
http://btzyjsxyzs.university-hr.com

DSP (XC2267) is the main control chip which does the increment PI algorithms and realizes the voltage and current double closed-loop control. Three-phase thyristor rectifier method based on the phase self-adjusting of FPGA is proposed. A method for swept-frequency start circuit is designed to implement the transition between the high-power and low-power. The invert system uses the compound control of improved PWM and frequency phase lock to improve the control accuracy and efficiency. Lastly, by using bench, the circuit is tested and the feasibility and effectiveness of the whole system are verified.

Keywords: Induction heating power system; DSP; FPGA; PLL; frequence tracking.

1. Introduction

The method which uses the APLL to realize the frequent tracking exists many problems, such as the circuit is complicated, the system upgrade is hard to carry out, and so on. With the development of FPGA and DSP, it is possible to realize the digital intermediate frequency heating power and to improve the power regulation speed and resonance frequency tracking. The ability to deal with data and algorithm of 16-bit single chip microcomputer makes the whole control system more simplify and control the algorithm of the mediate frequency heating power system efficiently.

2. Principle and Structure

2.1. *Principle of induction heating power supply*

According to the principle of electromagnetic induction, the induction heating power supply heats the work pieces up quickly in the alternating magnetic field. Through the work piece, the alternating magnetic field lines form the circuit and generate the induced current in the cross section. The induced current makes the part of work pieces generate heat instantaneously.

2.2. *Block diagram of the induction heating power system*

The induction heating power system consists of rectifier, inverter, filter, drive circuit, signal acquisition circuit, protective circuit, control circuit, PLL and so on. The three-phase full-bridge controlled rectifier circuit converts the three phase current to pulsating direct current which is to be a constant DC power supply through the large inductance filter. The constant direct current is inverted to a constant power of single-phase medium frequency voltage through the single-phase bridge inverter using SCR. The drive circuit mainly produces the drive signal to control the diode of Rectifier Bridge and SCR of Inverter Bridge. The intermediate frequency voltage signal which is gathered by the sensor is sent to the controller to do the improved PID and to track the frequency. The overall block diagram is shown in Fig. 1.

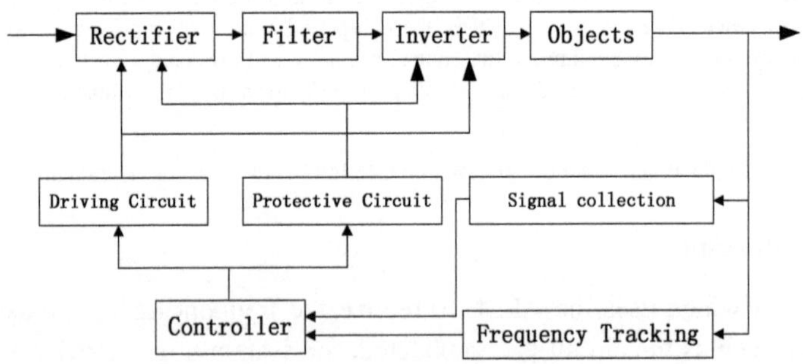

Fig. 1 The overall block diagram.

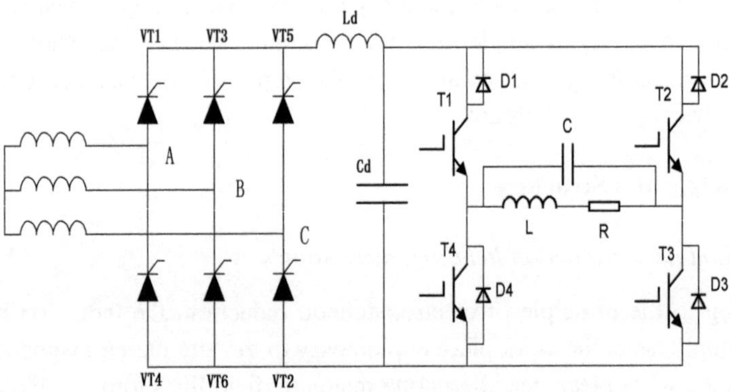

Fig. 2 Parallel-resonant inverter.

2.3. *Solution and hardware construction*

The paraller-resonant inverter structure is shown in Fig. 2. The large inductance filter is used to suppress the surge current and to reduce the impact of the power grid by circuit. The main controller of this system is XC2267 which does the algorithm. The FPGA is used to generate the signal of all the driver circuit and to design PLL, which is shown in Fig. 3.

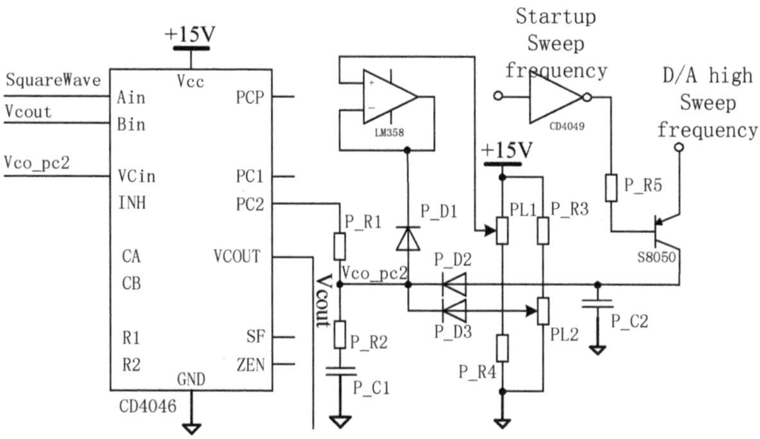

Fig. 3 Overall system structure.

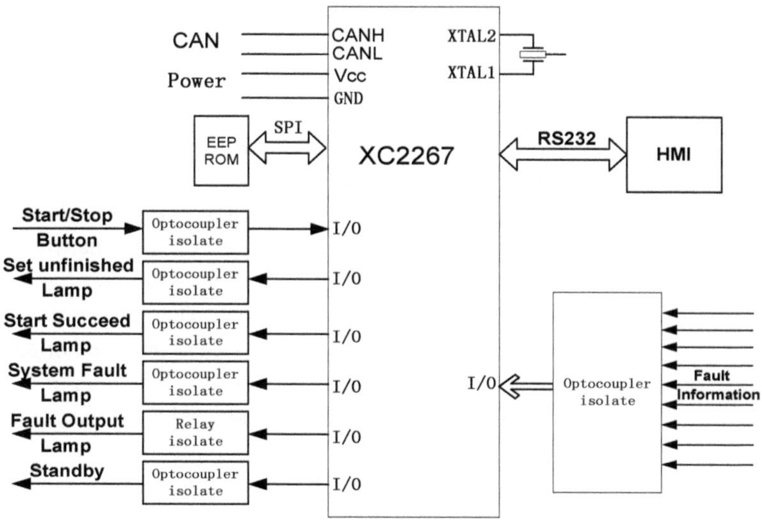

Fig. 4 Frequency tracking and control system.

3. Frequency Tracking and Control

There are two phase discriminator in CD4046, the phase discriminator 1 is exclusive-OR gate, where there are 90° phase shift between Ain and Bin, the phase discriminator 2 is edge triggered flip flop, where there is 0° phase shift between Ain and Bin. In this schedule, phase discriminator 2 is used. Frequency tracking and control system is shown in Fig. 4.

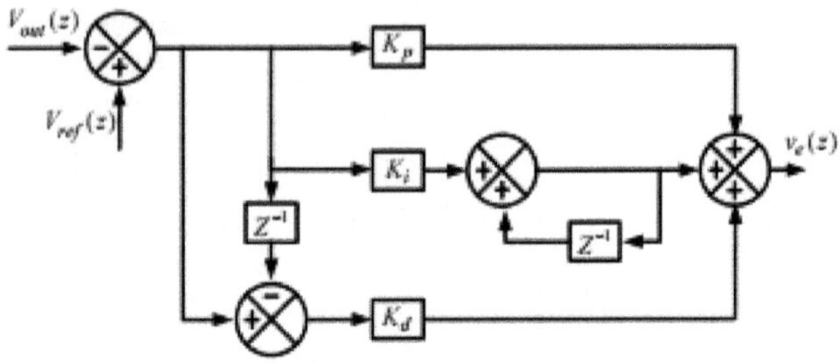

Fig. 5 Block diagram of a digital implementation of PID controller.

4. PID Control

In order to overcome the aforementioned limitations of conventional PID controller certain modifications of this kind of controller are proposed . The use of two different PID controllers is proposed resulting in two different bandwidth values, a lower bandwidth during steady state and a higher bandwidth which takes effect during transients. It might cause unnecessary oscillations due to a large sudden change in bandwidth. A nonlinear implementation of PID controller that behaves differently during load transient condition is proposed. Its implementation is not straight forward and requires calculation of many parameters. Moreover, the digital implementation requires more resources for the calculation of exponential terms. In order to make a smooth PID transition from steadystate to transient state, an adaptive PID controller method is presented in this paper. This paper proposes a control strategy that results in reduction in the overshoot/undershoot and the settling time for the power converter output voltage during dynamic transients. The proposed control method does not require sensing any additional parameters that are not already available in any conventional PID controller and is relatively simple to realize. The strategy of integral separation PID control is adopted. The basic idea of improved PID is as follow: When the deviation of controlled variable and set point is large, integral action is cancelled , on the other side, integral action is used to eliminate static error and improve the control precision. Follow the steps outlined below as Fig. 5:

5. Experimental Result and Conclusions

All the test is based on 160 KW/8 KHZ SCR medium frequency induction power supply. Controller board is shown in Fig. 4. The result of PLL test is as shown in Fig. 7–Fig. 11. The XOR gate is used as PD. When the system is stable, the output signal is 90 degrees ahead of input signal. The blue line is output signal and the yellow line is input signal. The middle line is the basic time of 90 degrees and the work frequency is 20 kHz. The controller board is shown in Fig. 6.

The result of the short-circuit test is as shown in Fig. 7. It shows that when there is a short circuit load, the current increases rapidly and appears overshoot. It turned out that improved PI can adjust the current effectively and protect the main circuit.

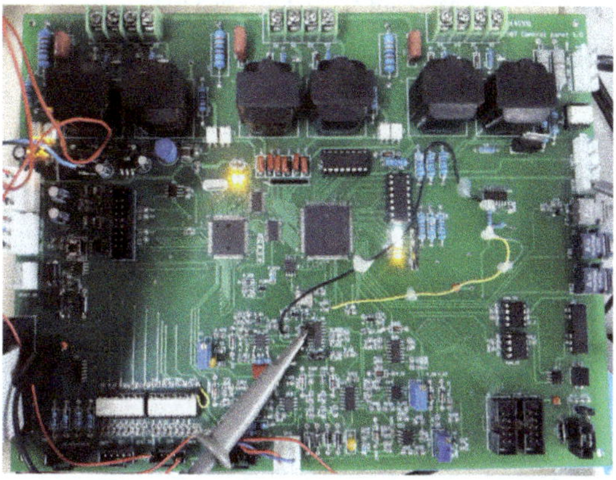

Fig. 6 Controller board.

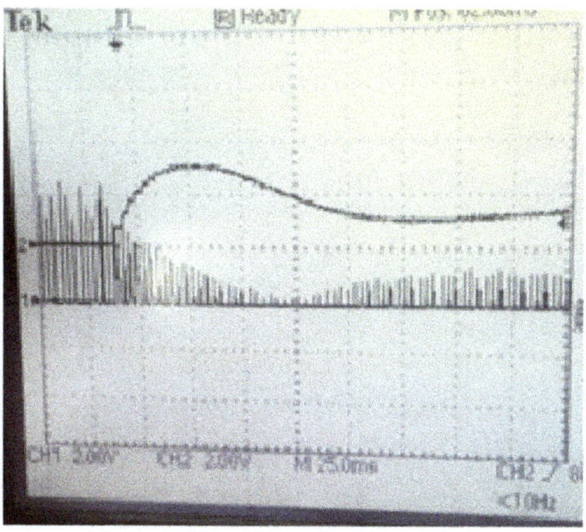

Fig. 7 Current loop response curve.

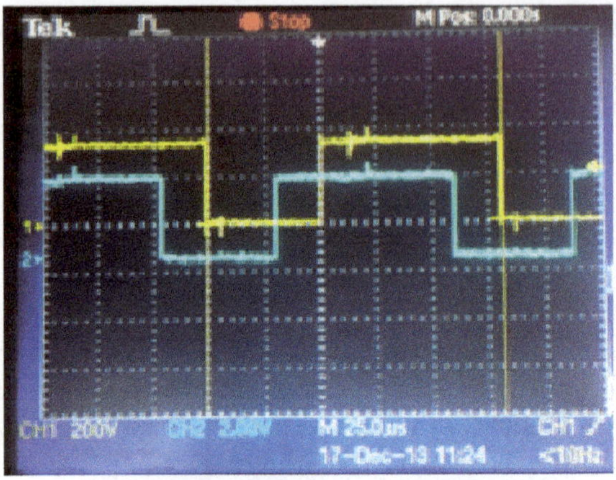

Fig. 8 Phase shift between Ain and Bin.

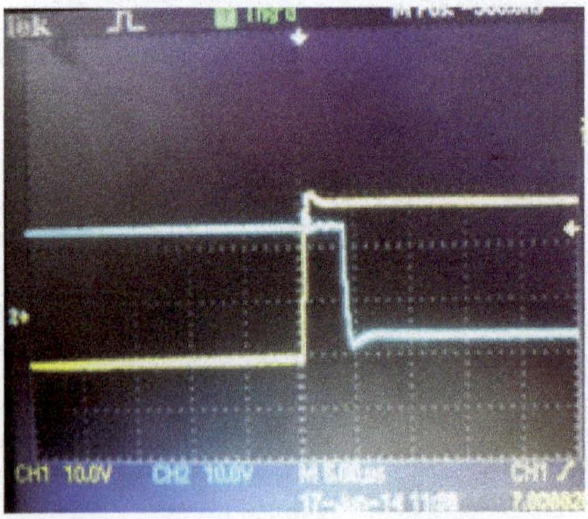

Fig. 9 Overlap time between upper and lower IGBT.

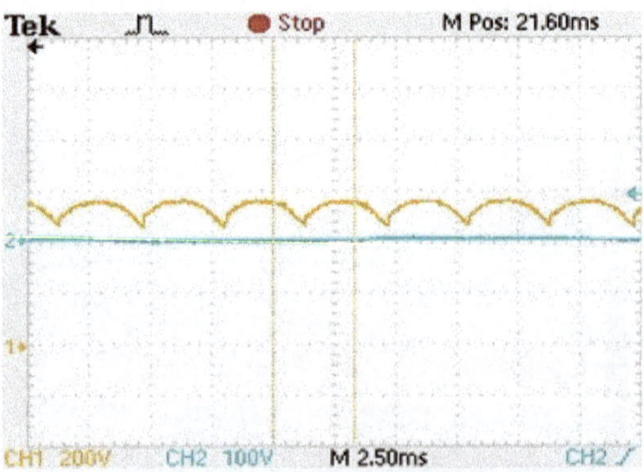

Fig. 10 DC bus voltage curve.

The waveform of Rectifier Bridge with pure impedance load is as shown in Fig. 9. The experiment steps are as follows: Remove the load of inverter, and connect a resistance of 500 Ohm with DC bus in series. As there is no feedback, the phase-shifting angle of Rectifier Bridge is zero.

The waveform of current and voltage of load is as shown in Fig. 11. After the load oscillation and given the intermediate frequency voltage, the waveform of current is square wave and the waveform of voltage is sine wave.

The experiment indicated that: the hardware designed in this thesis meets the design requirements; the digital phase-locked loop increases the range of phase, and improves the power factor; frequency tracking is realized; improved PID also achieves great control effect.

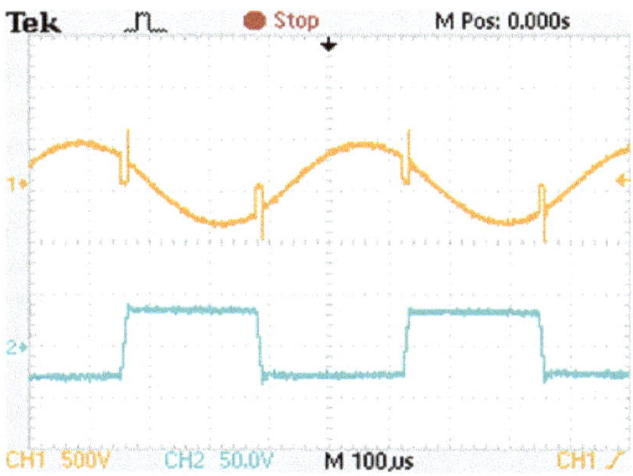

Fig. 11 AC side current and voltage curve.

References

1. Su Yanping, Cui Jianfeng: Design of digital phase shift trigger of induction heating power system. (International Conference on Electronic, 2011).
2. Li Heming, Li Yabin: FPGA-Based All Digital Phase-Locked Loop Controlled Induction Heating Power Supply Operating at Optimized ZVS Mode. IEEE 1-4244-0549-1/06 (2006).
3. Piao Xingzhe: The Research on 10kHz/150kW Mid-Frequency Heating Power Induction Heater. Shenyang University of Technology (2004).
4. Yang Xiaojing: The Key Technology Research of the Digital Intermediate Frequency Induction Heating PowerSupply. Xi'an University of Architecture and Technology (2012).
5. D.H. Wolaver: Phase-Locked Loop Circuit Design. Prentice Hall. Englewwood Cliffs. NJ (1991).

Modeling and Simulation of Powertrain and Control Strategy for a Series-Parallel Hybrid Electric Bus

Qin Dong-chen[a], Pan Shou-chen[b], Xie Yin-qian[c] and Pei Dong-jie[d]
School of Mechanical Engineering, Zhengzhou University, Zhengzhou, 450001, China
E-mail: [a]dcqin@zzu.edu.cn, [b]panshouchen1991@163.com, [c]1063328860@qq.com, [d]peidongjie@zzu.edu.cn

To research the development of hybrid powertrain and control strategy, the simulation model including its core components is established for a new type of series-parallel hybrid electric vehicle system; and the fuzzy logic control strategy is developed using the fuzzy control method, which is embedded into the vehicle model to achieve simulation analysis. The result demonstrates that the vehicle model can satisfy the requirements of speed and acceleration performance under the simulation conditions, and the fuzzy logic control strategy can allocate the power between engine and the traction motor reasonably according to the working condition , and the fuel economy is improved by 11.02% compared with the control strategy with motor assist, which proves the accuracy and efficiency of the simulation model and control strategy.

Keywords: Series-parallel; hybrid electric system; modeling; fuzzy logic control strategy; simulation.

1. Introduction

Series-parallel hybrid powertrain has both advantages of the series and parallel structure, which can realize the flexible control of allocating energy and power reasonably between the engine and traction motor, ensure the hybrid system to have a high efficiency in different conditions, and improve the economy of fuel and reduce the emission [1, 2]. Vehicle control strategy is the core part to realize the energy saving and emission reduction for hybrid electric bus, and it is also the key of energy management. From the current study situation, the species of control strategy in most studies are: the logic threshold control strategy [3], the control strategy based on instantaneous optimization [4], the control strategy based on global optimization [5] and the fuzzy logic control strategy [6].

The theoretical models of the engine, traction motor (TM) and other core components have been established in this paper for a new type of series-parallel hybrid electric bus (SPHEB). And the vehicle model is built in the software Advisor. With the best fuel economy as the control target, a fuzzy logic control strategy is developed to realize the reasonable distribution of power for powertrain. At last, the system simulation and analysis are conducted.

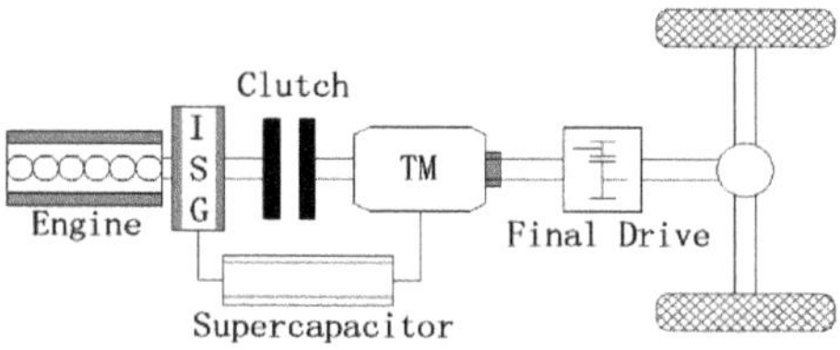

Fig. 1 The structure of the series-parallel hybrid system.

2. Hybrid Powertrain of the SPHEB

2.1. *Introduction of the hybrid powertrain*

The structure of hybrid powertrain is mainly composed by a six cylinder engine, a integrated/starter generator (ISG) motor, an automatic clutch, a traction motor, a single ratio transmission and an ultra capacitor group, as shown in Figure 1. This system uses coaxial arrangement, where ISG motor is installed at the back of the engine and the spindle connected to the engine crankshaft directly. The switch between series mode and parallel mode can be realized by opening and closing of the clutch installed between the two motors.

2.2. *Division of work modes*

According to the system structural characteristics, the following work modes can be achieved under the series and parallel modes combined with the power required in different driving conditions: pure electric mode, engine-only drive mode, engine and TM combined drive mode, engine driving and charging mode, energy recovery mode.

Table 1 Parameters of SPHEB and main components.

Projects	Parameters	Projects	Parameters
Curb weight [kg]	14000	Engine power rating [kW]	115
Wheel base [m]	0.68	Maximum speed of engine [min^{-1}]	2000
Height of mass center [m]	0.9	TM power rating [kW]	85
Final ratio	4.38	Maximum speed of TM [min^{-1}]	2700

3. Establish of Simulation Models

3.1. *Main parameters of the vehicle and powertrain*

The main parameters of the SPHEB and hybrid system studied in this paper are as shown in Table 1.

3.2. *Simulation models of the core components*

The main objective of study and control is the engine. Its working process is non-linear, and it's very complex to build a theoretical model of engine. However, the working process can be analyzed based on the method combined experiments and theories. According to the working conditions of engine, theoretical model is established in the SIMULINK environment. As shown in Figure 2.

The model has many sub-modules such as control interface, torque calculation, speed evaluation and fuel consumption/emissions and so on.

TM is a permanent magnet brushless DC motor rated at 85kW. It has characteristics as operating reliably, maintaining easily and simple structure, and it also has a larger output torque and higher power density. The theoretical model of TM in the SIMULINK environment is shown in Figure 3, which includes sub-modules such as speed evaluation, torque limit, available torque calculation.

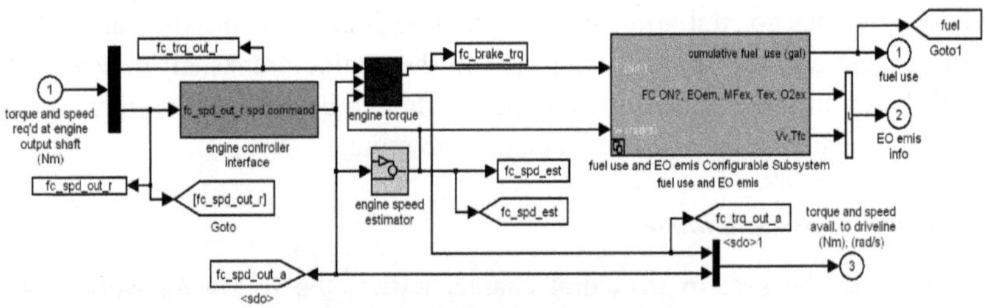

Fig. 2 Simulation model of engine.

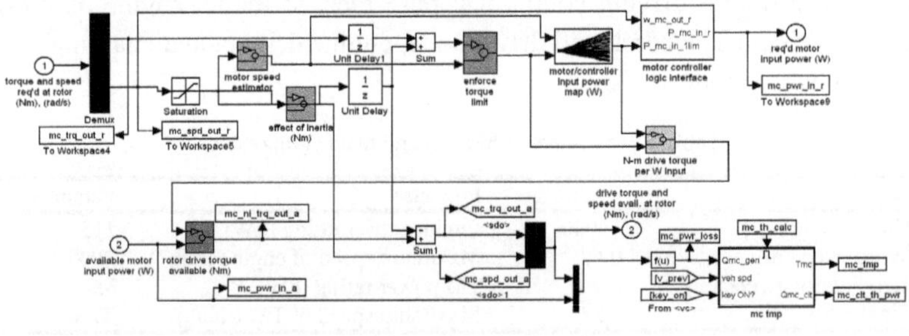

Fig. 3 Simulation model of TM.

3.3. *Vehicle simulation model*

Based on the secondary development of Advisor software, the vehicle simulation model is established.

Starting from the simulation conditions, in accordance with the backward simulation ideas, the backward simulation block diagram is established according to the required direction of power. Then the feedback information is added between the various modules to complete the forward simulation path and build. And then the vehicle simulation model is complete as shown in Figure 4. Finally, the secondary development of software will ensure that the model structures can run smoothly in Advisor.

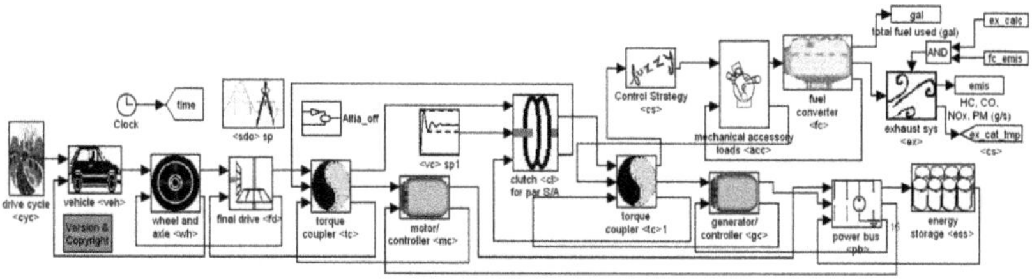

Fig. 4 Simulation model of vehicle.

4. Development of Control Strategy

A better control strategy is the guarantee to allocated power rationally between various components of the powertrain, and is the key to achieve a best fuel reasonably [7]. Using fuzzy control method, a fuzzy logic control strategy is developed to realize the reasonable distribution of power for powertrain.

The fuzzy logic controller is the core of the fuzzy logic control strategy [8]. According to the pre-defined membership function of the variables, the extent of membership will be determined.

State of charge (SOC) of the super-capacitor, current speed (spd) of TM and the difference ΔT between torque required (T_{req}) and current output torque (T_{out}) of engine are chosen to be input variables of the fuzzy controller, and the engine actual output torque (T_e) is the output variable.

The design of membership functions is divided fuzzy membership for each input and output variables after determining the fuzzy subset of the variables and their respective thresholds. The membership functions for the four control variables are shown in Figure 5.

Domain of the torque difference ΔT after fuzzy treatment is [-1,1]. It is divided into seven fuzzy subsets: {NM, NB, NS, Z, PS, PB, PM}. SOC's domain is [0,1], and divided into six fuzzy sets: {Z, VL, L, M, H, VH}. spd's domain is [0,1], and divided into three fuzzy sets: {L, M, H}. Domain of output variables Te is [0,1], and divided into six fuzzy sets: {Z, VS, S, NM, B, VB}.

The principles that control the engine working in the vicinity of optimal working area are used in the development of control rules to ensure that can get better fuel economy. Then the fuzzy logic control strategy is established in SIMULINK environment. Its structure diagram is shown in Figure 6. T_{opt} is the optimum output torque of the engine.

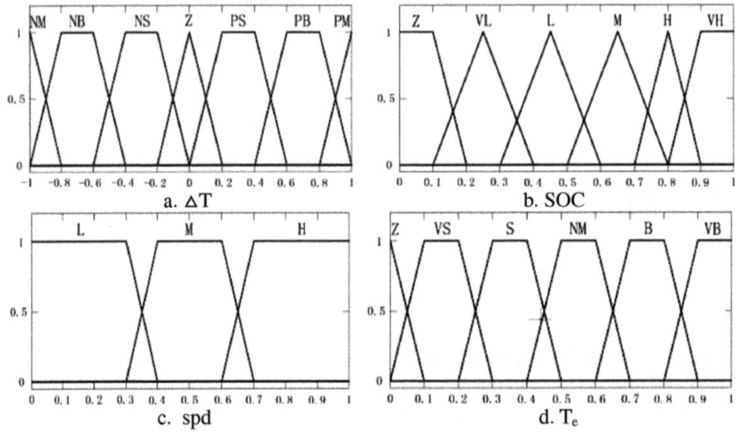

Fig. 5 Membership functions of the four control variables.

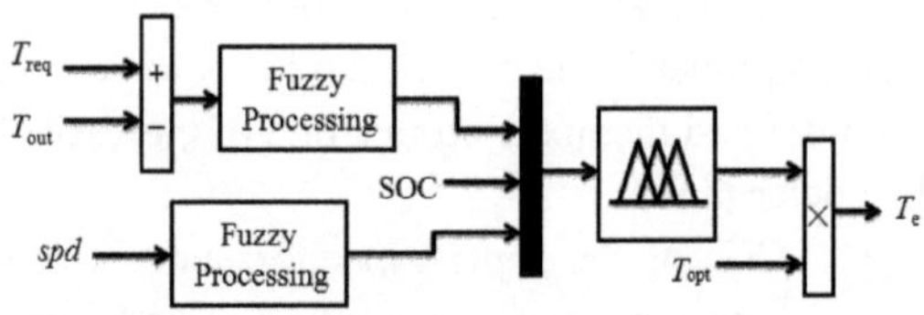

Fig. 6 Structure diagram of fuzzy logic control strategy.

5. Simulation Results and Analysis

The fuzzy logic control strategy is embedded into the established vehicle model. Then the correctness of the control strategy and model will be verified by simulations. According to the test method of specified by GB/T 19753-2005 [9], the China typical city bus simulation conditionis chosen to simulate, and the simulation results obtained are as follows.

The comparison results between the fuzzy logic strategy and control electric assist control strategy are shown in Table 2. From Table 2, the vehicle model can satisfy the speed and acceleration performance requirements of simulation conditions, which can verify the correctness of the vehicle simulation model. In addition, under the same road conditions, fuzzy logic control strategy can obtain 2.7L/100km less fuel consumption than the electric assist control strategy. The fuel economy is improved by 11.02%. It proves that fuzzy logic control strategy is more effective, and has a better control effect.

Power curves of different components are shown in Figure 7.

Figure 7 shows the power of engine and TM can coincide with the power required by system basically. The real-time working efficiency of engine can maintain at 38.5% basically through experimental verification. This simulation results show that the fuzzy logic control strategy can allocate the power of engine and the TM reasonably according to the power requirements and road condition, and can obtain a better fuel economy.

Table 2 The comparison of simulation results.

Strategy	Fuel consumption $[L\cdot(100km)^{-1}]$	Maximum speed $[km\cdot h^{-1}]$	0-50 $km\cdot h^{-1}$ accelerate time[s]
Fuzzy logic control strategy	21.8	77.2	14.9
Electric assist control strategy	24.5	77.8	15.3

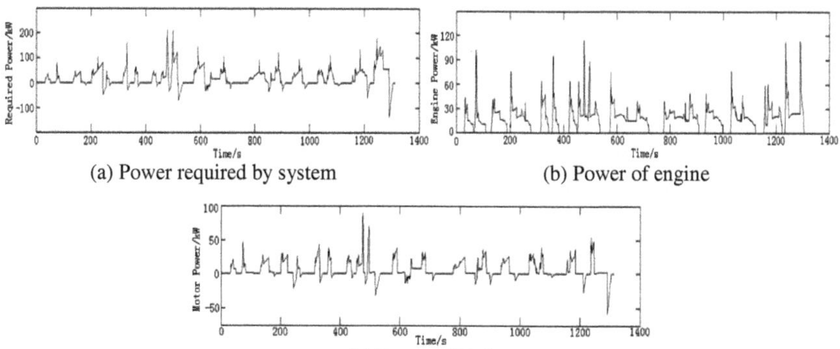

(a) Power required by system (b) Power of engine

(c) Power of TM

Fig. 7 Power curves of different components.

6. Conclusions

The models of core components and vehicle are established on the basis of system analysis and secondary development of the software Advisor for the new type powertrain SPHEB. And the fuzzy logic control strategy is developed by using the fuzzy logic method with the best fuel economy as the control goal.

The simulation result shows that the vehicle model can satisfy the speed and acceleration performance requirements of simulation conditions, which can prove the accuracy of the vehicle simulation model. In addition, the fuzzy logic control strategy can allocate the power between engine and the traction motor reasonably according to the working condition and power requirement, and the fuel economy is improved by 11.02% compared with the control strategy with motor assist. All of these verify the rationality of fuzzy logic strategy and efficiency for improving the fuel economy.

Acknowledgments

This study is supported by the Transformation Project of National Major Scientific and Technological Achievements: "Development and Industrialization of the Depth Hybrid Electric Bus", 2012, China.

References

1. Chen Qingquan, Sun Fengchun, Zhu Jiaguang. *Modern Electric Vehicle Technology* [M]. Beijing: Beijing Institute of Technology Press, 2004.
2. Lin Xinyou, XueRui, Sun Dongye. *Development of a Real-time Optimization Algorithm for a Series- parallel Hybrid Electric Bus Energy Management* [J]. China Mechanical Engineering, 2013, 24(18) pp. 2539- 2543.
3. B.Mashadi, S. A. M.Emadi. *Dual-mode power-split transmission for hybrid electric vehicles* [J]. IEEE Transactions on Vehicular Technology, 2010, 59(7) pp. 3223-3232.
4. Lin Xiao, Xu Xiao, Guan Cheng. *Subsection-typed Energy Management for a Plug-in Hybrid Electric Vehicle Based on Equivalent BSFC and Battery SOC Balancing*[J]. China Mechanical Engineering, 2012, 23(4) pp.493-498.
5. F. Payri, C. Guardiola, B. Pla, et al. *A Stochastic Method for the Energy Management in Hybrid Electric Vehicles*[J]. Control Engineering Practice, 2014, 29 pp.257-265.
6. Li Jun, Zou Faming, TuXiong, et al. *Simulation Research on PHEV Based on Fuzzy Logic Control Strategies* [J]. Journal of Chongqing Jiao Tong University (Natural Science), 2013, 32(2) pp. 329-333.
7. Wang Lei. *Research on Energy Management Strategy and Mode Transition Control for a Series-parallel Hybrid Electric Bus* [D]. Shanghai: Shanghai Jiao Tong University, 2013.
8. Wang Yunlong, Zhang Hongtian. *Research on Fuzzy Controller of Parallel-Series Hybrid Electric System* [J]. Journal of Wuhan University of Technology (Transportation Science & Engineering), 2013, 37(4) pp.733-736.
9. GB/T 19753-2005, *Test Methods for Energy Consumption of Light-duty Hybrid Electric Vehicles* [S]. 2005.

A Product Gene Based Approach for Conceptual Design of Mechanical Products

Li Pan[1,a], Yan Yan[1,b] and Wang Guoxin[1,c]

[1]*Beijing Institute of Technology, School of Mechanical Engineering, Beijing 100081, China*

[a]*lipanhappy1987@163.com,* [b]*yanyan331@bit.edu.cn,* [c]*wangguoxin@bit.edu.cn*

To solve the problem of low product design efficiency caused by information search difficulties under the environment of information explosion, product genes research was doneon the basis of analogy with biological genetic engineering ideas. The connotation of product genes was redefined, which is more consistent with biological genes so that it is benefit for deeper study on product genes drawing on biological genetic engineering advanced technology. Operating technologies of product genes were summarized. Based on this, a product gene based approach for conceptual design of mechanical products was presented. Take corn combine harvest stalks device as an example, the design approach was verified, and the results show that the conceptual design method based on product genes greatly improved the design efficiency and shortened the product design cycle.

Keywords: Genetic engineering; product genes; conceptual design; design methodology.

1. Introduction

Recently, the main target of product design is to meet customer's needs. Therefore, product innovation and rapid responses to customers' personalized needs largely determine the competitiveness of enterprises. According to surveys, about 75%-80% of the product design is based on existing product design, only about 20% of the product design belongs to new design [1-3]. Variant design realizes product innovation through changing part of component structures, size, parameters and so on, which is essentially as same as biological genetic engineering. Take principle, structure, functions and so on as the genetic information of products, the concept of product gene is presented. Utilizing product genes to control and inherit characters of products, and then recombining the product genes, we can finally realize product innovation.

Conceptual design is the initial stage of the product design process. It can decide the basic characteristics of the product design and product innovation to a large extent. This paper puts forward the concept of product gene and analyzes its related operating technologies. Based on this, a conceptual design method based on product genesis presented. In order to verify the feasibility of this method, corn combine harvest stalk device was used as an example, and the results show that this method can reduce the blindness and improve the efficiency of conceptual design.

2. Product Genes

Although product gene is researched both at home and abroad, its concept has not yet unified due to different study fields, methods and focus of different researchers. Some researchers define product gene as genetic knowledge about product function and its realization means [4-6,7]; or think product gene is a kind of standardized information sets, which determines the length of the product life cycle and processes of product knowledge delivery and restructuring [8-11]; other researchers think that product gene is the basic information unit determining product characters [12]. However, most of the definitions are abstract and not similar to the double helix structure of biological genes.

This paper defines product gene as a double helix structure consists of product design control elements, knowledge elements and relationships between them, as shown in Fig. 1. In this structure, product design control elements and knowledge elements are respectively amount to the two strands of DNA, and relationships between them are amount to the hydrogen bond connected the two strands of DNA. Product design control elements mainly include information of product components and parts, such as materials, size, surface roughness, accuracy and so on, knowledge elements consists mainly of related papers, patents, design handbooks, experiences and so on. Their classifications and forms are shown in Table 1.

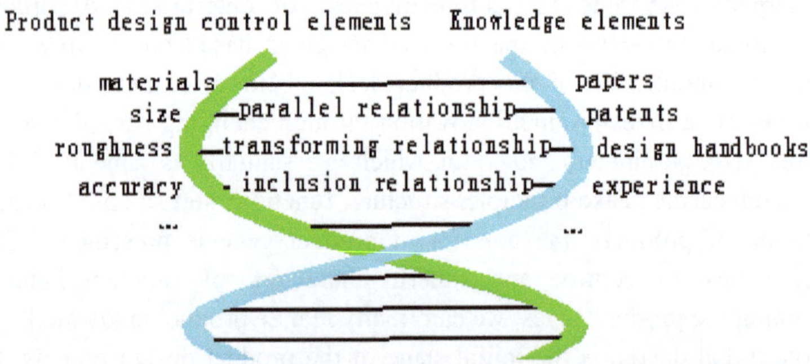

Fig. 1 Connotation of product genes.

Table 1 Classifications and forms of product design control elements and knowledge elements.

No.	product design control elements	forms	No.	knowledge elements	forms
1	materials	paper or electronic documents	1	regulations and system	electronic documents
2	size	paper or electronic documents	2	technical condition	electronic documents
3	roughness	paper or electronic documents	3	descriptive files	electronic documents
4	accuracy	paper or electronic documents	4	engineering report	electronic documents
5	structure parameter	paper or electronic documents	5	standard	electronic documents
6	technological parameter	paper or electronic documents	6	training documents	electronic documents
8	strength	paper or electronic documents	8	company standard	electronic documents
...	...	...	...	...	...

Product design control elements are one kind of information, while knowledge elements belong to the category of knowledge. So relationships between them can be described with the relationships between information and knowledge. According to recent research, relationships between information and knowledge include parallel relationship, transforming relationship and inclusion relationship. Through these relationships, product design control elements and knowledge elements have formed into product genes. This definition is not only more fit with biological gene structure, but also combined with product design control elements and knowledge elements, which is more conducive to the innovation of product design.

3. Conceptual Design Method based on Product Genes

3.1. *Operating technology of product genes*

Similar to biological genes, product genes also can undertake operations of transcription, translation, replication, and reverse transcription, and details for each operation respectively elaborated as follows.

3.1.1. *Transcription and translation of product gene*

Transcription and translation of product genesare expression process from product genes to product entities. Designers getproduct genes from existing products at first, and then through transcription they can attain the action mode of products, namely effect solutions, which is amount to the RNA of biological genes. And then, through process of translation, we can get principle solutions from effect solutions, which are amount to protein in biological genes. Finally, principle solutions are transformed into specific products.

3.1.2. *Product gene replication*

Product gene replication is the process of directly using the existing design knowledge in new product design through storing and matching process. Product gene replication greatly improves the efficiency of product design.

3.1.3. *Reverse transcription of product gene*

Reverse transcription of product genes is the process of obtaining product genes from existing products. Using reverse engineering knowledge, the action principle is deduced from existing products. Analyzing the action mode of the action principle, we can find out the corresponding product design control elements and knowledge elements, thus product genes are finally obtained.

3.2. *Conceptual design method based on product genes*

Product gene based conceptual design is conducted on the basis of product gene reuse, and its design process framework was shown in Fig. 2.

In product conceptual design, product functional requirements should be explicit at first. According to the functional requirements, we could find out corresponding existing products, abstract principle solutions of every sub-function from these products, and finally obtain product genes through the process of reverse transcription. In this method, product genes of existing relevant products were analyzed, and defective genes and their position in the whole product genes were found out. Then, better genes, which could improve product gene defects or replace the defective product genes, were found out from product gene pool, and then were respectively combined with the existing product genes. By this way, many feasible solutions would be obtained. According to function requirements and existing design conditions and other requirements, solutions best met the function requirements were optimized. After that, effect solutions were transcribed from product genes optimized, and then translated into principle solutions. Finally, action principle of products was obtained.

Conceptual design method based on product genes presented that product genes are bridges connecting product functions and specific product structures. Using product genes, map from function requirements to specific product structures is quickly realized, which greatly improves efficiency of product conceptual design.

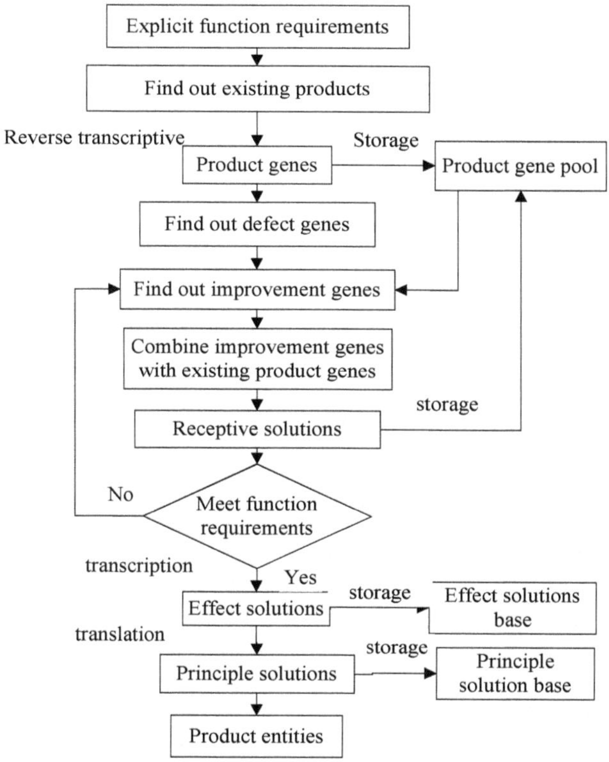

Fig. 2 Design process framework of conceptual design based product gene.

4. Example

In order to verify the feasibility of the conceptual design method based on product genes, conceptual design of corn combine harvest stalk device was used as an example. At present, corn harvest most adopts rotor milling cutter as stalk chopper devices. When it works, its rotation diameters is small and its rotating speed is high, which easily lead to problems of hitting ground, breaking knife, and high impurity rate of chopped stems. Therefore, combine harvest stalk device should be improved.

According to the conceptual design method based on product genes, we abstracted product genes of rotor milling cutter at first, as shown in Table 2. And then, through transcription and translation, we found out feasible solutions, the solutions included principle solutions and effect solutions, as shown in Table 2.

In Table 2, power consumption, cutting length and impurity rate of chopped straw are main design control elements to be considered when choosing stalk device.

Every type of stem cutters and its principle solutions are shown in Fig. 3.

Table 2 Corresponding product genes and feasible solutions of rotor milling cutter.

No.	function needed	product genes		
		design control elements	knowledge elements	relationships
1	cut off	power consumption	design handbook, papers, patents, parameter library, test data, etc.	parallel relationship, transforming relationship, inclusion relationship
2	cut off	efficiency	design handbook, papers, patents, parameter library, test data, etc.	
3	cut off	cutting force	design handbook, papers, patents, parameter library, etc.	
4	cut off	cutting length	technical conditions, standards, parameter library, specification, etc.	
5	cut off	impurities rate	standards, specification, regime, technical conditions, etc.	
6	cut off	grasping force of stems	design handbook, papers, patents, parameter library, etc.	
7	cut off	moving direction of cutting off stems	experiences, papers, patents, learning resources, etc.	

⇩ Transcription, translation ⇧ Reverse transcription

No.	feasible solutions	function	principle solutions	effect solutions
1	disc serrated knife	cutting off corn stems	figure 3 (a)	sliding cutting
2	straight edge hob cutter	cutting off corn stems	figure 3 (b)	sliding cutting
3	reciprocating type knife	cutting off corn stems	figure 3 (d)	shearing

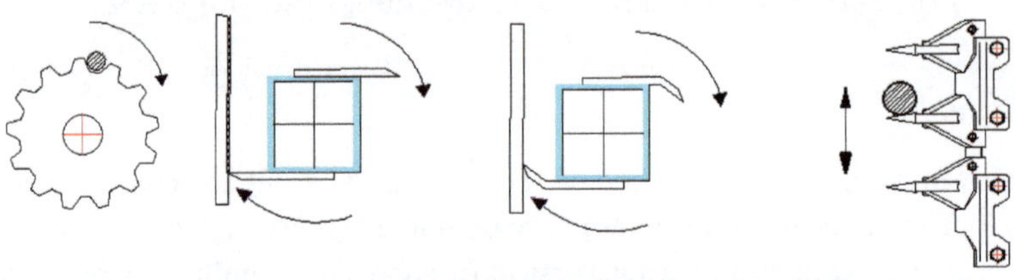

1. Disc serrated cutter 2. Straight edge hob cutter 3. Rotor milling cutter 4. Reciprocating type cutter

Fig. 3 Structure and principle solution diagrams of stem cutters.

In Figure 3, according to corresponding resources and experience, we know that in the four types of cutters, reciprocating type cutterhas simple structure and reliable work. When it works, the forces on it and impurity rate of chopped stalks collected is low [13]. Therefore, stem harvesting device with reciprocating type cutter was selected as the optimum solution, other parts of corn harvestgenes were directly copied into new product design. Next, through transcription and translation, effect solutions were obtained, and then translated into principle solutions through translation. Finally, principle solutions were transformed into product entities according to machinery handbooks and other related resources. This example suggested that conceptual design method based on product genes not only helps designers to quickly find required knowledge, but also greatly improves design efficiency through replication process of product genes.

5. Conclusion

In order to improve the product innovation efficiency and quickly response to the personalized needs of customers, product genes were redefined according to existing research and biological genetic engineering technics. A double helix structure of product genes was presented, consisting with product design control elements, knowledge elements and relationships between them. This definition is more consistent with biological genes. Then, operation technologies were summarized. On the basis of this, a product gene based conceptual design method design process framework was proposed, and an example of conceptual design of corn combine harvest stalk device was used to verify the feasibility of this method. The results show that the product gene based conceptual design method effectively shortened the product design cycle and supported new product innovation needs.

References

1. Baxter D., Gao J. Case K., et al. A framework to integrate design knowledge reuse and requirements management in engineering design [J]. Robotics and Computer-Integrated Manufacturing, 2008, 24(4): 585-593.
2. Goel A. K., Vattam S., Witgen B., et al. Cognitive, collaborative, conceptual and creative-Four characteristics of the next generation of knowledge-based CAD system: A study in biologically inspired design [J]. Computer-Aided Design, 2011, 12(6): 221-232.
3. VAREILLES E., ALDANONDO M. BOISSE A. C., et al. How to take into account general and conceptual knowledge for interactive aiding design: Towards the coupling of CSP and CBR approaches [J]. Engineering Applications of Artificial Intelligence, 2012, 25(1): 31-37.
4. FENG Peien, CHEN Yong, ZHANG Shuai, et al. Product gene based conceptual design [J]. Chinese Journal of Mechanical engineering, 2002, 38(10): 1-6.

5. HE Bin, FENG Peien, PAN Shuangxia. Conceptual Design Based on Product Ecological Model [J]. Computer Integrated Manufacturing Systems, 2007, 13(7): 1249-1267.
6. FENG Peien, ZHU Aihua, CHEN Yong, et al. Establishing Knowledge Base of Product Genes for Conceptual Design of Energy Transformation Systems [J]. Journal of Engineering Design, 2004, 11(3): 113-117.
7. CHEN Yong. A Bionics-based Methodology for Conceptual Design of Technical Products [D]. Hangzhou: Zhejiang University, 2004.
8. YANG Jinyong, HUANG Kezheng, SHANG Yong, et al. Summary of Study on Product Gene [J]. Journal of Mechanical Design, 2007, 24(4): 1-4.
9. Shang Yong. Research on Theory and Key Technologies of Conceptual Design Based on Product Gene [D]. Shandong: Shandong University, 2007.
10. ZHU Aihua. Summary of the Study on Mechanical Product Gene [J]. Journal of Beijing University of Civil Engineering and Architecture, 2009, 25(4): 58-61.
11. ZHAO Xiuyan, ZHAO Tingting, Wei Xiaopeng, et al. New Research for Optimized Variant Design [J]. Computer Engineering and Applications, 2009, 45(19): 68-71.
12. CHEN Hongwu, XuZhe, Cao Shouqi, et al. Research on Product Gene Growth Design [J]. Journal of Engineering Graphics, 2009, 3: 13-21.
13. WANG Wanjun, HU Zhong. Agricultural Mechanical Design Manual (I) [M]. China Agricultural Machinery Research Institute, 1988.

Supply Power Capacity Design Method of Active Heat Exchanger for Precision Machine Tool Structure*

Ning Wang[1,2,a], Weiguo Gao[1,b], Teng Liu[1], Yifan Zhang[3], Wentie Niu[1] and Dawei Zhang[1]

[1]*Tianjin Key Laboratory of Equipment Design and Manufacturing Technology, Tianjin University, Tianjin 300072, China*

[2]*School of Mechanical Engineering, Inner Mongolia University of Technology, Inner Mongolia, 010051, China*

[3]*School of Electrical Engineering and Automation, Tianjin University, Tianjin 300072, China*

[a]*thomasdarren@163.com*, [b]*Corresponding author: gaowg@tju.edu.cn*

To control thermal deformation of precision machine tool structure, a supply power capacity design method of Active Heat Exchanger (AHE) is provided in this paper. The supply power capacity can be adjusted through changing the inlet temperature and flow rate of coolant, some simulations have been completed, including the inlet temperature, flow rate of coolant and layout of the coolant channels. The simulating results illustrate that this method can be used to control and improve the thermal deformation of precision machine structure.

Keywords: Thermal deformation; precision machine tool; supply power capacity design; active heat exchanger.

1. Introduction

In the operation of machine tool, the machine accuracy will generally be disturbed by its internal generated heat and the changing ambient temperature, which result in geometric inaccuracies of the workpiece. To precision machine tools, thermal error can contribute up to about 75% of its comprehensive error [1]. It is necessary to investigate the appropriate method to cut down the machine thermal errors, and then to remain and improve the machine accuracy.

The traditional methods to deal with machine thermal error are mainly based on the error compensation. Chen [2] made the thermal error prediction and compensation of various kinds of precision machine tools based on the neural network theory. Wu [3] realized the off-line testing and compensating the thermal deformation of machine tool, using the linear regression method. Han

* This paper is supported by the state S&T projects for upmarket NC machine and fundamental manufacturing equipments of China (No. 2013ZX04005-013).

[4] introduced Fuzzy C-means clustering theory into the artificial neural network for the machine thermal error modeling. Yang [5] used the method of grey system theory and artificial neural network theory to make the thermal error modeling, improving the efficiency of machine thermal error compensation. These contributions can deal with machine thermal errors in some degrees, but the thermal error compensation has the negative factors such as the time-varying, hysteretic and poor robustness behaviors.

The authors provided a differentiated multi-loops bath recirculation system for precision machine tools [6], and this paper will present an Active Heat Exchanger (AHE). This innovative device is designed to be attached to the surfaces of machine tool structure to realize its real-time heat exchanging with machine structure. The reverse thermal deformation caused by the AHE is used to offset the machine thermal errors.

2. Supply Power Capacity Design Method of AHE

2.1. *Supply power capacity calculation of AHE*

When the AHE working, the coolant is supplied at its inlet, flowing along the internal coolant channel. Owing to the heat accumulation of the internal flowing coolant, there is generally a temperature difference between the coolant at inlet and outlet. The supply power of the AHE at any moment can be calculated in equation (1).

$$H = 1.67 \times 10^{-5} c\rho Q \Delta T \tag{1}$$

Where, H is the supply power of flowing at this moment (W); c is the special heat of coolant (J/(kg•°C)); ρ is density of coolant (kg/m^3); Q is the supply volume flow rate of coolant (L/min); ΔT is the coolant temperature difference between outlet and inlet (°C).

The maximum supply cooling power of AHE can be seen in its steady heat transferring state. If this maximum supply cooling power at steady heat transferring state is caused by the lowest supply temperature and highest supply volume flow rate of coolant, this maximum supply cooling power will stand for the supply power capacity of AHE.

2.2. *Simulation process of supply power capacity design of AHE based on heat-fluid-solid coupling FE simulation*

In order to simulate the supply power capacity of AHE, the heat-fluid-solid interaction FE method is adopted. In ANSYS, the CAE models of AHE structure and its internal flowing coolant are established and meshed. Then the fluid and solid material properties concerned are assigned to their respective model regions. The coolant material is oil, and the structure material of AHE is copper and aluminum. The properties of these materials are listed in Table 1.

As revealed in Fig. 1, the supply temperatures (20°C) and volume flow rates (5L/min) are exerted onto inlet surfaces of coolant models (flowing in Channels inside AHE shown in Fig. 1(a)-(b)) respectively; outlet surfaces of them are provided with 0 Pa pressure. To simulate the highest supply power of AHE, the consistent 20°C temperature load is exerted on its surface connecting with precision machine structure. Besides, the convection temperature 20°C of ambient air is exerted onto the outer surfaces of AHE structure model. When all heat loads, thermal boundary conditions, material properties are defined properly, the heat-fluid-solid coupling FE simulation for AHE can be performed in ANSYS.

Table 1 Material properties in FE modeling simulation of AHE.

	Cover (copper)	Channel support (Aluminum)	Coolant (Oil)
Density (kg/m^3)	8930	2793.6	910
Thermal conductivity (W/(m·K))	398	192.16	0.13
Specific heat (J/(kg·K))	386	963.74	2090
Young's Modulus (GPa)	128	73	—
Poisson's ratio	0.34	0.33	—
Linear expansion coefficient (K^{-1})	1.22e-5	1.28e-5	—

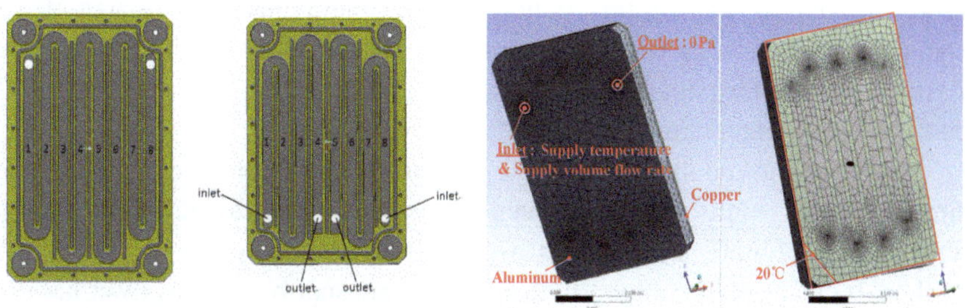

(a) single route (b) symmetrical double routes (c) CAE model

Fig. 1 CAD/CAE models of AHEs.

3. Supply Power Capacity Analysis of AHE

3.1. *Cross section design of coolant channel inside AHE*

The scale of cross section of channel inside AHE determines the volume flow rate of coolants, and then influences its supply power. The cross section design of coolant channel inside AHE is discussed in this section.

The flowing coolant has a big temperature difference between its outlet and inlet which can be seen in Fig. 2(a). This difference can be used in the supply power calculation of AHE. In order to analyze the supply power regulation caused by different cross section scale of AHE, the heat-fluid-solid coupling FE simulations are done.

The obtained supply power regulation caused by different cross section is shown in Fig. 3(a). It can be seen in it that, coolant supply power has an increasing tendency with the growing cross section area of AHE.

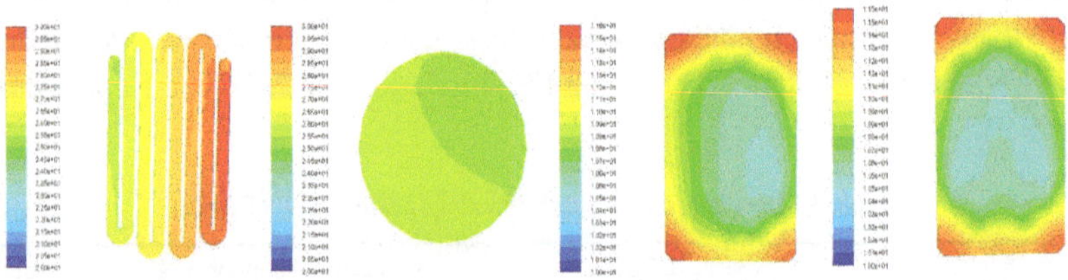

(a) (b) (c) (d)

(a) coolant in channel; (b) coolant in outlet; (c) surface of AHE with single channel (d) surface of AHE with symmetrical double channels

Fig. 2 Temperature field of AHE.

3.2. *Coolant supply temperature design of AHE*

Coolant supply temperature is one of critical factors determining the supply power of AHE as well. In this section, the maximum cross section area of the coolant channel is being taken, temperature fields of coolant and its outlet inside AHE are obtained by simulation method in Fig. 2(a) and Fig. 2(b), with the 30°C coolant supply temperature.

With various coolant supply temperatures, heat-fluid-solid coupling FE simulations of AHE are done. Supply powers caused by different supply temperatures of AHE are obtained by heat-fluid-solid coupling FE simulation method. It can be seen in Fig. 3(b) that, the coolant supply cooling power has the decreasing tendency with the increasing supply temperature. When the coolant supply temperature is higher than 20°C, the AHE has the supply heating power onto machine structure, and the power scale has increasing tendency with the increasing supply temperature.

3.3. *Supply coolant flow rate design of AHE*

Beside supply temperature, the supply flow rate is also the determining factor influencing the supply power of AHE. The supply power regulation caused by the varying supply coolant flow rate of AHE is studied in this section.

The varying tendency of supply power of AHE caused by its increasing supply volume rate is shown in Fig. 3(c): The coolant supply power has an increasing tendency with the increasing supply volume rate.

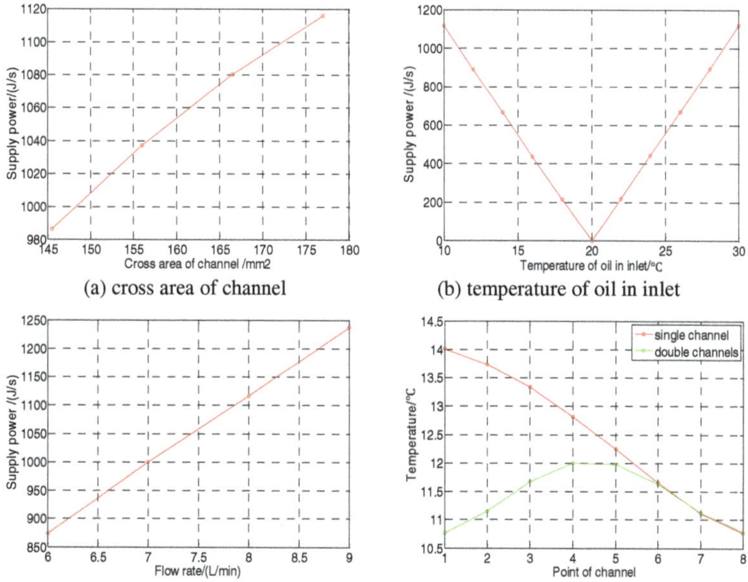

(a) cross area of channel (b) temperature of oil in inlet

(c) flow rate (d) temperature of oil in outlet with single and double channels

Fig. 3 Supply power capacity analysis.

3.4. *Layout design of coolant channels inside AHE*

The maximum scale of coolant channel cross section being taken, the temperature field of AHE above is obtained by FE simulation method shown in Fig. 2(c). As depicted in them, the temperature field of the AHE is almost symmetrical on vertical direction, but it is very unsymmetrical on horizontal direction.

This difference causes the heat transfer imbalance on the AHE as a whole. Therefore, another design of coolant channel layout of AHE is tried, which is shown in Fig. 1(b). The temperature fields of this kind of AHE above are also obtained by FE simulation method, and shown in Fig. 2(d).

In order to clearly expose the temperature field of flowing coolant, temperature values of 8 locations are extracted from the flowing coolant inside AHE with 2 kinds of coolant channel layouts.

It can be seen in Fig. 3(d) that, the coolant temperature values of symmetrical coolant channel layout are lower than the ones of unsymmetrical layout. For the further verification of the advantages of unsymmetrical coolant channel layout of AHE, the outlet/inlet coolant temperature differences and supply powers are calculated and listed in Table 2. It can be shown that the symmetrical channel layout has the higher supply power capacity of AHE than the other layout.

Table 2 Supply powers comparing between 2 kinds of channel layout of AHE.

Channel layout	Temperature difference of coolant outlet and inlet /°C	Supply power /(J/s)
Unsymmetrical	4.400	1115.781
Symmetrical	2.510	1273.005

3.5. *Analysis and discussion*

After the FE simulations above, some analyses and conclusions can be done: the supply power capacity of AHE can be intensified by the following methods: the increase of its cross section area of channel, the increase of the coolant supply temperature, the increase of supply volume flow rate and the usage of unsymmetrical coolant channel layout.

In order to clearly present the relationship between supply powers and coolant supply conditions (supply temperature and volume flow rate), the following nonlinear regression function is adopted in this paper.

$$z = 2176.8x - 4046.2y - 201.1x^2 + 826.2y^2 + 7.3x^3 - 72.2y^3 - 0.1x^4 + 2.3y^4 \quad (2)$$

In the equation 2, x is the coolant supply temperature, y is the coolant supply volume rate, and z is the supply power capacity of AHE. The obtained 3 dimensional graph is shown in Fig. 4.

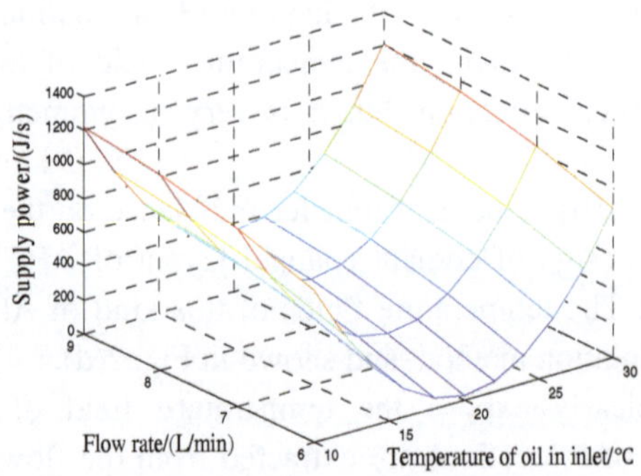

Fig. 4 Supply power capacity of AHE under different coolant supply conditions.

4. Conclusions

A supply power capacity design method of AHE is provided in this paper. The supply power capacity can be adjusted through changing the inlet temperature and flow rate of coolant, some simulations have been completed, including the inlet temperature, flow rate of coolant and layout of the coolant channels. The simulating results illustrate that this method can be used to control and improve the thermal deformation of precision machine structure.

References

1. M. Weck, P. McKeown, R. Bonse. *Reduction and compensation of thermal errors in machine tools*. CIRP Ann. - Manuf. Techn. 44 (1995) 589-598.
2. Y. Kang, C. Chang, Y. Huang. *Modification of a neural network utilizing hybrid filters for the compensation of thermal deformation in machine tools*. Int. J. Mach. Tool. Manu. 47 (2007) 367-387.
3. C. Wu, C. Tang, C. Chang, Y. Shao. *Thermal error compensation method for machine center*. Int. J. Adv. Manuf. Tech. 59 (2012) 681-689.
4. J. Han, L. Wang, H. Wang, N. Cheng. *A new thermal error modeling method for CNC machine tools*. Int. J. Adv. Manuf. Tech. 62 (2012) 205-212.
5. Y. Zhang, J. Yang, H. Jiang. *Machine tool thermal error modeling and prediction by grey neural network*. Int. J. Adv. Manuf. Tech. 59 (2012) 1068-1072.
6. T. Liu, W. Gao, Y. Tian, H. Zhang, W. Chang, K. Mao, D. Zhang. *A differentiated multi-loops bath recirculation system for precision machine tools*. Appl. Therm. Eng. 76 (2015) 54-63.

Research on the Modification Technology for Tapered Roller Bearing of Rotary Liner Hanger in Ultra-Deep Well Drilling*

Weiqing Li, Zhijun Niu and Guangshe Chen

School of Engineering and Technology, China University of Geosciences (Beijing)
Beijing, 10083, China
liweiqing@cugb.edu.cn

The bearing is a key part of the rotary liner hanger in the drilling engineering of ultra-deep wells and complex wells. However, the load capacity and service life of bearings are always the primary bottlenecks for the development of rotary liner cementing technology. The main failure form of rotary liner hanger bearing is roller end breakage. This paper put forward the improved modification methods of tapered roller to amend the classical modification theory. The improved methods were applied to thrust tapered roller of rotary liner hanger bearing and were analyzed by FEM. The analyzing result show that the improved modification methods are effective and accurate and the improved logarithmic generatrix is the best modification scheme of hanger bearing roller. The research result can provide a practical and theoretical basis for tapered roller bearings in ultra-deep well drilling engineering.

Keywords: Roller generatrix modification; rotary liner hanger bearing; FEM.

1. Introduction

In ultra-deep and complicated well drilling, well cementing is the most important step of drilling engineering. The bearing is a key part of the rotary liner hanger. In the liner drilling and cementing process, the bearing has to carry the weight of the entire liner [1]. Fig. 1 shows the bearing location in rotary liner hanger. However, the size of the bearing is small because of borehole size restrictions. A special bearing is needed that can function under heavy loads (more than 60 t axial force and more than 600 N•m torque) and extreme working conditions, such as high temperature (more than 120°C), high pressure, and mud. The load capacity and service life of bearing are the primary bottlenecks in the development of rotary liner cementing technology. Previous research [2] show that the main failure form of rotary liner hanger bearing is roller end

* This work is supported by the Fundamental Research Funds for the Central Universities (265201304)

breakage. One of the reasons is that Roller end appear stress concentration [3]. This paper apply roller generatrix modification to improve the stress concentration phenomenon of roller ends, so as to further improve the bearing capacity and prolong its service life [4].

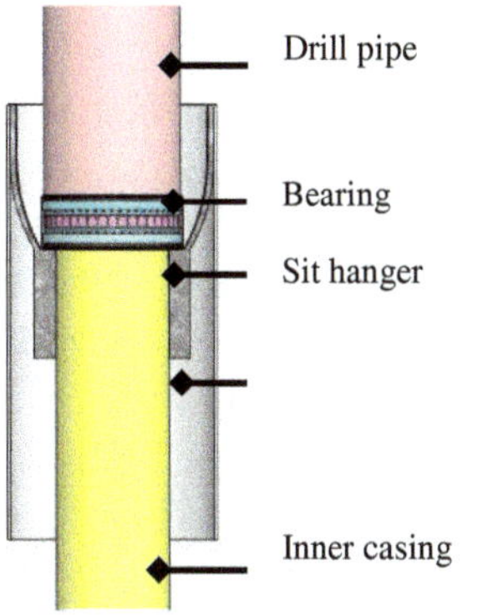

Fig. 1 Bearing location in rotary liner hanger.

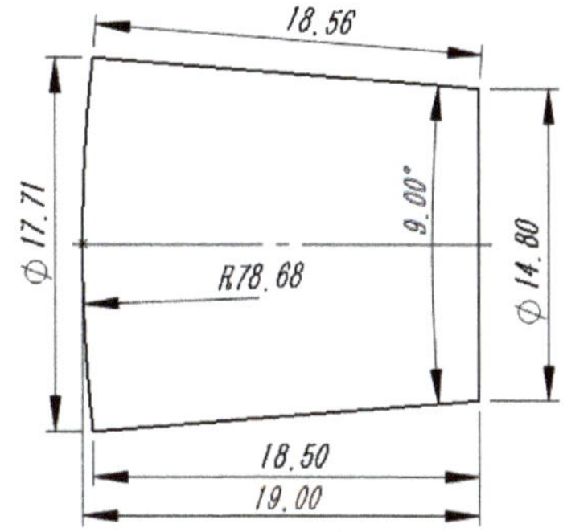

Fig. 2 Original shape of the bearing roller.

2. Modeling of Modification Generatrix for the Tapered Roller

Paper take rotating liner hanger bearing roller as an example to carry on the tapered roller modification research.

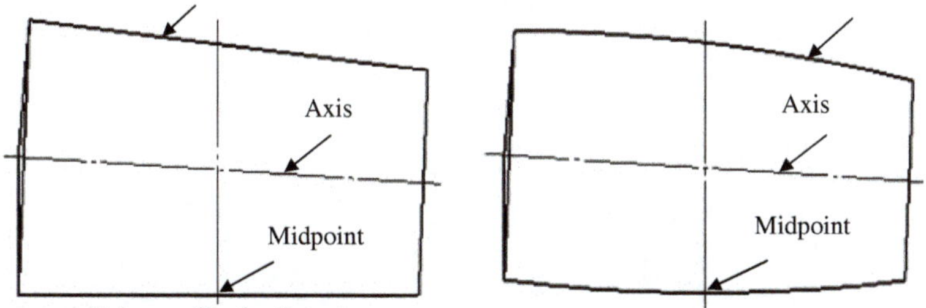

Fig. 3 Modeling of the modification tapered roller.

Fig. 2 is the original shape of its bearing roller. The modification generatrix modeling for the tapered roller is based on the following modification rules:

(1) keep the original axis and the midpoint of the generatrix unchanged before and after modification,
(2) put the generatrix of tapered roller in horizontal direction,
(3) set up new modification curve surrounding the original straight generatrix,

(4) rotate the new modification curve around the axis in 3D software modeling environment and the model is obtained.

Modeling process is shown in Fig. 3.

3. Improvement of Optimum Crown for Generatrix Modification of Intersecting, Cut and Convex Method

Four classic generatrix modification methods [5] are shown in Fig. 4. The generatrix modification curve formula for classic intersecting, cut, convex method show that the roller modification generatrix modeling is only based on geometric parameters of roller without involving the information of the load, material and other physical parameters. Generally, modification crown Z (L_{eff} / 2) (L_{eff} is the effective contact length) was defined by engineering experience. Z is the basis that calculate generatrix modification parameter R_c (the radius of the curve [6]). Then, based on the R_c, after roller was designed (select or define a certain material) and processed or modeled, actual experiment or Computer engineering analysis was done to verify the validity of the results. This method is difficult to be successful by one time and often need test or trial again and again which is inefficient and wasteful of resources, and the modification parameters may not be the best value.

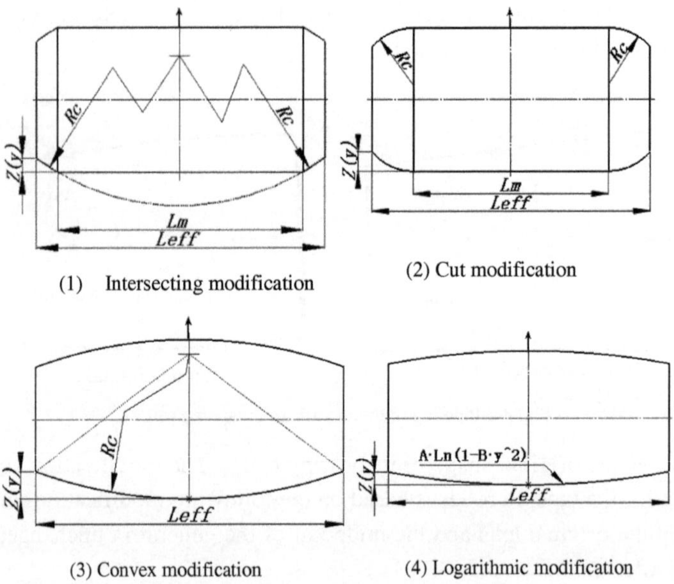

(1) Intersecting modification

(2) Cut modification

(3) Convex modification

(4) Logarithmic modification

Fig. 4 Four generatrix modification methods.

This paper gives improved modification formulas based on contact theory, which include comprehensive parameters for the tapered roller modification plan so that the modification is simple, accuracy and effective.

Contact problem research on the deformation in the contact area between two object that contact each other. Generally, the deformation is during the elastic range. Relative displacement will be produced because of the extrusion of the two contact objects. The relative displacement is called elastic approach (expressed by Palmgre formula [7]). Luo Jiwei [8] improved this formula by introducing the rate of roller length to diameter to it. This paper introduce the improved elastic approach into the tapered roller modification and obtain a general solution including geometric, material and load properties, as in Eq. (1).

$$\delta = 4.80 \cdot \left[\frac{1-\upsilon_1^2}{\pi E_1} + \frac{1-\upsilon_2^2}{\pi E_2} \right]^{0.9} \cdot \frac{F^{0.9}}{L_{eff}^{0.74} D_{we}^{0.1}} \tag{1}$$

Where, δ is the value of elastic approach of the roller and the ring. L_{eff} is the length of the straight generatrix. ν_1 and ν_2 respectively are the poisson's ratio of the roller material and ring material. E1 and E2 respectively are the young's modulus of the roller material and ring material. F is the vertical load of the roller generatrix. D_{we} is the equivalent diameter of the tapered roller, as in Eq. (2).

$$D_{we} = 0.5 \cdot (D1 + D2) / \cos\alpha \tag{2}$$

Where, D_1 and D_2 respectively are the big end and small end diameter of the tapered roller. α is the half cone angle of the tapered roller.

This paper made an assumption that the boundary value of the roller modification curve is equal to the elastic approach, as in Eq. (3). When the roller and raceway contact under load, roller ends and the raceway just contact and the stress values of the roller ends is almost zero [9]. This solution will greatly reduce the contact stress of the roller ends.

$$Z(\frac{L_{eff}}{2}) = \frac{\delta}{2} \tag{3}$$

Where Z is the modification crown.

Then, the best modification geometric parameter of the tapered roller can be obtained. Eq. (4), Eq. (5) and Eq. (6) respectively are the expressions of the radius for intersecting, cut and convex modification curve.

$$R_{c1} = \sqrt{\left[\frac{\left(1\text{-}a^2\right) L_{eff}^{\ 2}}{4\delta} - \frac{\delta}{4}\right]^2 + \frac{L_{eff}^{\ 2}}{4}} \tag{4}$$

$$R_{c2} = \frac{\delta}{2} + \frac{\left(1\text{-}a\right)^2 L_{eff}^{\ 2}}{4\delta} \tag{5}$$

$$R_{c3} = \frac{\delta}{4} + \frac{L_{eff}^{\ 2}}{4\delta} \tag{6}$$

The improved formulas not only include the geometry information, but also include the material and load information. In order to verify the result of this modification, finite element method was applied on both sides of the value from the improved formula and the result showed that the modification results is optimal value.

4. Improvement of Logarithmic Curve Modification Scheme

Classic Lundberg [10] logarithmic modification curve is Eq. (7) that contains the load, material parameters, geometric parameters of roller and etc. However, the modification curve has jumping discontinuous points which locate at the border point ($y=\pm L_{eff}/2$) and may produce stress and distortion. The measure in industry is that abandoned some curve outside the jump discontinuity point and expand the curve between two jump discontinuity points on the whole generatrix. Efficiency of this kind of design is low, and it is not able to fully apply the advantages of Lundberg logarithmic curve.

$$\begin{cases} Z(y) = \left(\dfrac{1\text{-}\nu_1^2}{\pi E_1} + \dfrac{1\text{-}\nu_2^2}{\pi E_2}\right)\dfrac{F}{L_{eff}} \ln\left[\dfrac{1}{1-\left(\dfrac{2y}{L_{eff}}\right)^2}\right] & \left(-\dfrac{1}{2}L_{eff} < y < \dfrac{1}{2}L_{eff}\right) \quad (7\text{-}1) \\ Z\left(\pm\dfrac{L_{eff}}{2}\right) = \left(\dfrac{1\text{-}\nu_1^2}{\pi E_1} + \dfrac{1\text{-}\nu_2^2}{\pi E_2}\right)\dfrac{F}{L_{eff}}\left(1.1932 + \ln\dfrac{L_{eff}}{2b}\right) & \left(y = \pm\dfrac{1}{2}L_{eff}\right) \quad (7\text{-}2) \end{cases}$$

Ma Jiaju [11] put forward a kind of measure for cylindrical roller logarithmic curve. This paper combined the measure of Ma Jiaju with the subject of the specific condition of tapered roller and established a successive approximation modification curve by curve fitting.

In order to unify the two formula form (Eq. (7-1) and Eq. (7-2)), the transformation was carried on, as in Eq. (8).

Given:

$$\left(1.1932 + \ln\frac{L_{eff}}{2b}\right) = Ln\frac{1}{1-\left(1-\frac{1}{e^{1.1932}}\frac{2b}{L_{eff}}\right)} \tag{8}$$

$$A = \left(1-\frac{1}{e^{1.1932}}\frac{2b}{L_{eff}}\right) \tag{9}$$

$$B = Ln\frac{1}{1-\left(1-\frac{1}{e^{1.1932}}\frac{2b}{L_{eff}}\right)\left(\frac{2y}{L_{eff}}\right)^2} \tag{10}$$

Where b is the contact width of roller and ring.

$$b = \sqrt{\frac{2FD_{we}}{\pi L_{eff} E'}} \quad \text{and} \quad \frac{1}{E'} = \frac{1-\nu_1^2}{E_1} + \frac{1-\nu_2^2}{E_2}.$$

A is almost equal to 1 because of $b \ll L_{eff}$.

So, B not only approximately equal to the behind item of Eq. (7-1) when $-\frac{1}{2}L_{eff} < y < \frac{1}{2}L_{eff}$, but also approximately equal to the behind item of Eq. (7-2) when $y = \pm\frac{1}{2}L_{eff}$

So the Lundberg logarithmic curve become the continuous form as Eq. (11) by curve fitting.

$$Z(y) = \left(\frac{1-\nu_1^2}{\pi E_1} + \frac{1-\nu_2^2}{\pi E_2}\right)\frac{F}{L_{eff}}\ln\frac{1}{1-\left(1-\frac{1}{e^{1.1932}}\frac{2b}{L_{eff}}\right)\left(\frac{2y}{L_{eff}}\right)^2} \quad \left(-\frac{1}{2}L_{eff} \le y \le \frac{1}{2}L_{eff}\right) \tag{11}$$

By the above transformation, unified expression to express the logarithmic modification was obtain and solved the problem of discontinuity for the logarithmic curve modification of tapered roller.

5. Verification

Applying the improved tapered roller modification formulas, this paper set up each corresponding modification scheme models in the Solidworks software and assembly with the axis ring and seat ring and simulate their effects by finite element simulation software [12].

Fig. 5 showed that the stress concentration appeared at both ends of the straight generatrix roller, which is the edge effect that is the main reason of the failure for the bearing.

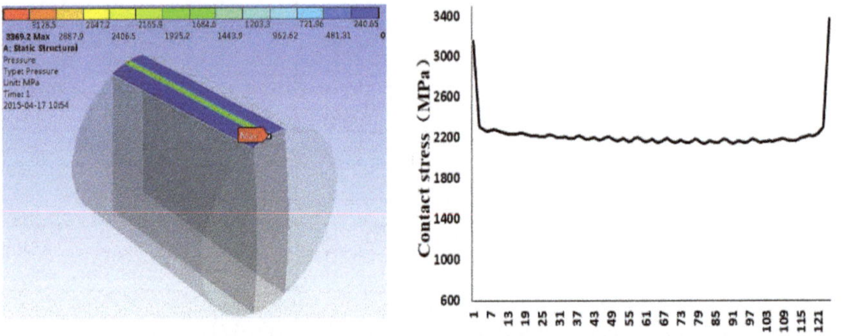

The edge effect showed in FEM Relative length along straight generatrix of the roller

Fig. 5 Distribution of contact stress of straight generatrix roller.

Fig. 6 show the modification effect of four improved modification methods.

(1) Improved intersecting medication: The edge effect at both ends disappear in the intersecting modification generatrix roller. However, relatively large stress concentration phenomenon appear at the junction of the intersecting curve and linear though the curve of the middle parts of the stress is relatively flat.

(2) Improved cut modification: The distribution of contact stress on improved cut modification generatrix roller is similar to the intersecting modification generatrix roller. The maximum stress value is slightly smaller than the maximum stress of intersecting modification roller.

(3) Improved convex modification: The edge effect at both ends disappeared on the improved convex modification generatrix roller. However, the distribution of the contact stress is arc form which is similar to the shape of the generatrix, and the maximum stress is in the middle of the roller generatrix.

(4) Improved logarithmic modification: The edge effect at both ends do not appear and there is not any stress concentration phenomenon in the improved logarithmic generatrix roller.

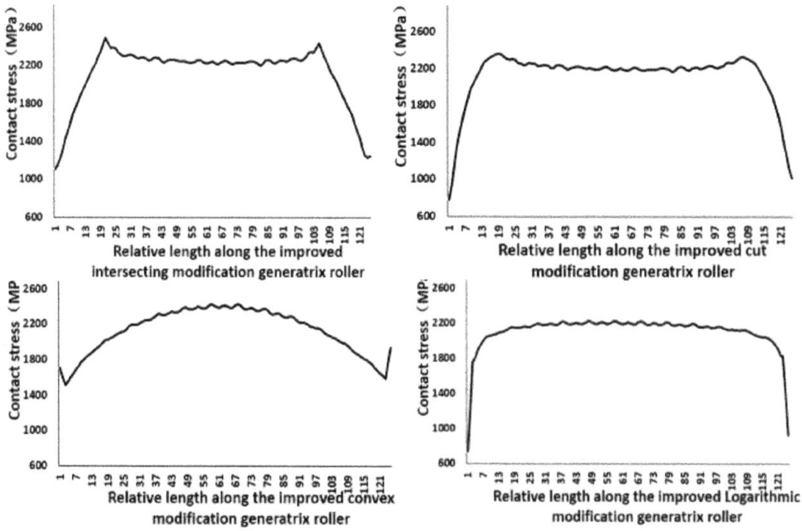

Fig. 6 Distribution of contact stress on improved modification generatrix roller.

Table 1 is a summary table of maximum stress and distribution of the four kinds of improved modification roller.

Table 1 Summary table of maximum stress and distribution of the four kinds of improved modification roller.

Schedule of improved modification	Value of the maximum stress (Mpa)	Edge effect	Stress concentration
Straight	3869.2	Yes	----
intersecting	2495.1	No	Yes
cut	2366.3	No	Yes
convex	2431.3	No	Yes
Logarithmic	2233.5	No	No

Table 1 showed that logarithmic modification method is the best way because its maximum stress is minimum and there is no edge effect and no stress concentration.

6. Conclusion

This paper improved the modification theory and applied the result to the hanger bearings for deep well drilling. The capacity and service of the bearing have been improved. The improved modification methods have certain universal significance in tapered roller bearing modification.

References

1. Wang Jianchong, *Finite Element Analysis of Rotary Liner Hanger Bearing in Ultra-Deep Well Drilling Based on ANSYS WORKBENCH, Master's Thesis*, China University of Geosciences for Master Degree (2014).
2. Weiqing Li, Jianchong Wang, *Analysis of Thermo-Mechanical Coupling Characteristics and Structural Design of Rotary Liner Hanger Bearing in Ultra-Deep Well Drilling.* Proceedings of IMETI 2014. P33-39, (Orlando Florida, USA), July 15-18, 2014.
3. Tedric A. Harris, Michael N. Kotzalas, *Essential Concepts of Bearing Technology, Rolling Bearing Analysis,* (Taylor & Francis Group, NW. USA, 2007), pp. 146-147.
4. Hertz H., *on the contact of elastic solids*, (J. Reine and Angew. Math. 1881).
5. Wei Yangang, Wang Zhongmin, Qu Rongjun, *Design of Roller Crowning of Cylindrical Roller Bearings*, Vol. 25, (Journal of Dalian Railway Institute, China, 2004), pp. 23-27.
6. Liu Jiajun, *Processing technology of bearing rollers and its Analysis,* metal processing, Vol. 1 (Metal Processing, China, 2014), pp. 47-49.
7. Palmgren, *Ball and Roller Bearing Engineering*, (Skf Industries Inc, Philadelphia, 1959).
8. Luo Jiwei, *Analysis Calculation and Application of Rolling Bearing*, (Mechanical Industry Press, China, 2009)
9. Weng Shixi, *Construction of Convexity Programs for the Tapered Roller Bearing*, Vol.35, (Harbin Bearing, China, 2014), pp. 82–84.
10. Lundberg G., Plangent A. *Dynamic Capacity of Rolling Bearings*, Vol. 1, (Alta Polytechnic a Mechanical Engineering Series, Swedish, 1974).
11. Ma Jiaju, Xu Wen, Liu Shuangbiao, et al, *Engineering design of logarithmic roller*, (Bearings, China, 1997), pp. 2-5.
12. Huang Zhixin, *Super Learning Manual of Workbench14.0 ANSYS*, (People's Posts and Telecommunications Press, China, 2013).

Design and Analysis on a Scalability Mechanism for Plug Seedling Transplanting and Separating

Xifeng Liang and Yangyang Cai
College of Mechanical and Electrical Engineering, China Jiliang University, Hangzhou, 310018, China
E-mail: lxfcjlu@163.com; cjlucyy@sina.com

In order to improve the operating efficiency and quality of the plug seedlings, a machine for seedling transplanting and separating with extensibility was developed. This machine is composed of end effectors and transplanting seedling mechanism. In the paper, we designed seedling transplanting and separating mechanism and analyzed the force on the machine. We adopted the upper two-dimensional X-Z mobile platform for initial position adjustment, and lower two-dimensional X-Y mobile platform for column and row adjustment. The end effectors take or put off the seedlings through cam mechanism. The simulation results of force analysis show that the maximum stress and the maximum error of ball screw are $3.40^{+07}N/m^2$ and 0.82mm respectively. The maximum stress and the maximum error of the finger are respectively $3.90^{+07}N/m^2$ and 4.1mm, which can meet the seedling transplanting and separating requirements.

Keywords: Seedling separating; transplanting; force analysis; end effector.

1. Introduction

When plug seedlings or pots are put into the greenhouse, lighting will be affected with seedling growing due to the fixed plug seedlings position. So it is necessary to transplant and separate the plug seedlings. At present, some researchers at home and board have studied many plug seedling transplanting machines, but it still in the initial stage in China[4]. For example, the robotic transplanter of bedding plants is invented by Kutz[1] and the XT616 transplanter is invented by Transplant Systems Corporation[2]. The main function of those transplanting machine are transplanting seedlings from the tray to the another tray. Most end effectors adopt pneumatic technology due to this technology has the advantages of high reliability, long service life and no pollution to the environment[3]. Many searchers are studying the transplanting machine to make it more comprehensive and perfect [5]-[9]. But there are some problems in the technology, such as it's difficult to determine the initial position and the number of end effectors is limited on many transplant machines. Column and row space adjustment is hard to achieve at same time. In this paper, we designed a seedling transplanting and separating machine which can adjust the column and row space of the plug seedlings simultaneously and transplant the seedlings from one position to another. At the time, force analysis and simulation is conducted on the machine.

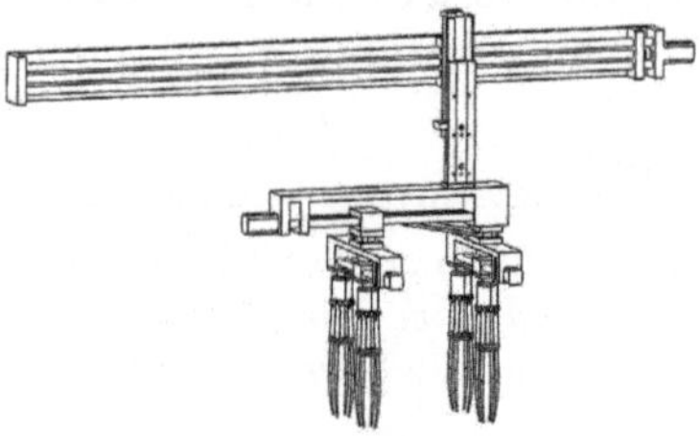

a. The Assembly Drawing

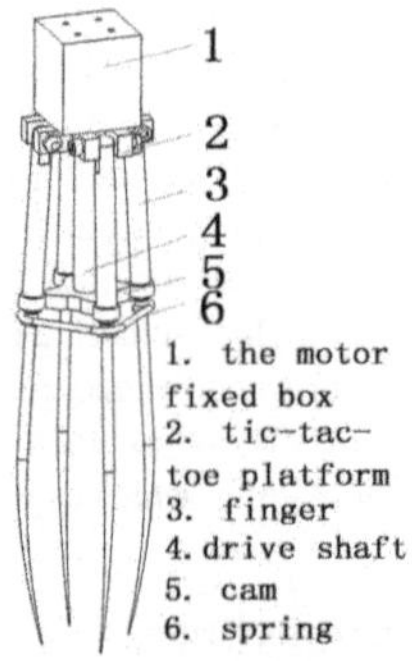

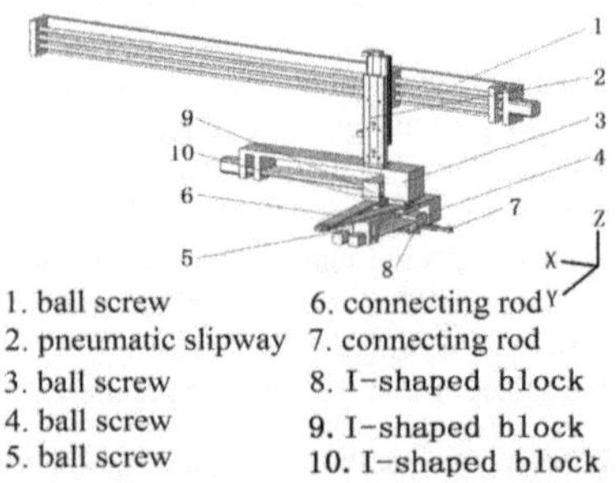

b. The End Effector c. The Transplanting and Separating Mechanism

Fig. 1 Seedling transplanting and separating machine and its constitutes.

2. Mechanical System Design of the Machine and the Principle of Seedling Transplanting and Separating

The seedling transplanting and separating machine (Fig. 3a) is composed of the end effectors (Fig. 3b) and the transplanting and separating mechanism (Fig. 3c). From Fig. 3b, we can see when the end effector works, the opening angle of the end effector is decided by the cam stroke. The spring is to control the end effectors grasping force. From Fig. 3c, the transplanting and separating mechanism is composed by the ball screw and pneumatic slipway. When the machine begins to take plug seedlings, all the sliders of the ball screw will be moved to the end of the ball screw. The cam will be kept at the maximum stroke. Then, the pneumatic slipway begins to decline and the cam will be turned 90 degrees. When the machine begins to put off plug seedlings, the sliders of the ball screw will be moved to the expected position. Then, the pneumatic slipway begins to decline and the cam will be turned 90 degrees. In order to improve the working efficiency, we can add the number of the no screw thread and end effector between the screw thread sliders and the end of the ball screw on the machine according to different specification plugs due to Sliders connect with M-shaped link mechanism.

3. Force Analysis on Seedling Transplanting and Separating Machine

3.1. *Force analysis of end effectors*

Insert the finger of the end effectors into the soil with a certain angle. When the end effectors grabbed the plug seedlings, the plug seedlings are subjected to adhesion K (include the adhesion K_{side} of the four sides and the adhesion K_{gorund} of the ground), the four fingers' support N and the friction F_f between one plug seedlings and finger. The plug seedling is kept balance state in the whole process of grasping. The four fingers are subjected to the well-distributed force and the force of the fingers can be simplified to the two mutually perpendicular planes. In the plane of two fingers, the balance equation of the various forces in the vertical direction is:

$$4F_f\cos\alpha + 4N_1\sin\alpha = K_{ground} + 4K_{side1}\cos\beta \tag{1}$$

Where, K is determined by the plugs' material, the size of the plugs, the weight of plug seedlings, the component and moisture content of the plug seedlings and other factors. The adhesion K measured by experiment is 5.6N. F_{f} is composed of two parts, the soil slip friction F_{a} and the slip resistance F_b due to the soil stickiness.

$$F_{f1} = F_a + F_b = \mu\left(N_1 + kS_1\right) \tag{2}$$

Where, μ is coefficient of soil friction, set as 0.5. N means grasping force. k is adhesion pressure, k=3×10^{3}Pa. S is the adhesion of the actual contact area between the soil and the finger, in this paper it means the buried area of the fingers, set S_1 as 90×10^{-6}m^2. Combining Eq. (1) and Eq. (2), we could get the relational model between the grasping force and the buried angle of the fingers:

$$N_1 = \frac{1.4 - 0.27\cos\alpha}{0.5\cos\alpha + \sin\alpha} \tag{3}$$

In simulation, we set the buried angle α=10° and select the materials of the effector is aluminum alloy. Then we can get N_1=1.7N and the reaction force of the plug seedling to the finger is N_2=1.7N. And we set the elastic force of the spring as F_{spring}=2N. The end of the finger is fixed on the tic-tac-toe platform. The stress and deformation variation of the finger are shown in Fig. 2a and Fig. 2b.

From Fig. 2a and Fig. 2b, we can see the maximum stress of the finger is 3.90^{+07} N/m^2 and the maximum deformation is 4.1mm. When the end effector do not grab seedlings, the maximum distance of the fingers is 31.6mm. So the final distance of the fingers is 39.8mm. And the distance between one plug seedling and another is 40mm. Therefore, the end effector meets the working requirements.

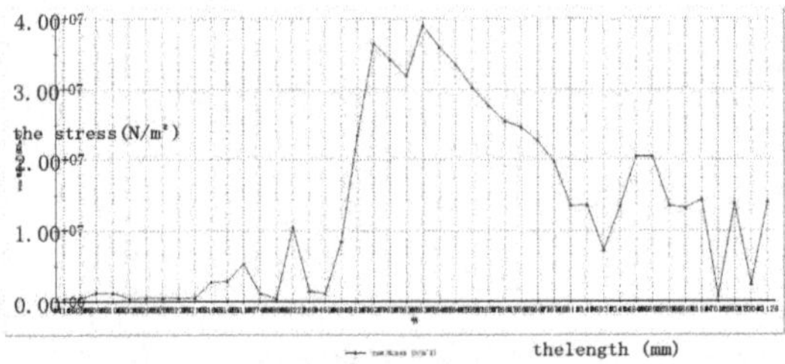

a. Stress Variation of the Finger

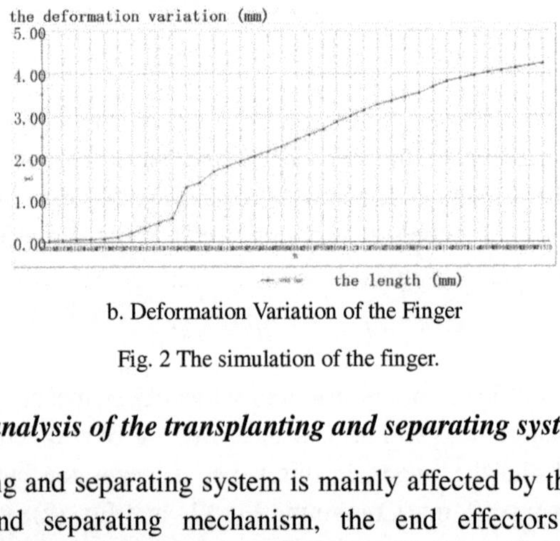

b. Deformation Variation of the Finger

Fig. 2 The simulation of the finger.

3.2. *The stress analysis of the transplanting and separating system*

The transplanting and separating system is mainly affected by the quality of the transplanting and separating mechanism, the end effectors and the plug seedlings. We analyzed stress and deformation of all the ball screws on the machine. Only taking the ball screw 1 (shown in Fig. 1c) for example in this paper due to the ball screw 1 is subjected to the maximum force. The simulation flow chart is shown in Fig. 3.

In simulation, we set the material of the ball screw 1 as Alloy steel. And the weight of the each end effector is 77g. The weight of the transplanting and separating mechanism is 14kg. So the pulling force of the ball screw 1 is

14.077kg. At the same time, we add support force in the both ends of the ball screw 1.

From Fig. 4a and Fig. 4b, we can see the maximum stress of the ball screw 1 is $3.40^{+07}N/m^2$ and the maximum deformation is 0.82mm. So the maximum load of the ball screws 1 is 27kg. The length of the ball screw 1 is 1100mm, so the ball screw 1 has super stiffness and the material of the ball screw 1 is rational. Therefore, the strength and stiffness of the ball screw 1 meets the operation requirements.

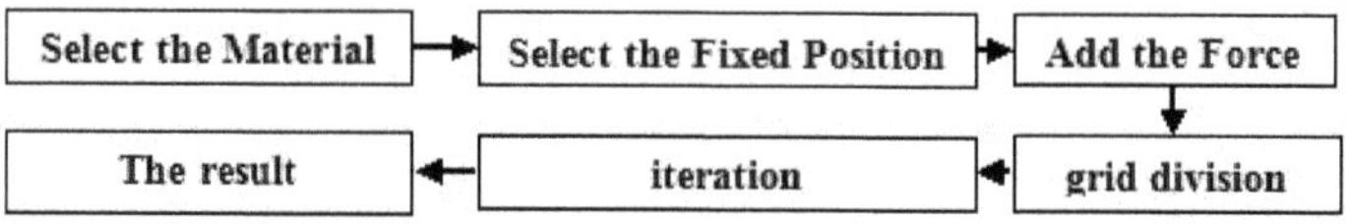

Fig. 3 The simulation flow chart.

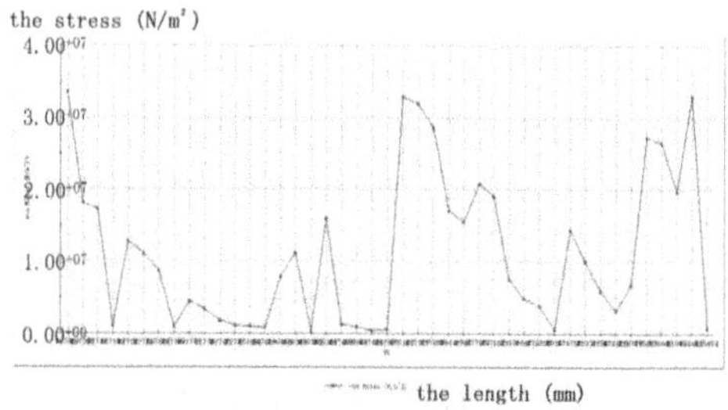

a. Stress Variation of Ball Screw 1

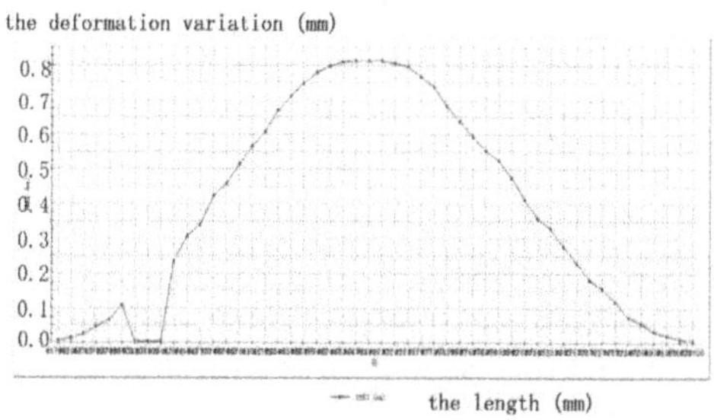

b. Deformation Variation of Ball Screw 1

Fig. 4 The simulation of the ball screw 1.

4. Conclusion and Discussions

We design the seedling transplanting and separating machine and build its 3D model in Solidworks. Stress and deformation of the end effector and the transplanting and separating mechanism of the machine are analyzed and simulated. The results show that The maximum distance of the end effector is

39.8mm. It shows that The maximum precision of the transplanting and separating system is 0.82mm. The strength and stiffness of the seedling transplanting and separating machine meet the working requirements.

The transplanting and separating machine's strength will be changed with the material change, so many experiments based on different materials should be conducted. In addition, the success rate of transplanting needs further research in the future.

Acknowledgment

This study is supported by Zhejiang Provincial Natural Science Foundation (LQ13E050010) and the National High-tech R&D Program (863 Program) (2012AA10A504).

References

1. W. Liu, J.Z. Liu, Review of End-effectors in Tray Seedlings Transplanting Robot, Journal of Agricultural Mechanization Research, 2013(7).
2. L.H. Zhang, L.C. Qiu, S.B. Tian, Progress in the Research of Manipulator of Transplanting Potted Tray Seedlings, Agricultural Science & Technology and Equipment, 2009(185).
3. H. Zhou, The Combination of Pneumatic and PLC in the Application of the Manipulator Design, Chinese Hydraulics & Pneumatics, 2004(3): 38-39.
4. H. Li, W.B. Cao, W.J. Gu, Design of New Roller－type Plastic Film Collector for Cotton Fields, Journal of Agricultural Mechanization Research, 2014(7).
5. W.J. Gu, W.B. Cao, W.M. Li, Q. Wang, Research on the Automation of Rod －type Pick up Device for Plug Seedlings, Journal of Agricultural Mechanization Research, 2013(12).
6. T. Zhou, X.C. Wang, C. Q. Wang, Design and Simulation Analysis of Transplanter for Potted tray Seedlings in Greenhouse, Machine Design and Research, 2009, 25(2).
7. H.P. Mao, W.Q. Ding, F. Liu, Structure Design and Simulation Analysis on the Plug Seedlings Auto-Transplanter, Proceedings of the 2010 International Conference of Agricultural Engineering, 2010.
8. Q.C. Feng, X. Wang, K. Jiang, Design and test of key parts on automatic transplanter for flower seedling, Transactions of the Chinese Society of Agricultural Engineering, 2013, 29(6).
9. G.H. Gao, W. Lv, S. Zhang, New Type of Seedlings Transplant Manipulator design in Greenhouse, Chinese Agricultural Mechanization, 2012(2).

Prediction of Vibration in Steam Turbine Shafting with Support Vector Machine

Tongtian Deng*, Jiasheng Wang, Xiaojun Li, Jingliang Zhong, Suobin Wang
Guizhou Electric Power Test and Research Institute, Guiyang 550002, China.
**E-mail: dengtongtian@163.com*

Dongxiang Jiang, Xiao Fu and Wenguang Yang
State Key Laboratory of Control and Simulation of Power System and Generation Equipments, Department of Thermal Engineering, Tsinghua University, Beijing 100084, China.

Prediction of vibration in steam turbine is beneficial for predictive maintenance. Based on vibration data in a practical steam turbine shafting, this work presents prediction of vibration parameters using support vector machine (SVM). Firstly, principle of SVM in parameter prediction is introduced. Secondly, the vibration data in the steam turbine is presented and the preprocessing is applied to get the deterioration trend. Finally, the prediction of the vibration is carried out with SVM, and the accuracy of the prediction is estimated. The results show that high accuracy is obtained with the proposed model.

Keywords: Vibration prediction; steam turbine; support vector machine.

1. Introduction

Prediction of vibration in steam turbine shafting is an important aspect in condition monitoring of steam turbine, where the vibration of the shafting is critical to the safety of the equipment [1]. Through analyzing the parameters that can indicate the statue of the steam turbine shafting, effective vibration parameters can be applied in prediction, to find out the deteriorating trend of the equipment and foresee the probable failure in an early stage. Historical data is usually applied in determining the failure feature and forming the prediction model.

In prediction of vibration parameters in steam turbine shafting, the amount of the historical data is a restrictive issue, where the prediction will be less accurate with insufficient data. And this is the situation in reality, where the prediction with statistical approaches is usually applied [2-4]. Prediction with small sample size is increasingly researched in the past decades, and support vector machine (SVM) is more and more applied due to its characteristics in obtaining optimal generalizing performance with minimal structural risk [5-6].

Based on vibration data in a practical steam turbine shafting, this work presents prediction of vibration parameters using SVM. Firstly, principle of SVM in parameter prediction is introduced. Secondly, the vibration data in the steam turbine is presented and the preprocessing is applied to get the deterioration trend. Finally, the prediction of the vibration is carried out with SVM, and the accuracy of the prediction is estimated.

2. Prediction of Time Series Data with Support Vector Machine

Based on minimal structural risk, SVM, proposed by Vapnik, is aimed to obtain optimal generalizing performance in small sample size [5]. SVM is proved with advantages in solving problems of nonlinearity, high dimensional, and local minimum. SVM can be applied in classification and regression. In prediction of parameters, Support Vector Machines Regression (SVMR) is used where the regression estimate is applied in SVM [7].

Given the training set, $D=\{(x_1,y_1),(x_2,y_2),\cdots,(x_n,y_n)\}\in(X\times Y)^n$, the regression is aimed to find out the minimal expectation of the risk:

$$R[f]=\int c(x,y,f)dP(x,y) \tag{1}$$

where the distribution of $P(x,y)$ is unknown.

For the linear regression, a regression function is defined:

$$y=f(x)=w\cdot x+b \tag{2}$$

To find out the minimal risk in Eq. (1), minimum of w is to be determined. Slack factors and Lagrangian multiplier are introduced, and the optimization equation is obtained,

$$\max W(\alpha_i,\alpha_i^*)=-\sum_{i=1}^{l}y_i(\alpha_i-\alpha_i^*)-\varepsilon\sum_{i=1}^{l}(\alpha_i+\alpha_i^*)-\frac{1}{2}\sum_{i,j=1}^{l}(\alpha_i-\alpha_i^*)(\alpha_j-\alpha_j^*)(x_i\cdot x_j). \tag{3}$$

subject to

$$\begin{aligned}&(1)\quad \sum_{i=1}^{l}(\alpha_i-\alpha_i^*)=0;\\ &(2)\quad \begin{cases}0\le\alpha_i\le C,\\ 0\le\alpha_i^*\le C.\end{cases} i=1,2,\cdots,l,\end{aligned} \tag{4}$$

With solutions of α_i,α_i^*, regression function is obtained from Eq. (2).

$$f(x)=\sum_{i=1}^{l}(\alpha_i-\alpha_i^*)(x_i\cdot x)+b \tag{5}$$

The linear regression is solved with Eq. (5). For the nonlinear regression in a lower dimensional space, kernel function is applied to get the linear problem in a higher dimensional space. The problem in the nonlinear regression is,

$$\max W(\alpha_i,\alpha_i^*)=-\sum_{i=1}^{l}y_i(\alpha_i-\alpha_i^*)-\varepsilon\sum_{i=1}^{l}(\alpha_i+\alpha_i^*)-\frac{1}{2}\sum_{i,j=1}^{l}(\alpha_i-\alpha_i^*)(\alpha_j-\alpha_j^*)K(x\cdot x_i). \tag{6}$$

where, $K(x,x_i)$ is the kernel function.

Then, the regression function is obtained with the kennel function,

$$f(x)=\sum_{i=1}^{l}(\alpha_i-\alpha_i^*)K(x\cdot x_i)+b. \tag{7}$$

RBF kernel function is widely applied and proved to be an optimal option.

3. Prediction of Vibration of Steam Turbine Shafting

Data collected from a steam turbine unit is applied in this work. During the operation, the vibration of the shafting increases from 50μm to 128μm. Historical data in a steam turbine shafting is shown in Fig. 1. Fluctuations are observed during the long term operation. In order to obtain the trend of the increasing vibration, data preprocessing is applied and the results are shown in Fig. 2.

With SVMR model, the prediction of the vibration is carried out, and the results are shown in Fig. 3.

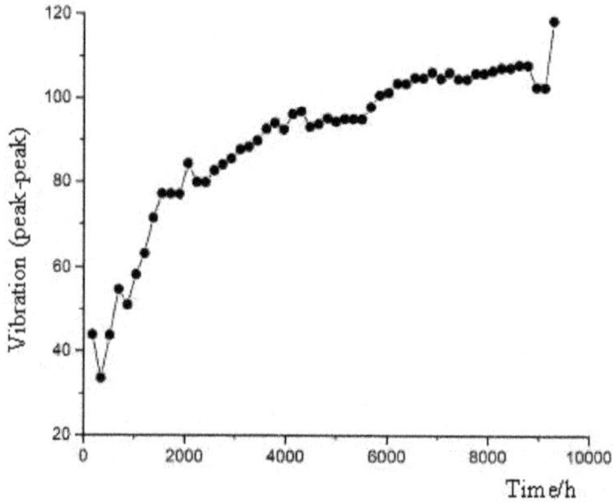

Fig. 1 Historical data of vibration in a steam turbine shafting.

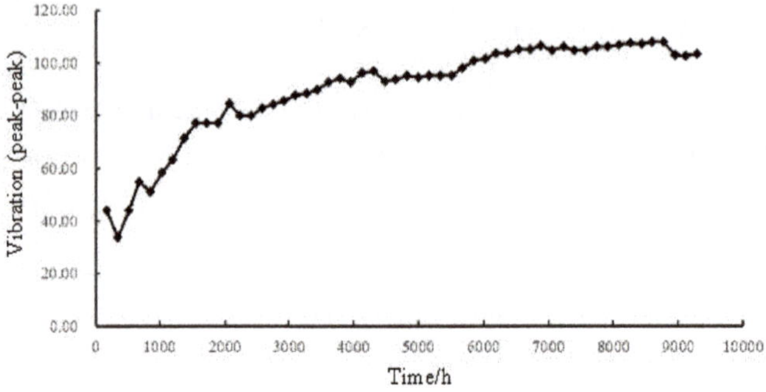

Fig. 2 Historical data of vibration in a steam turbine shafting (after preprocessing).

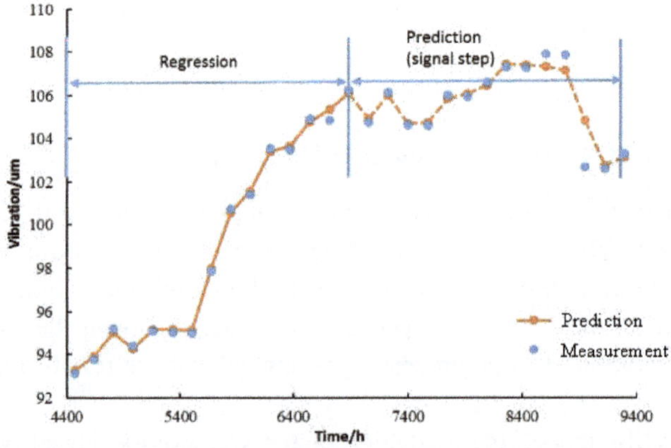

Fig. 3 Prediction results.

In order to estimate the performance of the prediction results with SVM, Mean Square Error (MSE) and correlation coefficient are defined:

$$MSE = \frac{1}{l}\sum_{i=1}^{l}(f(x_i) - y_i)^2, \tag{8}$$

$$r^2 = \frac{(\bar{l}\sum_{i=1}^{\bar{l}} f(x_i)y_i - \sum_{i=1}^{\bar{l}} f(x_i)\sum_{i=1}^{\bar{l}} y_i)^2}{(\bar{l}\sum_{i=1}^{\bar{l}} f(x_i)^2 - (\sum_{i=1}^{\bar{l}} f(x_i))^2)(\bar{l}\sum_{i=1}^{\bar{l}} y_i^2 - (\sum_{i=1}^{\bar{l}} y_i)^2)} \tag{9}$$

MSE in the prediction results is 0.41, and the correlation coefficient is 0.99. Also, the relative error is obtained and shown in Fig. 4.

Generally, the deterioration trend of the vibration in steam turbine shafting is predicted by SVM, and the MSE is below 2% in more than 90% of the cases.

High accuracy is obtained in the fitting results of the model, where the maximal MSE is 0.82%.

The maximal error in the prediction results lies in 8944h, where the MSE is 15.98%, and the relative error is 2.3%. The reason is that an obvious change is observed between the point and the previous point. It validates that, the accuracy is significantly decreased when the data presents quick changes.

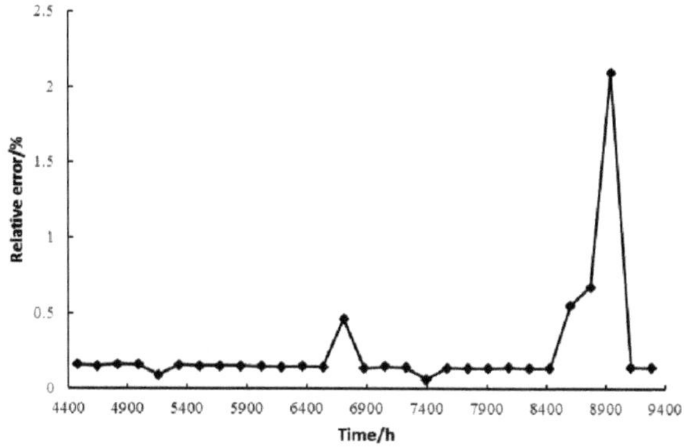

Fig. 4 Error estimate.

4. Conclusion

Prediction of vibration in steam turbine shafting is important for the fault diagnosis in an early state, which is beneficial for the predictive maintenance. Based on the operation data collected in the steam turbine unit, this work presents the prediction of vibration with support vector machine, where the support vector regression is applied. The results show that high accuracy is obtained with the proposed model. The prediction model can be applied in reality for condition monitoring, where the predicted results can be used for alarm setting. Further work is being carried out on problems of less accurate prediction when the data presents quick changes.

References

1. Beebe, Ray. "Condition monitoring of steam turbines by performance analysis." Journal of Quality in Maintenance Engineering 9, no. 2 (2003): 102-112.
2. Gençay, Ramazan, and Tung Liu. "Nonlinear modelling and prediction with feedforward and recurrent networks." Physica D: Nonlinear Phenomena 108, no. 1 (1997): 119-134.
3. Mirikitani, Derrick T., Lahcen Ouarbya, Lisa Tsui, and Eamonn Martin. "Improving forecasts of geomagnetic storms with evolved recurrent neural

networks." In Cybernetic Intelligent Systems (CIS), 2011 IEEE 10th International Conference on, pp. 44-49. IEEE, 2011.

4. Gao, You, and Yuli Shen. "Prediction of Aero-Engine Exhaust Gas Temperature Based on Chaotic Neural Network Model." In Advances in Mechanical and Electronic Engineering, pp. 145-150. Springer Berlin Heidelberg, 2012.
5. V.N. Vapnik, 'An overview of statistical learning theory', IEEE Transactions on Neural networks, vol. 10, No. (5), pp. 988–999, 1999.
6. S. Yuan, F. L. Chu, Support vector machine-based fault diagnosis for turbo-pump rotor, Mechanical Systems and Signal Processing, vol. 20, pp. 939-952, 2006.
7. Chang CC, Lin CJ: LIBSVM: a library for Support Vector Machines. [http://www.csie.ntu.edu.tw/~cjlin/libsvm] Tech. rep., Department of Computer Science, National Taiwan University; 2010.

The Application of Virtual Design in Packaging Carton Modeling in Combination

Wen Zhao[a], Zhang Xinrui[b], Zhou Kecheng[c] and Cai Huiping[d]
School of Printing and Packaging Engineering, Beijing Institute of Graphic Communication, Beijing, 102600, China
†E-mail: [a]wz315911@163.com; [b]1042142566@qq.com; [c]1607145593@qq.com; [d]caihuiping@bigc.edu.cn

Virtual design is an essential part of the folding carton design in packaging combination. In order to achieve the ideal result of the design, packing box type from 2D to 3D interface changes, in the process of transformation, by correction and adjustment of design parameters. In this paper, we analyzed the combination of triangles and non-triangular packaging carton design and molding, and given the appropriate combination of shaping design examples. In view of the virtual design application in the folding cartons combination, to find the different shapes of the structure of the forming and packing assembly in stack tile forming method of virtual design. According to the influence of the packaging combination modeling show, production and cost estimates, find out the optimal design. Not only for the convenience of the designer create a more beautiful and practical folding carton packing, but also to shorten production time packaging design, to save the cost of packaging design production, to reduce unnecessary loss of time, thereby to improve the production efficiency.

Keywords: Virtual design; carton model of the combination packing; triangular folding carton unit; non-triangular folding carton unit.

Virtual design is supported by the computer, on the premise of comprehensive simulation system. In the stage of product design, Virtual design based on virtual product design development and the whole process of simulation, and to modify related parameter model in the virtual environment, to start the simulation study of the manufacture of performance, cost, product design and production process. In product development and design process continuously improve product quality, at the same time to better estimate the product cost, reduce material waste. In today's sales package, folding carton packaging combination has become the most widely used in the production of the product packaging form. In order to save resources, protect the environment, virtual design in the packaging application combination box modelling design is particularly important. [1~4]

In the combination box packaging design, virtual design is an essential part in the design and production of packaging combination. Virtual design is applied to the packaging assembly modelling design. In order to achieve the ideal result of the design, packing box type from 2D to 3D interface changes, in the process of transformation, by correction and adjustment of design parameters. Virtual design can reduce the packaging waste of manufacturing costs, save material resources in the very great degree. In optimization design method, shorten the packing box production cycle, to improve the work efficiency. This article through to the different shapes of folding carton assembly modelling studies, looking for folding carton in virtual design optimization design approach, to discuss the triangular and non-triangular folding cartons basic structural units of the virtual design method.

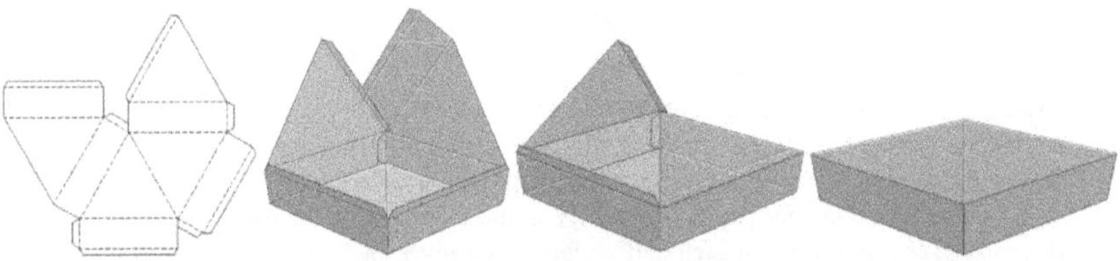

Fig. 1 Displays of the design of two triangular stack molding box.

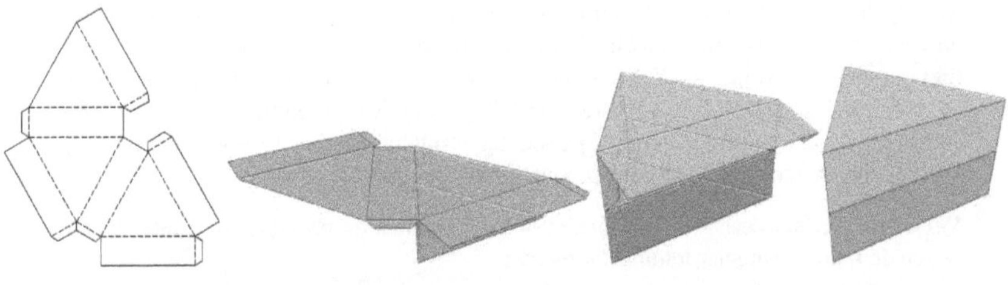

Fig. 2 Displays of the design of two triangular flat out into diamond shape.

1. The Combination of Triangular Folding Carton Unit

1.1. *The two symmetric combination model*

Two pieces of symmetric composite box based on triangle plate folding carton as the basic structural unit. Using surface connection between structural units formed the combination of two boxes. There are two kinds of forming method. Stack is a kind of two triangle box molding (Fig. 1), the other is a flat out into rhombus boxes (Fig. 2). Two symmetric combination boxes are suitable for the triangular two combination packing goods.

Horizontal combination of the bottom area is larger, can convenient observation content, but the display is covering. Vertical combination of the bottom area is lesser, display up to save space, but not convenient to observe the contents of each box.

1.2. *The three symmetrical combination model*

Three pieces of symmetric composite box based on triangle plate folding carton as the basic structural unit. Each structural unit with this part of the line connection thus formed the foundations of the three combination box. Also, this box has two kinds of forming method, the flat type (Fig. 3) and the stack type (Fig. 4). But stack type molding structure unit is used in plane connection. Three pieces of symmetric composite box is suitable for the three combination packaging of the triangle goods.

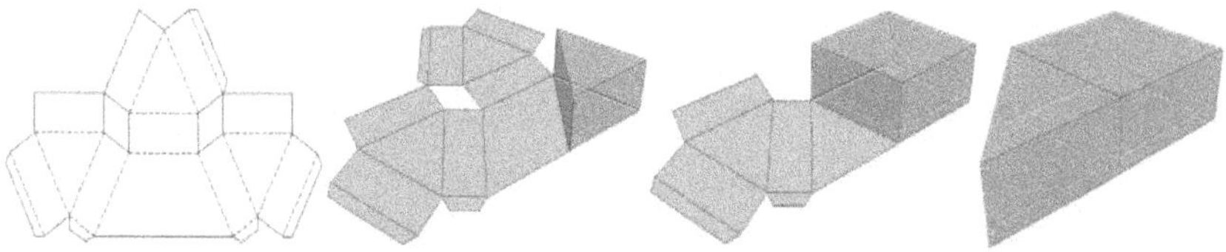

Fig. 3 Displays of the design of the flat shape molding.

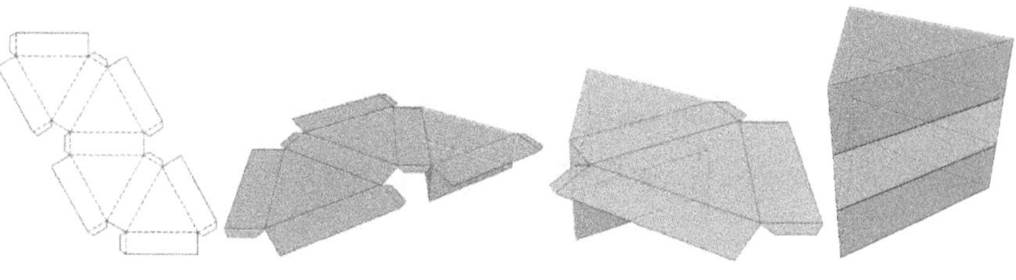

Fig. 4 Displays of the design of the stack type molding.

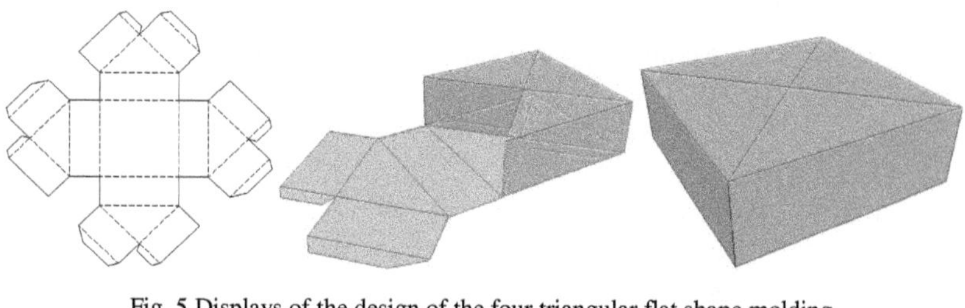

Fig. 5 Displays of the design of the four triangular flat shape molding.

1.3. *The four symmetrical combination model*

Four pieces of symmetric composite box based on triangle plate folding carton as the basic structural unit. Each structural unit with this part of the line connection thus formed the four a combo box. This box can be used in a four triangular tiling (Fig. 5). It can also be in the form of two stacked triangles (Fig. 6). Four symmetrical combination boxes are suitable for the triangle commodity combination of four pieces of packaging.

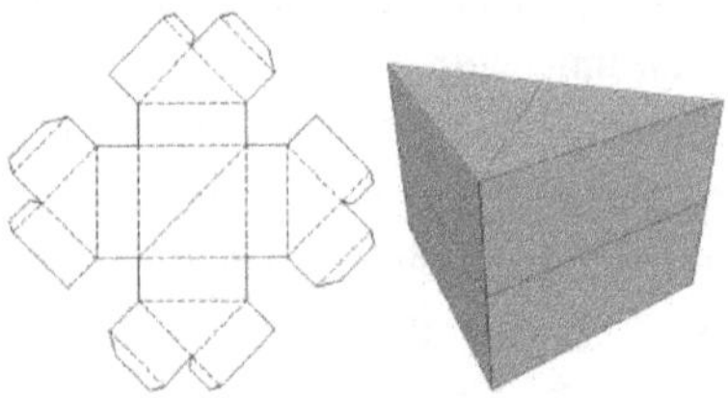

Fig. 6 Displays of the design of the two triangular stack type shape molding.

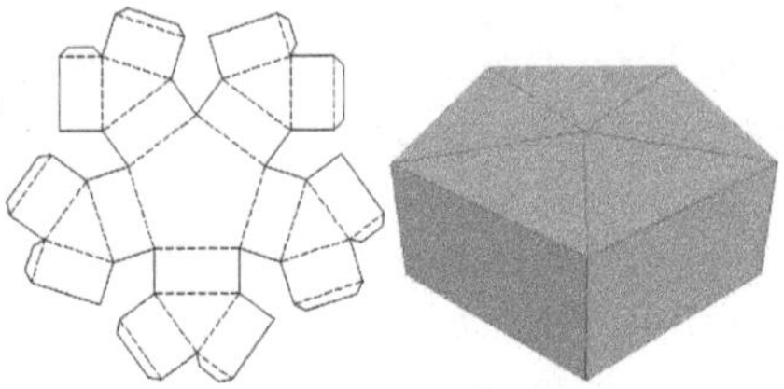

Fig. 7 Displays of the design of the five pieces of symmetric shape molding.

1.4. *The five symmetrical combination model*

Five pieces of symmetric composite box (Fig. 7) based on triangle plate folding carton as the basic structural unit. Each structural unit with this part of the line connection thus formed the five pieces of combo box. Five pieces of symmetric array combination box is suitable for the triangle of five pieces of goods packaging.

1.5. *The six symmetric combination model*

Six pieces of symmetric composite box based on triangle plate folding carton as the basic structural unit. Each structural unit with this part of the line connection formed the six combo box. This box with two forming modes, one is six triangular tiling is large hexagonal boxes (Fig. 8), another is three triangles stacked trapezoidal box (Fig. 9). Six pieces of symmetric composite box is suitable for the triangle commodity packaging six combinations.

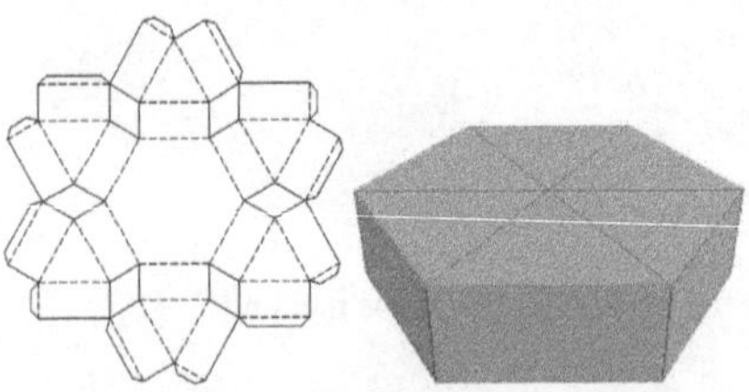

Fig. 8 Displays of the design of the flat shape molding.

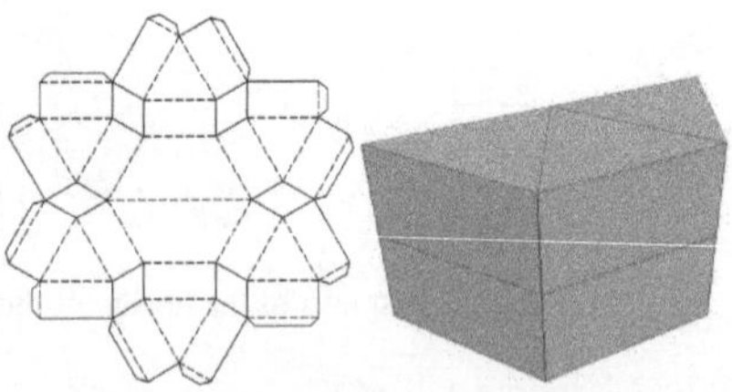

Fig. 9 Displays of the design of the stack type molding.

1.6. *The non-equilateral triangle carton combination of modeling*

All of the above is a combination of equilateral triangle folding carton. There can also be non-equilateral triangle folding cartons to combine (Fig. 10). This project is through the combination of the two folding carton right triangle, after forming the two right-angled triangle box consists of a four-prism box. And the two units are connected with line. The Non-equilateral triangle combo boxes are suitable for the two triangle commodity combination packaging.

The combination of two units has a change, can put the box type combination after forming the square into a parallelogram (Fig. 11). The two units are also connected with line. Parallelogram box is better than a square box can attract the consumers.

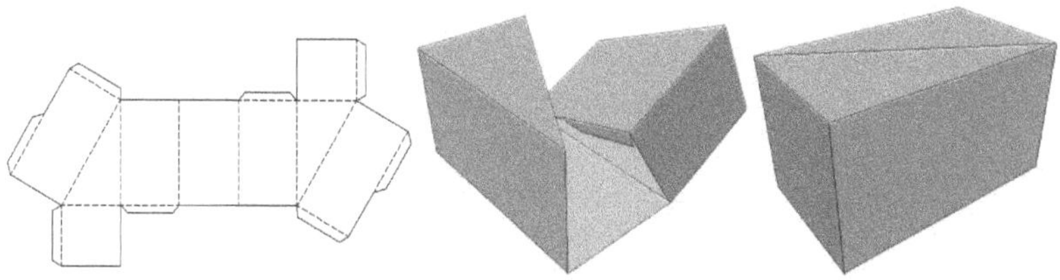

Fig. 10 Displays of the design of the non-equilateral triangle molding.

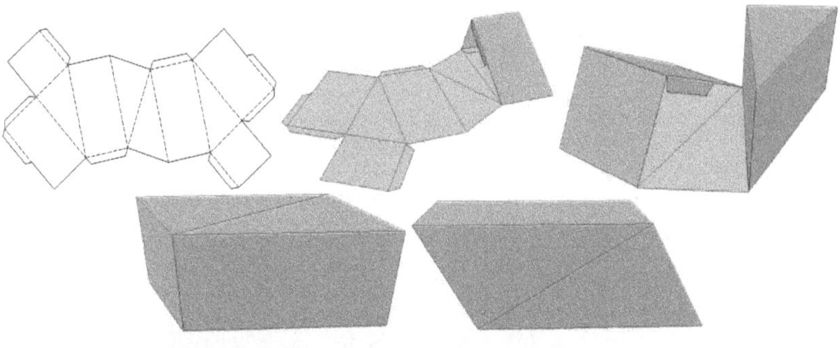

Fig. 11 Displays of the design of the Parallelogram box molding.

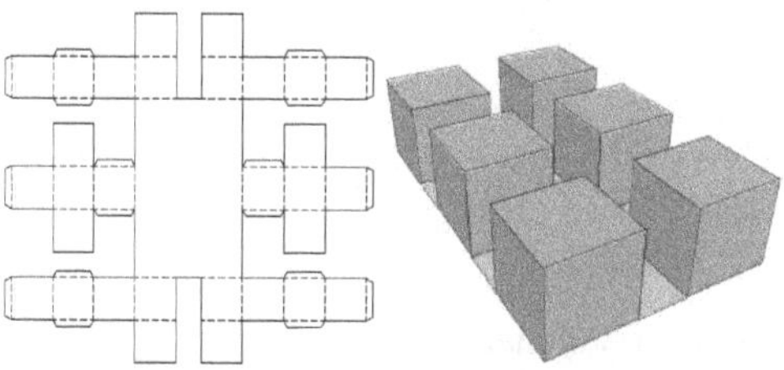

Fig. 12 Displays of the design of the square carton unit molding.

2. The Combination of Non-Triangular Folding Carton Unit

2.1. *The square box unit combination*

Six pieces of symmetric composite box based on square plate folding carton as the basic structural unit (Fig. 12). Each structural unit with this part of the line connection formed the six combo box. Six units are exactly the same, and join plate design, in order to convenient display and carton forming. If add some decoration in the diaphragm, the display effect is better.

2.2. *The frustum of a pyramid box unit combination*

Two pieces of symmetric composite box based on three frustum of a pyramid folding carton as the basic structural unit (Fig. 13). Each unit connected by lines. Molding, the bottom two triangles overlap together.

Two pieces of symmetric composite box based on six frustum of a pyramid folding carton as the basic structural unit (Fig. 14). Each unit connected by lines. Molding, the bottom two hexagons overlap together.

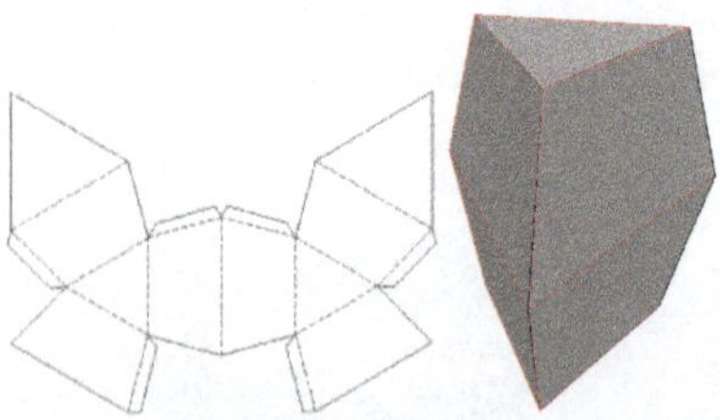

Fig. 13 Displays of the design of the three frustum of a pyramid type folding molding.

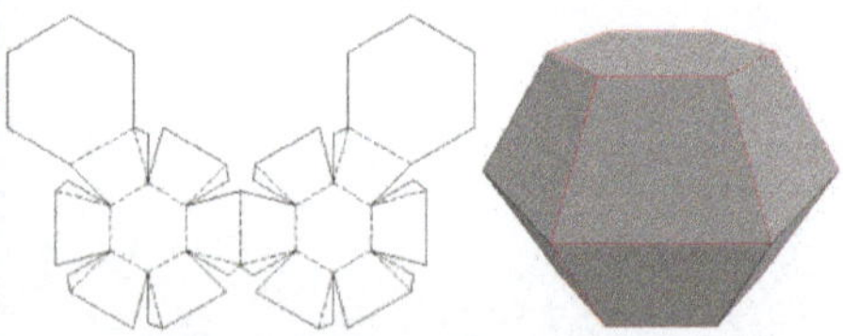

Fig. 14 Displays of the design of the six frustum of a pyramid type folding molding.

Fig. 15 Displays of the design of the three asymmetric combination boxes.

2.3. *Child-Mother combination box*

The three asymmetric combination boxes (Fig. 15), from left to right, respectively is mother-box, son-box 1 and the son-box 2. They are common tube type folding carton. And their structure of each unit of length, width and depth are not equal. Among them, the mother-box to son-box belongs to the box body is connected. Son-box 1 and 2 belongs to the box body is connected.

To sum up, this kind of child-mother box can be flexible according to the actual packing situation changes, in order to meet the need of commodity packaging. The child-mother box is suitable for supporting the commodity packaging box, such as cosmetics, clothes, toiletries, etc of form a complete set of packaging. This kind of packing is both beautiful and convenient, it is very practical.

2.4. *The carton with angle combination box*

This is the quadrangular columnar folding carton angular design (Fig. 16). Different from in front of three prism angle structure, quadrangular prism cartridge body angular part is integrally, however, in front of three prism Angle structure is the paste. So the quadrangular columnar folding cartons are more solid and practical.

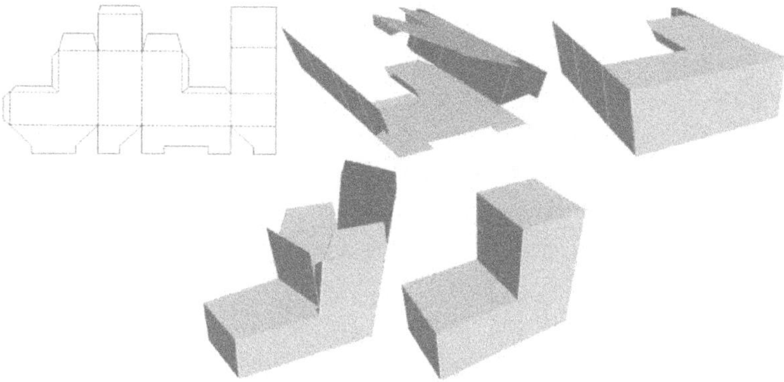

Fig. 16 Displays of the design of the carton with angle combination box.

3. Conclusion

Because of the folding carton assembly modeling in the process of structural design, virtual design is very necessary and meaningful. So, through the design of triangular and non triangular combination, give the analyzed to the corresponding combination of shape design example. Firstly, According to flat and stack type classification, the triangular folding carton composition unit to carry on the design, to study the forming process and characteristics. Tile forming, is advantageous to the contents of the display and observation, but the display area is larger, not easy to place. Stack molding, the display area is lesser, but it is not easy to put contents. In the second, When study the triangular folding carton unit combination, we studied the square type, frustum of a pyramid type, child-mother type and contains the angle type combinations, according to the corresponding structural unit and display content characteristics of box type design.

For virtual design in the application of combination folding carton, we can draw the following conclusions. Different shapes of the structure of the forming and packing assembly in stack tile forming method of virtual design, will affect their show in packing assembly modeling, production process and cost budget, etc. Virtual design, not only for the convenience of the designer create a more beautiful and practical folding carton packing, but also to shorten production time packaging design, to save the cost of packaging design production, to reduce unnecessary loss of time, thereby to improve the production efficiency.

References

1. WEI Li-min, The interesting design of the carton packaging, 25 June 2007.
2. ZHU He-ping, the Research of Modern packaging design Theory and Application. People's publishing house, December 2008.
3. YUAN Ming-song, CHI Yi-lin, ZHANG Miao, The Present Situation and Future Development Direction of Virtual Design, 15 March 2002.
4. CHEN Hao, LIU Chen, ZHANG Hai-qing. The application of CAD technology in the packaging structure design. 04 July 2008.

Research on the Wear and Protection of Agricultural Implements*

Xiong Liu, Lin Dong, Jie Yang, Zhi Wei Liu, Jingqing Tao, Qiao Wen
School of Mechanical Engineering, Xihua University, Chengdu, Sichuan 610039, China
†*E-mail: donglin11723@mail.163.com*
http://www.xhu.edu.cn/

The wear of agricultural machinery caused serious economic losses, environmental damage and resources consumption. The working conditions, wear sources, wear failure phenomenon and reasons, anti-wear and protective measures of agricultural machinery were studied by statistical method. The results put forward the reasonable choice method for wear-resistant materials, lubrication condition, surface treatment, anti-wear optimization structural design in the operation and maintenance of agricultural machinery. The research provides the scientific basis for solving tribological design and improving the service life of agricultural machinery.

Keywords: Agricultural implements; wear; protection; research prospects.

1. Introduction

There are many types of agricultural machinery, mainly including tillage equipment, planting machinery, field management machinery, irrigation and drainage machinery, harvesting machinery, etc. They are important parts of the machinery industry. The main working objects of agricultural machinery are the soil and crops. The damage characteristics of agricultural machinery have very great difference in different areas. Agricultural machinery works in severe environment, which are in the state of strong friction, vibration, impaction of sand, soil and crops. At the same time agricultural machinery operates under the corrosive medium such as fertilizer and corrosive water, these caused wear situation seriously. Abrasive wear, fatigue wear and corrosion are the worst failure problem. Therefore, it is vital significant to put forward effective anti-wear technology and protective measures.

* This work is supported by Key Scientific Research Fund of Education Department in Sichuan Province (No. 13ZA0021), Open Research Subject of Key Laboratory (Research Base) of Manufacturing and automation (szjj2015-081), the Science and Technology Fund of Ministry of Human Resources and Social Security of the P.R. China, Talent Fund of Xihua University (No. R0920203).

2. Wear Sources of Agricultural Implements

Agricultural machinery parts have the serious working condition, often service in wet or corrosive environment (fertilizer and manure, pesticide, etc.). Often friction and wear occurs with abrasive sand or crops in soil, but also by the vibration and impact. Those cause agricultural wear phenomenon more complex.

3. Force and the Wear Failure Phenomena of the Agricultural Implements

China is a large agricultural country, so agricultural machinery is widely used, but of differences in soil properties and changes around the actual working conditions of the environment, leading to the stress factors of agricultural machinery are more, stress is more complex and uneven, most components are subjected to contact fatigue of more intense stress, bending fatigue force, the impact load and wear serious impact, cause the service life shorter, the failure serious. Effectiveness of agricultural machinery common phenomenon and the main reason is as Table 1:

Table 1 Failure analyses of agricultural implements.

Agricultural Implements category	Failure phenomenon main reason
Power, Transportation (Agricultural vehicles, trailers, tractors, internal combustion engine)	Track shoe worn by silt and crops Tire wear by ground, as well as by the paddy field and corrosive
Tillage (Plough, rake, cultivator, seeder, etc.)	Bent or broken because of friction of the handle and the blade by the soil sand, roots.
Harvest (Cutter-Rower combine harvester).	The wear and fatigue wear by silica body in the crops, cutting edge blunt.
Irrigation, drainage (Large pumps, deep well pump, submersible pumps, sprinklers and other trenching machine).	Erosion wear and abrasive wear By the water contained a small amount of sand, impurities, generating micro cutting and deformation.
Plant protection, grain, cotton and economic crops processing (fluffing machine. Grinder, ect.)	Extrusion by Rice and rice husk and other impurities, wear become thinner, rupture.

4. Anti-Wear and Protection Measures

No matter what kind of wear sources and failure phenomenon is, will pose a threat on the service life of agricultural machinery, to bring certain difficulties and resistance. Therefore, according to the wear mechanism of agricultural machinery, anti-wear and protection method of the agricultural machinery are discussed and researched.

4.1. *Reasonable choice of materials and the development of resistant materials*

In the choice of agricultural materials, should consider the material hardness, toughness, solubility, heat resistance, corrosion-resistance, etc. Therefore, when choose the use of agricultural machinery and materials should according to the specific conditions and wear mechanism. When machinery is mainly adhesion wear, should choose the material side of miscible smaller. When is given priority to with abrasive wear, should choose high hardness materials or try to improve the hardness of the selected material, also can choose anti-wear material wear of materials. And if it is given priority to fatigue wear, the choice does not contain nonmetallic inclusion of high quality steel. Moreover, all kinds of wear resistance of the new material development work should be carried out, to adapt to the development of modern science and technology the demand for new agricultural machinery and wear-resistant materials.

4.2. *Reasonable choice of lubrication conditions*

We now commonly use lubricants including lubricating oil, grease and solid lubricant, etc., they are one important method to reduce agricultural machinery and wear in practical engineering, the good, the reasonable lubrication technology can make the wear failure of agricultural machinery and reduce to a minimum. But there are many types of agricultural machinery in China, have different structure, and working conditions is different also, so according to the concrete agricultural machinery and its working conditions to choose the appropriate lubricant correctly.

4.3. *Reasonable choice of surface treatment process*

In agricultural machinery and all kinds of failure, most characterized by excessive wear on the surface of the relative movement of friction and wear failure forms of different. From Figure 1 we can see the wear and friction at different experiment parameters. Therefore, the purpose of the surface treatment method is to change the surface properties, make its excellent physical, chemical and mechanical properties. For example, through the surface heat treatment, can improve agricultural machinery and material surface hardness and wear resistance, improving mechanical properties of the surface. And the surface chemical treatment, thermal spraying and different deposition method to join or sink and matrix material, can be further given by the substrate materials do not have the new performance, etc.

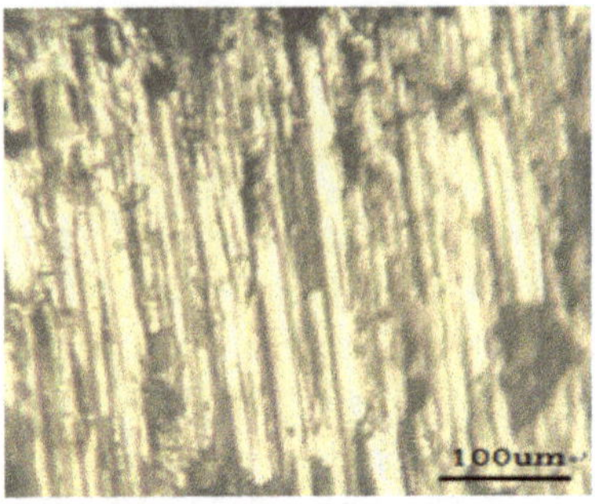

(a)

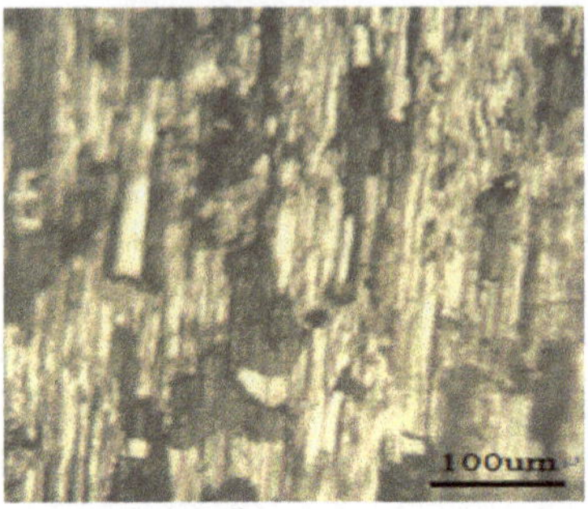

(b)

Fig. 1 Worn surface morphologies rotary of tiller dry-land blade under different experiment parameters.

4.4. *Reasonable structure design*

Correct structure design can reduce the wear of friction pair, the structure of the designed to benefit the formation of surface film and recovery, uniform pressure distribution, and is good for heat dissipation and chip discharge structure. Anti-wear optimized structure design of mechanical transmission mechanism is an important improvement measures, designers must consult the performance characteristics of transmission mechanism, strengthen the resistance to wear and tear of the structure of the improved processing.

4.5. *Using, repairing and maintenance*

Using, repairing, and maintenance of agricultural machinery and need to run in the process of wear and failure law of various quick-wear part, combining with the change of state in the agricultural machinery and technology of various environmental factors, such as on the fixed cycle of daily maintenance and maintenance, the main problems should be paid attention to in the process.

(1) Strengthen the filtering device maintenance. The air filter, fuel filter and oil filter, known as the "filter", is stopping the impurity, reduce mechanical producing abrasive wear mark, must strictly carry out cleaning and replacement of the filter core according to the maintenance requirements.

(2) The oil to add and change regularly. Engine oil in service besides there should be no drip loss, according to the rules to allow trace part of consumption, but not more than 5g/p s,h. So every time before the start of inspection, if necessary, according to the scale of oil feet up.

(3) Maintenance and repair farm vehicles, should choose environment clean and tidy, small dust content in the air and no dust on the ground, must

clean parts before assembly, pay special attention to remove oil and the corner of the material.

5. The Research Methods and Results

Research on agricultural machinery wear mainly includes two aspects of theoretical research and experimental research, respectively, through the theoretical calculation and experimental data to confirm two aspects, to study the mechanism and law of agricultural machinery and the wear and anti-wear technologies.

In China, The main direction of research focused on aspects of wear-resistant metal materials and surface engineering technology applications, research methods commonly used for farm machinery, such as ditching disc, hammer, harvester blade, rotary knife and ploughshare and other analyzes their working conditions, mechanical characteristics, failure modes and mechanisms proposed to optimize the design of new anti-wear, thus further improving the life of farm machinery.

In other countries, research in this area earlier than the start of the production and use of traditional agricultural resistant materials through the peak of years of research and development, has now stabilized, is now focused on the development of new wear-resistant materials and promotion of anti-wear technology.

6. Conclusion

Based on the current situation of agricultural machinery in China, during future works, on the one hand to problems of existing agricultural products to make scientific analysis on the basis of organizational strength of scientific research, to take measures to improve the content of science and technology, the degree of green products. Agricultural machine manufacturing enterprises should make products and high-tech compatible, improve agricultural intelligent, automation degree, improve product quality and efficiency. On the other hand to strengthen cooperation and exchanges with other agricultural research, constantly start from new types of agricultural materials, new anti-wear technology, optimize the structure, such as wear-resistant parts, developed in line with our own agricultural development of new agricultural products, so that China's farm machinery towards the full development life cycle to green, efficient, rapid development of automation direction.

Acknowledgments

The authors would gratefully thank for the Talent Fund of Xihua University (No. R0920203), Open Research Subject of Key Laboratory (Research Base) of Manufacturing and automation (szjj2015-081), the Science and Technology Fund of Ministry of Human Resources and Social Security of the P.R. China, Key Scientific Research Fund of Education Department in Sichuan Province (No. 13ZA0021).

References

1. GAO Lei, WEI Xinchun, Supporting Agricultural machinery situation analysis in our country present [J], Agricultural Machinery, 2010(07) : 102-104.
2. ZHOU Ping'an, Agricultural machinery tribology problems [J], Lubrication Engineering, 1983(02): 1-7.
3. ZHANG Jianlong, YU Longgang, Agricultural machinery to scientific and rational use of lubricants [C], 13th National Farm Machinery Repair Conference Proceedings, 2007: 85-90.
4. HANG Dong, Farm machinery maintenance and repair techniques [J], Agricultural Machinery Quality & Supervision, 2013(02): 34-36.
5. YIN Xianying, Discussion steel abrasive wear and tools [J], Cereals and Oils Processing, 1981(05): 44-53.
6. Li, D.Y., A new type of wear-resistant material: pseudo-elastic TiNi alloy [J]. Wear, 1998. 221(2): 116-123.

Research on Feature Correlation Dimension Extraction Method and Its Application on Rolling Bearing Fault Diagnosis

Siyuan Liu[a], Haosong Hu[b] and Linlin Ding[c]
Hebei Provincial Key Laboratory of Heavy Machinery Fluid Power Transmission and Control, Yanshan University, Qinhuangdao, 066004, China
Key Laboratory of Advanced Forging & Stamping Technology and Science (Yanshan University), Ministry of Education of China, Qinhuangdao, 066004, China
E-mail: [a]liusiyuan@ysu.edu.cn; [b]hsby@outlook.com; [c]31363353@qq.com

Aiming at the nonlinear and non-stationary characteristics of rolling bearing fault vibration signals, feature correlation dimension (FCD) extraction method combining phase space reconstruction (PSR) and fractal theory is proposed. The method reconstructs high-dimension phase space from one-dimension vibration signals of different fault states of the rolling bearing so that deep data mining is achieved. Then through analysis of varying correlation dimension of phase space feature signals, FCD that corresponds to each fault state is extracted. The experiment shows that feature correlation dimension extracted by the method is effective to fault diagnosis of rolling bearing. The method can provide reliable feature information for condition monitoring and fault diagnosis of complicated rotating machinery, and has a broad application prospect.

Keywords: Fault diagnosis; correlation dimension; fractal theory; phase space reconstruction; feature extraction.

1. Introduction

Feature extraction from non-stationary and nonlinear vibration signals is crucial to accurate diagnosis of equipment in the fault diagnosis field [1]. Correlation dimension (CD) can process different vibrations with fractal characteristics [2]. FCD was proposed as fault characteristics factor and used to diagnose mechanical equipment in different working conditions. Firstly measured vibrations were processed with PSR. One-dimensional vibration signal was reconstructed to high-dimensional phase space to form new feature sample set in order to obtain more feature information. Fault characteristic was qualitatively analyzed through three-dimension phase space graph. Secondly correlation dimensions of vibration signals were calculated via G-P algorithm. FCD was defined to quantitatively analyze different faults of rolling bearings. The effectiveness of FCD to rolling bearing fault diagnosis was verified by experiment.

2. Principles and Methods

2.1. *C-C method of PSR*

When reconstructing phase space by time series, how to determine embedding dimension m and time delay τ is crucial. C-C method assumes the two parameters are interdependent and could simultaneously obtain time delay and time window [3].

The correlation integral of embedding time series is

$$C(m,N,r,t)=\frac{2}{M(M-1)}\sum_{1\le i\le j\le M}\theta(r-d_{ij}),\ r>0. \tag{1}$$

where $d_{ij}=\|X_i-X_j\|_{(\infty)}$, $\theta(x)$ denotes Heaviside function, $\theta(x)=0$ when $x<0$, $\theta(x)=1$ when $x>0$, r denotes the hyper sphere radius of m-dimension space.

2.2. *Correlation dimension based on G-P algorithm*

G-P algorithm calculates correlation dimension directly from time series based on embedding theory and PSR technique [4,5].

Correlation dimension is defined as

$$D_R=\lim_{r\to 0}\frac{\ln(C(r))}{\ln(r)}. \tag{2}$$

Let $y_i=\ln(r)$, $z_i=\ln(C(r))$, and

$$E=\sum_{i=1}^{M}(z-z_i)^2=\sum_{i=1}^{M}(ky_i+b-z_i)^2. \tag{3}$$

where M is the effective points of curve fitting. Let $\frac{\partial E}{\partial k}=0$, $\frac{\partial E}{\partial b}=0$, then CD can be rewritten as

$$D_R=k=\frac{\left(\sum_{i=1}^{M}z_i\sum_{i=1}^{M}y_i\right)-M\sum_{i=1}^{M}z_iy_i}{\left(\sum_{i=1}^{M}y_i\right)-M\left(\sum_{i=1}^{M}y_i^2\right)}. \tag{4}$$

2.3. *FCD extraction*

Calculate CD differences of the same embedding dimensions of two signals

$$e_{DR} = \left| D_{Ri} - D_{Rj} \right|. \tag{5}$$

where D_{Ri} is the CD of first segment of signal and D_{Rj} the second segment. Find the embedding dimension point $m = k$ when e_{DR} takes the minimum. FCD is mean of two corresponding CDs.

$$CD_R = \left(D_{Ri} + D_{Rj} \right)/2, m = k. \tag{6}$$

3. Experiments

The bearing data is taken from Case Western Reserve University Bearing Data Center. Single point defects were set on the bearings with depth by 0.011 in and diameter by 0.007 in. The working conditions include healthy, inner race, outer race and ball defect. The rotating speed was set to 1750 rpm and the sampling frequency 12 kHz.

Table 1 Time delay in different conditions when $m = 3$.

Conditions	Healthy	Inner race defect	Outer race defect	Ball defect
τ	3	3	10	3

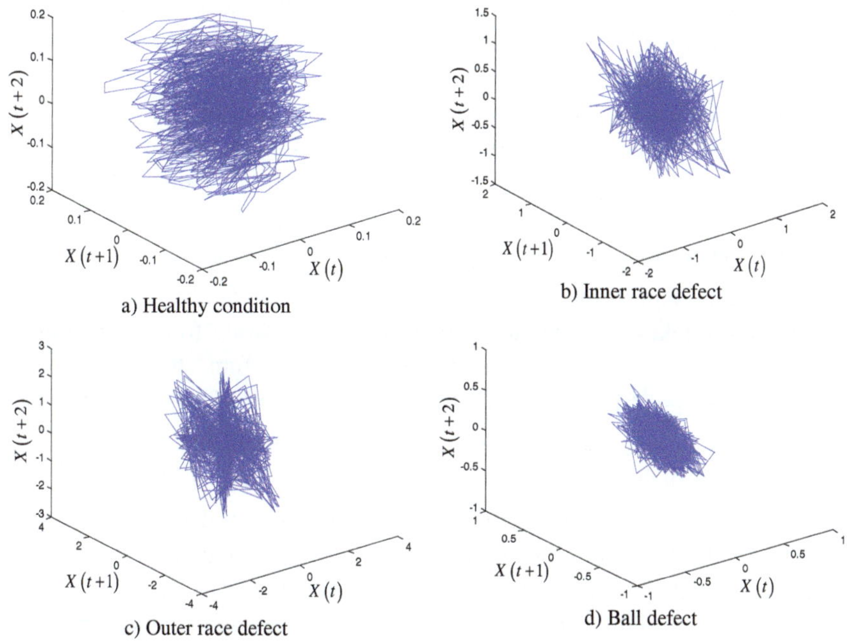

a) Healthy condition

b) Inner race defect

c) Outer race defect

d) Ball defect

Fig. 1 PSR graph of bearing vibrations.

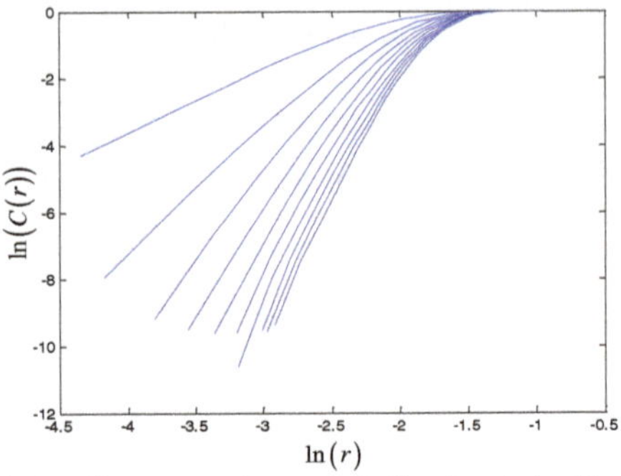

Fig. 2 Correlation dimensions of measured vibrations in healthy condition.

Set embedding dimension $m = 3$ and maximum time delay $\tau_{\max} = 20$. Perform PSR to bearing vibrations in different conditions and obtain 3-D phase space graph (Fig. 1). Fig. 1 shows that the attractors of bearing system concentrated to a group but the group shape differs between different conditions. It appears as a regular sphere in healthy condition. It tends to extend outward along some axis of the sphere in inner defect and the extension directions increases in outer defect. It appears as a regular ellipsoid in ball defect. Results show that the attractor is sensitive to the changes of bearing vibrations.

Set 10 searching radius and calculate CDs of the measured vibrations in healthy condition with G-P algorithm (Fig. 2). Fig. 2 shows that the CD is convergent.

Three samples for each condition were extracted from bearing data set with each sample containing 2000 points. Two samples were training set and the other testing set. Firstly calculate CDs in different embedding dimensions of the training set. D_{R0} denotes the CDs of healthy condition and D_{R1} inner race defect, D_{R2} outer race defect and D_{R3} ball defect. Table 2 shows all CDs when the embedding dimension varies from 12. Then find the dimension point when the difference takes the minimum which can be seen easily from the CD trend curve (Fig. 3). Thus FCD can be obtained from the CD mean, $CD_{R0} = 4.25(m = 36)$, $CD_{R1} = 1.76(m = 14)$, $CD_{R2} = 3.92(m = 36)$. To ball defect, trend is more stable when embedding dimension takes $m = 12 \sim 26$. Thus FCD of ball defect was calculated at $m = 18$, i.e. $CD_{R3} = 2.93(m = 18)$.

Calculate CDs of testing set (Table 3). Table 3 shows that CD at m=18 of testing sample D_1 is 2.91 which is close to FCD 2.93 of ball defect. Thus D_1 was diagnosed as ball defect. CD at m=36 of testing sample D_2 is 4.24 which is close to FCD 4.25 of healthy condition. Thus D_2 was diagnosed as healthy condition. CD at m=36 of testing sample D_3 is 3.90 which is close to FCD 3.92 of outer race defect. Thus D_3 was diagnosed as outer race defect. CD at m=14 of testing sample D_4 is 1.75 which is close to FCD 1.76 of inner race defect. Thus D_4 was diagnosed as inner race defect. Results conform to reality. Therefore, the proposed method is effective to rolling bearing fault diagnosis.

Table 2 CDs of different dimensions in different conditions.

Embedding dimension	Correlation dimension							
	D_{R0}		D_{R1}		D_{R2}		D_{R3}	
Sample number	1	2	1	2	1	2	1	2
m=12	2.9784	2.7250	1.6042	1.5382	1.9870	1.5624	2.0282	2.6487
m=14	3.2947	2.8788	1.7685	1.7530	2.1382	1.9457	2.2751	2.7874
m=16	3.2984	2.9646	2.0428	1.8887	2.3154	2.2523	2.4433	3.0033
m=18	3.4682	3.0984	2.3112	2.1128	2.5309	2.3840	2.6880	3.1657
m=20	3.5874	3.1404	2.2537	2.2700	2.7569	2.5313	2.9054	3.4638
m=22	3.7721	3.3401	2.4617	2.3435	3.0468	2.6440	3.1323	3.6679
m=24	3.9351	3.5151	2.6321	2.4136	3.1714	2.8189	3.2551	3.9433
m=26	4.0826	3.5705	2.7894	2.5718	3.3148	3.0389	3.4669	4.1729
m=28	4.2071	3.7152	2.9200	2.6760	3.4773	3.2014	3.1886	4.4429
m=30	4.2461	3.8422	3.0620	2.7656	3.6792	3.4924	3.3787	4.4359
m=32	4.3441	3.9594	3.2090	2.8840	3.7712	3.7022	3.5635	4.7059
m=34	4.2539	4.0691	3.2708	3.0047	3.7455	3.8302	3.4743	4.9669
m=36	4.3233	4.1700	3.4253	3.1803	3.8936	3.9405	3.1833	5.2507

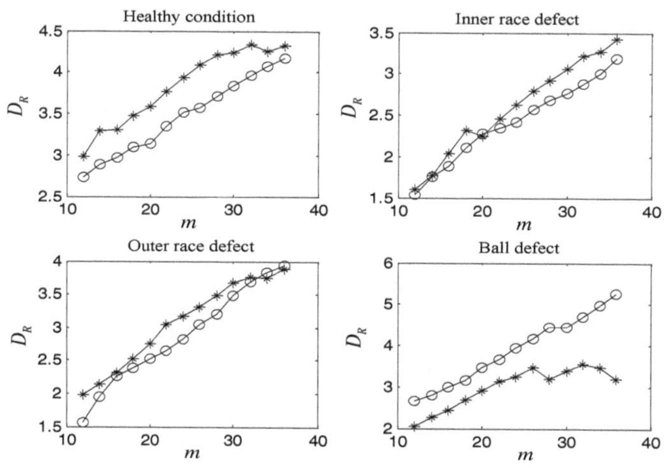

Fig. 3 Trend curve of correlation dimension.

4. Conclusions

(1) The proposed FCD is an effective factor to rolling bearing fault diagnosis. Various conditions have significant differences in fractal characteristic so can be distinguished from each other by CD. The proposed method simpli-

fies the diagnosis process by only taking FCD as diagnosis criterion.

(2) The attractor is sensitive to the changes of different bearing vibrations

Table 3 Correlation dimensions of testing samples and diagnosis result.

Embedding	Correlation dimension			
	D_1	D_2	D_3	D_4
m=12	2.2555	2.8324	1.8228	1.4283
m=14	2.4848	2.9522	1.9986	**1.7538**
m=16	2.5943	3.1615	2.3014	1.7799
m=18	**2.9106**	3.3917	2.5681	1.9734
m=20	2.9196	3.5710	2.7418	2.2172
m=22	3.1768	3.4519	2.8806	2.4370
m=24	3.2880	3.6242	3.0483	2.4700
m=26	3.5237	3.7465	3.2857	2.5140
m=28	3.7643	3.8826	3.3694	2.6625
m=30	3.7279	4.0063	3.2061	2.8128
m=32	3.9377	4.0698	3.3416	2.9026
m=34	3.8695	4.1637	3.4977	3.0451
m=36	3.5534	**4.2456**	**3.9049**	3.2016
Diagnosis result	Ball defect	Healthy	Outer race	Inner race

Acknowledgments

This work is supported by the National Key Basic Research Program (973 Program) of China (2014CB046405) and Natural Science Foundation of Hebei Province, China (E2013203114).

References

1. J. G. Wang, L. F. Wu, X. H. Wu, Rolling Bearing Vibration Signal Fault Feature Extraction Based on Autocorrelation Analysis and LMD, *China Mechanical Engineering*, 2014, 25(2):186-191.
2. W. L. Jiang, D. N. Chen, C. Y. Yao, Correlation Dimension Analytical Method and its Application in Fault Diagnosis of Hydraulic Pump, *Chinese Journal of Sensors and Actuators*, 2004, (1):62-65.
3. P. Grassberger, I. Procaccia, Measuring the Strangeness of Strange Attractors, *Physica D*, 1983, 9:189-208.
4. L. Li, Y. X. Zhang, T. T. Ming, Gear Fault Diagnosis Based on Correlation Dimension Pre-processed with EMD, *JVS*, 2009, 28(4):145-148.
5. N. Li, Y. J. Fang, Fault Signal Analysis of Mechanical System Based on Correlation Dimension, *JVS*, 2007, 26(4):136-139.
6. Z. S. Wu, W. Wang, M. Huang, et al, Analysis of Characteristic of Vibration Signals in High- voltage Circuit Breakers Based on Phase Space Reconstruction, *MEP*, 2006, 23(1):10-14.

Design and Analysis of the Smart Milling Tool Based on RFID

Yafei Yu[a] and Bo Tao[b]
Institute of Mechanical Science & Engineering, HUST, Wuhan, 430074, China
[a]hithust_yu@126.com, [b]taobo@mail.hust.edu.cn
www.hust.edu.cn

The machining quality controlling of the aeronautical thin-walled components is a problem hard and urgent to be solved in aeronautical industries. This problem seriously hinders the development of the aviation industry. Measuring and monitoring the condition of the cutting tool is an effective way to achieve good surface roughness and dimensional accuracy of the parts, as well as providing processing parameters for self-adapting machining. This article presents a novel smart milling tool based on RFID for real-time measurement and transmission of tool condition in precision milling operations. Contactless transmission channel is modeled by the Loos equivalent model and mutual inductance model. The effects that operational frequency, coupling size and different primary and secondary compensation topologies have on system transmission performance have been analyzed and validated.

Keywords: Smart milling tool; RFID; contactless transmission performance.

1. Introduction

At present, airframes are widely made of thin-walled components for the sake of weight reducing and strength ratio improvement. However, due to factors such as cutting force induced flexible deflection, dynamic vibration and high cutting temperature, precision machining of these thin-walled parts has been providing a serious challenge for engineers. As a result, the importance to measure and monitor the cutting tool in the machining process real-time has been well recognized by the machining research community and industry [1]. The change of cutting condition has direct effects on the machining outcome of thin-walled components. In order to take corrective action in the event of accidents, reliable and effective sensors can be equipped to monitor machine operation. However, the crucial problem of sensors data transmission must be overcome in the milling process. In modern manufacturing, some smart tools for milling characteristics have been developed and applied. Most of smart milling tools realize data transmission via Bluetooth, SAW technology. With some significant drawbacks, such as complex process, low availability and high cost. Moreover, the usage of battery results unsustainable run and increases the volume of system. Therefore, it is essential to develop a smart milling tool with the real-time and continuous monitoring and transmission of tool condition capability [2].

This article presents a novel smart milling tool, which employs RFID to transmit measurement data. At the same time, the smart milling tool can obtain required energy form RF field. It also achieves compatibility with existing smart tool management system by inquiring the tool identity information. It has the advantage of simple structure, easy to implement, sustainable run and manageable through tool identification. This article also analyses and optimizes system transmission performance through simulation and experiments.

2. Design of the Smart Milling Tool

The smart milling tool mentioned in this article employs RFID to solve the problem of data transmission in milling process. The contactless transmission system of the smart milling tool consists of the primary unit and the secondary unit together. Communication is bidirectional and secondary unit can obtain required energy from RF field in the contactless transmission system. Moreover, sensors are mounted in the tip region.

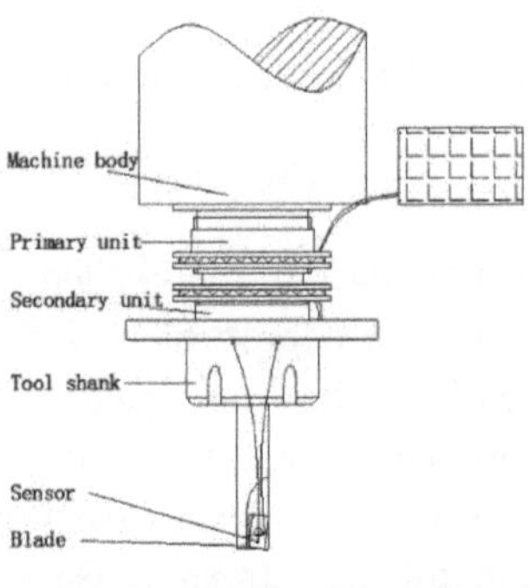

Fig. 1 The schematic diagram of the smart milling tool.

In the milling process, the secondary unit samples the real-time data of sensors. Primary unit can demodulate and decode the sensor data, which is modulated onto the carrier wave of contactless transmission channel. In order to ensure that the system can run sustainably, the secondary unit can obtain required energy from the RF field while communicating. The smart milling tool also achieve compatibility with a smart tool management system by inquiring the tool identity information stored in the secondary unit. As a result, the system possesses distinct advantages to adapt the today's industrial model of digital manufacturing. Fig. 1 shows the schematic diagram of the smart milling tool.

3. Modeling of the Contactless Transmission Channel

Due to the characteristics of RFID, the design of the system is quite complicated [3]. Furthermore the contactless transmission module plays a vital role in the smart milling tool. As a result, how to optimize the transmission performance at given operating conditions is one of the core problems. Current research on contactless transmission channel use separate transformer inductance equivalent model and ignore the influence of eddy currents [4]. However, the contactless transmission channel of smart milling tool works in metal environment. Therefore, it is necessary to establish an accurate model to lay theoretical grounds for engineering design.

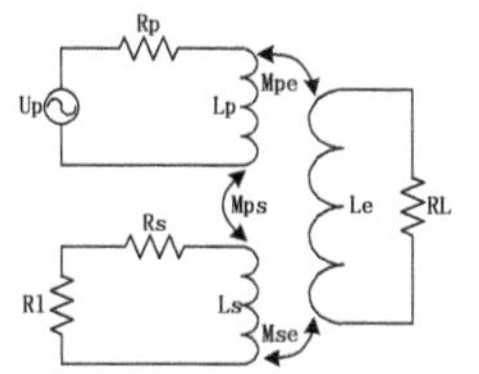

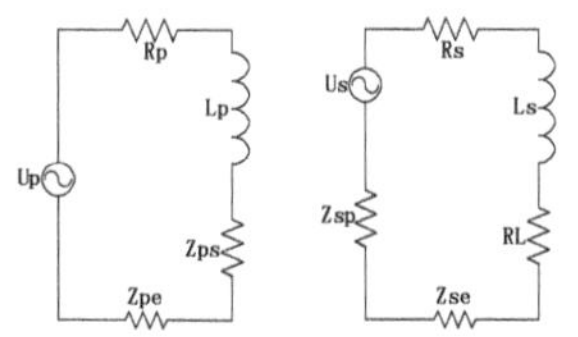

Fig. 2 Circuit model of transmission channel. Fig. 3 Equivalent circuits with reflected impedance.

According to LOOS equivalent model, the eddy current can be equivalent to a series of closed loop composed by an inductor and a resistor [5]. Considering the leakage inductance of the contactless transformer, mutual inductance model is adopted to simplify the analysis. The equivalent circuits of the primary, secondary and eddy current are as shown in Fig. 2. The primary is driven by high frequency voltage U_p with frequency of f. The resistance and inductance values of all three parts are respectively R_p, L_p, R_s, L_s, R_e, L_e. M, M_{pe}, M_{se} are the mutual inductance between the three parts. RL is the load resistance. Reflected impedance is introduced to reflect the interaction between circuits. The equivalent circuits with reflected impedance are as shown in Fig. 3. Z_{ps} and Z_{pe} are respectively the primary reflected impedance from secondary unit and eddy current. Z_{sp} and Z_{se} are respectively the secondary reflected impedance from primary unit and eddy current. U_s is induced voltage from the primary unit. They can be expressed as follows:

$$Z_{pe} = \frac{-j\omega M_{pe} I_e}{I_p} = \frac{(\omega M_{pe})^2}{R_e^2 + \omega^2 L_e^2} \mathrm{R_e} + j\frac{-(\omega M_{pe})^2}{R_e^2 + \omega^2 L_e^2} \omega L_e = R_{pe} + jX_{pe} \qquad (1)$$

$$Z_{pe} = \frac{-j\omega M_{pe} I_e}{I_p} = \frac{(\omega M_{pe})^2}{R_e^2 + \omega^2 L_e^2} \mathrm{R_e} + j\frac{-(\omega M_{pe})^2}{R_e^2 + \omega^2 L_e^2} \omega L_e = R_{pe} + jX_{pe} \qquad (2)$$

$$Z_{pe} = \frac{-j\omega M_{pe} I_e}{I_p} = \frac{(\omega M_{pe})^2}{R_e^2 + \omega^2 L_e^2} \mathrm{R_e} + j\frac{-(\omega M_{pe})^2}{R_e^2 + \omega^2 L_e^2} \omega L_e = R_{pe} + jX_{pe} \quad (3)$$

$$Z_{se} = \frac{-j\omega M_{se} I_e}{I_s} = \frac{(\omega M_{se})^2}{R_e^2 + \omega^2 L_e^2} \mathrm{R_e} + j\frac{-(\omega M_{se})^2}{R_e^2 + \omega^2 L_e^2} \omega L_e = R_{se} + jX_{se} \quad (4)$$

$$Z_{ps} = \frac{-\mathrm{j}\omega \mathrm{M}\dot{I}_s}{\dot{I}_p} = \frac{(\omega \mathrm{M})^2}{R_{s1}^{\ 2} + X_{s1}^2} R_{s1} + j\frac{-(\omega \mathrm{M})^2}{R_{s1}^{\ 2} + X_{s1}^2} X_{s1} = R_{ps} + jX_{ps} \quad (5)$$

$$Z_{sp} = \frac{-\mathrm{j}\omega \mathrm{M}\dot{I}_p}{\dot{I}_s} = \frac{(\omega \mathrm{M})^2}{R_{p1}^{\ 2} + X_{p1}^2} R_{e1} + j\frac{-(\omega \mathrm{M})^2}{R_{p1}^{\ 2} + X_{p1}^2} X_{p1} = R_{sp} + jX_{sp} \quad (6)$$

$$U_s = j\omega M I_p = \frac{j\omega M U_p}{Z_p} \quad (7)$$

Among which, $\omega = 2\pi f$, $R_{p1} = R_{pe} + R_p$, $R_{s1} = R_{se} + R_s + R_L$, $X_{s1} = X_{se} + \omega L_s$, $X_{p1} = X_{pe} + \omega L_p$.

The energy transfer efficiency and voltage gain are the most important performance parameters in the energy and data transmission system. The power absorbed by the reflected impedance is exactly the power transferred. So the energy transfer efficiency η and voltage gain γ can be expressed as follows:

$$\eta = \frac{Z_{ps}}{Z_{ps} + Z_{p1}} \cdot \frac{R_L}{Z_{s1}}, \gamma = \frac{R_L}{Z_{s1}} \cdot \frac{\mathrm{U}_s}{\mathrm{U}_p} \quad (8)$$

Among which, $Z_{p1} = R_{p1} + X_{p1}$, $Z_{s1} = R_{s1} + X_{s1}$.

As can be seen from the Eq. 1-8, the transmission performance is determined by many factors. But the main electrical parameters are selected according to the specific system requirements. Therefore, we can only optimize the operating frequency and the mutual inductance to improve the system performance. The mutual inductance is mainly influenced by geometrical parameters and material characteristics of the magnetic structure. Taking actual operability into consideration, we choose the operating frequency and geometrical parameters as the optimization parameters of this system.

4. Analysis and Optimization of Transmission Performance

According to the analysis in the previous section, the operating frequency and geometrical parameters of the system can be optimized to improve system performance. ANSYS is employed to analyze the contactless transmission channel to discover effect of operating frequency and coupling size. Because the smart milling tool has axisymmetric structure and considering employing 2D model can improve calculating efficiency and accuracy, the article use a 2D model for system performance analysis. Analysis model is as shown in Fig. 4.

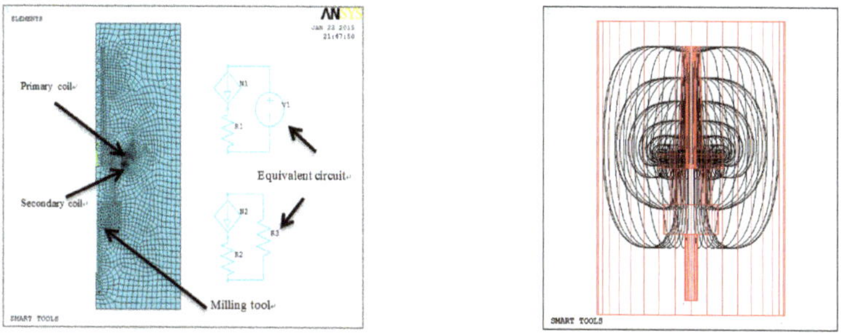

(a) 2D model of contactless transmission channel (b) Rotary stretch rendering of the 2D model

Fig. 4 Analysis model of contactless transmission channel.

4.1. *The coil inner diameter r and the coil spacing d*

Taking into account the limitations of the actual system, the *r* and *d* are selected as the key study parameters. Under the condition that the secondary coil remaining the same position, the *r* of two coils and the mounting position of primary coil are sequentially changed. The *d* is changed from 4 to 13mm and the *r* is changed from 16 to 31mm. By calculating the simulation data, the results are as shown in Fig. 5. Both energy transfer efficiency and voltage gain show increasing trend with the decrease of the *d*. However, with the *r* of the coil increasing the above two parameters show first increasing and then decreasing trend. Furthermore the *d* has a greater impact on system performance than the *r* of the coil. The system obtains the best performance when r=19mm and d=5mm.

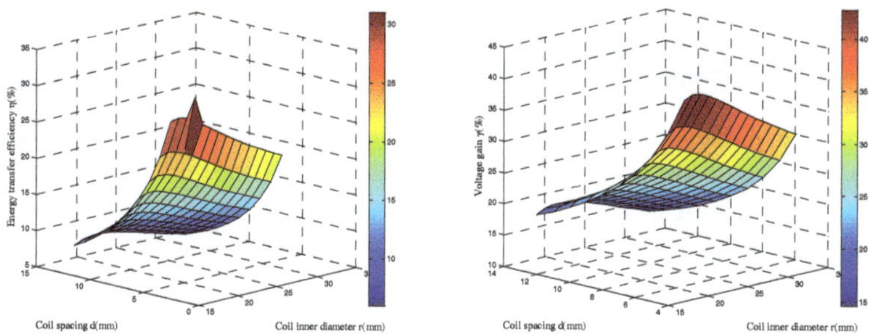

(a) Energy transfer efficiency η (b) Voltage gain γ

Fig. 5 System transmission performance with the spacing and inner diameter of coil.

4.2. *The relative size of coils Δr ($\Delta r = r_p$-r_s)*

The r_p and r_s are respectively the inner diameter of secondary coil and primary coil. The r_s is fixed to 19mm and Δr varies from -2mm to 7mm when changing r_p. Both energy transfer efficiency and voltage gain show first increasing and then decreasing trend. System obtain the best performance when $\Delta r = 0$. Therefore, we should use the same size coil to build our system.

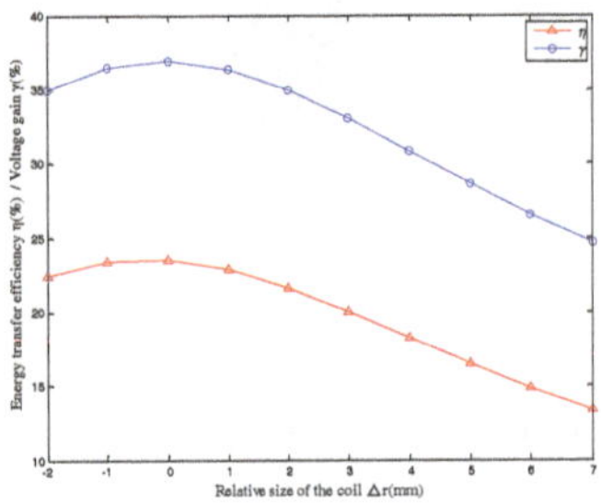

Fig. 6 Energy transfer efficiency and voltage gain with the relative size of the coil.

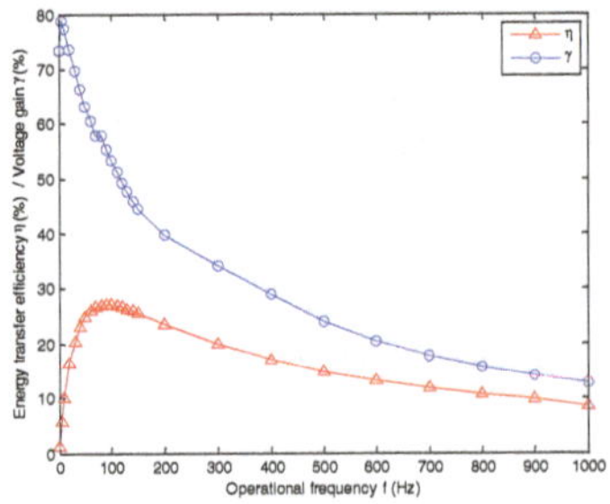

Fig. 7 Energy transfer efficiency and voltage gain with the operating frequency.

4.3. *The operating frequency f*

In non-metallic environment, the system show better contactless transmission performance with the increasing of the *f*. However, in metal environment, high-frequency electromagnetic fields can cause severe eddy current effects. So the analysis of this system shows a result different from those in the non-metallic environment, as shown in Fig. 7. Both energy transfer efficiency and voltage gain show first increasing and then decreasing trend. However, voltage gain has a smaller turning frequency than energy transfer efficiency. Due to the fact that the data transmission rate and the *f* was positively correlated, smaller operating frequency should be selected in the case of sufficient transmission rate.

5. Experimental Verification

Based on the above analysis, the article design an experiment platform of smart milling tool system showed in Fig. 8. Experiments were carried out to verify the above analysis results by the experiment platform.

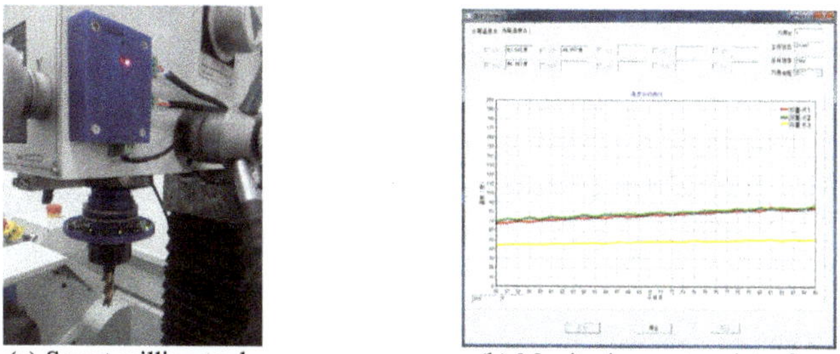

(a) Smart milling tool (b) Monitoring system interface

Fig. 8 Experiment platform of smart milling tool system.

As shown in Table 1, the trend reflected in the experimental data and simulation results are the same. Experiments 1-7 verify the effect of the coil size and spacing on the transmission performance. The effect of operating frequency on the performance can be reflected by the experiments 2 and 8-11.

Table 1 Experimental parameters and results.

Groups	r_p [mm]	r_s [mm]	d [mm]	F [kHz]	Compensation topology	η [%]	γ [%]
1	18	18	4	200	no	22.87	35.96
2	19	19	4	200	no	23.42	36.84
3	20	20	4	200	no	22.93	36.17
4	19	19	5	200	no	20.12	32.74
5	19	19	6	200	no	15.57	29.60
6	18	19	4	200	no	23.29	36.37
7	20	19	4	200	no	22.80	36.27
8	19	19	4	30	no	20.26	69.54
9	19	19	4	60	no	25.74	60.20
10	19	19	4	90	no	27.67	55.21
11	19	19	4	500	no	14.61	23.69

6. Summary

A novel smart milling tool based on RFID is proposed. The system is able to monitor and transmit tool condition in real time. Modelling and simulation is performed to analyse the performance and to obtain the optimal parameters of the system. The article also verifies the results by experiments.

Acknowledgments

This work is supported by the National Science and Technology Major Project under Grant 2012ZX04010-071 and the National Fundamental Research Program of China under Grant 2013CB035803.

References

1. Tlusty, J.: A critical review of sensors for unmanned machining. CIRP Annals-Manufacturing Technology, 1983.32(2): pp. 563-572.
2. Tönshoff: Developments and trends in monitoring and control of machining processes. CIRP Annals-Manufacturing Technology, 1988.37(2): pp. 611-622.
3. Ying, W, et al. Design of New Contactless Power Supply System. in CAS. Zhong guan cun, Beijing, China.
4. Hirai, J, T. Kim and A. Kawamura: Study on crosstalk in inductive transmission of power and information. Industrial Electronics, IEEE Transactions on, 1999. 46(6): pp. 1174-1182.
5. Le Bihan, Y: Study on the transformer equivalent circuit of eddy current nondestructive evaluation. NDT & E International, 2003. 36(5): pp. 297-302.

Research on Driven Function Experiment for Rigid-Flexible Lower Limb Rehabilitation Robot*

Wang Keyi†, Zhang Song,Wu Bosong, Fang Shuo and Di Chengbao
College of Mechanical and Electrical Engineering, Harbin Engineering University, Harbin, 150001, China
†E-mail: wangkeyi@hrbeu.edu.cn
www.hrbeu.edu.cn

Considering of the function requirement of the lower limb rehabilitation robot to achieve corrective walking, a mode of robot was proposed and a model machine was developed. Based on the control objective of according walking training, expected hip and knee angles and the load needed in strength training, the driving force on wires produced by the robot was calculated by giving known force on wire 1 to determine the other wires. A tension sensor calibration was done on the robot. And two wire driven function experiments were done under different condition based on it. It was indicated that the control system of the model machine was able to meet the required stability and controllability, and the accuracy and response rate of the wire output force were up to the control demand of rehabilitation training. The paper has a great significance on servo control of wire-driven parallel robot.

Keywords: Rehabilitation robot; rigid-flexible coupled robots; driven function.

1. Introduction

According to medical surrey, an half of disabled were limb disabled with rising proportion in China [1]. The data showed that the patient could recover effectively with the method of combining modern medical means with motortherapy [2]. Recently it has been gradually approved to replace traditional limb motortherapy with rehabilitation method by this robot.

International and domestics academics started to study the rehabilitation robot in mid 20th century. HOCOMA medical instrument company and Balgrist Medical rehabilitation center in Zurich Suit developed LOKOMAT, a walking rehabilitation training robot [3]. Free University of Berlin produced Haptic Walker robot in 2003 [4]. Basing on the exoskeleton model made by Lockheed Martin, the Berkeley bionic technology company in the United States improved

* This work is supported by National Natural Science Foundation of China (51405095); Technological Innovation Talent Special Fund of Harbin (2014RFQXJ037).

and successfully developed the eLegs, a kind of wearable lower limbs exoskeleton system [5]. There were some achievement on this robot in China, thought it began comparatively late. The PT-2-AM designed and produced by Beijing Bao da hua rehabilitation equipment technology company, is a rehabilitation robot integrated intelligent and application [6]. Basing on theoretical research of lower limb exoskeleton, Zhejiang University developed lower limb rehabilitation robot [7]. Paralysis of walking robot developed by Tsinghua University and Beijing Rui hai bo technology company cannot only walk independently driven by walking mechanism, but also coordinate with medical treadmill as main rehabilitation requirement for lower extremity impairment training [8]. In addition, Harbin Institute University and Zhejiang University developed a kind of lower limb exoskeleton device [9]. But compared with rigid mechanism, wire-driven manipulator has advantage of good flexibility and easy to achieve force/position control. The rigid-flexible lower rehabilitation was researched in this paper. And the wire-driven character was studied experimentally. These lay the function of robot's force and compliance control.

2. Rigid-Flexible Lower Limb Rehabilitation Robot

2.1. *Structural concept of robot model*

Based on the demand of motion space in walking rehabilitation training, a rigid-flexible robot with flexion and extension configuration is proposed. Its system was shown in Fig. 1. Patient and robot constituted a man-machine collaboration system with binding effect [10]. This robot presented a bilateral symmetry and each side was formed by three driving wires. The knot as high as patient's ankle joint was linked by the end of three wires, which were connected to a thin plate bound with patient's crus. The other ends (B2 and B3) of wire 2 and wire 3 around wheel fixed on frame were linked to torque motor 2 and torque motor 3 respectively. The other end (B1) of wire 1 around wheel fixed on screw-nut mechanism was connected with torque motor 1 and constituted rigid-flexible branch. During rehabilitation training, patient was pulled by treadmill and wires' knot of lower limb rehabilitation to realize the man-machine interaction and complete various training schedules.

2.2. *Solving wire force in robot*

As was shown in Fig.1, world coordinate system was built according to original point O. Based on wire-driven institution structure, the knot was set P(Px,Py), slider position of screw-slippery course was set B1(B1x,0), and the other fastening endpoint was set B2(B2x,B2y) and B3(B3x,B3y). It is necessary to solve the gait path (motion trial of P) as robot input during gait correction training.

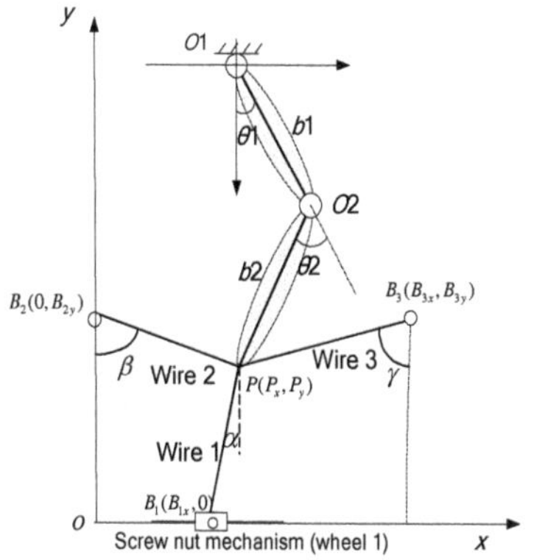

Fig. 1 Structure diagram of wire driving cell block.

In there, expected hip joint θ_1 and knee joint θ_2 can be approximated as followed:

$$\begin{cases} \theta_1 = 20\sin(2.7t) + 10 \\ \theta_2 = 30\cos(2.7t) - 30 \end{cases} \tag{1}$$

And then according to robotics, the location of knot P can be deduced as:

$$\begin{bmatrix} P_x \\ P_y \end{bmatrix} = \begin{bmatrix} O_{1x} \\ O_{1y} \end{bmatrix} + \begin{bmatrix} \sin\theta_1 \\ -\cos\theta_1 \end{bmatrix} \cdot b_1 + \begin{bmatrix} \sin(\theta_1 - \theta_2) \\ -\cos(\theta_1 - \theta_2) \end{bmatrix} \cdot b_2 \tag{2}$$

Where b_1 and b_2 were respectively indicated as the length of thigh and shank. Loading force F was generated by all wires' traction on P. Angle matrix A(η) would be solved by angles α, β, γ between wires 1,2,3 and plumb line. In terms of the relationship, of equilibrium $A(\eta)T=F$.

According to angular dependence, the force balance equation was obtained as follows:

$$\begin{bmatrix} \sin\alpha & \sin\beta & -\sin\lambda \\ -\cos\alpha & \cos\beta & \cos\lambda \end{bmatrix} \begin{bmatrix} t_1 \\ t_2 \\ t_3 \end{bmatrix} = \begin{bmatrix} -F\cos(\theta_2 - \theta_1) \\ -F\sin(\theta_2 - \theta_1) \end{bmatrix} \tag{3}$$

Where $\alpha = \mathrm{ac}\sin(\frac{P_x - B_{1x}}{l_1})$, $\beta = \mathrm{ac}\sin(\frac{P_x}{l_2})$, $\gamma = \mathrm{ac}\sin(\frac{B_{3x} - P_x}{l_3})$.

Therefore, coupled problem of driving force among three wires was turned into solving issues of nonhomogeneous equation set. Apparently, Eq. 3 had an infinite number of solution. Ambiguity was not allowed in control system, hereon, the solution of systematic wire traction was attained by setting the tensile force of wire 1 and keeping it tense in the process of traction.

3. Wire Driven Function Experiment

3.1. *Single-wire driven function experiment*

The stability of output force both in motor static and dynamic was demanded during rehabilitation training. Monopodium dynamic tracking experiment was shown in Fig. 2. Torque motor, tension sensor and pull-tab constituted the system. In experiment, set the motor output moment constantly. The trainer pulled the tab from forth to back in different speed. And use capture to record tension sensor force signal.

In order to observe and manage easily, the data generated in LabVIEW waveform was imported in MATLAB. The variation diagram of motor output force which was recorded in different cycles of motion was shown in Fig. 3.

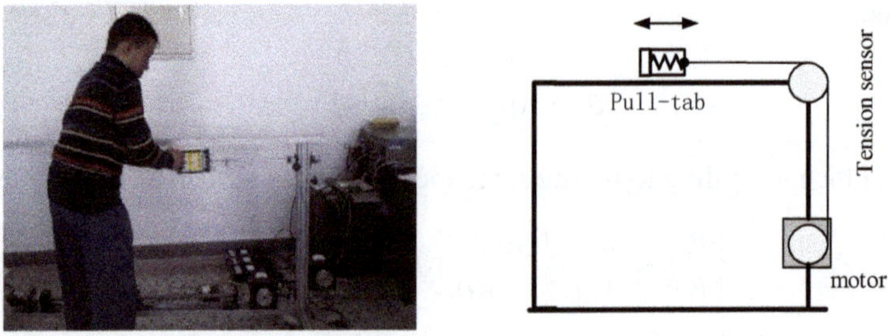

(a) Single-wire driven function experiment's image (b) Schematic diagram

Fig. 2 Single-wire driven unit output force experiment.

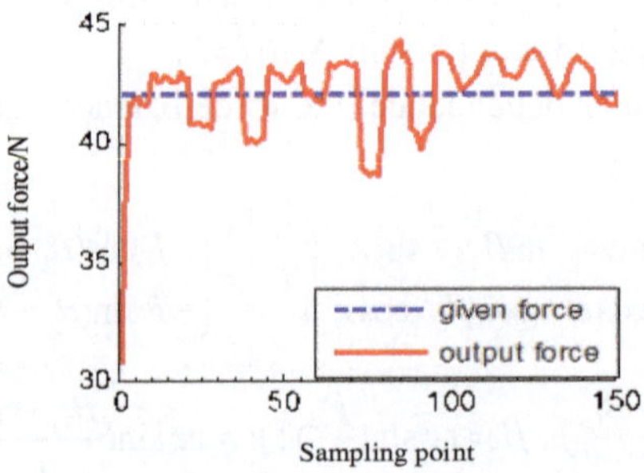

Fig. 3 The diagram of single-shaft's dynamic tracking cycle of 3s.

It was easy to find out that the output force fluctuated up and down in constant value depending on changing the pulling cycle and direction. The direction of motor and output force determined its direction and size. When the motor output force and the motor movement had the same direction, the output force was less than the expected value. The reason was that the counter electromotive force and the given voltage had the opposite direction, then weakened the effect of given voltage. On the contrary when they had the opposite direction, the output force was greater than the expected value.

3.2. *Two-wires driven unit output force experiment*

Sometimes two-wire driven unit output force was needed to meet requirement of multiple training modes during rehabilitation training. This experiment was designed to test the availability and cooperation between the two-wire driven unit output force. This experiment included two torque motors, two tension sensors, pull-tab and so on shown in Fig. 4.

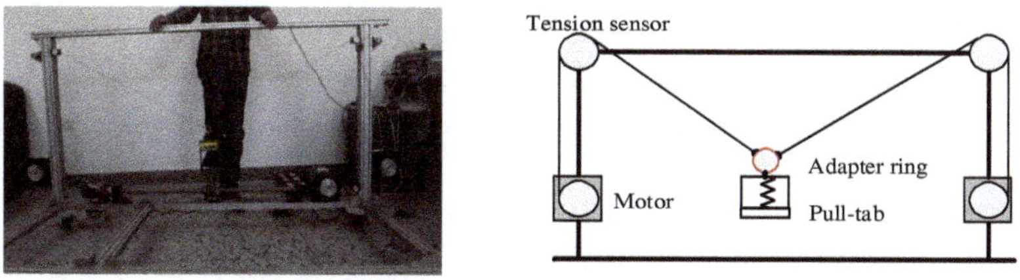

(a) The image of two-shafts' tracking (b) The schematic diagram of couple-shafts' tracking

Fig. 4 Two-wires driven unit output force experiment.

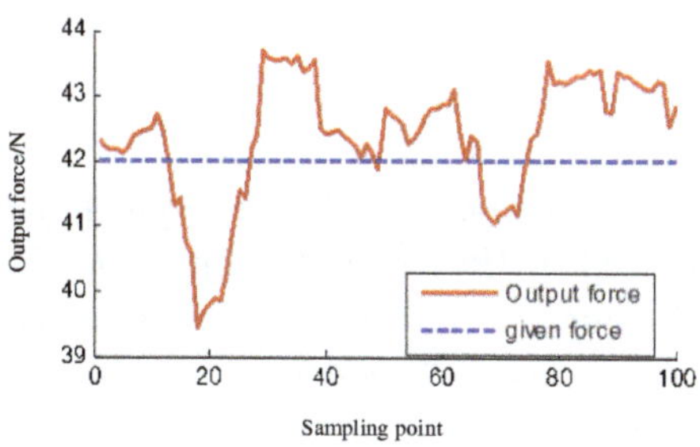

Fig. 5 The diagram of couple-shafts' dynamic tracking cycle of 3s.

Two torque motors exported the same constant force at the same time during experiment. The trainer took flexion and extension movement up and down with one foot on the pull-tab. The waveforms of output force shown in Fig. 5 under different velocity of movement were measured by changing the frequency of the flexion and extension.

4. Conclusion

Considering of the requirement of lower limb tread of rehabilitation training and the character of existing robot, a model of rigid-flexible robot was proposed. With enhancing the robot's flexibility, the system achieved better rehabilitation training effect. And its wires force were solved under the model of gait correcting training. Based on it, the robot machine was developed, on which the single-wire driven function and two-wires driven function had been done. The result of static and dynamic performance of wire output force in experiment verified the feasibility of this robot. This research has a great significance on servo control of wire-driven parallel robot.

References

1. Y.B. Wang, L.H. Ji and G.Z. Wang, *The process and prospect of research on brain rehabilitation robot,* in *Chinese Journal of Rehabilitation Medicine*, Vol. 18, pp. 230-231.
2. W. Han and J. Chang, *The development overview of modern rehabilitation engineering,* in *Medical Equipment*, 2007, pp. 13-15.
3. M.O. Charles, *Human visual orientation in weightlessness,* in *Levels of perception,* 2003, pp. 375-398.
4. H. Sehmidt, S. Hesse, R. Bernhardt and J. Kruger, *HaPticWalker—A Novel HaPtie Food Device,* in *ACM Transactions on Applied Perception,* Vol. 2, pp. 166-180.
5. A.M. Simon, G.R. Brent and D.P. Ferris, *Symmetry-based resistance as a novel means of lower limb rehabilitation,* in *Journal of Biomechanics,* Vol. 40, pp. 1286-1292.
6. W. Wang, *Control of Wire-Driven Walking Mechanism,* Master's thesis of Harbin Engineering University, 2011, pp. 12-15.
7. J. Zhang, *Study on the Exoskeleton Leg for training paraplegic patients*, Master's thesis of Zhejiang University, 2007, pp. 7-9.
8. A.M. Simon, G.R. Brent and D.P. Ferris, *Symmetry-based resistance as a novel means of lower limb rehabilitation*, in *Journal of Biomechanics,* Vol. 40, pp. 1286-1292.
9. Z.C. Zhang, *Researcher on Lower Extremity Exoskeleton of Power Assist Robot,* Master's thesis of Harbin Institute University. 2011, pp. 20-25.
10. C. Philip and B. Rafael and R. Thais, *The human body in a microgravity environment: long term adaptations and countermeasures,* in *Aviation in Focus–Journal of Aeronautical Sciences*, Vol. 4, pp.10-22.

Deep Learning and Its Application in Object Recognition and Tracking

Dan Hu
School of Computer Science, Northwestern Polytechnical University, Xi'an, 710072, China
School of Information and Navigation, Air Force Engineering University, Xi'an, 710077, China
E-mail: plahudan@126.com

Xingshe Zhou
School of Computer Science, Northwestern Polytechnical University, Xi'an, 710072, China
E-mail: zhouxs@nwpu.edu.cn

Xiaohao Yu
General Research Institute, Equipment Academy of Air Force, Beijing, 10076, China
E-mail: yxhtgxx@aliyun.com

Inspired by recent advances in deep learning, this paper reviews the deep learning methods and its applications to object recognition and tracking. First, the concept of deep learning is introduced. Then three main stream deep learning models and algorithms, in addition to some new progresses on the research frontier of deep learning algorithms in object recognition and tracking are illustrated. Finally, a discussion about the difficulties are presented. The motivation of this work is to offer help for the research community on applying the deep learning to object recognition and tracking.

Keywords: Deep learning; object recognition; object tracking.

1. Overview for Deep Learning

Deep learning, which was primarily introduced by Hinton in 2006 [1], is a machine learning algorithm inspired by brains, based on learning multiple levels of representation/abstraction. Thanks to the success on automatic feature extraction via multi-layer nonlinear transformations, deep learning models and algorithms have gained significant attention especially in computer vision [2], speech recognition [3] and natural language processing [4].

In this work, we briefly review the deep learning methods and its applications to object recognition and tracking to do our small gains for the researchers who want to apply this method to the object recognition and tracking fields.

2. Deep Learning Methodologies

There exists three well founded deep learning methodologies, including deep belief networks (DBN)[5], stack auto-encoder (SAE)[6] and convolutional neural networks (CNN)[7], which would be introduced in details.

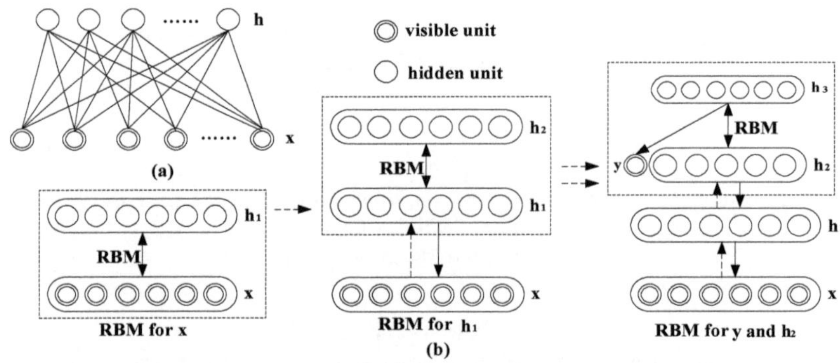

Fig. 1 (a) RBM model; (b) DBN generative process.

2.1. *DBN*

DBN is a generative model consisting of layers of Restricted Boltzman Machines (RBM), which is a two-layer, bipartite, undirected graphical model with full connection between visible units and respective units in the hidden layer, as shown in Figure 1(a).

The probabilistic semantics for an RBM is defined by its energy function, as in Eq. (1), in which $p(x)$ is the marginal probability density function of input x, and Z is a normalization factor.

$$p(x)=\frac{1}{Z}\exp(-freeEnergy(x)),$$
$$Z=\sum_x \exp(-freeEnergy(x)). \tag{1}$$

We can perform efficient block Gibbs sampling by alternately sampling each layer's units given the other layer. So this generative model is capable of estimating the probabilities of $p(sample\,|\,label)$ and $p(label\,|\,sample)$, in contrast to the traditional Neural Networks which can only estimate those of the second one.

The RBM model transforms its input vectors x to the output vectors h, which can be viewed as nonlinear representation of the input data and will be used as input for the next model. That is the DBN, as illustrated in Figure 1(b), combined a set of RBMs, in which the top two layers interact via undirected connections and all of the other connections are directed, can be learned derived a fast, greedy algorithm, the idea behind which is to allow each model in the sequence to receive a different representation of the input data [5].

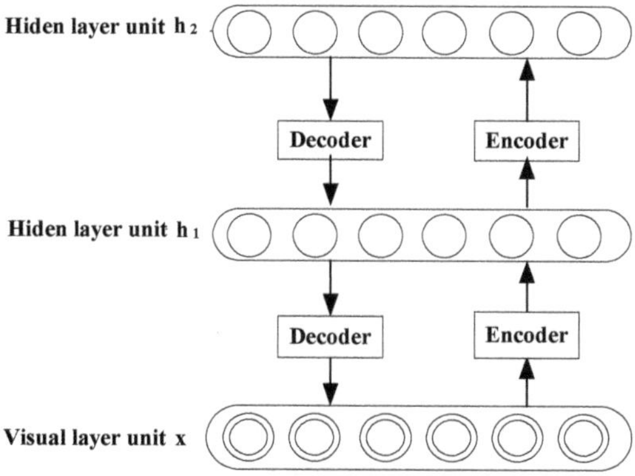

Fig. 2 The illustration of SAE.

2.2. *SAE*

Similar to DBN, a SAE is built by stacking two-layer neural network called Auto-Encoder (AE) which is trained to reconstruct its own inputs. The illustration of SAE is shown in Figure 2.

The SAE learns by minimizing the reconstruction error, as in Eq. (2).

$$\min_{W,W',b,b'} \sum_{i=1}^{k} \| x_i - \hat{x}_i \|_2^2 + \lambda(\| W \|_F^2 + \| W' \|_F^2). \tag{2}$$

Assumed there are k training samples, x_i and $\hat{x}_i$ are the input data sample and the output of the network, respectively. W and W' denote the weights for encoder and decoder, while b and b' are bias terms, λ is a parameter balancing the reconstruction error and weight penalty terms.

DBN and SAE are trained in an idiomatic manner proposed by Hinton et al.[5], involves greadily pretraining each layer (from lowest to highest) using the previous layer's activations as inputs, and then using back propagation algorithm to fine-tune the whole architecture subsequently. In that exact gradient of the log-likelihood is intractable, the contrastive divergence approximation for the deep neural network parameters optimization has been successfully applied in practice.

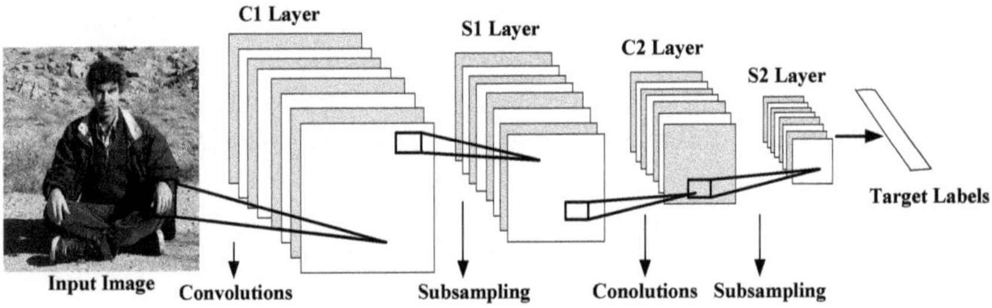

Fig. 3 The illustration of CNN.

2.3. *CNN*

Compared to the fully-connected and similarly-size layers architecture of DBNs and SAEs, CNNs leverage three important ideas that can help to improve a neural network: Local receptive fields, shared weights, and spatial or temporal subsampling. A typical convolutional network architecture is shown in Figure 3, which consists of sequentially placed pairs of convolutional and subsampling layers.

Each unit of a convolutional layer receives inputs from a set of units located in a small neighborhood in the previous layer using convolution in place of general matrix multiplication. The idea of connecting units to local receptive fields on the input goes back to the Perceptron in the early 60s, and was almost simultaneous with Hubel and Wiesel's discovery of locally-sensitive, orientation-selective neurons in the cat's visual system [7].

Weights sharing refers to each member of convolution kernel using on different parts of the image, which is in consideration that elementary feature detectors for one part may also be useful across the entire image. The outputs of such a single convolution kernel scanned the input image, computing one type of feature, constitute a feature map. And several feature maps with different weight vectors would extract multiple features at each location. Benefit from the weight sharing technique, CNNs have much fewer connections and parameters and so they are easier to train, while reducing the theoretically-best performance of the machine slightly and improving its generalization ability.

For most purposes, we care more about whether a feature's approximate position relative to other features is preserved than exactly where it is, which may vary caused by distortions or shifts of the input. Therefore, a subsampling layer applies a pooling mechanism over the local neighborhoods to reduce the resolution from the feature maps derived by the former convolutional layer, and obtain invariance to distortions and shifts.

3. Applications to Object Recognition

Current approaches to object recognition make essential use of deep learning methods. First, rapid developments of large scale parallel computing technique and high performance GPU make training a large deep neural network with millions of parameters and neurons possible. Then, large labeled datasets with millions of images has become available only recently, such as ImageNet [8], which consists of over 15 million labeled high-resolution images in over 22,000 categories, that can improve the deep learning models' performance dramatically.

Hinton has trained a large, deep convolutional neural network to classify the 1.2 million high-resolution images in the ImageNet LSVRC-2010 contest into the 1000 different classes, which achieved top-1 and top-5 error rates of 37.5% and 17.0% which was considerably better than the previous state-of-the-art at that time [2]. The record has been broken and has reached 11.2% by New York University, 12.5% by National University of Singapore, and 13.5% by Oxford on ImageNet 2013. In addition, the current best error rate on the MNIST digit-recognition task (<0.3%) approaches human performance.

Furthermore, all these records would be driven up by collecting larger datasets, learning more powerful models, and using better techniques for preventing overfitting.

4. Applications to Object Tracking

Object tracking is a fundamental problem in computer vision. The success of deep learning on automatic feature extraction also have captured attention of the research community in tracking field. However, the application of deep learning in visual tracking is challenging because it has only a few number of positive instances extracted from the first video frame, while the deep learning requires a large number of training samples to learn more powerful models and improve their performance.

In the recent work of Wang et al. [9], a stacked denoising auto-encoder (SDAE) has been applied for robust visual tracking, and promising results have been reported. As the first work on applying deep learning models to object tracking, it provides large room for further performance improvement. CNN, with distortions and shifts invariance properties, has shown better capability of image feature extraction. Thus employment of CNN in object tracking would be an promising and challenging direction.

5. Discussion

Although deep learning has reported satisfactory results, there remains many opportunities open for further research. Such as better configurations of existing techniques, that is hyper-parameter optimization problem, evaluation methods for extracted features, optimization methods for accelerated gradient descent and preventing overfitting etc., all of them provide more room for further performance improvement of the deep neural networks.

Acknowledgment

This work is supported by the National Natural Science Foundation of China (61175029, 61473309, 61403414).

References

1. G. E. Hinton and R. R. Salakhutdinov, Reducing the Dimensionality of Data with Neural Networks, *Science* **313**, 5786 (2006) pp. 504–507.
2. A. Krizhevsky, I. Sutskever and G. E. Hinton, ImageNet Classification with Deep Convolutional Neural Networks, in *NIPS* (2012).
3. T. N. Sainath, B. Kingsbury, G. Saon, H. Soltau, A. R. Mohamed, G. Dahl, and B. Ramabhadran, Deep Convolutional Neural Networks for Large-scale Speech Tasks, *Neural Networks* **64** (2015) pp. 39–48.
4. R. Socher, C. Liu, A. Ng, Parsing Natural Scenes and Natural Language with Recursive Neural Networks, in *ICML* (2011).
5. G. E. Hinton, S. Osindero and Y. W. Teh, A Fast Learning Algorithm for Deep Belief Nets, *Neural Computation*, **18**, 7 (2006) pp. 1527–1554.
6. P. Vincent, H. Larochelle, I. Lajoie, Y. Bengio and P. A. Manzagol, Stacked Denoising Autoencoders: Learning Useful Representations in A Deep Network with A Local Denoising Criterion, *Journal of Machine Learning Research* **11** (2010) pp. 3371–3408.
7. Y. LeCun and Y. Bengio, Convolutional Networks for Images, Speech, and Time-series, *Handbook of Brain Theory and Neural Networks* (MIT Press, 1995).
8. http://image-net.org/index.
9. N. Wang and D.Y. Yeung, Learning a Deep Compact Image Representation for Visual Tracking, in *NIPS* (2013).

Analysis of Constraint Condition on NC Cutting Parameter Optimization in Chemical Tower

Qingguo Chen* and Juncai Zhang
School of Mechanical Engineering, Hebei University of Science and Technology, Shijiazhuang, Hebei 050018, China
**E-mail: chenqg66@126.com*

Chemical tower, also known as column, is the important equipment to transfer liquid-liquid mass or gas-liquid mass. By UG secondary development, the CAM module of Bill of Materials (BOM) management for chemical tower is realized. Optimizing model must be confirmed firstly in design. It requires that objective function and constraint conditions are to be found. Constraint processing relates to algorithm's efficiency and calculate result. Based on the multi-objective function, constraint condition on NC cutting parameter optimization model in chemical tower has accomplished. It includes surface roughness of workpiece, cutter durability. Cutting power, speed, feed in maching tool are all involved too. These constraint conditions are inter-related and they interact with each other. Their relationship is nonlinearity. Constraint condition in optimization is processed by the combination of Genetic algorithm(GA) and simulated annealing algorithm. It will be theoretically and practically beneficial to construct NC mathematical model of BOM for chemical tower.

Keywords: Chemical tower, Bill of Materials (BOM), optimization design, NC cutting parameter, constraint condition.

1. Introduction

Chemical tower, also known as column, is the important equipment to transfer liquid-liquid mass or gas-liquid mass. Most manufacturing enterprise presently have adopted the traditional manual mode for technical data management. Aiming at the issues above, the paper develops CAM (computer aided manufacturing) on Bill of Materials (BOM) for chemical tower to improve the data management. In UG (Unigraphics) environment, computer aided design on BOM for chemical tower is developed using the development tools of VB. Mapping Algorithm is established to process all BOM data. BOM management module is created accordingly. In NC machining of CAM, cutting parameter library is firstly established to store information of cutting parameter, machining tool, blanks and so on. By taking highest production efficiency and lowest production cost as optimizing objective, a model of multi-objective optimal cutting parameters is founded. On information of engineering BOM and manufacturing BOM, taking manufacture equipment, cutting parameter as constraint conditions, GA and simulated annealing genetic algorithm of the model is solved to obtain the optimal cutting parameters. By UG secondary development, the CAM module of BOM management for chemical tower is realized, as demonstrated in Figure 1.

NC cutting is a complex process. The reasonable cutting parameter will cut cost, increase efficiency, reduce the enterprise cost. When the multi-objective function is solved by GA and simulated annealing genetic algorithm, constraint processing will relate to algorithm's efficiency and calculation result.

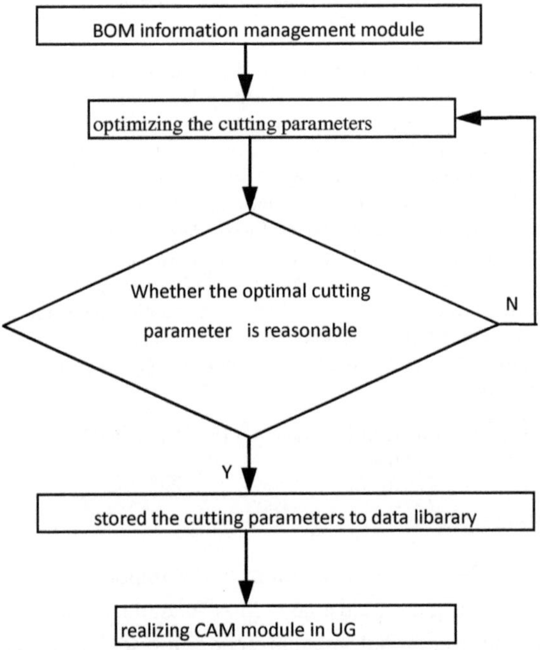

Fig. 1 Flow chart of realizing CAM module.

2. Limiting Factors in Selection Cutting Parameters

Optimization model must be determined firstly in optimizing. That means, objective function and constraint conditions are to be found. Cutting speed v, feed f, back engagement of the cutting edge a_p are the most active factors in machining. The multi-objective function with the cutting edge a_p, feed f, cutting speed v taken as independent variables relied on weighted sum approach to meet the highest production efficiency and the lowest production cost. Based on this evidence it will discuss limiting factors in this paper.

Selection cutting parameters is not a simple mathmatics. The selection will be limited by processing quality, calmp, cutter, machine tool and so on. These constraint conditions must be considered to optimize cutting parameters, to meet the actual production. Limiting factors for selection cutting parameter contribute to the following aspects: the characteristics of machine, processing techniques of part, cutting tools and fixture.

In machining, the above four constraint conditions haven't to be taken into account. The constraint conditions that have less impact on selection cutting parameter can be ignored. While in special processing, the additional constraint conditions are to be considered too. For example, chip shape and the vibration character of processing system are all limits to the cutting speed and feed.

3. Constraint Conditions to NC Machining Parameter Optimization Model in Chemical Tower

3.1. *Feed rate constraint in maching tool*

$$f_{\min} \le f_1 \le f_{\max} \tag{1}$$

Where $f_{\max}$ is the maximun feed rate. While $f_{\min}$ is the minimun feed rate.

3.2. *Cutting speed constraint in maching tool*

$$v_{\min} \le f_2 \le v_{\max} \tag{2}$$

Where $v_{\max}$ is the maximun cutting speed. While $v_{\min}$ is the minimun.

3.3. *Power constraint in maching tool*

$$f_3 = p_m = \frac{C_{F_Z} v^{n_{FZ}+1} a_p^{x_{FZ}} f^{y_{FZ}} K_{F_Z}}{6120} \le P_E \eta_m \tag{3}$$

Where P_E is the effective power in maching tool. P_m is the actual power required. The unit for power is KW. η_m is the transmission efficiency of machine, $\eta_m = 0.75 - 0.85$. y_{F_Z} is the feed index. C_{F_Z} is the cutting force coefficient. x_{F_Z} is the cutting depth index. n_{F_Z} is the the speed index.

y_{F_Z} , C_{F_Z} , x_{F_Z} and n_{F_Z} are all depended on the machined metal and machining conditions. K_{F_Z} is the product of correction coefficient of each influence factor to cutting force when the real conditions is different from the ideal in the experience formula of cutting force. P_E is motor power of machining tool.

3.4. *Constraint of cutter durability*

$$T_1 \leq \frac{C_T}{v^{\frac{1}{m}} f^{\frac{1}{n}} a_p^{\frac{1}{p}}} = T = f_4 \tag{4}$$

Where T_1 is the rational durability of cutter. T is the real durability of cutter. Then the following formula come into being.

$$v \leq \frac{C_V K_V}{T_1^m a_p^{x_v} f^{y_v}} \tag{5}$$

Where y_v is the feed influence index to cutter durability, $y_v = {}^m\!/_n$. x_v is the cut depth influence index to cutter durability, $x_v = {}^m\!/_p$. K_V is the product of correction coefficient of each influence factor to cutter durability when the real conditions is different from the ideal. C_V is the cutting speed influence index to cutter durability, which is depended on the workpiece materials and the other machining conditions.

T_1, the rational durability of cutter hadn't discussed so much in this paper. The constraint of cutter durability is to keep cutter not damage during machining. T_1 is not less than the actual time cutting, so taken $T_1 = t_m$.

3.5. *Surface roughness constraints on cutting parameter*

3.5.1. *The constraint on cutting of straight edge*

$$f_5 = R_{\max} = \frac{f}{\cot \kappa_r + \cot \kappa_r'} \leq 4 \times 10^{-3} \cdot R_a \tag{6}$$

Where κ_r' is tool minor cutting edgeangle. κ_r is tool cutting edgeangle. R_a is surface roughness, μm. $R_{\max}$ is the maximum remain height of area.

3.5.2. *The constraint on cutting of circular arc point ($\kappa_r > \kappa_r'$)*

When $f \le 2r_\varepsilon \sin\kappa_r'$

$$\frac{50f^2}{r_\varepsilon} \le R_a \tag{7}$$

Where r_ε is the corner radius, mm.

When $f > 2r_\varepsilon \sin\kappa_r'$,

$$R_{max} = r_\varepsilon(1-\cos\kappa_r') + \sin\kappa_r'(f\cos k_r' - \sqrt{2r_\varepsilon f \sin\kappa_r' - f^2 \sin\kappa_r'}) \le 3.5\times10^{-3} R_a \tag{8}$$

Formula (6), (7), (8) are the theoretical values on the condition of burr, flow measurement, built-up edge and remaine not occurring in metal cutting. But these common phenomena are inevitable in the real. The modifier can be determined concretely by physical simulation.

The solution of formula (8) is not exact. In this paper, the midpoint, 1/4 ~ 1/3 of the maximum remain height of area is set as the real surface roughness, R_a. In practical production process, R_a, R_{max} are related to the corner radius, r_ε. As r_ε gets smaller, the bigger of R_{max}'s value, the smaller percent of R_a in R_{max}.

Besides the constrained conditions discussed aboved, the other constrained conditions are added to meet the accuracy requirement of workpiece in accordance with the specific. The additional common constrained conditions include strength constraint of carbide chip, stiffness constraint of process system and so on.

4. Constraint Conditions Processing to NC Machining Parameter Optimization Model in Chemical Tower

These constraint conditions are inter-related and they interact with each other. Their relationship is nonlinearity. The choice of cutting parameter will be affected by a change of parameter value. The cutting optimization is a problem of multi-objective, nonlinear constrained one. The actual compute is very complex, to handle multi-objective, nonlinear constraints. The adopted algorithm must realize to search on cutting parameters in the global scope, not fall into the local optimal solution. It also has the ability of local search, to improve the convergence rate and optimize efficiency.

These demands make it difficult to achieve constraint conditions processing by single optimized algorithm. Genetic algorithm (GA), using parallel structure and self adaptive calculation principle, has the characteristics of global optimization. But it's inefficiency. It's global researching is limited as a result of premature convergence to local solutions. The simulated annealing algorithm has the performance of global optimum with probability. So the cutting optimization is solved by the combination of GA and simulated annealing algorithm in this paper.

5. Conclusion

In UG environment, computer aided design on BOM for chemical tower is developed. Constrained conditions have accomplished in setting multi-objective optimization function of NC cutting parameter for chemical tower. It includes surface roughness of workpiece, cutter durability. Cutting power, speed, feed in maching tool are all involved. These constraint conditions are inter-related and they interact with each other. Their relationship is nonlinearity. Constraint condition in optimization is processed by the combination of GA and simulated annealing algorithm. It will be theoretically and practically beneficial to construct NC mathematical model of BOM for chemical tower.

References

1. Wu Meiqing, Zhai Jianjun, Liao Hewen. Research on Parameter Optimization. China Mechanical Engineering [J], 2004,(3): 235-237.
2. Wang Yaodong, HeYuqiang, Cui Hongbing. Development Of BOM system based on UG three dimensional modeling. Manufacturing Technology & Machine Tool [J], 2012 (9): 32-35.
3. Huang Zongnan, He Lanlan, Shu Zhou. Constraints handling in Cutting Optimization by Genetic Algorithms. Mechine Design and Research [J], 2008, (4): 93-97.
4. Avanish umar Dubey et. al. Multi-objective optimisation of laser beam cutting process. optics & Laser Technology [J], 2008, (4): 562-570.
5. Ding Tongmei, Zhou Zhengwu, Wan Taiyong. Optimal Design of Multi-object for Cutting Parameters, Mechanical Engineering & Automation [J], 2006, (4): 38-40.

The Reactor Temperature Control of Pressurized Water Reactor in Nuclear Power Plant Based on RBF Neural Network

Li Haoran* and Yang Xuhong

Shanghai Key Laboratory of Power Station Automation Technology, Automatic Engineering of Shanghai University of Electric Power, Shanghai 200090, China
**Email:lhaoran1991@163.com*
www.shiep.edu.cn

Wang Hui

Guangdong Power Grid Yangjiang Power Supply Bureau, China
Email:1183232148@qq.com

The paper proposes the RBF neural network control method of reactor temperature, according to the PWR nuclear power plant units of 900MW. Firstly, the characteristic of control system of reactor temperature is tested on the simulation platform of PWR nuclear power plant; then, depending on the data from the experiment, the system is analyzed and transfer function fitted, and the transfer function of reactor temperature comes out. Basing on the traditional PID control, the RBF neural network combines with traditional PID control to achieve composite control, which has better control effect than traditional PID and fuzzy PID control.

Keywords: Reactor temperature control; RBF neural network.

1. Introduction

Since the 21st century, with the recovery of the world economy and the increasingly serious energy crisis, the nuclear power attracts attentions because of its advantage of clear energy. The types of nuclear reactor are various such as PWR reactor and boiling water reactor and heavy water reactor and fast reactor and so on. The PWR reactor has become the most widely used nuclear reactor in the world, for its advantages of compact structure and mature technology and low construction cost and short construction period. The point of this paper studies the temperature regulating system of PWR nuclear power reactor and the purpose is using intelligent controller like RBF neural network to optimize PID controller and the effect of reactor temperature control.

The temperature control of reactor cores is one of the most important control parameters in the nuclear power plant, which reflects the reactivity and power of reactor cores directly. And the effect of temperature control determines the safety of nuclear island. Therefore, the research and design of temperature regulating system of PWR nuclear power plant is very necessary.

2. Reactor Temperature Control

In recent years, there is a large number of research on temperature control system of PWR nuclear power plant at home and board with the development of nuclear power plant. An artificial neural network (ANN) technique has been developed to model the dynamic behavior of the considered temperature sensor, and ANN has been also combined with the discrete wavelet transform (DWT) [1-2]. A formula was derived for calculation of methodical error under stationary mode and within the stage of linear increase in temperature [3]. A real time modeling and simulation of core temperature monitoring system is developed. Combustion and ignition characteristics of a stoichiometric gaseous Primary Reference Fuel (blended fuel of n-heptane and iso-octane, PRF)/air mixture were investigated by using a micro flow reactor with a controlled temperature profile [3].

The reactor temperature control usually adopts traditional PI control in the production process of nuclear power plant. For the specially safe problem and significant nonlinear characteristics of itself of nuclear reactor, using traditional control like PI can hardly improve the rapidity of power change and the overshoot. In general, a compromise should be made between them. In order to improve the performance, advanced control strategy should be introduced. It is hard to control precisely using fuzzy control for the establishment of fuzzy rules depends on experiences. The paper tries to adopt RBF neural network to train PID parameters and control the reactor temperature and achieves a good effect.

3. RBF Neural Network Combined with PID Controller

The paper proposes the RBF neural network control method of reactor temperature, according to the PWR nuclear power plant units of 900MW. And the concrete steps are as follows:

1) First of all, the reactor temperature control system is tested on the simulation platform of 900MW PWR nuclear power units of the second three-loops. Then the response curve of reactor temperature is obtained under a variety of rod disturbances. The data from simulation can be considered as actual operation data of nuclear power plant for the data error between the simulation platform and actual operation data is less than 1%.

2) According to the data from the experiment, the system is analyzed and the transfer function fitted. By using the technique of system identification to fit the reactor temperature with transfer function, high precision mathematical model is built. The requirement of fitting is that the maximum deviation is less than 0.1%. The fitting result is shown in Fig. 1.

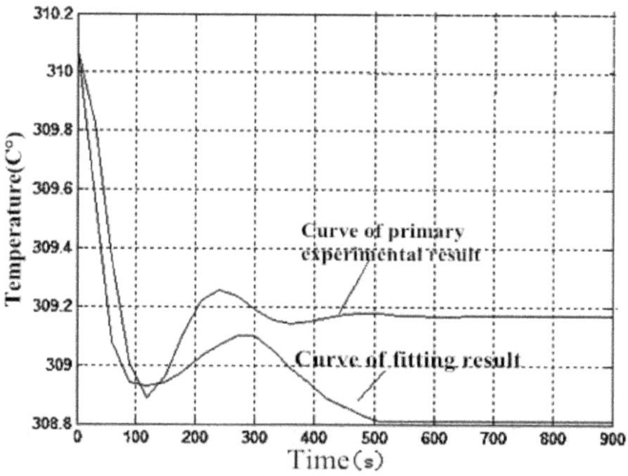

Fig. 1 The fitting curve of data.

Table 1 The fitting error.

Time(s)	0	30	60	90	120	150
Experimental data	310.07	309.57	309.08	308.94	308.93	308.94
Absolute value of error	0	0.00082	0.00091	0.00021	0.00013	0.00007
Time(s)	180	210	240	270	300	330
Experimental data	308.98	309.03	309.07	309.1	309.1	309.05
Absolute value of error	0.00040	0.00061	0.00060	0.00044	0.00029	0.00034
Time(s)	360	390	420	450	......	
Experimental data	308.99	308.94	308.86	308.83	......	
Absolute value of error	0.00049	0.00067	0.00088	0.00091	......	

Then a program is designed to compare and analyze the magnitude of error between the experimental data and the data of fitting transfer function. The error log are shown in Table 1 which analyses the error of fitting curve and actual curve. The maximum of absolute value of error is 0.00091, namely 0.09%, and the fitting precision is very high.

3) The traditional PID controller is designed and the parameters are repeatedly set to achieve the control. In the process of research, 3 groups of PID parameters are designed. The Fig. 2 shows the comparison of step response curves of 3 groups parameters. In the first group of K=0.3, T_i=0.03, T_d=100, the reactor temperature has overshoot and the system response is fast; in the second group of K=0.6, T_i=0.02, T_d=70, it has no overshoot and the system response is fast; in the third group of K=1, T_i=0.008, T_d=100, it has no overshoot but the system response is slow. Choosing the first group as the PID parameters, then they are K=0.3; T_i=0.03; T_d=100. The adjusting time t_s is 270s with no overshoot. Obviously, the controller meets the requirements of production process.

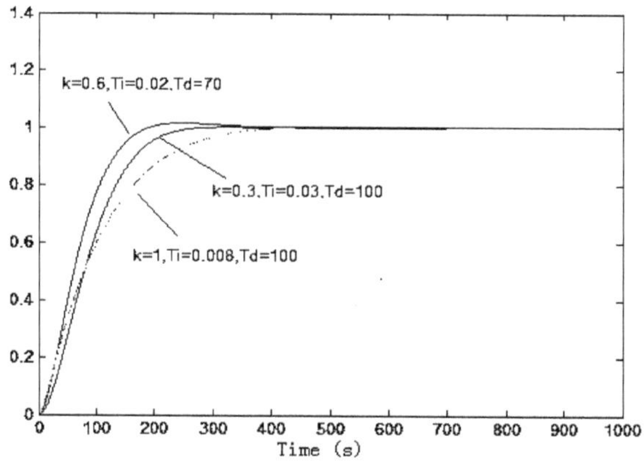

Fig. 2 The comparison figure of step response curve controlled by 3 groups of PID parameters.

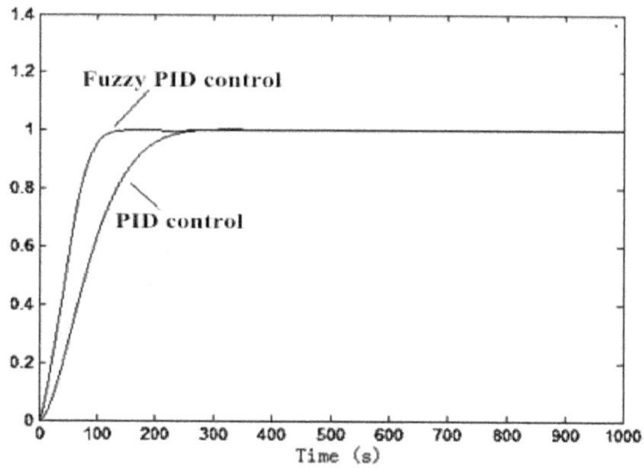

Fig. 3 The comparison of response curve between fuzzy PID controller and PID controller.

The algorithm of RBF neural network combined with PID control optimizes the traditional PID intelligently to achieve better quality of PID parameters and have more effectively control over controlled object. The comparison of response curve between fuzzy PID and PID control is shown in Fig. 3, and the adjusting time ts of fuzzy controller is 140s.

The comparison of control effect between RBF network combined with PID controller and PID controller is shown in Fig. 4, and the adjusting time is 75s. Obviously, the adjusting time of composite control is much shorter than traditional PID and fuzzy PID. Therefore, the control of RBF neural network is feasible.

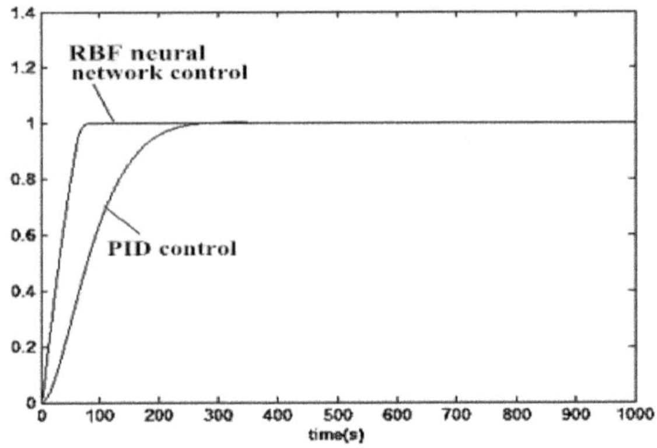

Fig. 4 The comparison of control effect between neural network combined with PID controller and PID controller.

4. Summary

In the production process of nuclear power plant, the reactor temperature control has strict requirements and the recent control is unable to adopt a large range of system parameters. Aiming to solve the problem, the paper proposes RBF neural network control of reactor temperature in PWR nuclear power plant. When the reactor operates in stable conditions and the parameters change in a small range, the control effect of usual PI or PID controller is better, but it can hardly fit for a large range of parameters. This paper combines the RBF neural network with traditional PID control to achieve composite control, and the control effect is better than traditional PID control and fuzzy PID control.

Acknowledgments

This paper is supported by National Natural Science Foundation of China (Project Number: 61203224), Shanghai Science and Technology Commission Key Program (No. 14511101200), Shanghai Natural Science Foundation (13ZR1417800), The Foundation of Shanghai Key Laboratory of Power Station Automation Technology (No. 13DZ2273800), project of Science and Technology Commission of Shanghai (project number: 12510500800).

References

1. Vasanthi, D; Pranavamoorthy, B; Pappa, N. Artificial Neural Network tuned cascade control for temperature control of polymerization reactor. 2011 IEEE International Symposium on Intelligent Control, 1367- 1372.

2. A. Messai, A. Mellit, I. Abdellani and A. Massi Pavan. On-line fault detection of a fuel rod temperature measurement sensor in a nuclear reactor core using ANNs. Progress in Nuclear Energy 79 (2015) pp: 8-21.
3. P. A. Zaytsev, S. V. Priymak, V. B. Usachev, P. P. Oleynikov and D. M. Soldatkin. Features of Temperature Control of Fuel Element Cladding for Pressurized Water Nuclear Reactor "WWER-1000" While Simulating Reactor Accidents. Its Measurement and Control in Science and Industry, Volume 8, 2013, 845-850.

The Research of the Key Techniques and Design for the Cutting Head of Roadheader

Xuemei Zong[1,2,a], Bing He[1,b], Yudong Xu[1,c]
[1] *Construction Machinery Research Institute*
Xuzhou, Jiangsu, China
[a]*zongxm@xcmg.com*, [b]*hebing5280@163.com*, [c]*xuydxcmg@126.com*

Lijie Zhang[2]
[2] *Hebei Provincial Key Laboratory of Heavy Machinery Fluid Power Transmission and Control, Yanshan University, Qinhuangdao, Hebei, China*
zhangljys@126.com

The main design parameters of roadheader cutting head include tooth top envelope surface, helix number and helix lift angle, circumferential angle, maximum cutting thickness, cutting angle and torsion angle. Due to more design parameters, and it interacts among these parameters, therefore, it have to be meet a certain matching relation. Considering influence of these design parameters comprehensively and finding best matching relation can obviously improve the cutting efficiency, reduce cutting specific energy, and ensure the operation reliability.

Keywords: Cutting head; envelope surface; helix lift angle; circumferential angle; maximum cutting thickness; cutting angle; torsion angle.

1. Introduction

Cutting head is roadheader working mechanism for cutting coal and rock, its performance directly affects the work efficiency and reliability and life of the whole machine, is the key of the roadheader parts. The design of the cutting head is very complex, and there are many design parameters, and design degrees of freedom is very big, how to reasonably determine the size and shape of the cutting head and cutting tooth arrangement have become a key problem in the design of the cutting head. These parameters need to modify repeatedly in the design, and workload is big, and the design efficiency is low, through establishing good cutting head parameterized design theory, it make selecting design parameters more reasonable, and improve the design efficiency of cutting head.

Many experts and scholars studied the design of the cutting head. Fanyong Meng determined the basic parameters of the cutting head and designed the cutting tooth arrangement [1]; Lanyan Wu studied on the life of the cutting tooth through analyzing the parameters of the cutting tooth [2]; Mengqi Zhang studied influence of the cutting tooth arrangement for spiral line on longitudinal cutting head performance [3], Xiaoyue Xu designed a method for installing and locating the cutting tooth of the cutting head [4]; Li Yang, Zhebo Zhou explored the distribution of the cutting tooth of the roadheader cutting head [5]. Xin, Zhang, Mei Yang studied the cutting tooth arrangement of the roadheader cutting head[6]. Jinwen Kui, Xiaohuo Li, Guixuan Li discussed the best cutting line spacing of the roadheader cutting head [7]. Guoshun Li, You Zhou, Jinyuan Tang researched the cutting tooth arrangement of the roadheader cutting head [8]; Jianwei Yan studied the installation angle of the roadheader cutting tooth [9]; Xiang Wang, Jinyao Zhang designed spiral of longitudinal roadheader cutting head [10]; On the basis of predecessors' achievements, the cutting tooth top envelope surface, helix number and helix lift angle, circumferential angle, maximum cutting thickness, cutting angle and torsion angle, these key design parameters were given solution.

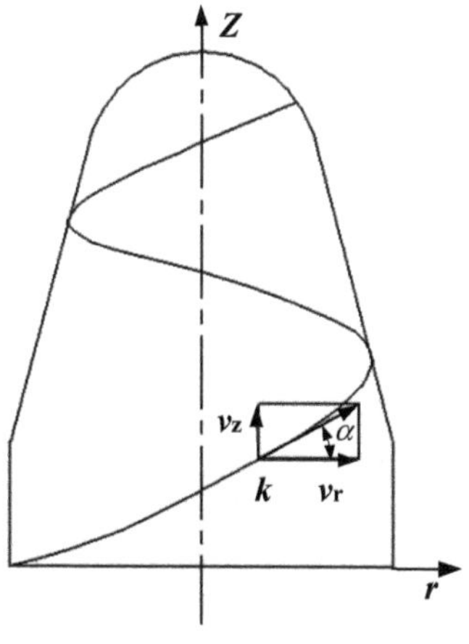

Fig. 1 Helix lift angle diagram.

2. Helix Number and Helix Lift Angle

Helix lift angle diagram as shown in Figure 1, the size of the blade spiral numbers and helix lift angle influence the chip removal effect of the cutting head. The more helix have, the more difficult to ensure cutting tooth orderly cut and cutting tooth number doesn’t change. Test shows, helix number should be less than or equal to 3, cutting tooth arrangement in a spiral angle of helix can make the cutting tooth distribution is uniform, and the chip removal efficiency increase. The helix number of the longitudinal roadheader generally choose 2 or 3, double-head helix cutting head is adopted in the small and medium-sized roadheader.

The best helix lift angle have something to do with the cutting head shape size and working styles. The best helix lift angle increase with increasing every turn drilling depth and transverse cutting distance. When to design cutting head, under the precondition of the cutting head shape size and working styles had be gained, the best helix lift angle could be determined.

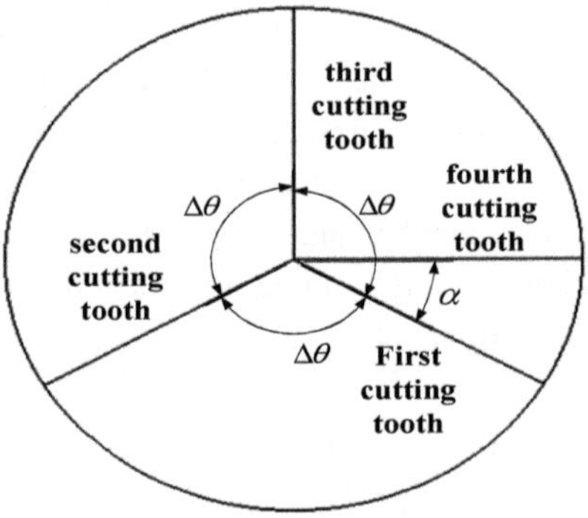

Fig. 2 Circumferential angle distribution diagram.

3. Circumferential Angle Distribution

Circumferential angle is the main factor to impact on the cutting vibration. When cutting teeth enter and exit orderly to cut, the valid cutting teeth of participated in the cutting process will change, it can cause the cutting head of load torque to change, so it leads to the vibration of the cutting head. Circumferential angle also affects the tooth wear. In order to make the cutting teeth of participated in the cutting process tooth in the meantime number is equal, the cutting tooth on the same helix circumferential distribution should be a progression arithmetic, it makes each cutting teeth stress is relatively uniform, wear is reduced. Circumferential angle distribution diagram is shown in Figure 2, take four adjacent cutting tooth on the different helix as an example, The two cutting tooth circumferential angle θ is equal.

$$\Delta\theta = \frac{360° + \alpha}{m}$$

Where α——adjacent cutting tooth circumferential angleon the same helix;
m——helix number.

4. Maximum Cutting Thickness

Maximum cutting thickness diagram as shown in Figure 3, cutting thickness is a depth which the cutting head take a turn to cut transversely into coal and rock. Cutting tooth maximum cutting thickness h_{max} is in direct proportion to the transverse velocity v of the cutting head and is inversely proportional to the number of teeth z and rotate speed n. Maximum cutting thickness changes between $0 \sim h_{max}$.

When cutting tooth cut coal and rock, it will cause coal and rock to avalanche at the front of the cutting tooth, at the same time coal and rock on both sides of the cutting tooth will avalanche because of the strong compression of the cutting tooth. on both sides of the cutting tooth avalanche to form two caving lines, one of the caving line and the center line of the cutter tooth forming angle is called the caving angle φ. Research shows that the rock caving angle not only relates to the nature of the coal and rock, also relates to the cutting thickness of the cutting tooth. As shown in Table 1.

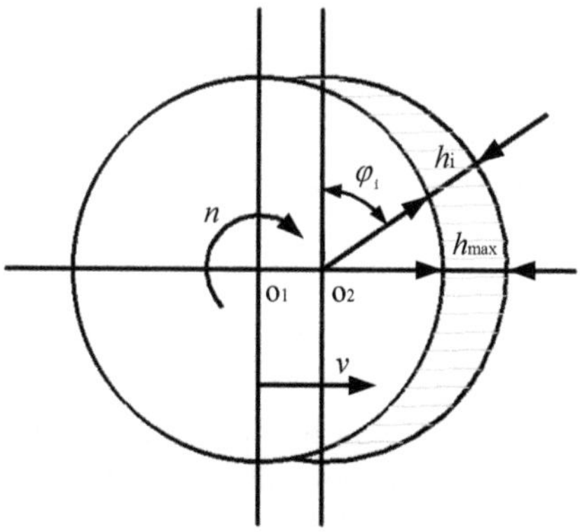

Fig. 3 Maximum cutting thickness diagram.

Table 1 Cutting tooth which cut brittle or viscosity coal and rock create the average caving angle.

The coal characteristic	cutting thickness (cm) $\varphi/(°)$								
	0.5	1.0	1.5	2	2.5	3	4	5	6
brittle	82	77	73	71	68	65	61	58	55
viscosity	69	63	63	55	52	49	45	42	41

The condition parameters of the roadheader determines the cutting thickness of cutting tooth, it affects the cutting resistance of the cutting tooth, cutting line spacing, cutting specific energy and production efficiency. It is important to research the roadheader cutting head.

5. The Best Cutting Line Spacing

Cutting line spacing is the distance of the adjacent cutter tooth which participate in cutting coal and rock. Different coal and rock and the installation method of the cutting tooth will impact on the coal and rock caving angle, and it leads to cutting line spacing too closeor too large. Cutting line spacing is too close can make less amount of broken, and increase dust quantity, and increase cutting specific energy. Cutting line spacing is too large cause coal and rock to cave difficultly, and jam guide plate easily, and reduce the cutting efficiency. When each kerve caving line overlap, each cutting tooth will cut coal and rock between adjacent kerve, which make full use of the coal and rock avalanche effect. It make cutting specific energy low and efficiency high. So the best cutting line spacing should be determined by this condition.

6. Cutting Angle

When cutting tooth cut coal and rock, the stress on the carbide head of the cutting tooth mainly concentrates on the top of the carbide head, and the carbide head bears large stress for along time. It is the main reason that the cutting tooth becomes dull. Some stress concentrates on affecting the weld of the carbide head, it cracks weld and looses the carbide head easily.

If cutting angle is bigger, the cutting tooth bear larger cutting torque, it increases the risk that the carbide head fall off. If cutting angle is smaller, it makes tooth holder and rock, tooth holder and chip participate in cutting, which make tooth holder wear quickly and the load of the cutting head increase, it doesn't lead to roadheader work normally. Therefore, cutting angle should consider the nature of coal and rock and the cutting tooth installation angle. After considering comprehensively, the cutting angle should be chosen from 45° to 55°, which ensure the cutting resistance of cutting tooth is small, and cut into coal and rock easily, but also avoid the tooth participate in cutting.

7. Torsion Angle

The effect of torsion angle is to make the cutting tooth to create a axial torque. The axial torque can let cutting tooth rotate around the cutting tooth axis, and change the contact position between the carbide head and coal and rockconstantly. The cutting tooth wear uniformly as far as possible and improve its working life.

If cutting tooth torsion angle is too large, the cutting tooth axial torque become large, and the contact area between the cutting tooth and rock is larger, and bearing the load on cutting tooth is very big too, which increase the wear of the cutting tooth. If cutting tooth torsion angle is too small, the cutting tooth axial torque become small, which cause the eccentric wear of the cutting tooth. Therefore, considering the torsion angle effect the cutting tooth auto rotation, the cutting tooth torsion angle should be chosen within 5°~12°. Selecting the cutting tooth torsion angle should consider different cutting head position, for example, when to select torsion angle on the spherical cap of the cutting head, it should guarantee the carbide head can contact the rock during drilling.

8. Conclusion

The envelope surface design is beneficial to reduce the uneven load of cutting tooth in process of cutting, it reflect the changing rule of the tooth top in the radius direction. Helix lift angle affects directly the chip removal effect of the cutting head, and make the cutting tooth arrangement more uniform. Circumferential angle is the main factor to influence cutting vibration, and it also affects wear of cutting tooth, it determines installation position of toothholder. Cutting tooth maximum cutting thickness h_{max} is in direct proportion to the transverse velocity v of the cutting head and is inversely proportional to the number of teeth z and rotate speed n. The rock caving angle associated with it. Cutting line spacing determines chip size, dust quantity and cutting specific energy. The nature of coal and rock, the installation method of the cutting tooth and the maximum cutting thickness all influence the best cutting line spacing. Cutting angle influence the stress of the cutting tooth and the cutting torque, and it plays an important role on the cutting performance. The torsion angle effect the cutting tooth autorotation. When the torsion angle selection is unreasonable, the bearing load of the cutting tooth is larger, and it causes cutting tooth serious wear, or it leads to cutting tooth not rotate and causes the eccentric wear of cutting tooth and reduces its working life.

References

1. Fanyong Meng. *Design EBZ315 roadheader machine head* [J]. Coal Mine Machinery, 2010, 31(07): 18-20. (In Chinese)
2. Lanyan Wu. *Research on Equal Life of the Longitudinal Roadheader Conical Bit* [C]. AnHui: AnHui University of Science Technology, 2010.

(In Chinese)
3. Mengqi Zhang. *Influence of Pick Arrangement for Spiral Line on Longitudinal Cutting Head Performance* [J]. Core Science and Technology, 2013, (12): 84-88. (In Chinese)
4. XiaoyueXu. *A Design Method for Attaching Bits Onto Cutting Head* [J]. coal mine and electromechanical, 2005, (4): 11-13. (In Chinese)
5. Li Yang, Zhebo Zhou. *Study on Pick Arrangement on Cutting Head of Roadheader* [J]. Coal Mine Machinery, 2008, (12): 71-73. (In Chinese)
6. Xin Zhang, Mei Yang. *Study of Bit Arrangement on Cutting Head of Roadheader* [J]. Coal mine and electromechanical, 2004, (04): 33-36. (In Chinese)
7. Jinwen Kui, Xiaohuo Li, Guixuan Li. *Study on the best cutting line spacing on Cutting Head of Roadheader* [J]. Coal Mine Machinery, 1993, (4): 13-16. (In Chinese)
8. Guoshun Li, You Zhou, Jinyuan Tang. *Study on the Pick Arrangement of a mining using longitudinal cutting head* [J]. Modern Manufacturing Engineering, 2011, (3): 103-107. (In Chinese)
9. Jianwei Yan. *Pick Assembly Angle Research of Roadheader Cutting Rock* [D]. LiaoNing: Journal of Liaoning Technical University, 2010. (In Chinese)
10. Xiang Wang, Jinyao Zhang. *Spiral Design of Longitudinal Roadheader Cutting Head* [J]. Coal Mine Machinery, 2011, (09): 6-8. (In Chinese)

Multiscale and Multidisciplinary Analysis of Deformation and Damage in the Case of Oligocrystalline Structures

Marijo Mlikota[a], Siegfried Schmauder[b] and Ulrich Weber
Institut für Materialprüfung, Werkstoffkunde und Festigkeitslehre (IMWF), Universität Stuttgart, Pfaffenwaldring 32, 70569 Stuttgart, Germany
E-mail: [a]marijo.mlikota@imwf.uni-stuttgart.de,
[b]siegfried.schmauder@imwf.uni-stuttgart.de
www.imwf.uni-stuttgart.de

Bojan Mitevski and Sabine Weiß
Lehrstuhl für Metallkunde und Werkstofftechnik (MWT), Brandenburgische Technische Universität (BTU) Cottbus – Senftenberg, Konrad-Wachsmann-Allee 17, 03046 Cottbus, Germany
E-mail: [b]bojan.mitevski@uni-due.de
www.tu-cottbus.de/fakultaet3/de/metallkunde

This paper serves as an overview of the ongoing research in the field of multiscale and multidisciplinary analysis of deformation and damage in the case of oligocrystalline structures. The research focuses on experimental measurement and numerical calculation of ductile failure in the X2CrNiMo18-15-3 (AISI 316L) stainless steel. An embedding numerical technique is employed where crystal plasticity theory is used to represent plastic deformation in the material and element removal technique based on Rice&Tracey damage model for ductile void growth to simulate damage initiation inside the material, which is observed in the experiments. Additionally, the crystal plasticity model is supported by a hierarchical multiscale approach connecting nano-, micro- and meso-scales.

Keywords: Oligocrystalline structures; FEM; crystal plasticity theory; Rice & Tracey damage model.

1. Introduction

Micro components, or miniaturized machines and tools, are used for a multitude of applications. Some examples in the multidisciplinary fields of medicine (e.g. minimally invasive surgery) and materials science are metal vessel scaffolds (coronary artery stents) which are inserted in the blood vessel to prevent the vessel wall from collapsing. The dimensions of these components are far below the dimensions of conventional test specimens. As available from literature, the mechanical behavior of such oligocrystalline components is much different from the one of polycrystalline. Therefore the common knowledge about polycrystalline materials is not able to describe the mechanical behavior of those micro components. The focus of the work is fundamental research on the deformation mechanisms of oligocrystals by means of crystal plasticity simulation. Based on experimental data a continuum mechanics model will be developed to predict the durability of oligocrystalline structures under defined deformation conditions.

2. Modelling – Theoretical Background

2.1. *Crystal plasticity (CP) theory*

The CP constitutive theory used in this work is a rate dependent plastic, finite deformation, crystallographic theory. The theory has been presented in full in [1–4] and thus the details are not given here. The essential point to note is that the theory is physically based and that plastic deformation of a single crystal is described solely in terms of continuum shear flows that occur along the various slip systems of the crystal. The plastic material description can be combined with an elastic material description to generate an elastic–plastic constitutive law, in the form of nonlinear rate equations. Slip system strain hardening is specified by the hardness function [2, 4]:

$$g(\gamma_a) = g_o + (g_{oo} - g_o)\, tanh\left|\frac{h_o\gamma_a}{g_{oo} - g_o}\right|. \tag{1}$$

where γ_a is the accumulated slip and the material hardening parameters g_o, g_{oo}, and h_o are the initial hardness of a slip system, the maximum slip system hardness when $\partial g/\partial\gamma_a = 0$, and the value of $\partial g/\partial\gamma_a$ when $\gamma_a = 0$, respectively. A quantity of importance in Eq. 1 is the accumulated slip, γ_a, which is a measure of the total crystallographic plastic strain at a point.

The above constitutive theory is implemented in the finite element code ABAQUS/Explicit as a user-defined subroutine (VUMAT), an explicit version of the subroutine coded in [4]. The development of the code is detailed in [1, 3, 4].

2.2. *Rice &Tracey damage model*

The model used in the present work to simulate material failure is the Rice&Tracey continuum damage mechanics model. The theory behind the model has been presented in full in [5–8] and thus the details are not given here. The model characterizes material failure in terms of a damage parameter in which a relationship between the stress triaxiality, η, and the equivalent plastic strain, ε_{pl}, determines the volume fraction of voids in the material; when the volume fraction of voids at a point in the material reaches a critical level immediate failure at that point is assumed. The damage parameter can be written as [8]:

$$D = \frac{1}{A} \cdot \int_{0}^{\varepsilon_{pl}} e^{B\eta} d\bar{\varepsilon}_{pl}. \tag{2}$$

The point of failure initiation happens at the critical damage parameter value of $D_c = 1$. In Eq. 2, A and B stand for two material dependent parameters.

Failure of a point in the material is numerically represented by reducing the stiffness of a finite element from the model, i.e. by eliminating the element and redistributing the load to the surrounding elements. For numerical implementation, the Rice&Tracey damage model is coded as an extra module in the CP numerical formulation.

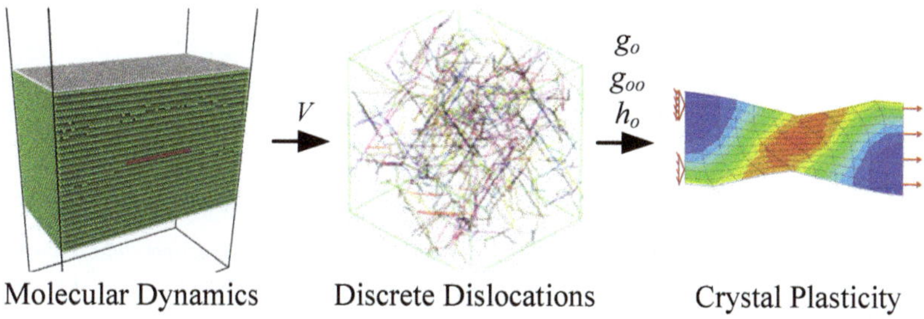

Figure 1 A scheme of a multiscale methodology that was used to calculate the material parameters of the hardening law needed at the CP level to predict the mechanical response of a single crystal [9].

2.3. *Multiscale modeling supported determination of the CP parameters*

Groh et al. [9] proposed the multiscale methodology, illustrated in Fig. 1, which presents the three different length scales and corresponding simulation tools used to bridge the respective scales and predict the mechanical response of a single crystal of meso-scale dimensions.

Five material parameters are needed at the CP level to numerically predict the stress-strain behavior. The two parameters of the flow rule (a, the reference strain rate and n, the rate sensitivity exponent [4]) can be estimated from published literature, while the three parameters in the hardening rule, i.e. g_o, g_{oo} and h_o (Eq. 1), can be calculated directly using discrete dislocations (DD) simulations and then transferred hierarchically to the CP level. At the DD level, the drag coefficient V needs to be quantified as well, either from experimental data or a lower length scale molecular dynamics (MD) analysis. In [9], this coefficient is calculated numerically using MD and then transferred hierarchically to the DD length scale level.

3. Experiments

For the experiments (MWT), the solution annealed stainless steel X2CrNiMo18-15-3 (AISI 316L) cut from plates was used. Fig. 2a shows the initial condition of a notched axially symmetric tensile flat specimen with a notch radius of 0.6 mm. The specimen was strained in three-step tensile tests. The tests were stopped at the beginning of plastic deformation at the notch ground (> yield strength) (Fig. 2b) and at maximum technical stress (Fig. 2c). An increasing elongation of the specimen (Fig. 2c) leads to a further deformation to thicker parts in-between the notch.

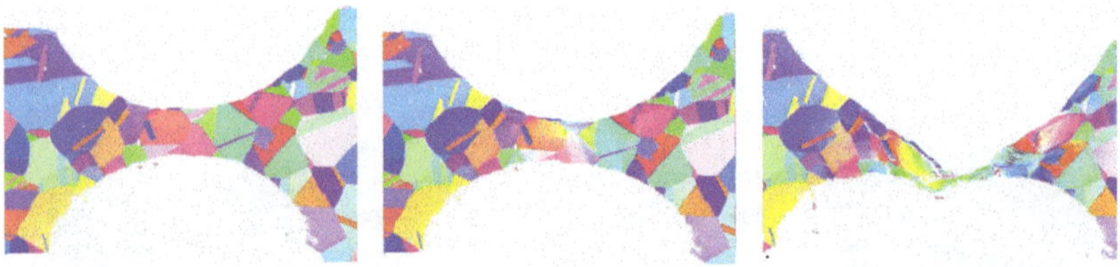

a) b) c)

Figure 2 Inverse Pole Figure Mappings (IPF || RD) of one notched flat specimen with increasing plastic deformation: a) before testing, b) at the beginning of plastic deformation (> yield strength) and c) and at tensile strength [10].

4. Modelling – Results

Fig. 3 shows a single crystal benchmark 2D model meshed with 100 CPE4R elements (IMWF). The element name CPE4R describes continuum first-order reduced integration plane strain quadrilateral elements. In a first step, the model was enriched by the CP formulation. Although the geometry is based in 2D, the crystal has a full 3D FCC crystallographic description – described using the generalized plane strain formulation. An externally applied displacement causes the activation of a preferred glide plane (system) in the system, which is usually somehow inclined with respect to the loading direction. However, the model enriched with the CP theory solely is not able to provide the valuable information on the moment of material failure, therefore, it is necessary to extend the model further by applying appropriate techniques, similar as in [11].

Thus, the Rice&Tracey damage model together with the element removal technique (ERT) was implemented. After a certain stretching (strain of about 60%) of the model, the Rice&Tracey damage criterion (A = 1.65, B = 0.4 [4]) was reached and a set of elements in the preferred glide system was eliminated from the model mesh (blue elements). Activation of a preferred glide plane (system) and succeeding damage show similarity with the experimental observations (see Fig. 2c).

The mechanical response has been obtained by applying the following CP material constants for the X2CrNiMo18-15-3 stainless steel: g_o = 150 MPa, g_{oo} = 360 MPa, h_o = 270 MPa, a = 0.0106 s^{-1} and n = 50, taken from [4].

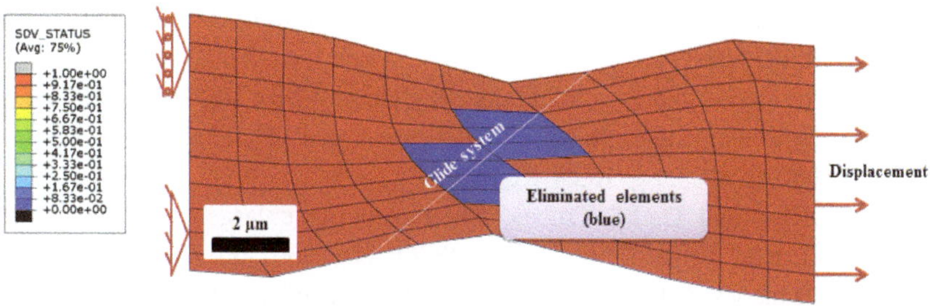

Figure 3 Status of the elements in the single crystal model.

5. Summary and Outlook

The presented modelling framework allow for the explicit representation of the metallic grains (crystals) and prediction of microstructural deformations until failure. Even though it is in the benchmark variant, the capability of the modelling framework allows to model polycrystalline structures with real microstructural geometries investigated experimentally (e.g. Fig. 2). In terms of model improvement, real microstructural morphologies need to be taken into account in the following stage of the research. Inclusion of these features will provide more information about the origins of material failure. Additionally, the multiscale modeling approach used to determine the material parameters of hardening law in the CP model will be applied in the next steps.

Acknowledgment

This work was financially supported by the German Science Foundation (DFG) in the frame of project SCHM 746/130-1 “Messung und Simulation der monotonen Verformung oligokristalliner Strukturen am Beispiel koronarer Stents".

References

1. D. F. Quinn, P. J. Connolly, M. A. Howe and P. E. McHugh, Simulation of void growth in WC–Co hard metals using crystal plasticity theory, *Int. J. Mech. Sci.* **39**, 2 (1997), pp. 173–183.
2. D. Pierce, R.J. Asaro and A. Needleman, Material rate dependence and localized deformation in crystalline solids, *Acta Metall.* **31** (1983), pp. 1951.
3. Y. Huang, *A user-material subroutine incorporating single crystal plasticity in the ABAQUS finite element program*, Harvard University Report, MECH 178.
4. F. J. Harewood and P. E. McHugh, Modeling of Size Dependent Failure in Cardiovascular Stent Struts under Tension and Bending, *Ann. Biomed. Eng.* **35**, 9 (2007), pp. 1539–1553.
5. J. R. Rice and D. M. Tracey, On the ductile enlargement of voids in triaxial stress fields, *J. Mech. Phys. Solids* **17** (1969), pp. 201–217.
6. J. W. Hancock and A. C. Mackenzie, On the mechanisms of ductile failure in high-strength steels subjected to multi-axial stress-states, *J. Mech. Phys. Solids* **24** (1976), pp. 147–169.
7. J. L. Mishnaevsky, M. Dong, S. Hönle and S. Schmauder, Computational mesomechanics of particle-reinforced composites, *Comput. Mater. Sci.* **16**, 1–4 (1999), pp. 133–143.
8. J. Arndt, H. Majedi and W. Dahl, Influence of Strain History on Ductile Failure of Steel, *J. de Physique* **IV**, 06 (1996), pp. 23-32.
9. S. Groh, E. B. Marin, M. F. Horstemeyer and H. M. Zbib, Multiscale modeling of the plasticity in an aluminum single crystal, *Int. J. of Plasticity* **25** (2009), pp. 1456–1473.
10. B. Mitevski and S. Weiß, Influence of the Notch Geometry and Microstructure of Thin 316L – Plates on the Mechanical Behavior: An In-Situ Study, Poster at DGM BioMat (Weimar, 2015).
11. A. Siddiq, S. Schmauder and Y. Huang, Fracture of bicrystal metal/ceramic interfaces: A study via the mechanism-based strain gradient crystal plasticity theory, *Int. J. Plasticity* **23** (2007), pp. 665–689.

Research the Influence of Asymmetry Radiation on the Thermal Environment of Plane Radiation Air-Conditioning Based on CFD

Liu Xue Lai†, Li Yu Ping and Li Yong An
Institute for thermal power engineering, Shandong Jianzhu University, Ji Nan, Shan Dong, China
†E-mail: liuxuelai147@163.com
www.sdjzu.edu

In this paper, large span and open type office space is selected as the research object. Established the mathematical physics model of planar radiation air conditioning, gives a simulation analysis steps of asymmetric radiant heat environment, and based on CFD and coupling of the human body thermal regulation model, simulation analysis of the applicability of the indicators asymmetric radiation temperature, asymmetric, radiating surface radiation temperature field of the aspect ratio changes, the change of indoor design temperature on the influence of asymmetric radiant heat environment.

Keywords: Radiation air-conditioning; asymmetric radiation; thermal environment; CFD.

1. The Physical Model

In this paper, a business office building radiation in air conditioning room is selected as the research object. Select 5~9 layers of large span and open type office space as the research object. Simplified construction model: room size (length x width x height) for 40 m * 17.6 m * 4 m; South the exterior wall, using a large area of glass curtain wall as the maintenance structure, window wall ratio is 73.6%, interior wall, east, west, north to the east, the west wall on the other side of the space and the room with the same thermal environment, north to the other side of the wall inside the space of corridor.

2. Mathematical Model

For quality control, energy and momentum conservation equation general form are represented according to the type of 1.1, specific form can see literature [1].

$$\frac{\partial(\rho\phi)}{\partial t}+div(\rho U\phi)=div\left(\Gamma_{\phi}grad\phi\right)+S_{\phi} \tag{1.1}$$

The particular form of radiation integral equation is as follows:

$$\frac{dI(\vec{r},\vec{s})}{ds}+(a+\sigma_s)I(\vec{r},\vec{s})=an^2\frac{\sigma T^4}{\pi}+\frac{\sigma_s}{4\pi}\int_0^{4\pi}I(\vec{r},\vec{s})\Phi(\vec{s},\vec{s}')d\Omega' \quad (1.2)$$

discrete equation as the following form:

$$a_p\phi_p = a_E\phi_E + a_W\phi_W + a_N\phi_N + a_S\phi_S + a_T\phi_T + a_B\phi_B + S_c\Delta x\Delta y\Delta z \quad (1.3)$$

Mathematical expression is as follows:

$$\mu_t = 0.03874\rho vl \quad (1.4)$$

Indoor air turbulent flow control differential equation is expressed as:

$$\frac{\partial}{\partial t}(\rho\varphi)+\mathrm{div}\left(\rho u\varphi-\Gamma_\varphi\cdot \mathrm{grad}\varphi\right)=S_\varphi \quad (1.5)$$

2.1. *The choice of radiation heat transfer model*

At present, the main radiation model includes surface (S2S) radiation model, P-1 model, discrete heat transfer (DT) radiation model and discrete-ordinate (DO) radiation model, Roseland radiation model [2]. Integrated the advantages and limitations of each radiation model [3], and the characteristics of the research problem, this paper adopts the DO radiation model, in the understanding of the human body surface and radiation Angle coefficient between surface, using S2S model.

Table 2.1 Outdoor temperature of summer air conditioning.

time	8	9	10	11	12	13	14	15	16	17	18
dry-bulb temperature(°C)	31.4	32.3	33.2	34	34.5	34.8	34.7	34.2	33.9	33.1	32.2

2.2. *Set of model boundary conditions*

(1) Outdoor calculated parameter

(2) the palisade structure boundary conditions

Capillary network radiating surface in this article are set to constant heat flux boundary condition and capillary spacing set of 20 mm, capillary net radiation device in the supply and return water temperature set at 18 °C / 20 °C, the average temperature for 19 °C within the capillary network, according to references [4], when the average temperature for 19 °C, the relationship between the capillary net heat transfer per unit area and indoor design temperature is shown in Table 2.2.

Table 2.2 Capillary net heat transfer per unit area.

Indoor air temperature(°C)	22	24	26	28	30
Heat transfer per unit area (W / m^2)	35.22	52.54	70.92	90.18	110.23

3. Numerical Simulation

3.1. *The human body thermal regulation model and CFD coupling*

The human body thermal regulation model and CFD numerical simulation analysis algorithm solving process can be divided into: (1) First surroundings to the human body parameters, including temperature, relative humidity and velocity, again according to the body's energy transport model, boundary conditions on the surface of the skin; (2) The body surface temperature and relative humidity are obtained by CFD simulation, and put it to the human body thermal regulation model as a known quantity, until the final simulation results to achieve convergence.

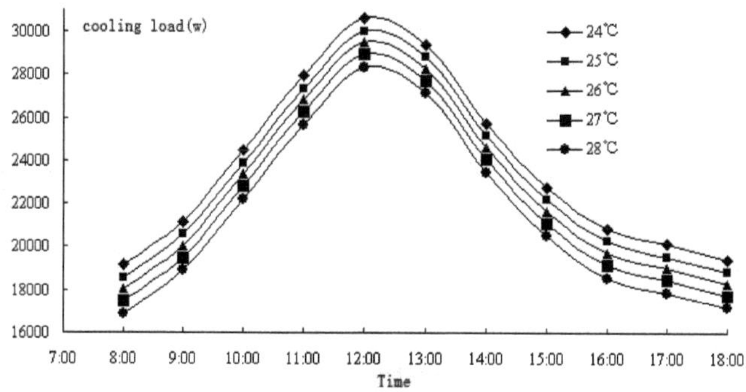

Figure 3.1 Cooling load under different temperature.

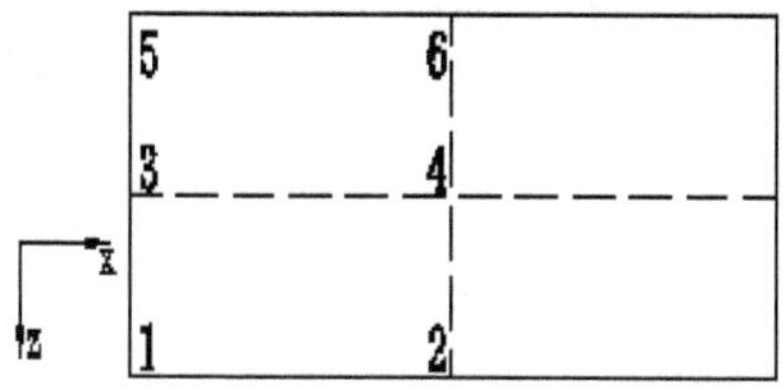

Figure 3.2 Schematic plan view of model room.

3.2. *The simulation analysis procedures*

Specific simulation steps as follows: (1) the D-est energy consumption simulation software to calculate the Jinan area typical design, as shown in

Figure 3.1. (2) Calculation of the different parts of the surface temperature of human body (3) The calculation of the weighted PMV [5].

4. The Numerical Simulation Analysis

4.1. *Analysis of asymmetric radiation temperature field*

In simulation analysis, indoor design temperature and laying modes of radiating surface is the same with what in Section 4.1. Indoor personnel in Figure 3.1 the position of the 2, 4, 6, section temperature field as shown in Figure 4.1.

Inside surface temperature of the envelope is 33 °C, and the temperature of inner wall of the structure is 25 °C, and the capillary network radiating surface temperature is about 19 °C.Personnel in the interior, especially in a nearby envelope, in one-side is hot directional radiation from the envelope surface about 33 °C hot, the other-side is cold directional radiation mainly from capillary network radiating surface about 19 °C. T

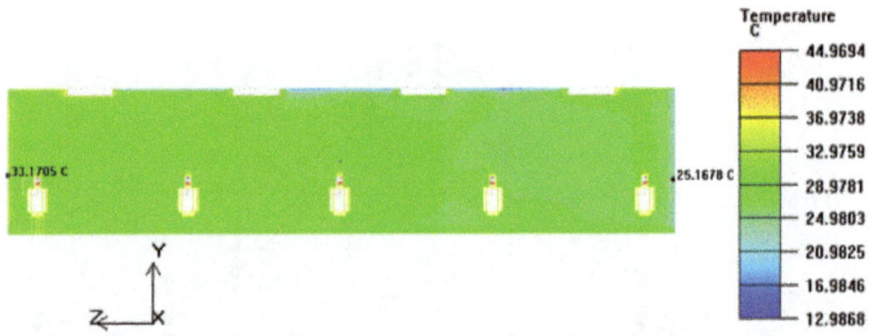

Figure 4.1 Temperature field of 2, 4, 6, location.

4.2. *The influence of radiating surface aspect ratio on heat environment*

Radiating surface under different length-width ratio, the indoor personnel in 2 ~ 6 different locations, the weighted PMV varied with the change of the distance between the envelope personnel and as shown in Figure 4.2, the selection of the location of vertical between graphs, near the envelope, to take a step per 0.5 m, 2.8 meters away from the envelope, take a step length per 2m.

The analysis of Figure 4.2 and Figure 4.3 shows that on the length direction of the model room, the weighted PMV in the same cross section changed a little, and in the width direction of model room, the weighted PMV in the same cross section changes greatly. In these three aspect ratio, when the radiating surface width is the same with the width of the room, the influenced on indoor personnel by asymmetric radiation is minimum, the thermal comfort zone is the largest.

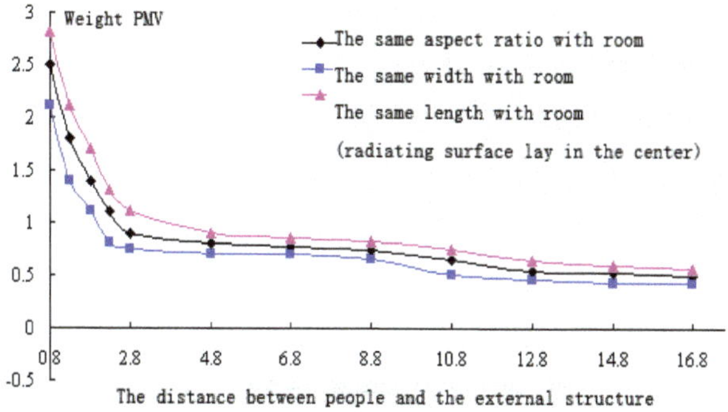

Figure 4.2 Weighted PMV varied with the change of personnel' position in point 1 to 5.

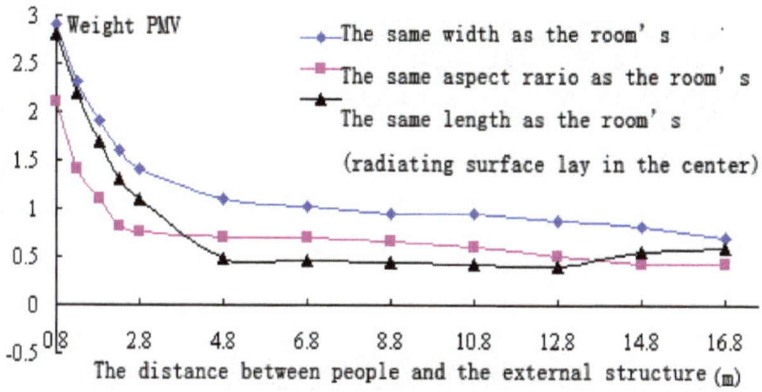

Figure 4.3 Weighted PMV varied with the Change of personnel' position in point 2 to 6.

4.3. *Influence of design temperature change on asymmetric radiant environment*

According to the load of different indoor design temperature in Figure 3.1, the corresponding of radiating surface area is calculated. According to, the change of the indoor personnel weighted PMV value of point 2 to 6 in Figure 3.2, analyze heat environment in different indoor design temperatures asymmetric radiant. Through lay in the middle of the model room roof, aspect ratio is the same with the room's. Simulation results are shown in Figure 4.4.

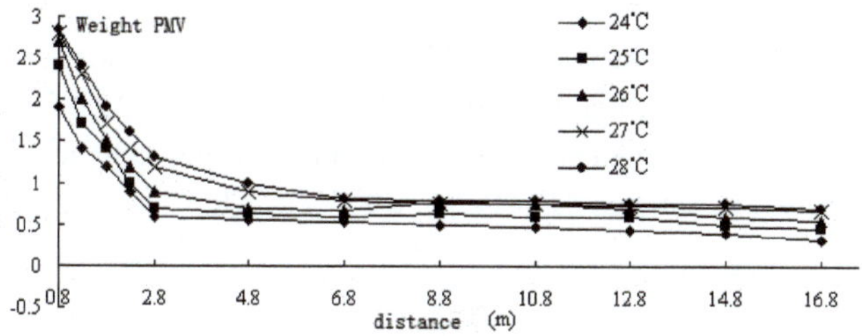

Figure 4.4 The change of weighted PMV along with interior staff position.

As you can see from the Figure 4.4, with the increase of indoor design temperature, thermal comfort zone is smaller, the effects of asymmetric radiation on indoor thermal environment is greater.

5. Conclusion

Along the length direction room, the weighted PMV in the same cross section changes little, and along the width direction of the model room, the weighted PMV in the same cross section changes greatly, and in these three aspect ratio, the width of the radiating surface is the same with the width of the room. From the view of thermal comfort and making full use of the point of architectural interior space, the installation method that radiating surface width is the same with the room width is better than other two methods, it can reduce indoor radiation field asymmetric effect on the human body thermal comfort, but from the point of energy saving, according to the inner surface of envelope thermal equilibrium relations, when the installation is adopted, heat flux of the envelope is the biggest.

References

1. Juanjuan Sun, Capillary plane radiant dynamic simulation and control system [D]. Jinan: Shandong Jianzhu University, 2011.
2. S.V. Patanker, D.B. Spalding. A calculation procedure for heat, mass and momentum transfer in three dimensional parabolic flows [J]. Int. J. Heat Mass Transfer, 1972, 15 (10): 1787-1806.
3. Xianchen Zheng, Several radiation model in FLUENT in [J]. Modern science and technology, 2009, 8(11): 67-69.
4. Xinyang Cu, Capillary plane thermal properties of air conditioning systems and hydraulic calculation method [D]. Jinan: Shandong Jianzhu University, 2010.
5. Yuan Jun Wei. Study [D] asymmetric impact of radiation on the air conditioning mechanism plane radiation. Jinan: Shandong Jian Zhu University, 2010.
6. P.O. Fanger, B.M. Ipsen, G. Langkilde, et al. Comfort limits for asymmetric thermal radiation [J]. Energy and Buildings, 1985, 8(3): 225–236.
7. Xiaomei Feng, Yongquan Xiao. Low temperature radiant floor heating characteristic parameters [J]. HVAC, 2004(1): 1-4.

Study on the Flexure Hinges Shape Design of The Uniaxial of Nanopositioning Stage Using ANSYS

Jen-Ching Huang†, Feng-Chin Tsai and Pei-Shiang Liao

Department of Mechanical Engineering, Tungnan University,
New Taipei City, Taiwan
†E-mail: jc-huang@mail.tnu.edu.tw
www.tnu.edu.tw

In this study, in order to make a wide range displacement amount of nanopositioning stage and precision positioning, so design a flexible nanopositioning stage structure to meet this requirement. In this study, three different shape of the spring with four different shapes of the rib to analyze various combinations of, seen from the analysis results, when spring appearance as a cross-type (S1 type), the displacement of the shape of a wave-shaped rib (R1 type) portfolio the minimum amount of errors, and successfully analyze its spring constant and the resonant modal. The results were available for follow-up production when the reference platform.

Keywords: Nanopositioning stage; spring constant; resonant modal.

1. Introduction

Recently, as the result of rapid developments in various fields of precision engineering, there has been a big increase in the need for precision positioning. In the precision positioning applications, it is often required that actuators have nanometer resolution in displacement.

Therefore, the advances in micro/nano technology are stimulating the research and development of the micro/nanopositioning stage, the related applications can be found in the fields of functional biomolecular assembly, biological cell automatic micro-injection, and integrated circuit (IC) packaging [1, 2]. Nanomanipulation could be defined as the manipulation of nanometer size (0.1–100 nm) objects using a nanometer size end-effector with (sub) nanometer precision via devices offering high positioning accuracy and dexterous motion of the end-effector, which has been enabled by the invention of scanning tunneling microscopes (STM), atomic force microscopes (AFM), and other types of scanning probe microscopes (SPM) [3].

So far, some nanopositioning stages have been proposed and commercialized [4, 5]. But, it also has some disadvantageous characteristics such as: hysteresis behavior, drift in time and temperature dependence. The disadvantageous characteristics of hysteresis are usually nonlinearities and uncertainty. Therefore, it is difficult to obtain an accurate trajectory tracking control [6]. As well known, the compliant mechanisms, i.e., flexure hinge-based mechanisms can be employed into parallel mechanisms for high precision applications thanks to their excellent characteristics in terms of vacuum compatibility, no backlash property, no nonlinear friction, and easy to manufacture, etc [7, 8]. Several parallel manipulators employing flexure hinges have been designed to perform the manipulation in micro/nano meter scales with high accuracy [9].

In this paper, ANSYS software was used to simulate the output characteristics of flexure hinges uniaxial nanopositioning stage of solving the displacement of the input and output of nanopositioning stage. And to investigate the effect of stage performance parameters, such as nanopositioning stage guide rib thickness, the shape of the plate spring, plate spring thickness. And calculated in accordance with ANSYS, select the appropriate combination of improved design and get the best nano-stage patterns.

2. The Design Nanopositioning Stage

In this study, a flexible hinge nanopositioning stage for object to really convey the amount of displacement caused by the actuator as the goal, ANSYS software to simulate the output characteristics of this nanopositioning stage and solving the ratio of input and output positioning platform ends displacements.

2.1. *Platform design*

In this study, the precision nanopositioning stage appearance is based on the literature [4-9], combined with the auxiliary spring designed and carried out with the observation which best meet what combination displacement ratio of input and output of the closest to the 1:1 case, the and cannot cause plastic strain.

In Figure 1, the ribs is the S-type shape and the auxiliary spring (Spring) is the X-type shape. The appearance of a variety of spring and rib according to Table 1 of the experimental design which consists of various combinations, and select the best combination of them by using ANSYS finite element analysis.

And observe the best combination, the displacement of its input and output terminal if equal (1:1), and the horizontal displacement, that has to meet the requirements of this study. Conversely, if the demand has not yet reached its displacement ratio, the structure further improved.

Table 1 The experimental design of various combinations.

Rib \ Auxiliary spring	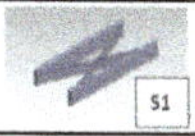	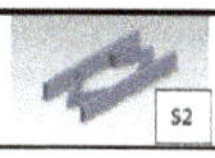	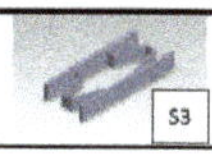
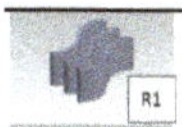	R1S1	R1S2	R1S3
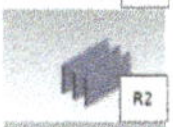	R2S1	R2S2	R2S3
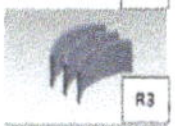	R3S1	R3S2	R3S3
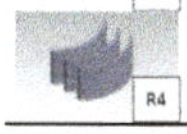	R4S1	R4S2	R4S3

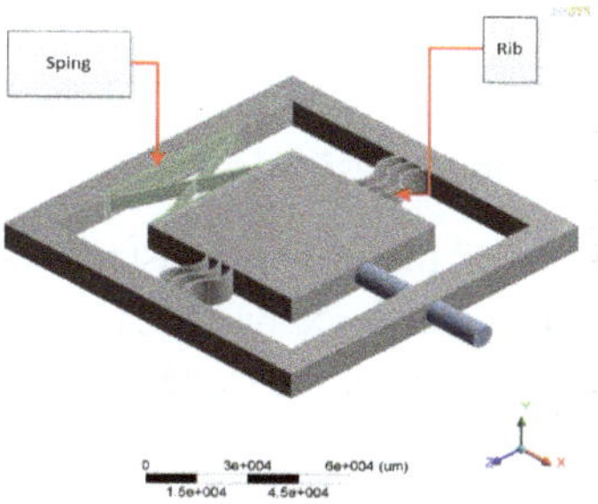

Fig. 1 This appearance of s nanopositioning stage.

3. Results and Discussion

3.1. *Displacement characteristics analysis*

Input displacement of nanopositioning stage is set 1000 μm in the horizontal direction, in order to observe the output displacement of the nanopositioning stage after each combination. This study analyzes the R1S1 to R4S3, a total of 12 combinations, the results shown in Table 2. The resulting simulation of the appearance shown in Figure 2. It can be found in Table 2, the best combination of the ribs and spring is R2S1.

3.2. *Spring constant platform analysis*

This study further analyzes of the spring constant R1S1 stage to follow the application. Applying a horizontal force on the stage inputs 1 N, with ANSYS analysis of the output displacement of the stage. Figure 3 can know its platform displacement of about 0.4 μm, the spring constant availability platform approximately 2.5×10^6 N / m.

Table 2 The output displacement of various combinations.

Combination Type	Output displacement (μm)
R1S1	1000.2
R2S1	1000
R3S1	1000.1
R4S1	1000.1
R1S2	1011.1
R2S2	1010.7
R3S2	1006.3
R4S2	1011.7
R1S3	1011.9
R2S3	1011.3
R3S3	1007.2
R4S3	1012.3

3.3. *Spring constant platform analysis*

This study further analyzes of the spring constant R1S1 stage to follow the application. Applying a horizontal force on the stage inputs 1 N, with ANSYS analysis of the output displacement of the stage. Figure 3 can know its platform displacement of about 0.4 μm, the spring constant availability platform approximately 2.5×10^6 N / m.

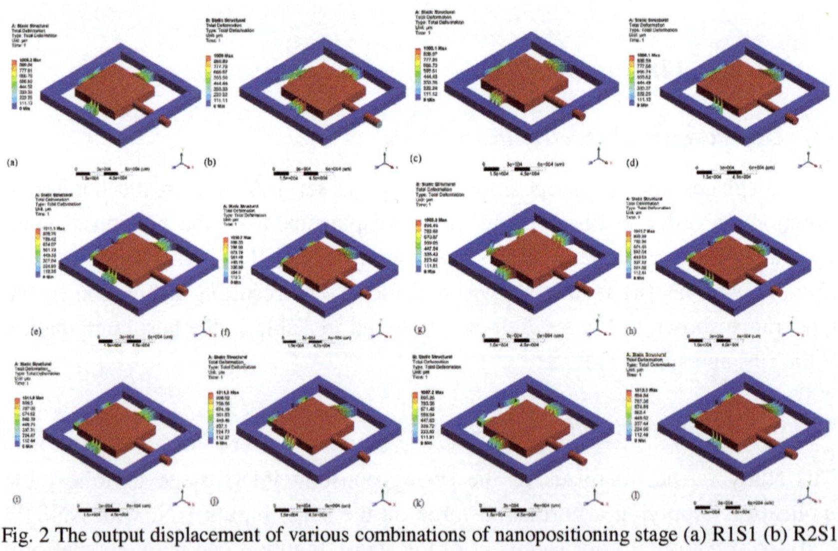

Fig. 2 The output displacement of various combinations of nanopositioning stage (a) R1S1 (b) R2S1 (c) R3S1 (d) R4S1 (e) R1S2 (f) R2S2 (g) R3S2 (h) R4S2 (i) R1S3 (j) R2S3 (k) R3S3 (l) R4S3.

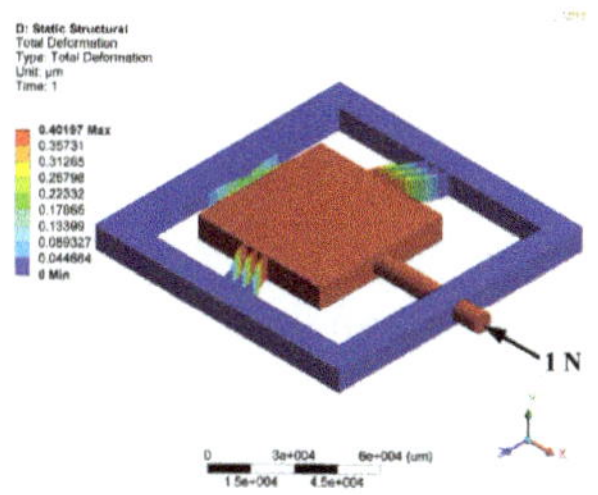

Fig. 3 The spring constant analysis of nanopositioning stage.

3.4. *Natural frequency analysis*

This article also made nanopositioning stage modal analysis and modal frequency value, in order to understand its dynamics characteristic.

Figure 4 is the first six modal of nanopositioning stage. From Figure 4, it can be found that the first order modal resonance frequency is 1078.2Hz; the second order modal resonance frequency is 1155.5Hz; the third order modal resonance frequency is 1296Hz; the 4th order modal resonance frequency is 1754.2Hz; the 5th order modal resonance frequency is 2225.7Hz; the 6th order modal resonance frequency is 2295.8Hz.

From this analysis that six groups of frequencies that can be found, in this study, designed to meet the needs nanopositioning stage use it.

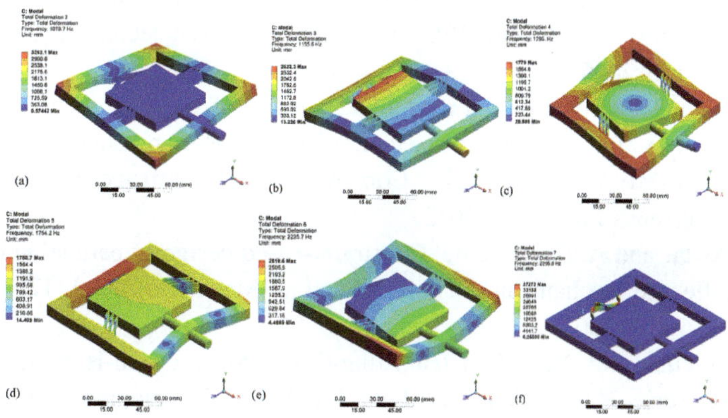

Fig. 4 The first six modal of nanopositioning stage.

4. Conclusion

In this study, three different shape of the spring with four different shapes of the rib to analyze various combinations of, seen from the analysis results, the nanopositioning stage when spring appearance as a cross-type (S1 type), the displacement of the shape of a wave-shaped rib (R1 type) portfolio the minimum amount of errors, and successfully analyze its spring constant and the resonant modal.

In this study, finite element analysis software analysis and design by ANSYS software, the good results were obtained and can available for follow-up production when the reference platform.

Acknowledgment

Work partially supported by grant 2-4570.5 of the Swiss National Science Foundation.

References

1. S. K. Kufer, E. M. Puchner, H. Gumpp, T. Liedl and H. E. Gaub, "Single-molecule cut-and-paste surface assembly", *Science*, Vol. 319, No. 5863, pp. 594-596, 2008.
2. H. Tang, Y. Li and X. Zhao, "Cell immobilization and contour detection for high-throughput robotic micro-injection", in *Int. Conf. on Fluid Power and Mechatronics*, August 17-20, 2011, Beijing, China, pp. 935-940.
3. Yangmin Li and Qingsong Xu, Design and Analysis of a New 3-DOF Compliant Parallel Positioning Platform for Nanomanipulation, Proceedings of 2005 5th IEEE Conference on Nanotechnology, Nagoya, Japan, July 2005.
4. Hui Tang and Yangmin Li, Optimal Design of the Lever Displacement Amplifiers for a Flexure-based Dual-mode Motion Stage, The 2012 IEEE/ASME International Conference on Advanced Intelligent Mechatronics July 11-14, 2012.
5. S. Awtar and A. H. Slocum, "Constraint-based design of parallel kinematic XY flexure mechanisms", Trans. ASME, J. Mech. Des., Vol. 129, No. 8, pp. 816-830, 2007.
6. Wen-Yuh Jywe, Yeau-Ren Jeng, Jing-Chung Shen, Chien-Hung Liu, Yun-Feng Teng, Yu-Te Jian and Hung-Shu Wang, Development of a novel multi-axis nano-positioning and the spiral tracking control, Journal of the Chinese Society of Mechanical Engineers, Vol. 30, No. 4, pp. 343~350 (2009)
7. L. L. Howell and A. Midha, "A method for the design of compliant mechanisms with small-length flexural pivots," *ASME J. Mech. Des.*, Vol. 116, No. 1, pp. 280–290, 1994.

8. B. H. Kang, J. T. Wen, N. G. Dagalakis and J. J. Gorman, "Analysis and design of parallel mechanisms with flexure joints," in *Proc. of IEEE Int. Conf. on Robotics and Automation*, 2004, pp. 4097–4102.
9. T. Tanikawa, T. Arai and N. Koyachi, "Development of small-sized 3 DOF finger module in micro hand for micro manipulation," in *Proc. of IEEE/RSJ Int. Conf. on Intelligent Robots and Systems*, 1999, pp. 876–881.

Research on Autonomous Cruise Garbage Collection System*

XU Yuting and LONG Ling[a]
College of Electrical & Information Engineering, Southwest University for Nationalities, Chengdu, 610041, China
[a]E-mail: long_ling_ll@163.com
www.swun.edu

This paper presents a new autonomous cruise garbage cleaning intelligent system, it is an independent garbage cleaning robot. The system has four functions: collecting garbage, waste identification, obstacle avoidance and autonomous cruise, it can help the cleaners clean up the garbage in public places. Compared with the traditional cleaning tools, it has the characteristics of intelligence, autonomy, efficiency etc., and well meets the cleaning needs.

Keywords: Garbage recognition; autonomous cruise; path optimization.

1. Introduction

City is the home of our lives, a city's sanitation has been the focus of attention. The sanitation of public places, such as squares, parks, railway stations, is the epitome of urban health, but also the priorities and challenges in urban health. We can often see fruit rind, paper, packaging bags in public places, plus the garbage in public places have mobility characteristics, which will irregularly appear in uncertain places. This has made a difficult problem for sanitation workers, They need to work constantly to keep clean. This paper proposes an intelligent trash cleaning system, which can share the heavy work of cleaning staff, so not only can reduce the demand for labor, reduce costs in public places, but also can greatly improve the efficiency of the cleaning work. It is a good solution for solving health problem in public places.

2. The Design Scheme of Garbage Cleaning System

In recent years, the smart home has got rapid development, Cobos and other companies introduced a smart vacuum cleaner for household cleaning, which

* This work is supported by the Fundamental Research Funds for the Central Universities of Southwest University for Nationalities (NO. 2014NZYQN10), College Students' innovation and entrepreneurship training plan of Southwest University for Nationalities (NO. S201410656018).

has brought a revolution of science and technology.[1] We put forward the concept of the garbage cleaning intelligent system by the design of intelligent vacuum cleaner, and made a lot of improvement and enhancement on this basis, because the smart vacuum cleaner has a small amount of garbage collection, which filled the vacancies of cleaning equipment in public places.

The proposed autonomous cruise garbage cleaning intelligent system mainly includes the following modules: intelligent obstacle avoidance module, refuse recognition module, navigation and route optimization module and human-computer interaction module. Hardware design scheme of the system is shown in Figure 1.

The system can be divided into garbage cleaning part and motion control section. The garbage recognition module uses ultrasonic wave to detect the presence or absence of garbage in the road ahead and transmit information to the microprocessor, then the microprocessor will control motor to finish cleaning the garbage; The obstacle avoidance module detects whether there is an obstacle around the robot in real time, meanwhile the navigation module controls the forward direction of the robot, after the microprocessor finish analyzing and processing these information.

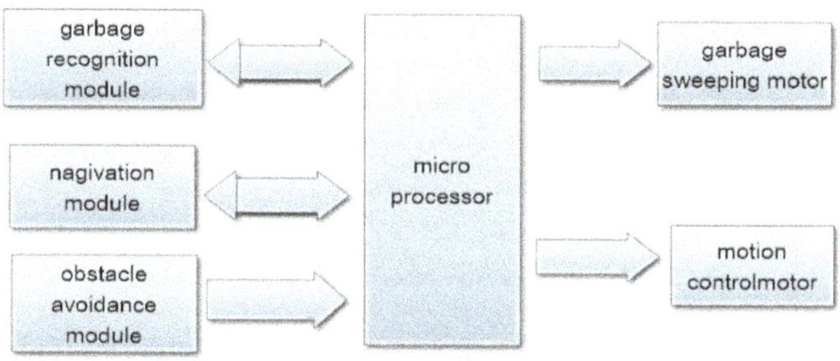

Fig. 1 Hardware scheme of the system.

2.1. *Intelligent obstacle avoidance*

Because public places have flower beds, stairs, pedestrians and other obstacles, which requires us to design an intelligent garbage cleaning system with intelligent functions of avoiding obstacles.[2] Our design uses a distance-sensitive sensor to realize this functionality. In fact, we are no stranger to the distance inductive sensor, it has been used a lot on our smart phones, when the user calls, the phone close to the head, the distance sensor can measure the distance.[3] We successfully applied this principle to the obstacle avoidance capabilities of the smart garbage cleaning system. We install the distance inductive sensors around the robot, when the distance is less than 20 cm between the robot and the obstacle, it will turn at an angle to bypass obstacles. In addition, we also added a human infrared sensor that can sense the faint far-infrared radiation, which can successfully avoid pedestrians.

2.2. *Recognition of garbage*

Garbage recognition is the emphasis and difficulty in the design, which not only can thoroughly clean the garbage, but also helps to optimize the path, so that the cleaning process has emphasis, and improves the work efficiency.[4]

This system eventually uses ultrasound to identify garbage.[5] as shown in figure 2, the ultrasonic module launch a ultrasonic wave about 45 degree angle with the ground, it will receive the reflection of the ultrasonic wave when the ground is not clean, we can achieve the identification of garbage through simple signal processing.

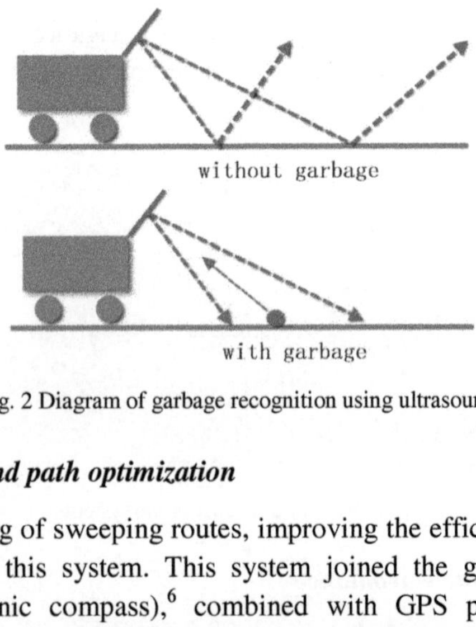

Fig. 2 Diagram of garbage recognition using ultrasound.

2.3. *Navigation and path optimization*

Reasonable planning of sweeping routes, improving the efficiency of cleaning is another feature of this system. This system joined the geomagnetic sensors (known as electronic compass),[6] combined with GPS positioning system.[7] Geomagnetic sensors have a much higher positioning accuracy, up to one meter, especially suitable for the occasions of parks, squares and stations which require high-precision positioning applications. Electronic compass will be able to identify the direction, recording the travel routes while moving, and forming a vector diagram of route in the adjacent matrix. At the same time, we divide the area which need to clean into a small grid, so as to optimize the cleaning path by artificial intelligence algorithms, which greatly improves the efficiency of the cleaning work.[8]

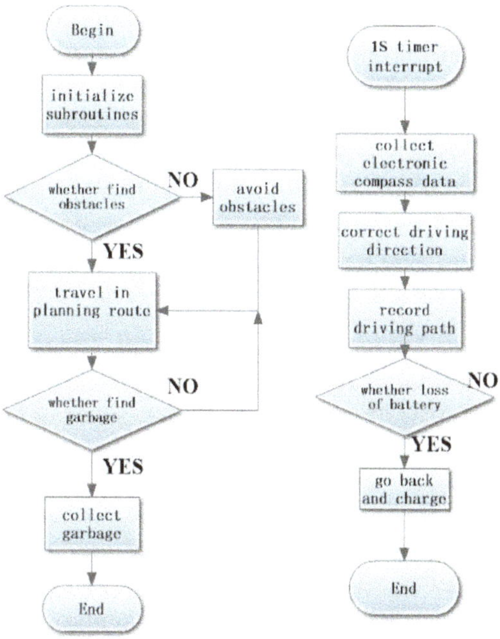

Fig. 3 Flow chat of the program.

3. Software Design of the Garbage Cleaning System

In order to realize the functions of this system, we have adopted a standardized, modular programming methods.[9] The software system is divided into five modules: obstacle avoidance module, garbage recognition module, navigation module, power detection module, motion control and cleaning control module. As shown in figure 3,when the system starts, MCU firstly initialize each subroutine, and then start the timer once per second to test each module, taking appropriate measures to solve problems according to the different test results.[10]

As an important part of modern intelligent trash cleaning system, system's compatibility and portability has become an important symbol of modern intelligent system. Intelligent garbage cleaning system, presented in this paper uses modular designing method, greatly reduces the complexity of the program, making the program designing, debugging and maintaining easy to operate, what's more, and provides great convenience for future system upgrades.

4. Conclusions

In this paper, the autonomous cruise garbage cleaning intelligent system has the function of garbage recognition, garbage collection, intelligent obstacle avoidance, autonomous cruise and path optimization. Which liberate the cleaning staff from the heavy work, at the same time greatly improving the work efficiency and reducing the cost of maintaining the public places clean. At present, the development of intelligent cleaning equipment in China is still in its infancy, but what is certain is that in the next several years, our country will be more attention to the development of intelligent cleaning equipment, this paper puts forward the intelligent garbage cleaning system which will be applied to the public places is an inevitable trend. It is believable that in the future various robots with artificial intelligence will appear and better serve the People's Daily life.

References

1. AI Yanting, YANG Mingsui, etc., *Software Design of the Robot Cleaner Controlling System*, in *Measurement & Control Technology*, Vol. 26 (2007), pp. 73–75.
2. Du Longyin, *Study on Obstacle Avoidance of Intelligent Vacuum Cleaner Based on Chaos Genetic*, in *Computer Measurement & Control*, Vol. 21 (2013), pp. 762–765.
3. JING Huashuiyue, *MTK Mobile Phone Calibration Distance Sensor,* in *Computer enthusiasts*, Vol. 10 (2007), pp. 75.
4. CHENG Yongmei, PAN Quan, etc., Computer *Intelligent Image Recognition Algorithm,* in *Journal of Computer Applications*, Vol. 24 (2004), pp. 65–68.
5. LI Qiang, YANG Keli, *The Means of Plotting DAC Curve Quickly and Exactly in Digital Ultrasonic Flaw Detection*, in *Group Technology & Production Modernization*, Vol. 31 (2014), pp. 56–58.
6. ZHOU Jun, GE Zhilei, etc., Key *Technique and Development for Geomagnetic Navigation*, in *Journal of Astronautics*, Vol. 29 (2008), pp. 1467–1472.
7. LIU Shaojie, *Speed Distance Induction Type GPS Car Alarm*, in *Technological innovation and application*, Vol. 7 (2014), pp. 50.
8. SUN Lingyu, LENG Ming, etc., Research *on Path Planning of Mobile Robot*, in *Journal of Jingangshan University,* Vol. 31 (2010), pp. 56–59.
9. DENG Dexiang, *Structured Control Flow Graph (fig. N-S) Improvement and Idea of Modular Programming Flowchart*, in *Journal of Computer Research and Development,* Vol. 32 (1995), pp. 21–26.
10. MA Zhenghua, LI Min, etc., *Full Coverage Traversed Path Planning and Simulation of Intelligence Cleaning Robot*, in *Measurement & Control Technology*, Vol. 31 (2012), pp. 99–102.

Drag Coefficients of Orchard Sprinkler Boat

Chatchai Marnadee
Department of Mechanical Engineering, Faculty of Engineering, Thammasat University, Khlongluang, Pathumtani 12120, Thailand
mchat@engr.tu.ac.th

Small boats have, for many years, been used for showering the canopies of orchards in The Central Plains of The Kingdom of Thailand. Little is known, however, about the exact workings of their mechanisms. This study discusses some of the physical processes that govern the functions of the boat. During the showering operation, the boat moves forward by a reactive force associated with the ejection of the water showered from two nozzles. A one-fifth scale model was used to study the mechanisms of the small boat. The apparent drag coefficient of the model, determined by measuring the total drag, was found to be inversely proportional to the Froude number and effectively applicable for predicting the drag on a planned prototype.

Keywords: Boat; showering; nozzle; thrust; model test; drag; drag coefficient.

1. Introduction

1.1. *Background*

The Kingdom of Thailand has developed its irrigation network and fluvial system by excavating numerous canals in The Central Plains for more than 120 years. The canals fed by the Chaophraya River are used to irrigate paddy fields [1]. In recent years, most of the paddy fields have been converted to orchard farming areas, which continue to increase annually, because of seawater damage sustained by littoral orchards. Consequently, farmers needing to move their orchards to The Central Plains have found orchard farming more profitable than rice culture. A general view of such orchard farming is shown in Fig. 1. The level of underground water in this area is high; consequently, farmers need to convert their flat paddy fields into high banks on which to plant trees, by excavating numerous small parallel channels where underground and irrigation water collects. The average height and width of the banks is 1.2 m and 3.8 m, respectively, at intervals of 7.0 m to one another. The water in the channels is stagnant, without currents and approximately 0.4 m deep. A typical orchard has

16 to 20 banks, each 400 to 800 m long, where citrus, guava, papaya trees, oil palms, and such are planted.

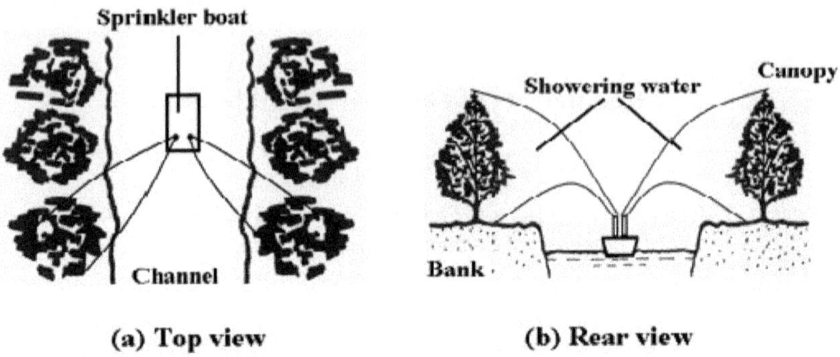

Fig. 1 An orchard on the banks and a sprinkler boat on the irrigation channel.

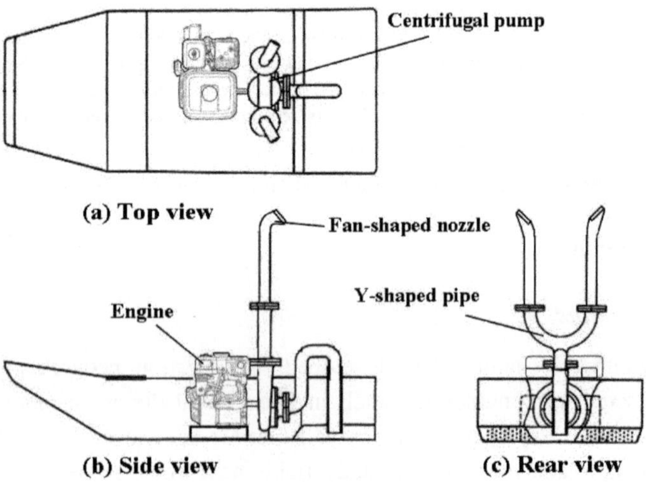

Fig. 2 Schema of typical sprinkler boat.

Despite the presence of water in the channels adjacent to these banks, farmers have to shower water on the tree canopies because of the shallow tree roots and the high diurnal temperatures. Generally, the farmers use a small boat (Fig. 2) to shower the tree canopies, usually twice a day, at approximately 12×10^{-3} m^3/s. Agricultural substances generally used for the trees result in chemical residues in the channels.

The small boat, hereby referred to as "sprinkler boat", is equipped with showering and thrusting devices consisting of a centrifugal pump, and two fan-shaped flat nozzles mounted on a Y-shaped discharging pipe with an angle to the horizon and to the centerline of the boat. The height of flat nozzles from pump outlet is 600 mm. The sprinkler boat, usually made of welded stainless steel plates, is approximately 1.8 m long and 0.8 m wide. While sprinkling water, the farmer on board steers the boat which is propelled forward by the thrust exerted by the water jet from the flat nozzles through which the water is directed to the tree canopies. The boat was driven by only the reaction force of the flat nozzles. The pump, connected directly to a 3.0 to 5.0 kW-gasoline engine, draws water through a strainer installed at the bottom of the boat. For large-scale orchard farming, the sprinkling may take more than two hours [2].

1.2. *Objectives*

The objectives of this study are to investigate fluid resistance to the forward motion of the boat and to clarify the propulsive force associated with the water jet from the nozzles during the sprinkling. In conventional sprinkler boat, the flat nozzles are used not only for driving the boat but also for showering. Therefore maximization of its showering efficiency is required. One countermeasure is to compose another independent propulsive system. The results will further our prospective studies for the development of a novel unmanned driving and steering system of the boat by employing a jet deflection fluidics, a fluid element without moving parts, installed at the bottom of the boat. Our final goals are the saving of human labor and, in particular, the protection of the farmer from exposure to agricultural chemical residues contained in the channels during the showering operation.

2. Theoretical Considerations

2.1. *Fluid resistance*

A boat is a body moving in two different fluids: water (the submerged portion below the waterline) and air (the portion above the waterline). Consequently, while moving forward, the boat experiences drag from both fluids. In this study, the aerial drag is disregarded, and the boat is considered a semi-submerged body in the moving fluid; consequently, the drag on the boat is calculated by the following equation:

$$D = C_D \cdot \frac{1}{2} \rho v^2 S \tag{1}$$

where D is the total drag; ρ the density of water; v the mean velocity of the boat relative to the water; and S the total area below the waterline of the stationary boat. C_D, a dimensionless constant of proportionality called "apparent drag coefficient", is measured for a given set of geometric and hydraulic conditions. Generally, the drag on the boat consists mainly of frictional drag and wave-making drag from the water, which make up the main proportion of total drag that is calculated by the product of dynamic pressure and the area below the waterline of the boat [3]. Nonetheless, the total drag on the boat comprises complicated drags and is related to the total submerged area of the boat [4]. In evaluating the resistance on the boat, generally the total submerged area of the boat, more than the projected submerged area, is used as one of parameters [5, 6]. The application of typical values for the steady motion of a submerged body in infinitely large volumes of fluid, as stated in most textbooks on fluid mechanics [7], may not be quantitatively valid in this case for several reasons: a free surface interacting with both the flow and the boat, the influence from Karman's vortex and the roughness of the boat skin. Moreover, the configuration of the boat investigated here is unique in that the aspect ratio (length-to-width ratio) is kept small to facilitate turning at the end of each bank, thus necessitating the determination of the apparent drag coefficient experimentally. From Eq. 1, when drag D is measured directly, the apparent drag coefficient of the boat is calculated by the following equation:

$$C_D = \frac{2D}{\rho v^2 S} \tag{2}$$

3. Experimental Methods

3.1. *Model test and apparent drag coefficient*

While the boat is being propelled forward in the channel, the drag on the boat is not readily measurable directly. A one-fifth scale model of the boat was therefore constructed for the investigation, with the use of a circulating water channel (Fig. 3) 5 m long with the working section 300 mm wide and 450 mm deep. The mean velocity of the flow was varied and measured by a hot-wire-type flow velocity meter installed 10 mm (the mean submerged depth of the model) below the surface of the water.

The specifications of the model compared with those of the prototype of the sprinkler boat are shown in Table 1. The submerged area and meta-centric height of the model were obtained by geometric similitude and the mass with operator by dynamic similitude. The model was mounted on a rectangular-beam-type transducer made of an S45C steel bar 250 mm long with a cross section of 3 mm × 11 mm and submerged to a depth of 20 mm below the surface of the water. The clearance from each side of the model to each side wall of water channel is 70 mm and the depth of water in the channel was 200 mm. The velocity of water flow was varied from 0.00 m/s to 0.30 m/s and slow enough that there is no effects from the side wall. One bridge of four strain gauges (2 each 100 mm apart) was attached to the steel bar. The transducer detected the drag exerted on the model and the signal was amplified by a dynamic strain amplifier (DPM-711B; Kyowa Co., Ltd.).

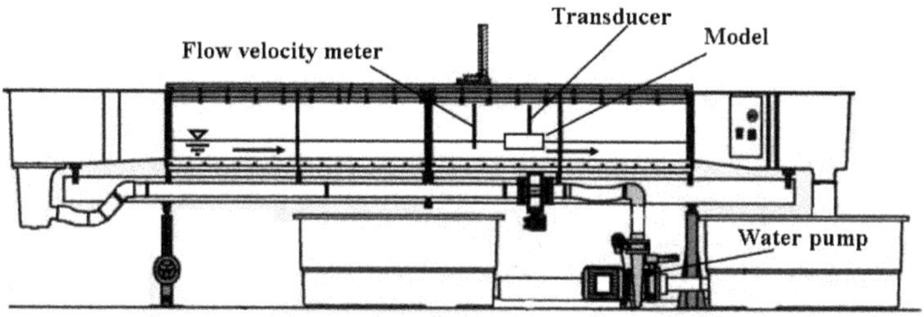

(a) General view of testing apparatus in a water channel

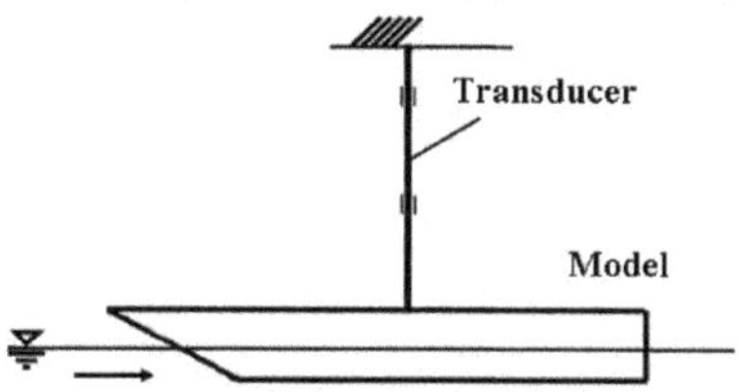

(b) A model mounted onto transducer

Fig. 3 Model test for fluid resistance.

Table 1 Specifications of prototype and model of sprinkler boat.

	Prototype	*Model*
Length l (m)	1.80	0.36
Width b (m)	0.80	0.16
Aspect ratio (l/b)	2.25	2.25
Submerged area S (m^2)	1.96	0.0784
Mass with operator m (kg)	140	1.12
Meta-centric height (m)	0.55	0.11

4. Results and Discussions

4.1. *Total drag on the model*

The relation between the Froude number and the total drag is shown in Fig. 4. To simplify comparison between the model and the prototype, the flow velocity is replaced by the Froude number. The drag on the model boat was 0.4 N at Fr = 0.15, corresponding to 50 N t 0.6 m/s, a typical operating speed of the prototype.

Nonetheless, from the equation of regression on total drag to the Froude number, the total drag contained a linear component which was attributed to the intense vortex in the wake of the model.

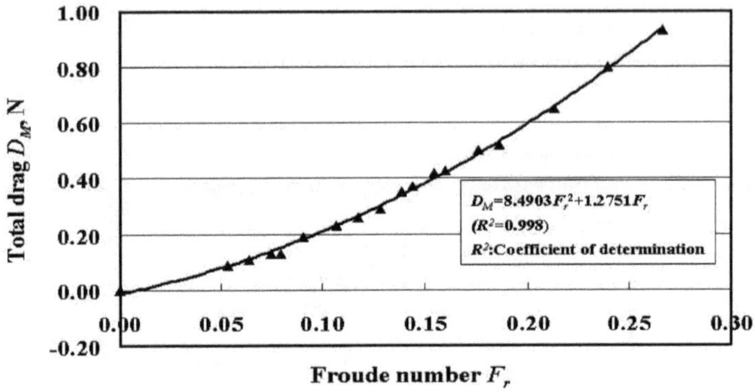

Fig. 4 Relation between drag and Froude number.

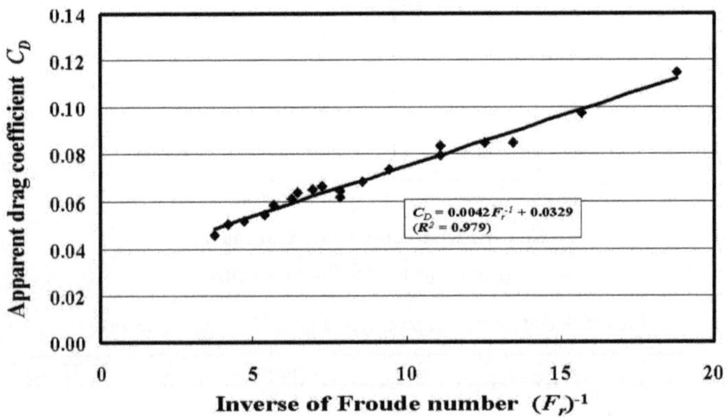

Fig. 5 Relation between apparent drag coefficient and the inverse of the Froude number.

4.2. *Apparent drag coefficient*

The regression line in Fig. 5 shows the relation between the apparent drag coefficient of the boat and the inverse of the Froude number. It increases gently from 0.045 to 0.115 while the inverse of the Froude number increases from around 4 to 18. The linear line was calculated from the result shown in Fig. 4 using Eq. 2. Thus, the apparent drag coefficient is closely related to the inverse of the Froude number.

5. Conclusions

The characteristics of the sprinkler boat, namely, the drag and the apparent drag coefficient were studied with the use of a model. The propulsive parameters, such as the thrust obtained from the flat nozzles and the traveling speed of the boat were determined by the use of a prototype. The results of the investigations led to the following conclusions.

The test of fluid resistance on the model boat showed that the fluid resistance to the total submerged area of the boat played a crucial role in the forward motion of the boat. Fluid resistance increases approximately 150% for every 0.20 m/s increase in boat speed. Fluid resistance to the prototype was predictable from the results of the model. With the velocity of the water jet of the prototype around 8.0 m/s, the mean traveling speed of the boat was 0.6 m/s and the fluid resistance approximately 40 N.

The apparent drag coefficient of the model clearly increased with increments in the inverse of the Froude number, leading to the speculation that the length of the boat has an affect on the decrease in the apparent drag coefficient. Moreover, the apparent drag coefficient obtained from the model test was applicable for predicting the drag on the prototype.

References

1. Asawai, S., History of Rangsit Canal (in Thai language). Thammasat University Press, Bangkok, Thailand, 1987, pp. 25-26.
2. Marnadee, C., Horio, H., Study on Fluidics as a Driving and Steering Control Unit of Orchard Sprinkler Boat. Proceedings of International Symposium on Automation and Mechatronics of Agricultural and Bioproduction Systems (ISMAB), Chiayi, Taiwan, (2002) 486-492.
3. Kunikiyo, Y., Kimoto, T., Nagao, T., Fluid Dynamics (in Japanese). Morikita Press, Tokyo, 2006, pp. 174-175.
4. Yamagata, M., (Nippon Kaiji Kyokai) The Collections of Papers of Dr. Masao YAMAGATA Part 2 (in Japanese), Toppan Press, Tokyo, 1984, p. 217.
5. Hayashita, S., Ikeda, Y., Katayama, T., Suzuki, K., An Experimental Method to Evaluate Resistance and Attitudes of Planning Craft Using Very Small Models (in Japanese), Journal of the Society of Naval Architects of Japan, 191 (2002) 1-7.
6. Kodama, S., Skin Friction Reduction of Ships by Microbubbles (in Japanese), Nagare, 20 (2001) 278-284.
7. Yunus A. C. and John M. C., Fluid Mechanics: Fundamental and Applications, McGraw-Hill Press, New York, 2006, pp. 565-568.

Comparative Study and Optimizaion of Traffic and Granular Merging Flow*

Mao-Bin Hu†, Wang-Ping Sun, Qi-Yi Liu, Rui Jiang and Qing-Song Wu
School of Engineering Science, University of Science and Technology of China
Hefei, Anhui 230026, P.R. China
†*Email: humaobin@ustc.edu.cn*

This paper compares the experiment and simulation results of vehicular traffic merging flow and granular merging flow. The flow rate behavior and the phase diagram of the two systems are reported and compared. Although the two systems show different flow rate behavior and phase transition phenomenon, they can be optmized with similar methods.

Keywords: Granular and traffic flow; merging flow; optimization.

1. Introduction

Traffic and granular flows are ubiquitous in natural and daily environments. The study of traffic and granular flows has attracted much attention [1-7]. Traffic flow system is composed of many self-driven cars which are not allowed to collide. Granular flow system is composed of many Newtonian particles colliding with each other. Although they are different in their driven modes and technical applications, they often show similar phenomena.

The scenario of merging flow are very important for the two system. In the traffic flow system, three distinct dynamic phases are observed on highways: the free traffic flow, the traffic jam, and the synchronized traffic flow. Recent experiments show that, synchronized traffic is often observed localized near bottlenecks like the on-ramps [7, 8]. Similarly, in a granular flow system, the merging of particles can trigger different flowing patterns in the upward channels, such as dilute flow and dense flow [9].

In this paper, we compare the results of traffic and granular merging flow. The two system's flow rate behavior is compared, together with their phase

* This work is funded by National Basic Research Program of China under Grant No. 2012CB725404, the Natural Science Foundation of China (NNSFC) under Key Project No. 11034010, and Project Nos.71171185, 71371175.

† Corresponding Author.

diagrams. The results show that the two systems behave quite differently, but they can be optimized by similar methods. Based on the findings of our experiments and simulations. We propose some optimization remarks for the two systems.

2. Experiment Setup and Simulation Model

We show simulation result for traffic merging flow, together with experimental results for granular merging flow. We emphasize that the results of traffic and granular merging flows presented here are different from our previous work (see Ref. [8-9]) in that we study a wider side channel.

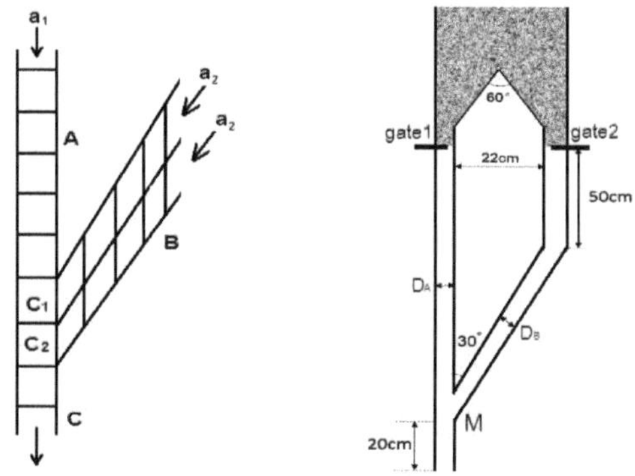

Fig. 1 Illustration of the modeled traffic merging system (a) and the experiment granular merging system (b).

2.1. *Simulation of traffic merging flow*

We adopt the Nagel-Schreckenberg (NaSch) cellular automata (CA) model to simulate the merging system, as shown in Fig. 1a. The merging system is composed of road A, road B and road C. Road B has two lanes. In each road, the dynamics obeys NaSch rules. Define Vi and Di as the velocity of car i and the number of empty cells in front of car i, respectively. In the NaSch model, the update rules are: (i) Acceleration: Vi→min (Vmax, Vi+1); (ii) Braking: Vi→min (Di; Vi); (iii) Randomization: Vi→max (0; Vi-1) with probability p; (iv) Moving: car i moves Vi cells. Here the maximum velocity is Vmax=1, and the slowdown parameter is p=0. The insering rates for road A and B are a_1 and a_2. The conflicts at cells C_1 and C_2 are handled by the rule similar to reference [4] but road A is privileged over road B. The control variables are a_1 and a_2.

2.2. *Experiment of granular merging flow*

The granular channels A and B merge at M, as shown in Fig. 1b. Channel A has a width of 20cm, while channel B has a width of 50cm. The channels are mounted on a plate with 30° to the horizion. We use steel beads of diameter 2.5mm as granular particles. The channel is designed to ensure one layer flow of particles in the system. Beneath the final exit, the flow rate is measured by an electronic balance with the sensitivity of 0.1g and the weighing frequency of 5Hz. The inflows from both channels are controlled by a gate with opening width of D_1 and D_2. Thus the controlling/adjustable variables in this system are D_1 and D_2, which plays a similar role as a_1 and a_2 in the traffic system.

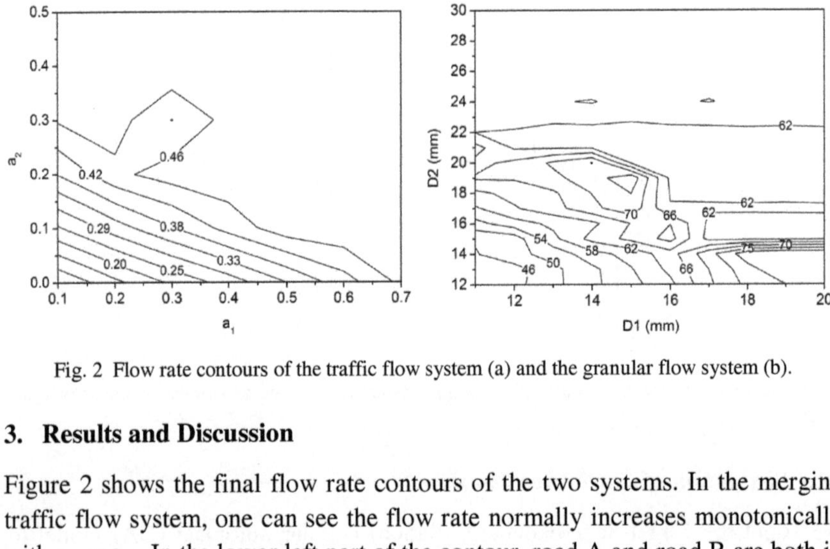

Fig. 2 Flow rate contours of the traffic flow system (a) and the granular flow system (b).

3. Results and Discussion

Figure 2 shows the final flow rate contours of the two systems. In the merging traffic flow system, one can see the flow rate normally increases monotonically with a_1 or a_2. In the lower left part of the contour, road A and road B are both in low density free flow state. This flowing state can be denoted as low density-low density state (or LL state). In the upper right part, road A is in low denstiy free flow, while road B is in high density congestion. This flowing state can be denoted as low density-high density state (or LH state).

Fig. 3 shows a typical flow rate behavior of Ja, Jb, Jc against a_1 with a fixed $a_2=0.2$. One can see that road A is always in free flow state, and Ja increases monotonically with a_1. When $a_1>0.2$, road B enters congestion, and Jb decreases correspondingly. Of course we have Jc=Ja+Jb. The maximal flow rate is 0.5. The theoretical prediction of maximal flow rate of NaSch model is:

$$J_{max} = \frac{V_{max}}{V_{max}+1}. \tag{1}$$

Considering Vmax=1, one can see that the simulation and theoretical prediction are in agreement.

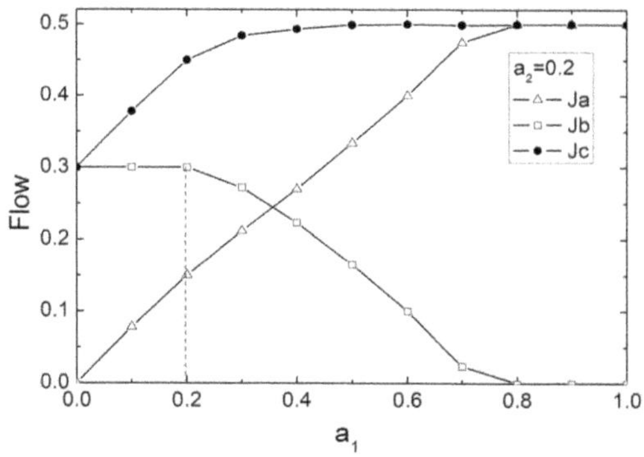

Fig. 3 Flow rates of road A, B and C vs a_1 for the traffic flow system (a_2 is fixed to 0.2).

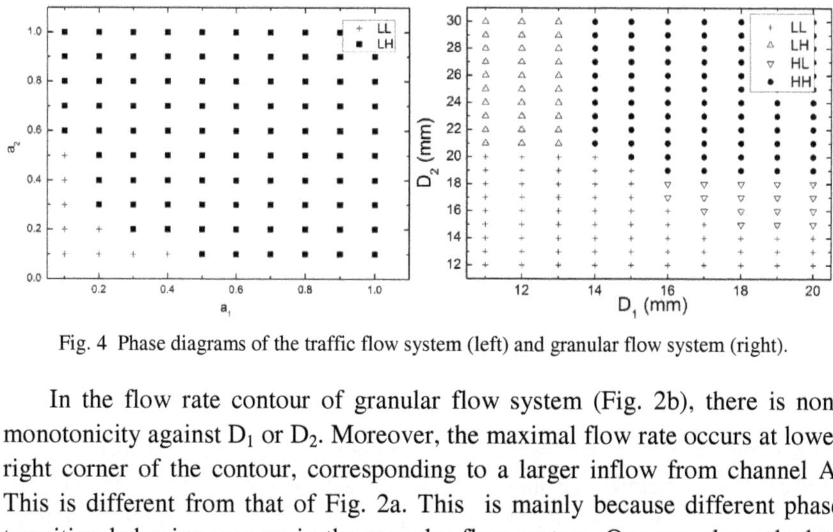

Fig. 4 Phase diagrams of the traffic flow system (left) and granular flow system (right).

In the flow rate contour of granular flow system (Fig. 2b), there is non-monotonicity against D_1 or D_2. Moreover, the maximal flow rate occurs at lower right corner of the contour, corresponding to a larger inflow from channel A. This is different from that of Fig. 2a. This is mainly because different phase transition behavior appears in the granular flow system. One can also calculate the flow rate by:

$$J = \rho VD = (\frac{\phi m_0}{S_0})VD \, , \qquad (2)$$

where V is the mean velocity of particles, D is the channel width, m_0=0.06g and S_0=4.9x$10^{-6}$$m^2$ is the mass and area of one particle, ρ is granular density, Φ is solid fraction. We find that the calculation results are in agreement with the experiment.

Figure 4 shows the phase diagram of the two systems. One can see that the traffic flow system shows two states of LL state and LH state. However, the granular flow system shows four states of LL, LH, HL and HH states. Compared with the flow rate contour of Fig. 2b, one can see that the boundaries of the states cannot be simply determined by the flow rate. The flow state should be determined by the local density in the channels. If the solid fraction is above 0.65 in the channel, the channel is in high density flow (or dense flow). If the solid fraction is below 0.65 in the channel, the channel is in low density flow (or dilute flow). The critical solid fraction of 0.65 agrees with literature [1, 9].

Figure 5 shows the illustration of the LH and HL state of the granular flow system. One can see that in both cases, the flow is blocked at the merging point. Therefore, the flow rate can not increase in both cases. This explains why the maximal flow rate occurs at the lower right corner of Fig. 2b, corresponding to the LL state and with a larger inflow from channel A.

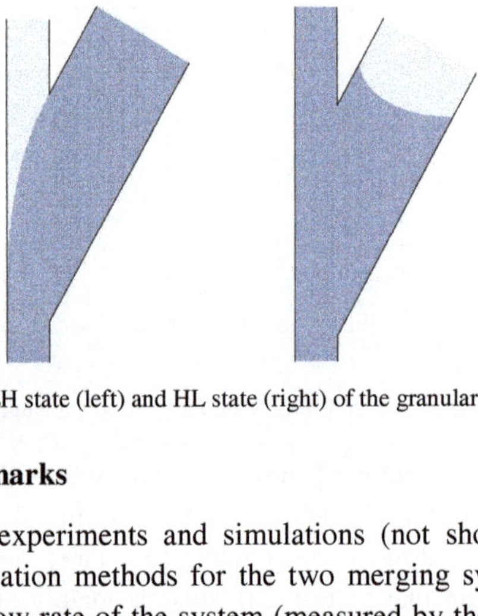

Fig. 5 Illustration of the LH state (left) and HL state (right) of the granular merging flow system.

4. Optimization Remarks

With comprehensive experiments and simulations (not shown here), we put forward some optimization methods for the two merging systems. In order to enhance the overall flow rate of the system (measured by the flow rate of Jc in traffic system, or the final exit flow rate in granular system), one should consider the following issues.

- The main road/channel should be privileged in the control. For traffic system, the main road should be given privilege when conflicts happen. For granular system, the main channel gate should be open first.
- It is important to keep a low density flow in the main road/channel. If the main road/channel is congested, the system's performance will greatly decrease.
- The flow rate can be further enhanced if the outlet size can be enlarged, regardless the inflow rate from the two channels.

5. Conclusion

In summary, we have studied and compared the behavior of traffic and granular merging flow. The flow rate behavior and the phase diagram of the two systems are reported. Base on the data, we propose some optimization issue for the two systems. Although the two systems can show quite different phases and phase transition behaviors, they can be optimized with similar methods.

The outcome of this work can be useful for the control and management of related systems, such as pedestrain flow, debris flow and land slides.

References

1. M. Hou, W. Chen, T. Zhang, K. Lu, and C. K. Chan, Global Nature of Dilute-to-Dense Transition of Granular Flows in a 2D Channel, *Phys. Rev. Lett.* **91**, 204301 (2003).
2. M. Hou, H. Tu, R. Liu, Y. Li, K. Lu, P.-Y. Lai and C. K. Chan, Temperature Oscillations in a Compartmentalized Bidisperse Granular Gas, *Phys. Rev. Lett.* **100**, 068001 (2008).
3. Y. Li, R. Liu and M. Hou, Gluing Bifurcation and Noise-Induced Hopping in the Oscillatory Phenomena of Compartmentalized Bidisperse Granular Gases, *Phys. Rev. Lett.* **109**, 198001 (2012).
4. R. Jiang, M. B. Hu, H. M. Zhang, Z. Y. Gao, B. Jia, Q. S. Wu, B. Wang and M. Yang, Traffic experiment reveals the nature of car-following, *PLoS ONE* **9(4)**, e94351 (2014).
5. M. B. Hu, Q. Y. Liu, W. P. Sun, R. Jiang, Q. S. Wu, Packing induced bistable phenomenon in granular flow: analyzed from a complex network perspective, *Applied Mathematics and Mechanics (English Edition)* **35**, 1565 (2014).
6. G. Hu, Y. Li, M. Hou and K. To, Traveling shock front in quasi-two-dimensional granular flows, *Phys. Rev. E* **81**, 011305 (2010).
7. R. Jiang, M. B. Hu, B. Jia and Z. Y. Gao, New mechanism for metastability of under-saturated traffic responsible for time-delayed traffic breakdown at the signal, *Comp. Phys. Comm.* **185**, 1439-1442 (2014).
8. R. Jiang, Q. S. Wu and B. H. Wang, Cellular automata model simulating traffic interactions between on-ramp and main road, *Phys. Rev. E* **66**, 036104 (2002).
9. M. B. Hu, Q. Y. Liu, R. Jiang, M. Hou and Q. S. Wu, Phase transition and flow-rate behavior of merging granular flows, *Phys. Rev. E* **91**, 022206 (2015).

Vibration Testing and Structural Optimization of EDM Spindle Head by Using Modal Test Combined with ODS*

Min Da WANG[a], Min WANG[b] and Huan Huan NIU[c]
Advanced Manufacturing technology of the Key Laboratory of Beijing Municipality, College of Mechanical Engineering and Applied Electronics Technology, Beijing University of Technology, Beijing, 100124, China
[a]wmd2007@163.com, [b]wangm@bjut.edu.cn, [c]1551646204@qq.com

Jian Yong LIU
Beijing Institute of EDM, Beijing, 100191, China
251643806@qq.com

Er Yang PEI
Machinery Industry Federation, Beijing, 100823,China
edept@mei.net.cn

ODS (Operating Deflection Shapes) and modal testing are used to analyze vibration frequency and working deformation of EDM machine tool spindle head for finding the weak part of the structure and the target modal through test results in actual conditions. A more accurate finite element model of the spindle head is obtained by modifying the original model based on the comparison between analysis result of the original model and the result of the real modal test. The target modal frequency of spindle head is increased by 30.93% by using optimization method, which utilizes the ISIGHT optimization software to integrate SolidWorks and ANSYS to optimize the dynamics of the weak part. The test and optimization method presented in this paper can be used to provide a convenient and effective way to improve the structural dynamics of the machine.

Keywords: ODS; modal parameters; ISIGHT; optimization.

1. Introduction

EDM is a special forming techniques, by removal of the spark discharge machining a workpiece. A lot of research had been done in the micro-EDM, but also achieved fruitful results [1-4].

* Innovation Project Ⅱ-3: Research on the integration of large depth-diameter ratio micro-hole ultra-precision EDM equipment of Aero-engine (project number: PXM2014_178102_000006), Natural Science Foundation of Beijing, Grant No. 3122005, KZ201410005010 and Important National Science & Technology Specific Projects of China, Grant No. 2012ZX04010021-001-004.

Experimental modal analysis is widely used in various engineering fields. Schwarz BJ [5] and Mchargue PL [6] researched the relationship and differences between ODS and modal shape through the traditional testing methods and ODS testing methods. The results of Cheng Heng [7] indicated, ODS can not only show the relative deformation of structural vibration, and can visually identify the failure location. Wu Feng [8] recognized the inherent characteristics of the rack in forced vibration response spectrum by ODS analysis.

To get the maximum deformation corresponding operating frequency and the weak parts of structure by EDM spindle head ODS and modal testing in B&K instrument, a more accurate finite element model of the spindle head is obtained by modifying the original model based on the comparison between analysis result of the original model and the result of the real modal test. The used of ISIGHT optimize finite element model by integrating SolidWorks and ANSYS. This method can improve the EDM vibration frequency and machining precision of workpiece.

2. The Principle and Testing of ODS

ODS (Operating Deflection Shapes) means running deformation modes, also often referred to as the deformation of work. For frequency-domain of ODS, the structure of the displacement at any point i ODS $X_i\left(jw_0\right)$ available excitation force and structure of the system frequency response function is expressed as [9]:

$$\left\{X_i\left(jw_0\right)\right\} = \sum_{k=1}^{n}\left\{H_{ik}\left(jw_0\right)\right\}F_k\left(w_0\right) \tag{1}$$

Where: i—The number of measuring point. $F_k\left(w_0\right)$—Linear spectrum of k DOF excitation force. n—The total number of exciting force.

From the above equation, ODS reflects both the effect on the structure of the incentive properties, but also reflects the dynamic characteristics of the structure itself. For a certain type of EDM in the actual process, the spindle motor speed is 100r/min, the discharge gap is 0.3mm, the electrode is copper, the material of the workpiece is $45^{\#}$ steel, continuous regular "carrying tool action" frequency of 1Hz. Adding electrode as the reference point, the measuring point distribution use of effective independent method [10] to optimize the measuring point, the sensor is arranged on the key components, B&K and 4507 accelerometer was used to test ODS in actual test shown in Figure 1 and a-point distribution shown in B&K in Figure 2. The work status of ODS test got frequency deformation curve of spindle head, and then analyzed large deformation frequency of 149Hz corresponding work deformation in Figure 3.

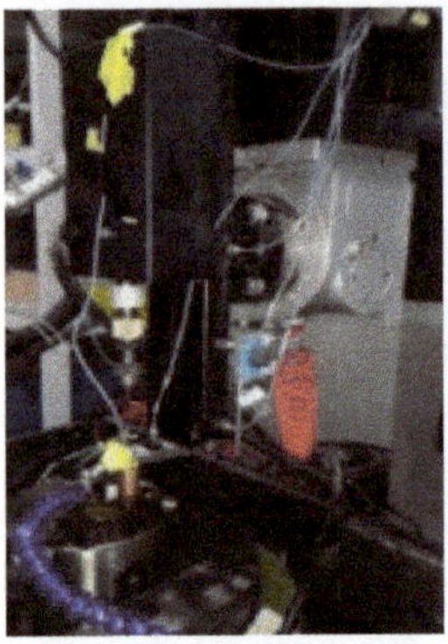

Fig. 1 The actual measuring point of ODS.

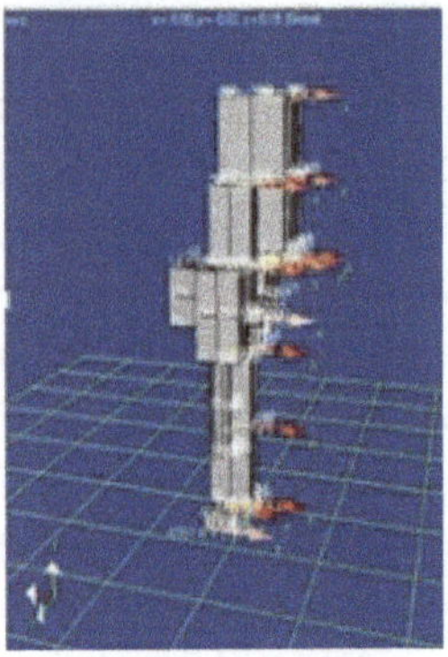

Fig. 2 Measuring point distribution of ODS.

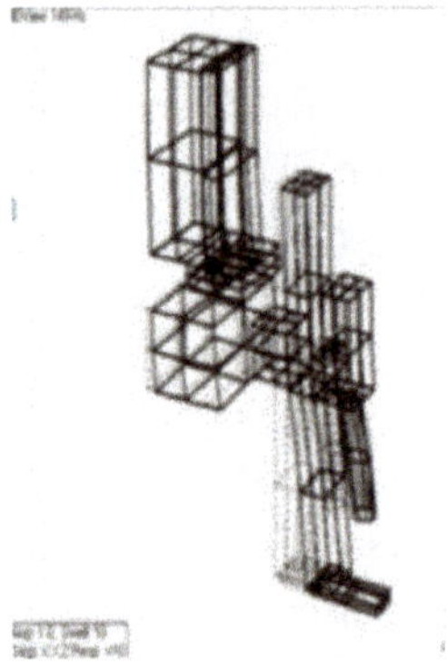

Fig. 3 Work deformation of 149Hz.

Table 1 Modes of the first three.

Experimental modal	Finite element modal	Modal description
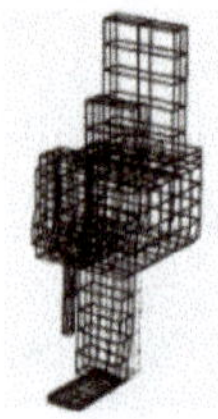	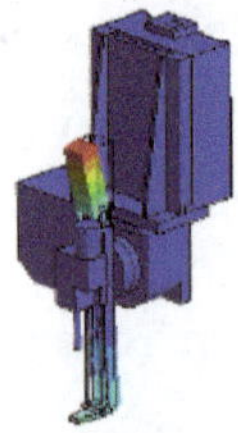	Linear module electrode side and the motor side reverse oscillating in the Y-direction
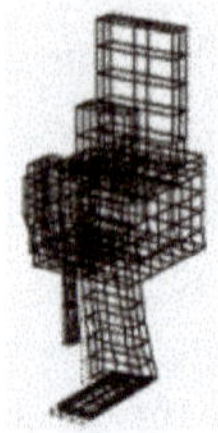	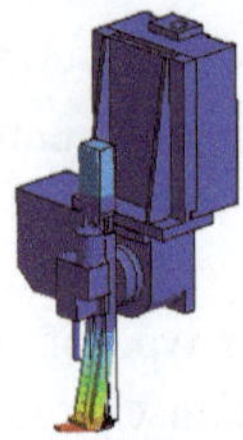	Linear module with the electrode side and the motor side in the Y direction to swing
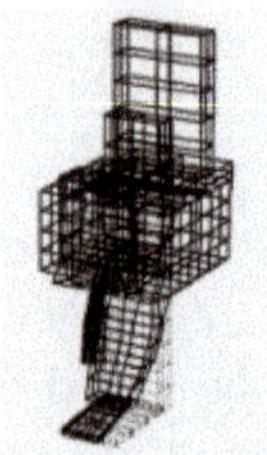	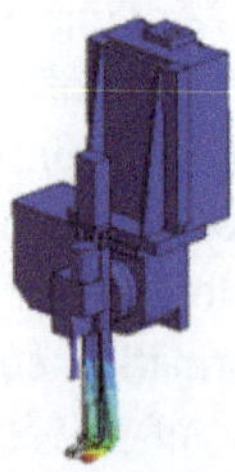	Bending and around the Z-axis linear module electrode side in the X direction of the torsion

3. Contrast Modal Experiments and FEM

Experimental modal parameter is identified process called experimental modal analysis method. Single-point vibration knowledge and multi-point excitation was used in the modal test.

A simplified three-dimensional model of EDM spindle head structure of modal was analyzed in ANSYS Workbench, The experimental results and the theoretical error of the finite element analysis results were 15% or less, for the first three tests of finite element modal compare Table 1.

By deformation analysis in frequency of 149Hz, the deformation and modal experiments of the second-order modes consistent with the natural frequency and modal experiments 129Hz relatively were close, so the second-order of the spindle head natural frequency determines the operating frequency.

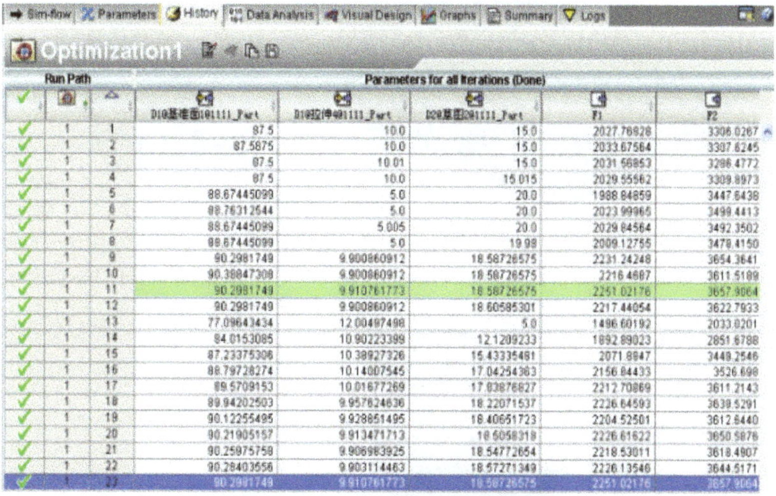

Fig. 4 Optimization results of the Isight.

4. Structural Optimization

Through the above analysis, linear modules are less rigid and larger vibration in working condition. Therefore, the key is to add the optimization of spindle head back and increase the stiffness of the linear module. ISIGHT integrated SolidWorks and ANSYS to optimize the size of connection plate structural, the results of optimization in Fig. 4 and Table 2.

Connecting plate model optimized in Figure 5, because of the vibration motor has little effect on the process, and the linear module is purchased standard parts, in order to increase the stiffness of the linear modules, the need to increase the secondary structure in Figure 6. The optimized plate and the spindle head back assemble to the model shown in Figure 7.

View optimization through simulation analysis results are shown in Table 3.

Table 2 Optimization results.

	Before optimization	Optimized
The center plane	87.5mm	90.29mm
Rib thickness	10mm	9.91mm
Base thickness	15mm	18.59mm
First Order	2027Hz	2251 Hz
Second-order	3306 Hz	3657 Hz

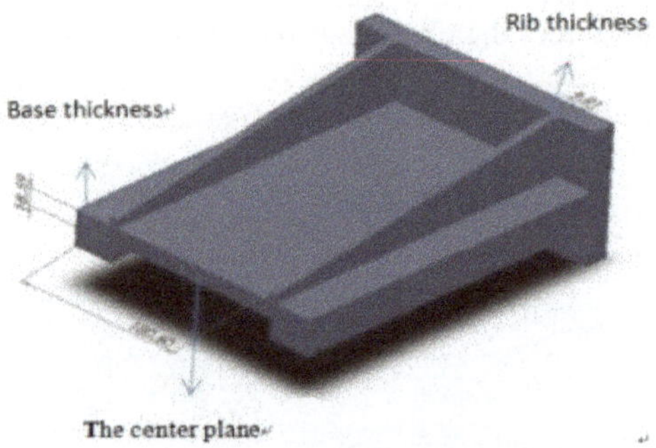

Fig. 5 The optimized size of connecting plate model.

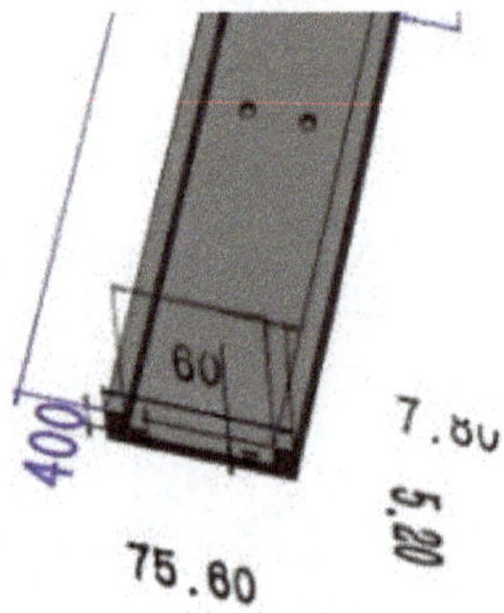

Fig. 6 The spindle head back.

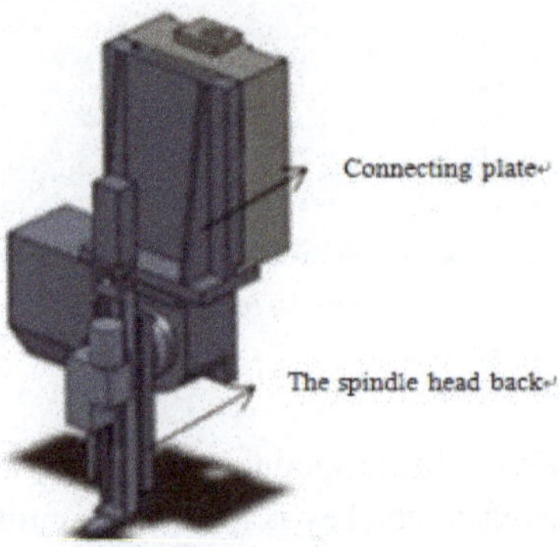

Fig. 7 The assembly diagram.

Before and after optimization of the spindle head of the natural frequencies and mode shapes showed that the optimized second-order natural frequency of the spindle head was increased by 30.93%, and the most value of vibration distortion decreased by 0.08mm.

Table 3 The natural frequency comparison between before and after.

Second-order natural frequency	
Before optimization 140.37Hz	Optimized 183.79Hz
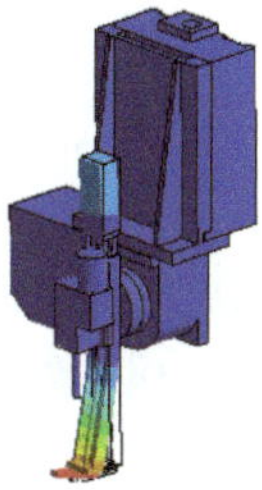	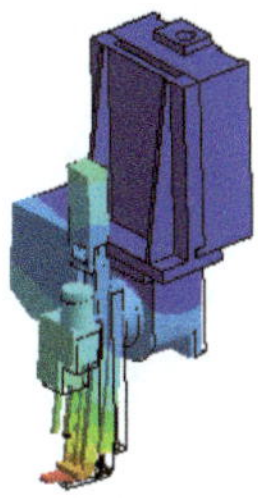

5. Conclusion

Based on modal analysis theory, obtaining the natural frequencies and mode shapes of EDM machine spindle head by modal tests and getting work frequency and distortion of the spindle head by ODS test, identifying the weak parts of the structure vibration in the conditions. The spindle head of natural frequency was increased by 30.93% by optimization. This way avoided the natural frequency of resonance frequency range and improved the machining accuracy of workpiece.

References

1. TANG Zhi-bin, TANG Xiao-qi. Research and implementation of high speed and high accuracy motion control method in CNC [J]. Manufacturing Technology & Machine Tool, 2003(3): 32-35.
2. Erkorkmaz K, Altinatas Y. High speed CNC system design. Part 1. Jerk limited trajectory generation and quantic spline interpolation [J]. International Journal of Machine Tools and Manufacture, 2001, 41: 1323-1345.
3. Hu Jun, Xiao Ling-jian, Wang Yu-han, et al. An optimal feed rate model and solution algorithm for high-speed machine of small line blocks with look ahead [J]. International Journal of Advanced Manufacturing Technology, 2006, 28(9): 930-935.
4. ZHANG De-li, ZHOU Lai-shui. Adaptive algorithm for feed rate smoothing of high speed machine [J]. Acta Aeronautica Et Astronautica Sinica, 2006(1): 125-130.

5. Schwarz BJ, Richardson MH. Introduction to operating deflection shapes. CSI Reliability Week, Orlando, FL, 1999.
6. Richardson MH, Mchargue PL. Operating deflection shapes from time versus frequency-domain measurements. Proceedings of the 11th International Modal Analysis Conference, 1993, 1923: 581-587.
7. Cheng Hang, Zhao Yuan. Application of Operational Modal Analysis to the Reducer Monitoring and Diagnosis[J]Journal of Vibration, Measurement & amp; Diagnosis Vo1. 30 No. 2 Apr. 2010,197-200.
8. Wu Feng, Zhang Sheng-bi. Dynamic Analysis of Loom Frame Structure and Vibration Analysis of Loom Frame under Operating Condition [J]. MECHANICAL SCIENCE TECHNOLOGY, Vol. 16 No. 3 May 1997, 91 : 96.
9. Zheng Chuan-rong, Cao Fa-hai. Study on the Application of ODS Method in the Dynamic Characteristics Analysis of Automobile Gear box [J]. CHINESEAGRICULTURAL. MECHANIZATION, 2008, 80-82.
10. Bai Xiang-he. Optimal Placement of Excitations and Sensors For CNC Machine Tools [D]. Huazhong University of Science and Technology, 2012.

Optimization Design of High Speed Hydraulic Chuck Structure

Tao Defei, Chen Jian and Wang Guicheng
School of Mechanical Engineering, Jiangsu University, Zhenjiang, 212013, China
E-mail:1256427455@qq.com

Li Zhufeng
Mechanical and Electrical Engineering College, Nantong Institute of Technology
Nantong, 226000, China
E-mail:782330954@qq.com

High speed chuck is an important part of high speed machining tooling system, the performance of which directly affects the property and processing quality of advanced computer numerical control machine tools. In this study, ansys optimization analysis module is used to optimize chuck/tool model. The results show that structural optimization improves chuck/tool contact stress distribution and decreases the concentrated stress in hydraulic chuck cavity corner transition region and contact pressure peak. In addition, it also improves the reliability and stability of high speed hydraulic chuck.

Keywords: High speed machining; hydraulic chuck; structural optimization; reliability; finite element method.

1. Introduction

As one of the key components of computer numerical control machine tools, high speed machining tooling system performance has a direct impact on the quality and efficiency of high speed machining [1]. Because of alternating loads, fatigue wear arises in chuck clamping hole wall and oil cavity cracks, which have an impact on chuck clamping performance and fatigue life [2]. Apply transition arcs to hydraulic chuck oil cavity corners and utilize finite element structural analysis techniques to optimize hydraulic chuck structure parameters and transition lines to obtain chuck reasonable sizes, so that the contact stress distribution is improved and stress concentration value is decreased.

2. Analysis of Hydraulic Chuck/Tool Contact State

Hydraulic expansive tool holder structure is shown in Fig. 1.

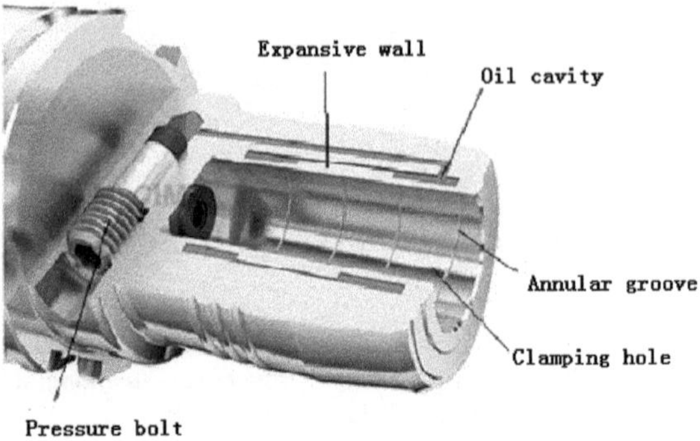

Fig. 1 Hydraulic expansive chuck structure.

With the pressure bolt tightened, oil pressure rises and cavity inner wall expand evenly and symmetrically in the axial direction to clamp tool. While the pressure bolt is loosened, oil pressure drops.

2.1. *Establishment and solution of hydraulic chuck finite element model*

Select TENDOHSK-C63 type of hydraulic chuck, which has a large clamping diameter range from 32mm to 16mm while using a reducing sleeve.

(1) Establishing the solid model

Ansys is utilized to build finite element model. According to actual situation, the chuck and tool physical characteristics are set.

(2) Defining model element and setting mating parameters and boundary degrees of freedom

Axisymmetric element is defined to mesh the chuck and tool. Establish target and contact element. According to the literature [3], the gap between chuck and tool is 16 um. For chuck/tool axisymmetric contact model, chuck and tool axial degree of freedom should be restrained and so is the radial degree of freedom of tool centerline.

(3) Loading and solving

Apply 65Mpa load to oil cavity and solve. And the results could be gained.

2.2. *Hydraulic chuck/tool contact problems*

(1) Contact pressure distribution is uneven. As can be seen from the relevant research, the contact pressure of chuck and tool distributes like a saddle.

(2) There is stress concentration in chuck oil cavity. The four corners are stress concentration areas and the maximum equivalent stress reaches 595.644Mpa.

3.Structural Optimization Design of Hydraulic Chuck

3.1. *Chuck optimization scheme*

It is shown in Fig. 2 that to reduce the stress of chuck oil cavity transition zone, based on hydraulic cylinder flange transition line and combining actual machining, single arc transition line is applied to chuck corner.

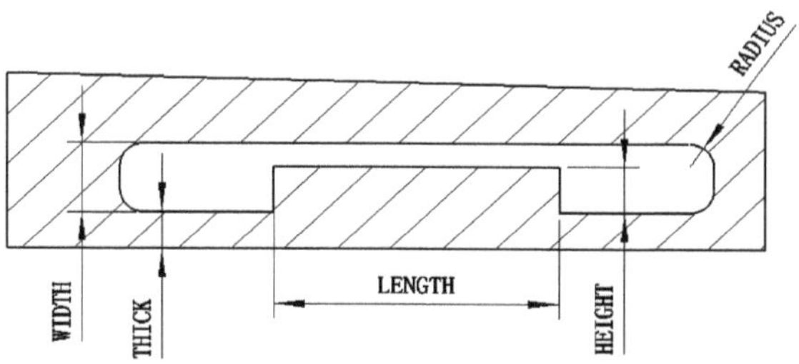

Fig. 2 Chuck single arc transition line.

3.2. *Establishment of the parametric analysis process of chuck/tool finite element contact model*

Ansys finite element optimization design technique needs the help of ansys parametric design language (apdl). With the application of apdl programming language and macro technology in managing ansys finite element analysis commands, parametric modeling can be achieved, parametric loads can be applied and parametric solving can be performed [4].

Ansys analysis file contains a complete cycle. In the iterative calculation process of optimization solution, optimization control file forces design variables constantly to change in each iteration until the design requirements are met.

3.3 *Establishment of the mathematical model of hydraulic chuck structure*

(1) Design variables

Seen from the formal, chuck oil cavity transition line fillet radius radius, chuck expansive wall thickness thick, expansive wall protrusion height height, protrusion length length and oil cavity width width are defined as design variables.

(2) State variables

Set up formulas, which are DH1=WIDTH-H and DH2=WIDTH-2R. Take the following formulas: DH1>0 and DH2≥ 0 as size constraints namely state variables. The maximum peak pmax of finite element analysis contact pressure and chuck/tool clamping torque T should be extracted and set to performance constraints.

(3) Objective function

Extract the maximum equivalent stress value mvonmises in finite element analysis and consider it as the objective function of structural optimization.

In summary, the establishment of hydraulic chuck optimization mathematical model is presented as Eq. (1) below.

$$\begin{cases} 0 < RADIUS \le 3 \\ 0.5 \le THICK \le 5 \\ 3 \le WIDTH \le 6 \\ 0.5 \le HEIGHT \le 6 \\ 5 \le LENGTH \le 45 \\ DH_1 = WIDTH - H > 0 \\ DH_2 = WIDTH - 2R \ge 0 \\ PMAX \le 65 \\ T \ge 450 \\ MVONMISES = Min\ \sigma_d \end{cases} \tag{1}$$

3.4 *Hydraulic chuck optimization results*

Ansys provides two optimization methods: first-order and zero-order. This research adopts sub-problem optimization of zero-order method.

(1) The optimal sequence of design optimization

It is about 20 optimization iterations to get the best design sequence: height=1.4343mm, radius=1.9730mm, thick=1.5982mm, width=4.9170mm, length=39.265mm, pmax=55.052Mpa, T=479.37N.m, mvonmises=480.59Mpa.

According to the actual machining, the design variables of chuck best optimization design sequence are rounded. Table 1 shows the comparison of chuck optimization design rounding sizes and the structural parameters of original design parameters.

(2) Chuck performance comparison before and after optimization

Fig. 3 shows chuck / tool contact stress distribution and the variation curve of contact pressure after optimization. Fig. 4 presents chuck/tool equivalent stress VONMISES distribution after optimization.

As can be seen from analysis results, structural optimization makes contact stress distribution more even and reduces stress concentration value of oil cavity transition area. Hydraulic chuck performance before and after optimization is presented in Table 2.

Table 1 Dimension comparison of chuck optimization design and original design.

Chuck dimension	Design variable(mm)				
	RADIUS	THICK	HEIGHT	LENGTH	WIDTH
Original design	0	2	2	22.9	3
Optimization design	2	1.6	1.5	39	5

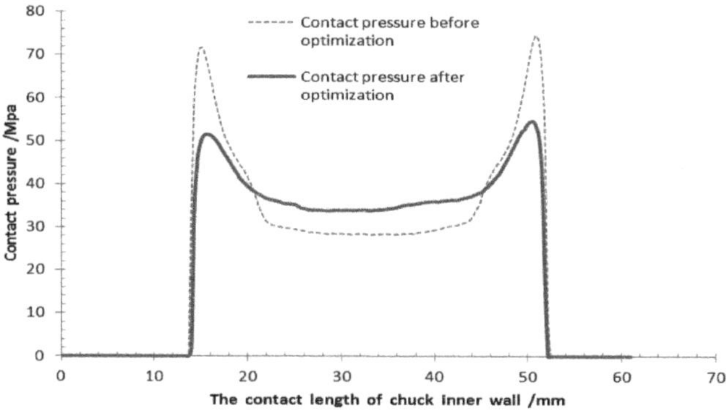

Fig. 3 Comparison of contact pressure variation curve before and after optimization.

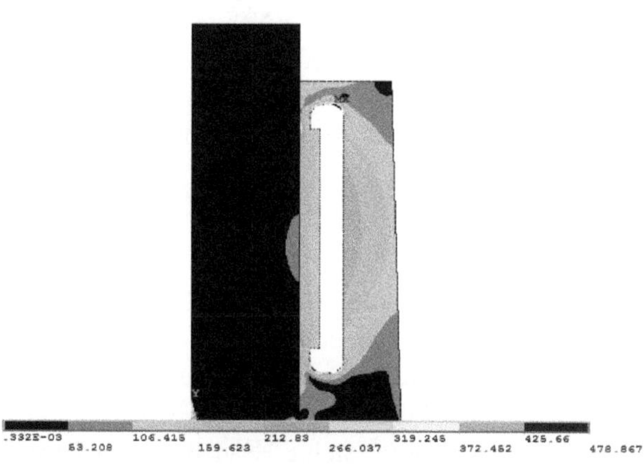

Fig. 4 Distribution of chuck / tool equivalent stress VONMISES after optimization.

Table 2 Hydraulic chuck performance comparison before and after optimization.

Chuck performance	Before optimization	After optimization	Difference	Amplitude of increase
Clamping torque (N.m)	453.200	473.630	20.430	4.51%
The contact stress peak (Mpa)	74.771	54.863	-19.908	-26.63%
The maximum equivalent stress (Mpa)	595.644	478.867	-116.777	-19.61%

From the table, the following results can be drawn. The delivered clamping torque T and the mean contact pressure is raised slightly. So that the chuck clamping performance is ensured. The contact stress peak pmax and chuck maximum stress mvonmises have different degrees of decrease, of which the margins are 26.63% and 19.61%. Chuck performance has been enhanced after optimization.

4. Conclusions

Based on structural optimization theory and optimization methods, Ansys optimization analysis module is applied to optimize hydraulic chuck structural parameters and transition lines. Compared with the original design, structural optimization decreases chuck/tool contact pressure peaks and makes contact stress distribution more reasonable. In addition, the concentrated stress of chuck oil cavity transition corner region is reduced, which has greatly improved chuck fatigue life.

Acknowledgments

This research is based upon work by the National Natural Science Foundation of China (No. 51075192, 51275217), National key projects of P.R. China (2013ZX04009031), A Project Funded by the Priority Academic Program Development of Jiangsu Higher Education Institutions and Nantong key laboratory (CP12014002).

References

1. Wang Guicheng. High Speed Machining Tooling System[M]. Beijing: National Defense Industry Press, 2005.
2. Li Zhufeng. Reliability Research on Clamping Performance of Hydraulic Expansion Toolholder [D]. Jiangsu University, 2014.
3. Shen Jian. Precision Tool Clamping Head Based on Hydraulic Expansion [J]. Tool Technology, 2005, 39(9): 55-57.
4. Game workshop. APDL Parametric Finite Element Analysis Techniques and Application [M]. Beijing: China Water Power Press, 2004.

Mechanical-Hydraulic Co-Simulation on Work Device of Hydraulic Excavator

Xiaohui He[a], Jian Luan[b] and Qiang Wang[c]
College of Field Engineering, PLA Univ. of Sci. & Tech.
Nanjing 210007, China
[a]hxhjcy@163.com, [b]yimudetian@163.com, [c]wangqiangjs@sohu.com

In order to get the hydraulic excavator mechanical-hydraulic coupling characteristics, the models of hydraulic and mechanical system are built in AMESim and Virtual Lab Motion. By the joint simulation interface, mechanical and hydraulic models can exchange data in time. The characteristics of excavator work device are analyzed in the aspects of cylinder movement situations and pressure changes as shown in Fig. 4 and Fig. 5. The max pressure exists in the arm cylinder and the value is 29.2MPa, which is smaller than the relief pressure. The excavator can work normally under the design load.

Keywords: Hydraulic excavator; work device; co-simulation.

1. Introduction

Hydraulic excavator is widely used. The performances of hydraulic excavator work device decide the mining efficiency and precision [1]. The work device is mainly composed with mechanical system and hydraulic system. Nowadays, the research for work device of hydraulic excavator concentrates on mechanical and hydraulic dynamic characteristics separately, which make it impossible to consider the coupling characteristics of mechanical and hydraulic system [2-4]. The physical prototype must been made to test the coupling characteristics, which will take a long time and it is easy to find problems [5]. Thus, this article use the method of mechanical-hydraulic co-simulation to research the characteristics of hydraulic excavator work device. The co-simulation method provides a way to consider the coupling characteristics in early design stage and a basis for optimization design of work device.

2. Mechanical-Hydraulic Co-simulation Model

2.1. *Hydraulic system model*

The hydraulic system of work device is composed with main oil circuit and pilot control circuit. The main oil circuit includes tank, the main pump, liquid control multi-valve, boom cylinder, arm cylinder, bucket cylinder and etc. the pilot control circuit includes tank, pilot pump, pilot control valve and etc. The simulation model is built with the help of AMESim hydraulic library and hydraulic component design library. The simulation model is shown in Figure 1.

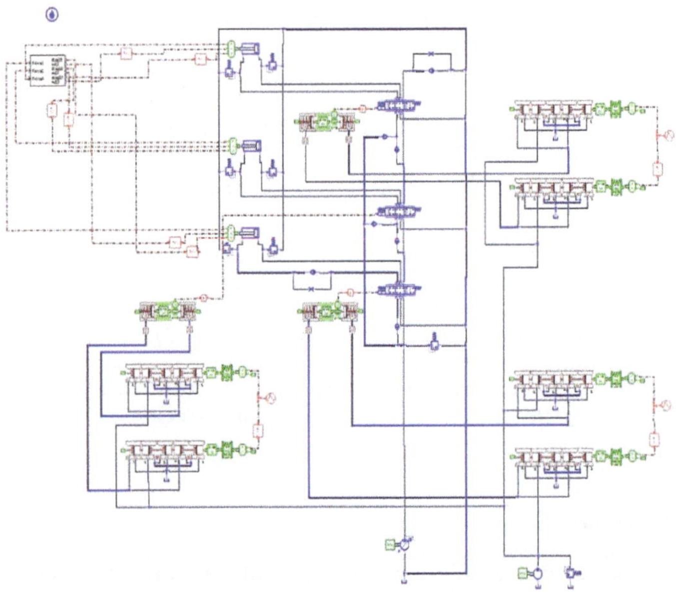

Fig. 1 Simulation model of hydraulic system.

In this hydraulic system of excavator work device, the simulation parameters are as follows. (1) Pilot control valve: TH40K1269, k=7.7N/mm, m=80mg, pressure of relief valve is 4MPa. (2) Liquid control multi-valve: UX28-57, k=30N/mm, piston bore is 15mm, rod diameter is 7.8mm, m=125g, d=1.5mm, spool stroke is -2mm to 2mm, pressure drop is 1.9MPa, and the flow of maximum opening is 380L / min. (3) The pump: A8V104. The parameters of hydraulic cylinders are shown in Table 1.

Table 1 Parameters of cylinders.

	type	Cylinder diameter	Rod diameter	stroke
Boom	JPG-7	120mm	85mm	1119mm
Arm	JPG-8A	140mm	90mm	1430mm
Bucket	JPG-50	110mm	80mm	1050mm

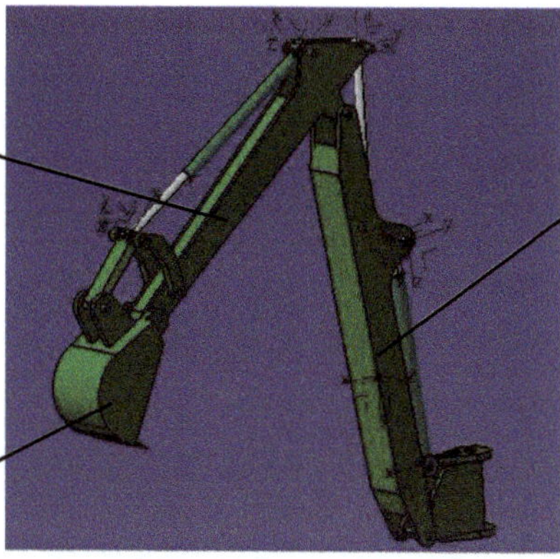

Fig. 2 Mechanical model of work device.

2.2. *Mechanical system model*

According to the dimensions of hydraulic excavator, the 3D model of work device is built in Virtual Lab Motion, as shown in Figure 2.

2.3. *Simulation conditions*

The main working process of hydraulic excavator is as follows: (1) boom down and adjust arm and bucket to a suitable location. (2) Digging operation with arm or bucket. (3) Raise the boom. Therefore, the control signals of liquid control multi-valve are shown in Figure 3.

During the digging process, the loads of excavator include gravity and digging resistance. The gravity is consisted of mechanical itself and the earthwork. The gravity of earthwork increase and the max is 1816N because of dipper capacity q is $0.8m^3$. The digging resistance includes tangential resistance and normal resistance [6].

$$F_t = \frac{K_0 q}{0.01745 R \phi K_s} \tag{1}$$

$$F_n = \lambda F_t \tag{2}$$

where $K_0 = 2.1\times10^5 N/m^2$, q=$0.8m^3$, R=1.47m, ϕ=42°, K_s=3.4, λ=0.4.

Substitute the data and the max digging resistance can be calculated as follows: F_t=45863.6N, F_n=18345.4N. Because digging process begins at 3.5s and ends at 6s, the force of bucket during digging process is shown in Table 2.

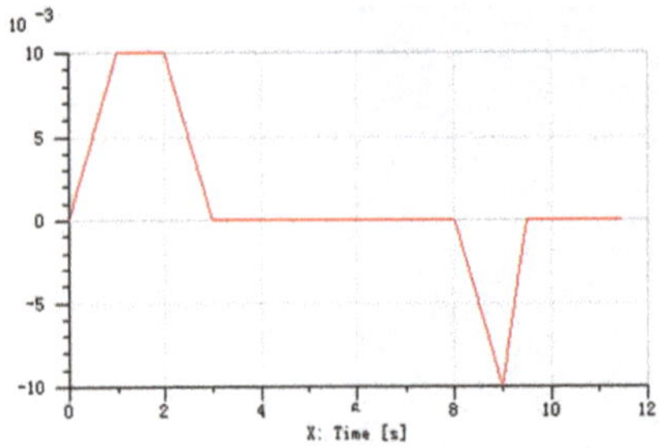

(a) Control signal of boom

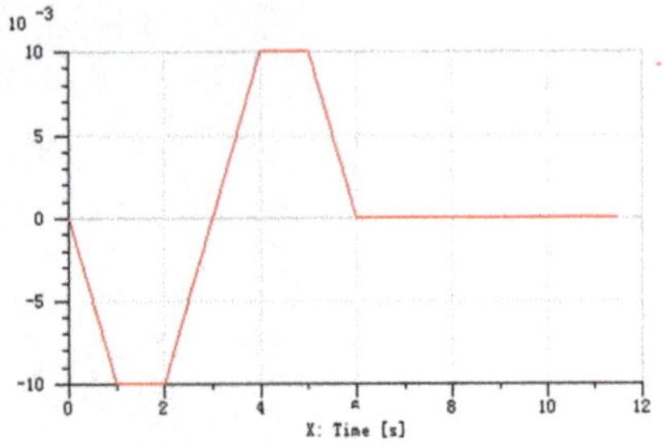

(b) Control signal of arm

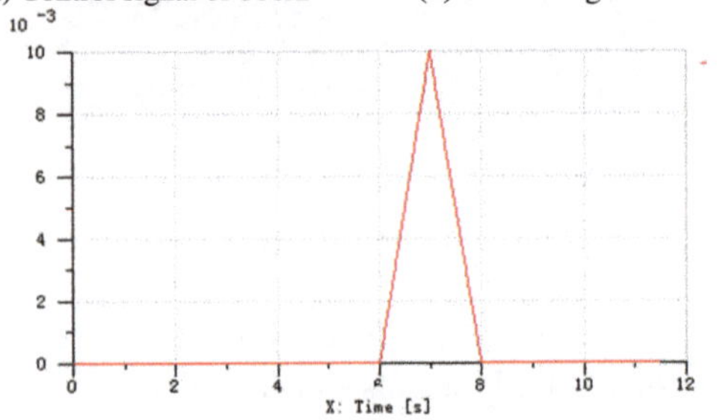

(c) Control signal of bucket

Fig. 3 Control signals of liquid control multi-valve.

Table 2 The force of bucket.

type	expression
tangential resistance	step(time ,3.5 ,0 ,4.5 ,45863.6)+step(time ,5 ,0 ,6 ,-45863.6)
normal resistance	step(time ,3.5 ,0,4.5,18345.4) +step(time ,5,0,6,-18345.4)
earthwork gravity	step(time ,3.5,0,6,1816)

3. Results Analysis of Co-Simulation

3.1. *Analysis of cylinder movement situation*

The movement situations of hydraulic cylinder are important and decide the motion trail of work device. Figure 4 gives the movement situation of boom cylinder, arm cylinder and bucket cylinder.

As been seen from Figure 4, the movement situations of boom, arm and bucket cylinder are steady and work device of excavator can complete the digging process according to the pilot control circuit. During the digging process (3.5-6s), the displacement of boom cylinder and bucket cylinder exist decrease, which of the boom cylinder is more obvious. This is because the force of two cylinders is so great that there will be leakage of hydraulic oil. Besides, the displacement of the cylinders exist fluctuation while the work status changes, which fit well with the accrual situation.

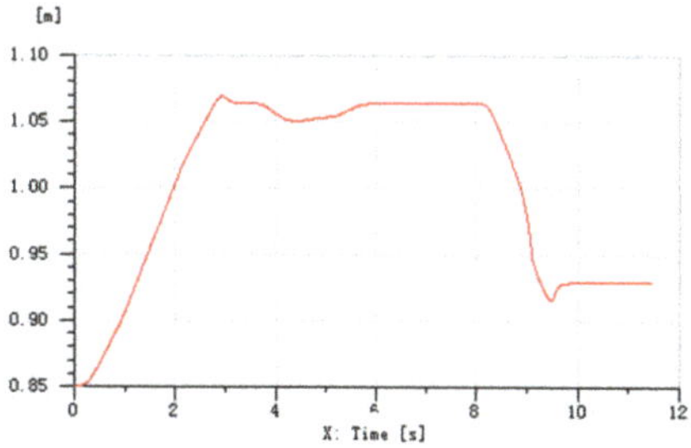

(a) Movement of boom cylinder

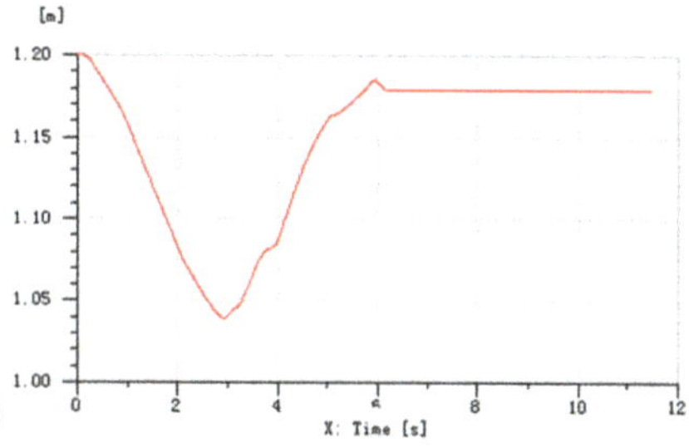

(b) Movement of arm cylinder

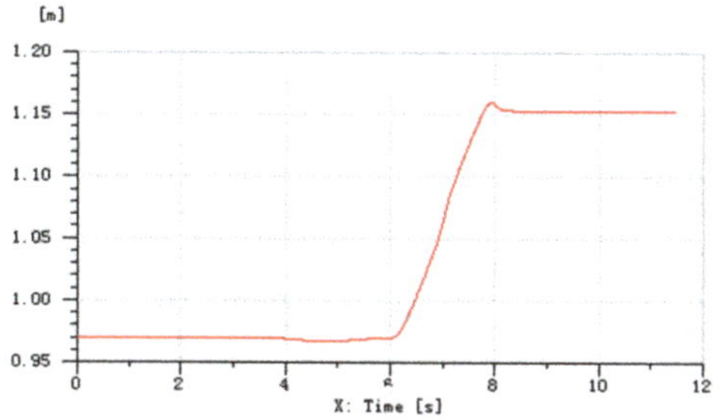

(c) Movement of bucket cylinder

Fig. 4 Movement situation of cylinders.

3.2. *Analysis of cylinder pressure*

The change of cylinder pressure decides whether the hydraulic system meet the design requirement. The pressure change of boom, arm and bucket cylinders is shown in Figure 5.

As been seen from Figure 5, the max pressure of boom, arm and bucket cylinder is smaller than the relief pressure 30MPa of relief valve. Thus, the excavator can work normally under the design load. The max pressure exists in the arm cylinder and the value is 29.2MPa. The pressure of bucket cylinder is smaller than others, so we need choose cylinder type according to the pressure.

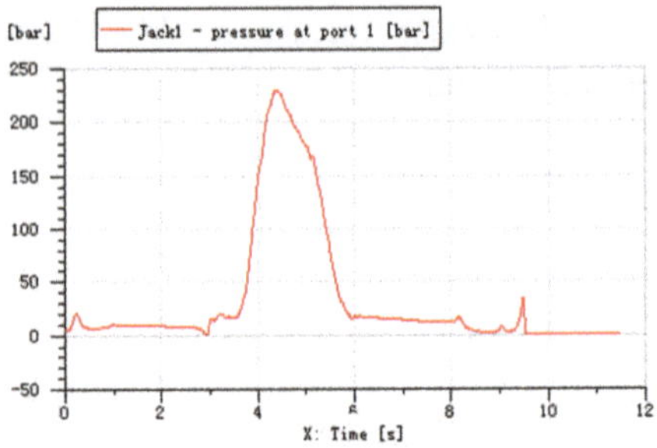

(a) Pressure of boom cylinder

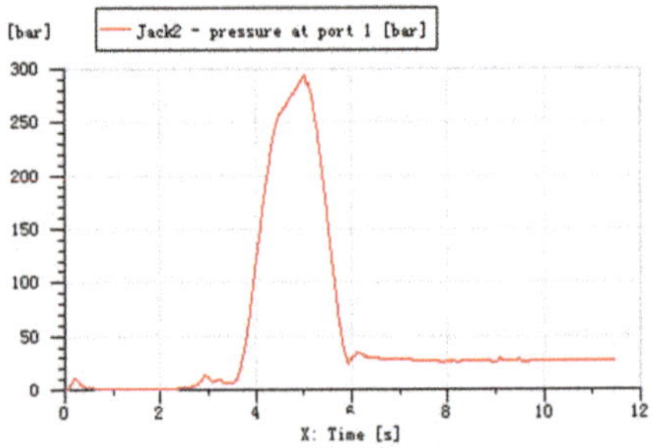

(b) Pressure of arm cylinder

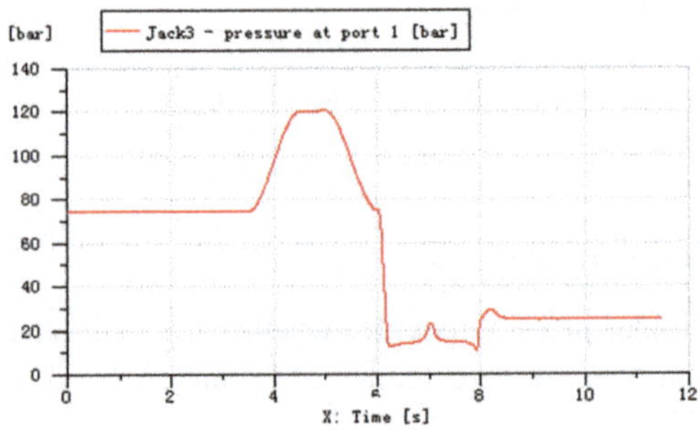

(c) Pressure of bucket cylinder

Fig. 5 Pressure change of cylinders.

4. Conclusions

(1) The method of mechanical-hydraulic co-simulation can accurately get the pressure changes of cylinders, which can improve the simulation accuracy.

(2) The movement situations of boom, arm and bucket cylinder are steady. And the displacement of the cylinders exist fluctuation if the work status changes. This can provide the basis for optimization design of work device.

(3) The max pressure exists in the arm cylinder and the value is 29.2MPa, which is smaller than the relief pressure. Therefore, the excavator can work normally under the design load.

References

1. Zhu Xiaojing, Quan Long, Wang Xinzhong. *Co-simulation Analysis of Working Characteristic for Large Hydraulic Excavator*. Transactions of the Chinese Society for Agricultural Machinery, 2011, 04: 27-32
2. Soonyoung Yang, Soonkwang Kwon, Sungmin Jin. *Hydraulic simulation and remote control system of field robot*. Control, Automation, Robotics and Vision, 2008: 2303-2308.
3. S Md Rozali, MF Rahmat, N Abdul Wahab. *PID Controller Design for an Industrial Hydraulic Actuator with Servo System*. IEEE Student Conference, 2010: 218-223.
4. Mouftah M. Mohamed, Moussa A. Hamdan. *Development of Control System for Two Degree of Freedom Hydraulic Motion Base*. International Conference on Mechanical and Electronics Engineering, 2010: 166-170.
5. Chen Jinguo, Jin Shaoxun, Chen Huipeng. *Coupled simulation study on working device of loader based on VL Motion*. Journal of Mechanical & Electrical Engineer, 2012, 10: 1135-1138.
6. Lin Muyi, Shi Qinglu. *Hydraulic excavator Construction and Design*. Beijing: Metallurgical Industry Press, 2011.4.

A Lorentz Force Powered Controllable Micro-Jet Injection System*

Kai Chen† and Laiwu Miao
School of Mechanical Engineering, Hangzhou Dianzi University, Hangzhou, 810008, China
†E-mail: kchen@hdu.edu.cn
www.hdu.edu.cn

A medical device of micro-jet injection for drug delivery is described in this paper. The device is powered by a Lorentz force driver (or voice coil motor, VCM) and is able to perform pulsed injection through controlling the direction of the current passing through the device. The driving force and the resulting injection pressure are also controllable through the control of the current intensity of VCM. A physical model was established by combining the existing jet injection model with the relationship of the driving force obtained from a FEM analysis. The numerical calculation of the physical model reveals the relationship between the injection pressure and the current intensity of VCM under system conditions. In a variable dose situation, the relationship between the current intensity of VCM and the dose value was obtained under the condition that the maximum injection pressure is kept above a threshold value. The calculation results can be used for optimization of the device.

Keywords: Jet injection; micro-jet; transdermal drug delivery.

1. Introduction

Over the years, conventional hypodermic needle is an effective way of subcutaneous drug delivery. However, the process of needle piecing into the skin will produce pain, cause panic and extra pressure. The needle-free jet injection technology which employs a high-velocity liquid stream to penetrate into the skin has a number of advantages such as simpler operation, better absorption, elimination of infection, etc. Most commercial jet injectors complete the injection in one shot, and are not able to achieve sustained and controlled release of drug delivery. The driving force that powers the jet injector is often fixed so that the injection depth is uncontrollable. When the injection depth is too deep and the jet touches nerves under the skin, it is often accompanied by a strong sense of pain. In addition to spring and compressed air, alternative

* This work is supported by China's National Natural Science Foundation (Program No. 51275142).

driving forces have been explored in order to transform the one-time jet injection into an intermittent micro-jet injection. For example, piezoelectric stack actuators have been used in jet injection technology. Owing to the small displacement of the piezoelectric actuator output, the single injection dose is very small and the injection depth is effectively controlled [1–3]. A pulsed micro-jet can also be produced using high-voltage electrode discharged in the liquid. Bubbles are created to drive the liquid out of the nozzle [4]. A recent study applied a pulsed laser irradiation into the liquid to generate driving bubbles to achieve micro-jet drug delivery [5]. This kind of continuous pulsed micro-jet injection for transdermal drug delivery has such features as less invasiveness, sustained drug delivery, controlled drug release and so on.

Taberner *et al.* reported a jet injector powered by a voice coil linear actuator which is composed of rare earth permanent magnets as the core and a winding pack of coil as the moving actuator [6]. A high power density of capacitor was used to discharge electricity that passes through the coil to produce the electromagnetic force (Lorentz force) high enough to obtain a high velocity jet. Because the driving force (Lorentz force) can be controlled and regulated through the current intensity and the time passing through the coil, the resulting impinging pressure of the jet and also the penetration depth are controllable through manipulating these parameters applied on the coil. Recently, Taberner et al. demonstrated a control strategy that can change and optimize the jet speed through feed back control of piston displacement during the course of jet injection [7]. However, the jet injection systems based on the Lorentz force actuator so far can only implement a single-shot injection. A continuous micro-dosing is thus necessary for controlled release of drug delivery in clinical applications. This paper presents a continuous micro-injection system based on the Lorentz force actuator. The relationship between the jet impinging pressure and the driving current intensity was established for different injection volumes, using a previous established mathematical model as well as results from FEM analyses of magnetic field.

2. The System Structure and Working Principle

Generally, a needle-free jet injection system includes an ampoule, a driving device and its fixture. The ampoule is mainly used for inhaling, reserving drugs and accomplishing flow ejection. The driving device provides driving force to the piston in the ampoule to expel the liquid out of a small orifice at the front end of the ampoule. As shown in Figure 1, the current continuous micro-jet injection system includes an injector, an ampoule, a VCM (voice coil motor) drive, a control system, a power supply and some moving and support structures. The VCM consists of a core pack of permanent magnets and a moving coil, both of which are surrounded by a shell. The piston inside the ampoule connects to the plunger of VCM through a coupler. 2 precision check valves on the ampoule function as pump valves to suck the liquid from the drug storage and expel the liquid from the front end of the ampoule, and then out of the orifice at the front end of the injector, through a hose that connects the front end of the ampoule to the back end of the injector.

In operation, the control system triggers the power supply to add high voltage on the VCM for a preset time period, after accepting the signal from the actuator of the injector. The moving coil in the VCM under Lorentz force pushes the piston inside the ampoule. The check valve on the orifice opens while the other check valve that connects to the drug storage closes. The high-pressure liquid flows through the hose into the injector and forms a high speed jet after coming out of the orifice. After injection, the control system provides a reverse direction current for the VCM. The piston then moves back. The two check valves operate just in opposition of the injection, and the liquid flows from the drug storage to the ampoule, in preparation for the next injection.

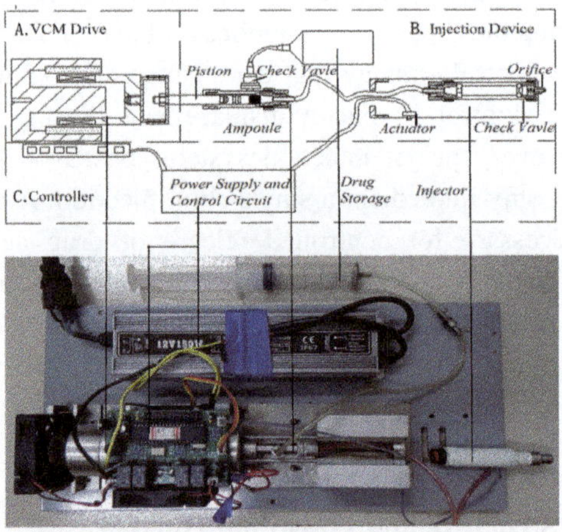

Fig. 1 The structure diagram of the continuous micro-jet injection system.

3. The Physical Model and Calculation

The injection pressure plays an important role in the performance of the jet injection process. It is reported that the maximum injection pressure in the initial moment needs to reach above a threshold value before the jet is able to erode and penetrate into the skin. The authors have developed a quasi-steady physical model to calculate the dynamic injection pressure for a given driving force [8]. Equation (1) was obtained to express the piston movement and the injection pressure as coupled functions of time.

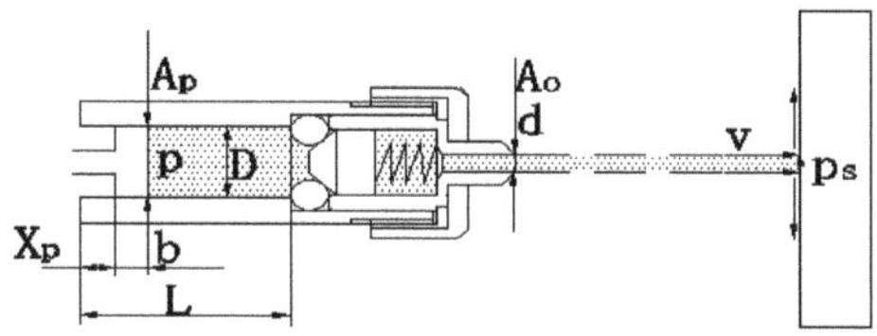

Fig. 2 The physical model of the injection flow.

$$\begin{cases} \dfrac{d^2x_p}{dt^2} = \dfrac{F}{m_p} - \dfrac{A_p p}{m_p} - \dfrac{\pi D b \theta (p + p_c)}{m_p} \\ \dfrac{dp}{dt} = \dfrac{(E+p)\dfrac{dx_p}{dt} - \dfrac{EA_0}{A_p}\sqrt{\dfrac{2p\dfrac{dx_p}{dt}}{\rho_0 \dfrac{dx_p}{dt} + \dfrac{64\mu L}{D^2}}}}{L - x_p} \end{cases} \tag{1}$$

Where x_p is the total displacement of the piston, F is the electromagnetic driving force of the VCM, p is the hydraulic pressure on the surface of the piston, others will be introduced in Table 2 of next section.

The injection pressure of the jet in the surface of skin can be calculated according to Bernoulli Principle, as shown in Equation (2), where v is the speed of jet out of the ampoule.

$$p_s = \frac{1}{2}\rho v^2 \tag{2}$$

In a separate paper, the authors have calculated the electromagnetic force through FEM simulation done on the commercial software Maxwell 3D for each separate displacement of the coil movement, and for different current values that pass through the VCM [9]. The following relationship was established that approximates the electromagnetic force F as a function of piston displacement x and the current intensity I.

$$F = -(0.01I + 0.06)x^2 + 4x + 10I \tag{3}$$

The Equations (1) to (3) are combined to create an Equation (4) which derives the injection pressure varies with time under certain system conditions.

$$\begin{cases} \dfrac{d^2x_p}{dt^2} = \dfrac{-(0.01I+0.06)x_p^{\ 2}+4x_p+10I-A_p p-\pi Db\theta(p+p_c)}{m_p} \\ \dfrac{dp}{dt} = \dfrac{(E+p)\dfrac{dx_p}{dt}-\dfrac{EA_o}{A_p}\sqrt{\dfrac{2p\dfrac{dx_p}{dt}}{\rho_0\dfrac{dx_p}{dt}+\dfrac{64\mu L}{D^2}}}}{L-x_p} \\ p_s = \dfrac{1}{2}(\dfrac{A_p}{A_o}\dfrac{dx_p}{dt})^2\rho_0 \end{cases} \qquad (4)$$

4. The Calculation Results

Equation (4) can be solved by the classical Runge-Kutta integration method. The main parameters of the VMC used for calculation and also for the device are shown in Table 1. The other system parameters used for calculation are listed in Table 2.

Table 1 The main parameters of VMC.

Parameters	Value
Coil stroke	40 mm
Diameter of permanent magnets	25 mm
The resistance value	3.7 ohms
Diameter of coil	34 mm
Width of coil	40 mm
Inductance coefficient	5 mh
Type of permanent magnets	Nd-Fe-B (N50)
The maximum temperature	428.15K

Fig. 3 shows the calculated injection pressure vs. time starting from the point of the injection (t=0). The current intensity (I) of the VCM was set as 17A. The injection pressure oscillates in the first 5ms due to the impact of the piston that causes intermittent behavior of the jet. The pressure gradually decreases in the following 10-100ms. It is seen that the maximum injection pressure occurs at the first peak of the oscillating curve. It is reported that the maximum injection pressure needs to reach a threshold of 14MPa before the jet is able to penetrate into human skin [8]. The VCM with the current intensity of 17A will produce a maximum injection pressure of 16MPa, which is bigger than the threshold value.

Table 2 The system parameters of the device.

Parameters	Numerical Value
The weight of the piston and moving coil, m_p	1.2×10^{-1} kg
The bulk modulus of elasticity of the drug, E	2.18×10^{9} Pa
The initial length of liquid, L	2.8×10^{-2} m
The cross-sectional area of the micro orifice, A_o	4.91×10^{-8} m^2
The cross-sectional area of the piston, A_p	1.79×10^{-5} m^2
The diameter of the chamber in ampoule, D	4.77×10^{-3} m
The initial density of the drug, ρ_0	1×10^{3} kg/m^3
The friction coefficient between ampoule and piston	2×10^{-2}
The conventional hydraulic pressure, p_c	3.5×106 Pa
The contact width between the ampoule and piston, b	1×10^{-3} m
The dynamic viscosity of the drug, μ	1.005×10^{-3} Pa·s

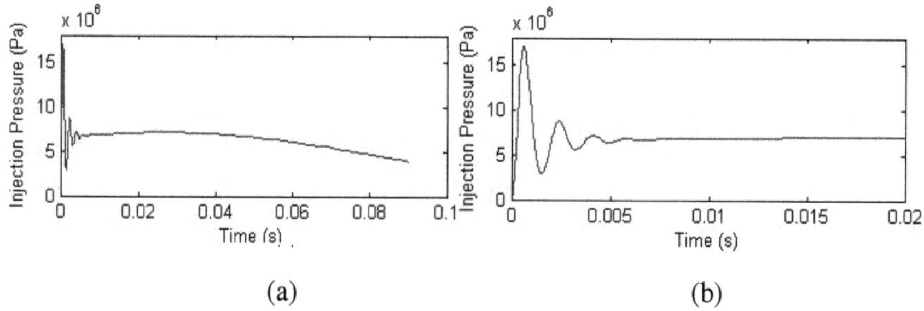

Fig. 3 Calculated injection pressure vs. time (a): first 100ms; (b): first 20ms.

Fig. 4 shows the calculated maximum injection pressure increases with increasing current intensity. Its relationship can be expressed in quadratic as Equation (8).

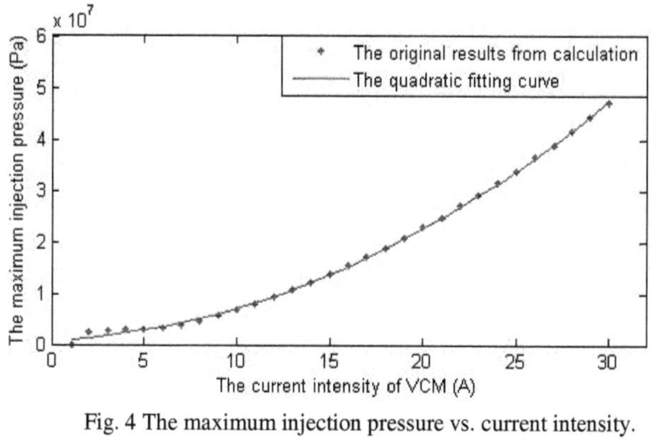

Fig. 4 The maximum injection pressure vs. current intensity.

$$P_{s,\max} = 46400I^2 + 156910I + 862040 \quad (1.05 < I < 35) \tag{8}$$

In clinical applications, each dose of pulsed jet injection can vary according to usage. The variable dose can be achieved either by fixing the ampoule chamber while changing the piston moving distance, or by fixing the piston distance while switching the ampoule. The later approach was chosen for the device and for the calculation. For each dose (V), a try and error method was used to calculate the current intensity (I) needed to keep the maximum injection pressure just above 16Mpa, so that the jet has the capability of penetrating into the skin. Fig.5 shows the calculated injection pressure vs. time for a different dose of 0.2ml, 0.3ml, 0.4ml and 0.5ml and their corresponding current intensity values so that the maximum injection pressure is above 16Mpa.

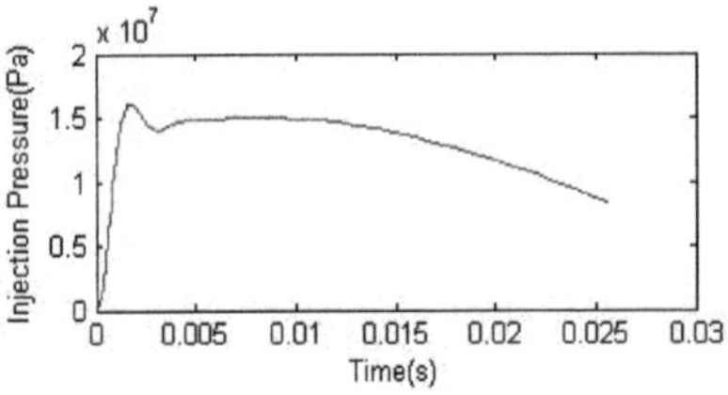

a. V=0.2ml, I=16.85A.

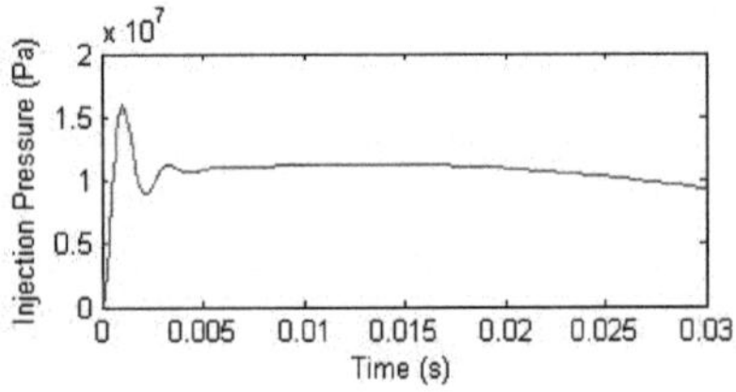

b. V=0.3ml, I=17.46A

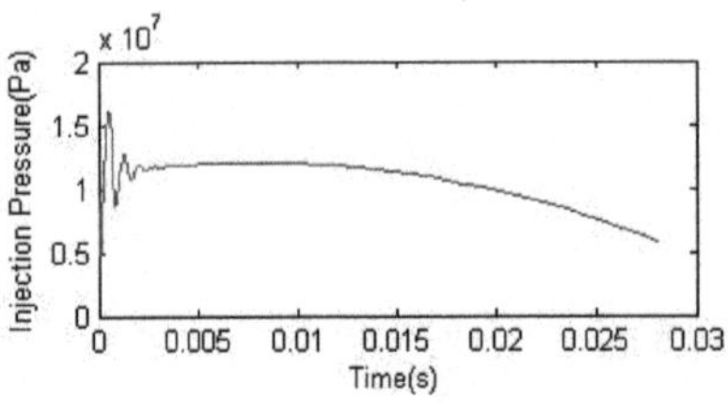

c. V=0.4ml, I=17.03A.

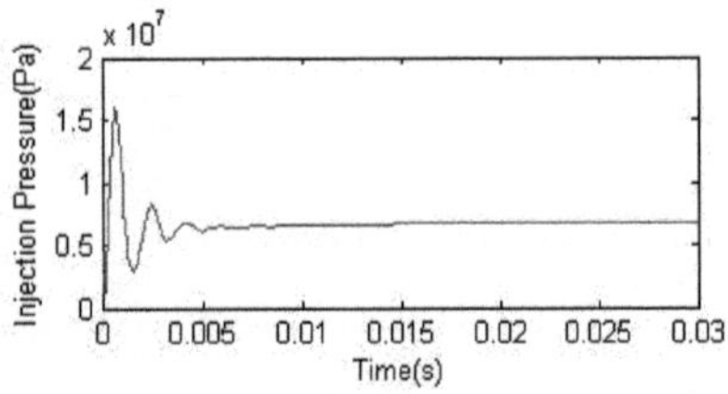

d. V=0.5ml, I=16.37A

Fig. 5 The injection pressure vs. time with different dose and current intensity.

The relation between the current intensity of VCM and the varying injection dose can be obtained by calculating each discrete value of injection dose and its corresponding value of the current intensity to maintain the maximum injection pressure right above 16Mpa. Fig. 6 shows its relationship. The current intensity first increases with the injection dose, before reaches a maximum value, and then decreases gradually. The increasing inertia due to increasing dose needs more current intensity to drive the liquid. However, the increasing cross sectional area of the ampoule due to a bigger dose will also increase the initial injection pressure, resulting in a compromising effect. The calculation results can be further expressed as a piecewise curve fitting Equation (9).

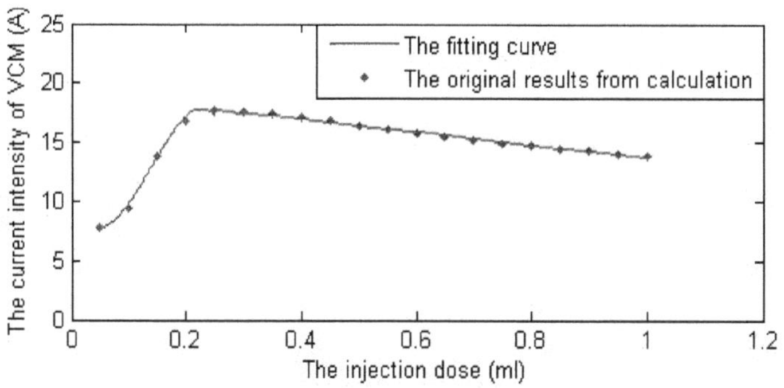

Fig. 6 The relation between the injected dose and the current intensity.

$$\begin{cases} I = -3348.8V^3 + 1374.1V^2 - 104.8V + 9.9 & (0.05 \le V \le 0.25) \\ I = -5.3856V + 19.0666 & (0.25 < V \le 1) \end{cases} \tag{9}$$

Equation (8) and Equation (9) can be used for the optimization of the current device to accurately control the value of the current intensity of VCM for different injection doses. Experiments will be carried out in the future to verify the calculation results and the injection effects of the device.

5. Conclusions

A controllable micro-jet injection system powered by a Lorentz force driver (or voice coil motor, VCM) was present in this paper. The device is able to perform a continuous pulsed jet injection through the control of electrical current passing through the VCM. The analysis of the jet mechanics was carried out based on the existing physical model in order to establish the relationship between the controllable current intensity and the injection pressure under different system parameters. The following conclusions can be obtained:

i) The driving force (Lorentz force of VCM) was simulated by FEM and can be represented through a function of current intensity under fixed system conditions. It can be substituted into the existing physical model to obtain the injection pressure under different system conditions.

ii) The physical model was solved numerically. The relationship between the maximum injection pressure that characterizes the jet performance and the current intensity was established, and can be represented through a curve fitting function.

iii) In a variable-dose situation, the relationship between the current intensity and the value of dose was obtained from calculation to keep the maximum injection pressure above a threshold. The above relationships can be used for optimization of the micro-jet injection device.

References

1. Arora A, Hakim I, Baxter J, Rathnasingham R, Srinivasan R, Fletcher DA, Mitragotri S. Needle-free delivery of macromolecules across the skin by nanoliter-volume pulsed microjets, J. Proc Natl Acad Sci U S A. (2007) Vol. 14, No. 11, 4255-4260.
2. Arora A, Prausnitz MR, Mitragotri S. Micro-scale devices for transdermal drug delivery, J. International Journal of Pharmaceutics. (2008) Vol. 364, No. 2, 227-236.
3. Chen K. A Novel Micro-jet Transdermal Drug Delivery System. Proc. ASME 4th Frontiers of Biomedical Devices (BioMed 2009), Irvine, CA, USA. 2009.
4. Fletcher DA and Palanker DV. A pulsed liquid microjet for ocular microsurgical applications, J. INVESTIGATIVE OPHTHALMOLOGY & VISUAL SCIENCE. (2001) Vol. 42, No. 4, S717.
5. Han TH and Yoh JJ. A laser based reusable microjet injector for transdermal drug delivery, J. Journal of Applied Physics. (2010) Vol. 107, No. 4, 103110-103113.
6. Taberner AJ, Ball NB, Hogan NC, Hunter IW. A Portable Needle-free Jet Injector Based on a Custom High Power-density Voice-coil Actuator, J. Conf Proc IEEE Eng Med Biol Soc. (2006) Vol. 2006, 5001-5004.
7. Taberner AJ, Hogan NC, Hunter IW. Needle-free jet injection using real-time controlled linear Lorentz-force actuators, J. Medical Engineering & Physics, (2012) Vol. 34, 1228–1235.
8. Chen K, Zhou H, Li J, Cheng G. Stagnation Pressure in Liquid Needle-Free Injection: Modeling and Experimental Validation, J. Drug Delivery Letters, (2011) Vol. 1, No. 2, 97-104.
9. Quan-wei Xu, Kai Chen and Yong-gui Lv. FEM Modeling and Validation of a Voice Coil Powered Jet Injector, Proceedings of the 2015 Asia-Pacific Biological Engineering and Biomedical Conference, Jan. 2015, Shanghai, China.

A Simple PFC Control Y- Rectifier AC/DC Conversion for LED Lamp

Narin Watanakul

Department of Electrical and Computer Engineering, Faculty of Engineering, Thammasat University of Thailand, Thailand

E-mail: wnarin@engr.tu.ac.th

The paper was to study ac/dc three phase PFC rectifier for LED lamp. The performance normally of the rectifier having is current low quality and low power factor and high total harmonics distortion current. Therefore, the objectives in this a paper going to improving power factor and reduce harmonics current. In this paper to propose power factor correction (PFC) with phase-modular Y-rectifier, boost type converter circuit using by one cycle control (OCC). For high performance method and tested of the result for realize that can solve power factor and reduce harmonic current. The research papers, conclusions for study and evaluate the circuit can be operation and suitable for use with LED 50 W (LED lamp). The data collected by MATLAB Simulation are used in comparison with the experimental tester of results.

Keywords: LED lamp, Phase-modular Y-rectifier, harmonics reduction, power factor correction, switch-mode rectifiers (SMRS), improved power quality converters (IPQCs).

1. Introduction

In 1990's ultra-bright LEDs using Aluminum Indium Gallium Phosphide (AlInGaP) to produce orange-red, orange, yellow and presently green light has become available. The first significant blue LEDs also appeared at the start of the 1990's, once again using Silicon Carbide - a throwback to the earliest semiconductor light sources, although like their yellow Russian ancestors the light output was very dim by today's standards. Ultra bright blue Gallium Nitride (GaN) LEDs arrived in the mid-1990s, with Indium Gallium Nitride (InGaN) LEDs producing high-intensity blue and green shortly thereafter (e.g. [1]-[3]). In Fig. 1, shows the current range of LED, which can take many forms and depending on the manufacturer. The package tube LED (LED package) Surface Mouth Type rated 50 watt, 30 volt level rang and the current rating of the LED about of current use 20-50 mA, 50-150mA and current 150mA-1000mA.

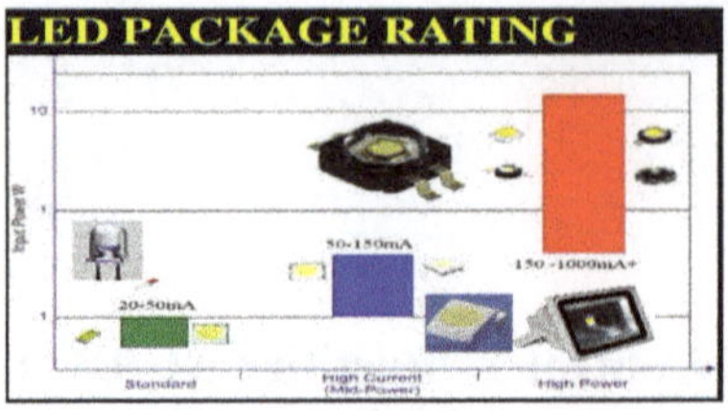

Fig. 1 Example, the current range of LED on type of production.

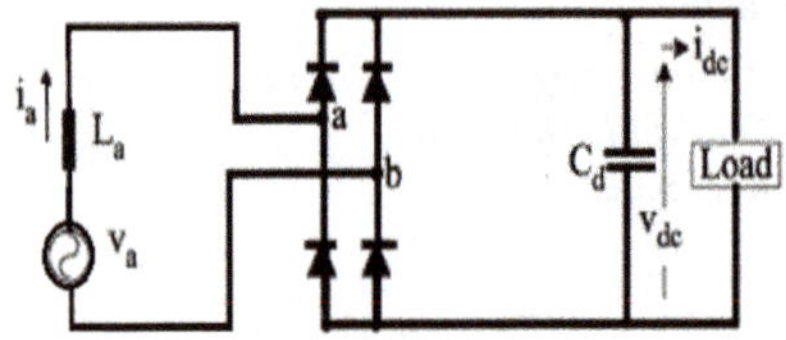

(a)

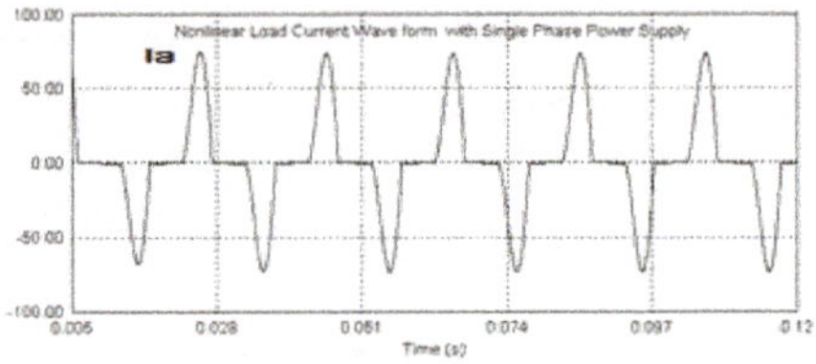

(b)

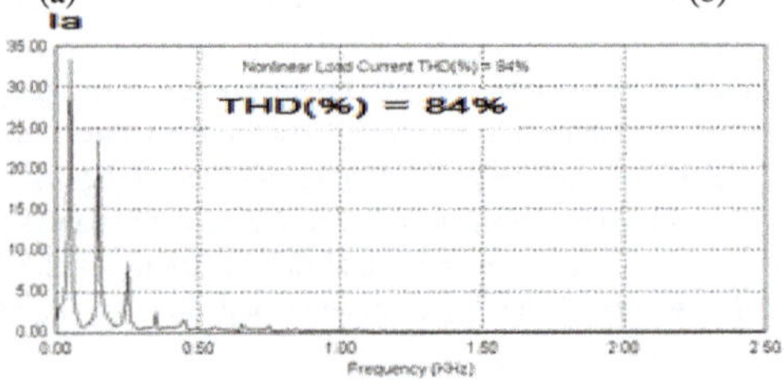

(c)

Fig. 2 Depicts the effects of current quality this circuit with the single phase rectifies (4-pulses) being delivered to a power factor corrected supply for a non-PFC unit.

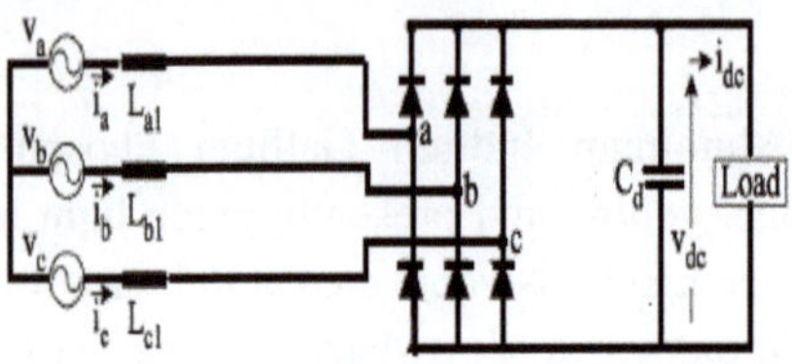

(a)

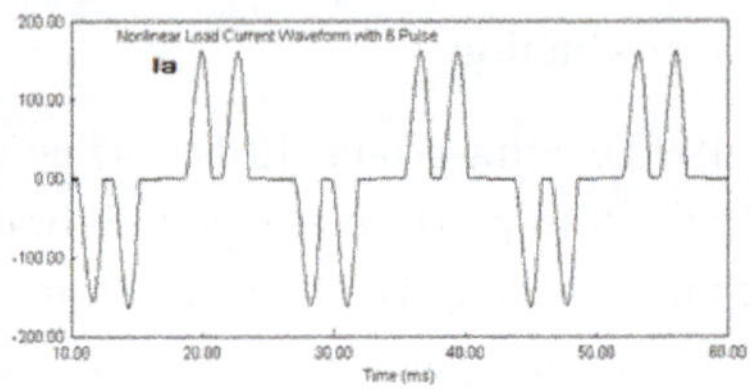

(b)

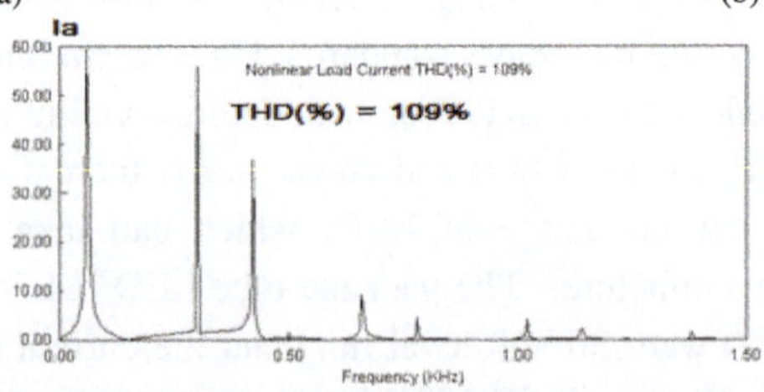

(c)

Fig. 3 Depicts the effects of current quality this circuit with the three phase rectifies (6-pulses) being delivered to a power factor corrected supply for a non-PFC unit.

In a theoretical case where output current can be estimated as clean DC current. As was shown in Fig. 2 and Fig. 3. Depicts the effects of this circuit with the same power being delivered to a power factor corrected supply for a non-PFC unit. This paper to propose Y-Rectifier in a three phase star connection technique based power LED driver topology. The three phase balance phase current AC/DC rectifier with the control can make it the input line current of power converter with the unity power factor, and the current waveform distortion results increase of the lower harmonics distortion.

2. Power Factor and THD

Conventionally, AC/DC converters, which are also called rectifiers, are developed using diodes and thyristors to provide controlled and uncontrolled dc power with unidirectional and bidirectional power flow. They have the demerits of poor power quality in terms of injected current harmonics, caused voltage distortion and poor power factor at input ac mains and slow varying rippled dc output at load end, low efficiency and large size of ac and dc filters.

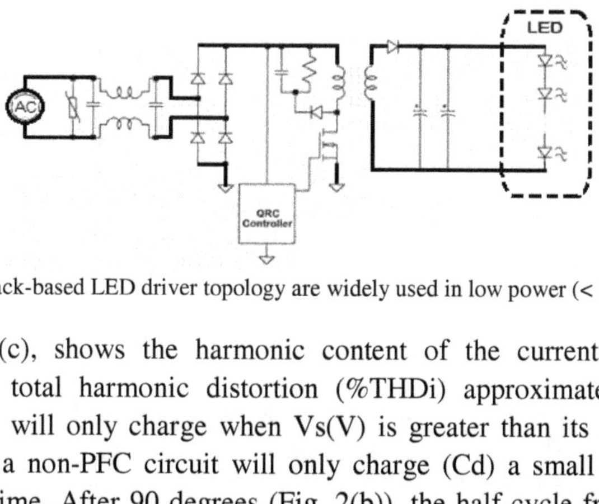

Fig. 4 Fly back-based LED driver topology are widely used in low power (< 100W) LED.

In Fig. 2(c), shows the harmonic content of the current waveform is percentage of total harmonic distortion (%THDi) approximately 84%. The capacitor (Cd) will only charge when Vs(V) is greater than its stored voltage ,meaning that a non-PFC circuit will only charge (Cd) a small percentage of overall cycle time. After 90 degrees (Fig. 2(b)), the half cycle from the bridge drops below the capacitor voltage (Cd), which back biases the bride, inhibiting current flow into the capacitor (via Vs). In Fig. 3(c), shows the harmonic content of the current waveform is percentage of total harmonic distortion (%THDi) approximately 109%. The Power Quality (PQ) in electrical systems is regulated by IEC and EN standards, used as reference by the utilities (e.g. [4]-[6]). Therefore, a good understanding of the LEDs harmonic production characteristics becomes necessary. Many studies about the PQ issues related to the lighting devices have been addressed to analyze these problems as in [7]. In Fig. 4, Show diagram Fly back-based LED driver topology are widely used in low power

(<100W) LED lighting applications primarily because of their low cost, simplicity (low part count), and acceptable performance. At higher power levels, however, these topologies become impractical, forcing designers to increase the complexity of their designs (e.g., increasing switch count), as in reference [8].

3. Phase-Modular Y-Rectifier

Owning to prevalence of power electronics system, many problems with regard to diode rectifiers, one of problems is a low input power factor, and another is current harmonics. These are reasons reduce the harmonic component of the input current, as in reference (e.g. [9]-[11]. The requirement placed on active PFC rectifier system can thus be summarized as follows: the Standard EN 6100-3-2 if < 16A and EN 6100-3-4 if > 16A,The harmonics <5% at rated power is often required, ohmic fundamental mains behavior (cos(ϕ)>0.99), compliance with specifications regarding electromagnetic, especially conducted interference emissions by means of suitable EMI filtering. The output dc voltage relative to the main voltage, a system with boost type, buck type, buck-boost-type characteristic has to be provided.

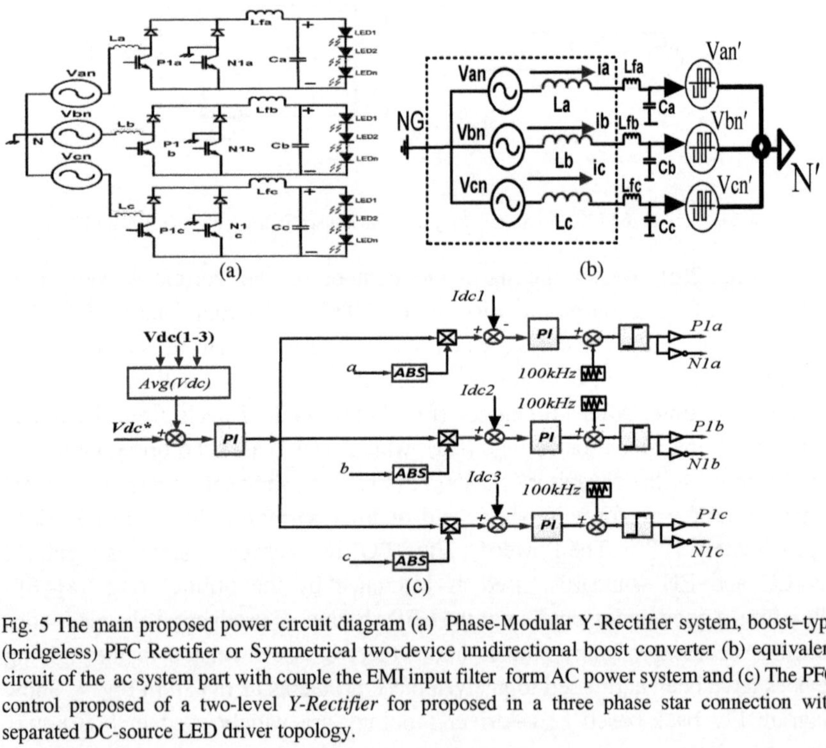

Fig. 5 The main proposed power circuit diagram (a) Phase-Modular Y-Rectifier system, boost–type (bridgeless) PFC Rectifier or Symmetrical two-device unidirectional boost converter (b) equivalent circuit of the ac system part with couple the EMI input filter form AC power system and (c) The PFC control proposed of a two-level *Y-Rectifier* for proposed in a three phase star connection with separated DC-source LED driver topology.

As shows in Fig. 5(b), the equivalent circuit of the ac system part with the EMI input filter (Lf , C) form connection power spurce, the ac currents is via the differences of the mains phase voltages to formed at the input of the rectifier stages shows in Eq (1). An offset of the reference phase voltage values (Va,Vb,Vc) is formed which, however, cannot be set by the phase current controllers because of the free star-point N, ia + ib + ic = 0 is unalterable. The phase currents thus keep their sinusoidal shape and the symmetry to the time axis.

$$\frac{d}{dt}(Ia + Ib + Ic) = 0 \tag{1}$$

The star-point voltage u(N′ GN) with consideration of and the star-point N′ is not connected to an artificial star-point, which could be formed e.g. by filter capacitors, a switching frequency voltage U(N′ GN) occurs between N′ and the mains star-point GN consideration of results shows in Eq (2) and Eq (3), Remark, voltage drop in the EMI filter (Lf, C) is three phase not shows equation due to not take in to consideration.

$$\mathrm{U}\left(\mathrm{N'GN}\right) = -\frac{1}{3}(Ua\mathrm{N'} + Ub\mathrm{N'} + Uc\mathrm{N'}) \tag{2}$$

$$\begin{aligned} La\frac{d}{dt}Ia &= UaGN - (Ua\mathrm{N'} + U\mathrm{N'}GN) \\ Lb\frac{d}{dt}Ib &= UbGN - (Ub\mathrm{N'} + U\mathrm{N'}GN) \\ Lc\frac{d}{dt}Ic &= UcGN - (Uc\mathrm{N'} + U\mathrm{N'}GN) \end{aligned} \tag{3}$$

The dimensionless index of the total harmonic distortion (THD) present and it is defined, The total harmonic distortion of a signal is for current and voltage respectively.

$$THD_V = \frac{\left(V_2{}^2 + V_3{}^2 + V_4{}^2 + \ldots Vn^n\right)^{1/2}}{V_1}, \quad THD_i = \frac{\left(I_2{}^2 + I_3{}^2 + I_4{}^2 + \ldots In^n\right)^{1/2}}{I_1} \tag{4}$$

The apparent power is decomposed into fundamental apparent power (*S1*), current distortion power *(DI)*, voltage distortion power *(DV)*, and harmonic apparent power (S_H).

$$S_1 = V_1.I_1\,,\; P_1 = V_1.I_1\cos\varphi_1\,,\; Q_1 = V_1.I_1\sin\varphi_1\,,$$

$$D_I = V_1.\left(I_2^{\,2} + I_3^{\,2} + I_4^{\,2} + ...In^n\right)^{1/2},\ D_V = \left(V_2^{\,2} + V_3^{\,2} + V_4^{\,2} + ...Vn^n\right)^{1/2}.I_1 \quad (5)$$

$$S_H = \left(V_2^{\,2} + V_3^{\,2} + V_4^{\,2} + ...Vn^n\right)^{1/2}.\left(I_2^{\,2} + I_3^{\,2} + I_4^{\,2} + ...In^n\right)^{1/2} \quad (6)$$

Combining them Eq (5), Eq (6) consist of, current distortion power, voltage distortion power and harmonic apparent power are related to the voltage and/or current distortion, it is possible to define the non-fundamental apparent power (S_N).

$$S_N = \left(D_I^{\,2} + D_V^{\,2} + S_H^{\,2}\right)^{1/2} \quad (7)$$

In Fig. 5(a), as shows the few circuit diagrams of Phase-Modular Y-Rectifier DC-link and the control strategy Phase-Modular Y-Rectifier SPWM rectifiers. This new breed of AC/DC converters gives excellent power quality indices like nearly unity input power factor, negligible THD in source current, reduced ripple factor of load voltage and fast-regulated load voltage. It is employed to reduce the dc-link voltage ripple supply currents, even in the case of unbalanced as reference in (e.g. [12] - [14]). The control technique proposed used in the rectifier is the One Cycle Control, consideration in Fig. 5(c). In the negative half cycle of the line voltage where P1a is turned on, the current will flow in the reverse direction through the switch itself, and when P1a is turned off, the current will flow in the reverse direction through the antiparallel diode. In the positive half line, when N1a is turned on, the current will flow in the reverse direction through itself and, when N1a is turned off the current will flow in the reverse direction through the antiparallel diode. In Fig. 5(a) and Fig. 5(c), The proposed the control of a two-level *Y-Rectifier* in a three phase star connection with separated DC-source for power driver power LED .

4. Study Results

One method to consider begins with plotting the I–V data on a semi-log graph, indicative of the exponential nature of the current voltage relationship as shows in Fig. 6.

The parameter tester consist of the AC power about rated power 500VA, frequency 50 Hz, and Phase-Modular Y-Rectifier system with the parameter consist of switching 100kHz, EMI, L-Filter (300uH), EMI, C-Filter (1uF), the output voltage (Vdc) for power LED about (30VDC), Output (Inductor) about 0.6mH and Output (capacitor) about (470uF) and PI-controller (kp=4, ki=0.084ms). The program simulation using by MATLAB and PSIM for Power

Electronics, for realize that can solve the current power factor and reduce harmonic current.

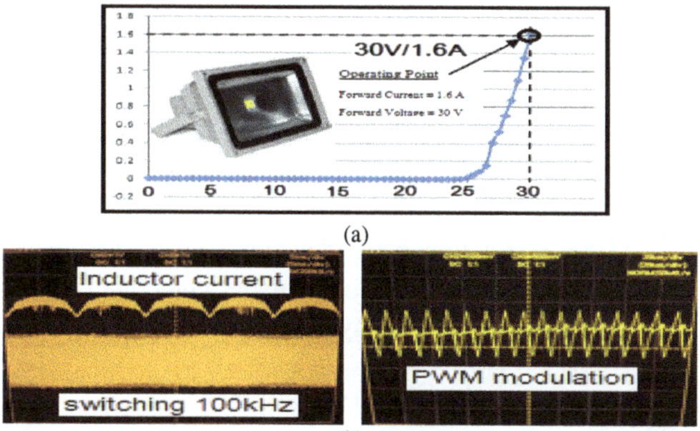

(a)

(b)

Fig. 6. (a) A typical Characteristics of operation voltage and current for a typical power LED (30V / 1.6A), current–voltage curve for an LED. Note that once the LED turns on, the current increases very quickly with increasing voltage and (b) For high performance and tested prototype in the laboratory, with continuous mode with inductor (line) current and switching frequency (on-off) about 100kHz

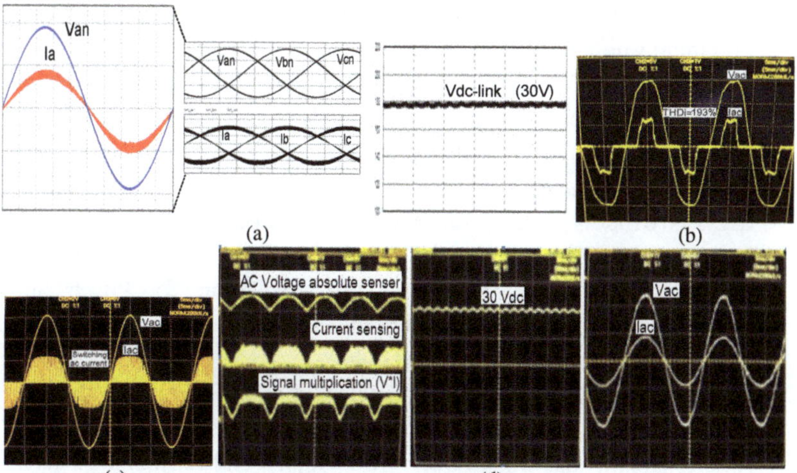

(a) (b)

(c) (d)

Fig. 7. Phase-Modular Y-Rectifier system, boost–type (bridgeless) PFC Rectifier Data collected by MATLAB and PSIM simulation are used in comparison with the experimental tester of results. (a) Results of Simulation, voltages and line current and output voltage (Vdc-link), (b) Before implements with experimental of results of depicts the effects of current quality this circuit with the single phase rectifies (4 - pulses) being delivered to a power factor corrected supply for a non-PFC unit (c) Experimental of results switching ac current with continuous mode with inductor (line) current and switching frequency (on-off) about 100kHz and (d) this sensor consist of feed forward voltage (ABS), and current feedback (Idc), the output voltage (Vdc-link) per set and AC input current power factor and harmonic current reduced vie voltages (Phase) and current (line).

5. Conclusion

This work presents described proposed Phase-Modular Y-Rectifier system, boost–type (bridgeless) PFC Rectifier. The control can make it the input ac line current of LED driver topology. For high performance method and tested of the result for realize that can solve power factor and reduce harmonic current. The research papers, conclusions for study and evaluate the circuit can be operation and suitable for use with power LED 50 W(LED lamp) per phase, the LED package Surface Mouth Type rated 30 Vdc/1.65A (phase-Phase) The data collected by MATLAB Simulation are used in comparison with the experimental tester of results. In addition, this study also provides guideline to further analyze and improve power quality in electrical system.

References

1. Availabal,http://www.uctv.tv/shows/Unleashing-the-Light-Lightingthe-World- Ep-3-24740.
2. Light Emitting Diode, Available:http://en.wikipedia.org/wiki/Light-emitting_diode.
3. Bessho, M. and Shimizu, K., Latest trends in LED lighting, Electronics & Communication in Japan, Vol. 95, Issue 1, Dec 2011.
4. IEC EN 61000-3-2: Electromagnetic Compatibility, Part 3, Section 2, Limits for Harmonic Current Emissions (Equipment Input Current ≤16 A per Phase), ed. 3; International Electro technical Commission (IEC), Geneva, Switzerland, 2011.
5. IEC EN 61000-4-7: Electromagnetic Compatibility (EMC), Testing and Measurement Techniques, General Guide on Harmonics and Interharmonics Measurements and Instrumentation, for Power Supply Systems and Equipment Connected Thereto; International Electrotechnical Commission, Geneva, Switzerland, 2002.
6. Voltage Characteristics in Public Distribution Systems, EN 50160; CENELEC, Brussels, Belgium, 1999.
7. Alberto Dolara and Sonia Leva, Power Quality and Harmonic Analysis of End User Devices, *Energies* 2012.
8. Pantaleone, G. Power electronics in public lighting systems: Are LEDs the only viable solution. *Power Syst. Des. Eur.* 2007, *4*, 42–44.
9. T. Noguchi, H. Tomiki, S. Kondo, and I. Takahashi, "Intantaneous Active and Reactive Power Control of PWM converter by using Switching Table", IEEJ Trans. onInd. App., Vol. 116, No. 2, 1996.

10. Bhim Singh, Brij N. Singh, Ambrish Chandra, Kamal AI-Haddad, Ashish Pandey and Dwarka P. Kothari, "A Review of Three-Phase Improved Power Quality AC-DC Converters" IEEE Transactions on industrial electronics, Vol. 51, No. 3, June 2004.
11. J.W. Kolar, T. Friedli and M. Hartmann, "Three-phase PFC rectifier And ac-ac converter systems – Part I, Tutorial," in *presented at 26th IEEE Applied Power Electronics Conf. and Exposition APEC'11.*, APEC'11, Mar. 6–10, 2011.
12. Bhim Singh, Brij N. Singh, Ambrish Chandra, Kamal Al-Haddad, Ashish Pandey, Dwarka P. Kothari, "A Review of Single-PhaseImproved Power Quality AC–DC Converters" IEEE Transactions on Industrial Electronics, Vol. 50, No. 5, October 2003.
13. Bhim Singh, Brij N. Singh, Ambrish Chandra, Kamal Al-Haddad, Ashish Pandey, Dwarka P. Kothari, "A Review of three-phase Improved Power Quality AC–DC Converters" IEEE Transactions on Industrial Electronics, Vol. 51, No. 3, October 2004.
14. T. Noguchi, H. Tomiki, S. Kondo and I. Takahashi, "Intantaneous Active and Reactive Power Control of PWM converter by using Switching Table", IEEJ Trans. on Ind. App., Vol. 116, No. 2.

Undermine Intelligent Gas Detection Car Based on INS/WSN and Algorithm Implementation

Zhe Yan[1,a], Yuting Zhu[1,b], Hualin Huang[1], Changwang Yuan[1] and Xiyuan Chen[1,2,c]

[1]*School of Instrument Science and Engineering, Southeast University,*
[2]*Key Laboratory of Micro-Inertial Instrument and Advanced Navigation Technology of Ministry of Education*
Southeast University, Nanjing, China
[a]*seuyanzhe@163.com*, [b]*zhuyuting940826@gmail.com*, [c]*chxiyuan@seu.edu.cn*

This paper introduces a design of smart car which is used for gas detection and positioning under coal mine. The smart car uses INS/WSN integrated technology based on extended Kalman filter, thus overcoming the drawbacks of INS/WSN separate navigation and improving the positioning accuracy. Both the hardware and the software of this smart car will be described. The actual simulation results show that compared with INS and WSN, the INS/WSN integrated navigation system has an obvious improvement in positioning precision. In the simulated condition, the measurement of mine gas concentration and the accurate location of the system can be achieved.

Keywords: Gas detection and positioning; INS/WSN integrated navigation; extended kalman filter.

1. Introduction

Nowadays, all kinds of unexpected production safety accident occur frequently. Among them, the mine gas leakage and explosion attracts people's attention especially. People desperately hope to know the real-time gas concentration under the mine so that when a danger occurs, relevant measures can be taken quickly around the danger position.

In this paper, a kind of smart car designed to detect the gas concentration and position itself under mine is introduced. The INS navigation technology cannot navigate precisely for a long time because the error accumulates over time. [1-5] Though GPS/INS integrated navigation technology is quite common and mature now, the GPS signal cannot be sent or received undermine. [2]

Wireless sensor network (WSN) shows great advantages in indoor area. However, the range and precision of WSN navigation are often limited by the layout of network nodes. Therefore, INS/WSN integrated navigation method based on extended Kalman filter can effectively solve the problem above and realize accurate positioning undermine.

2. Working Principle and Construction

In this system, a Freescale smart car model is used as a mobile platform. And a SS5100 gas sensor is used as the core of detection module. INS/WSN integrated navigation technology is used to realize the complementary advantages of these two kinds of navigation technology. Besides, to convey the concentration and position of gas undermine, both ZigBee and GSM are used [3, 5-6]. Figure 1 shows the system construction and Figure 2 shows the communication system.

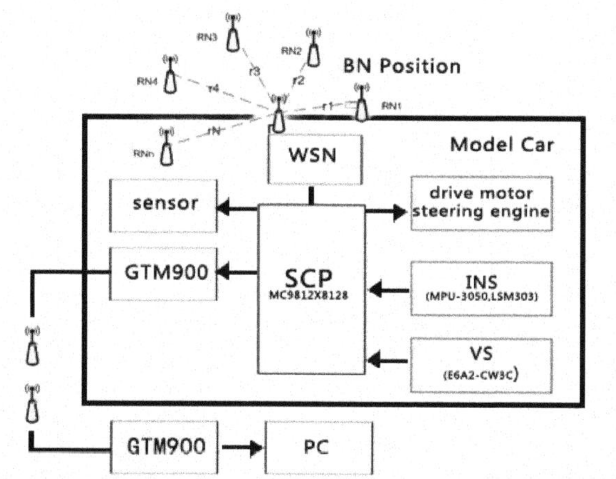

Fig. 1 System construction.

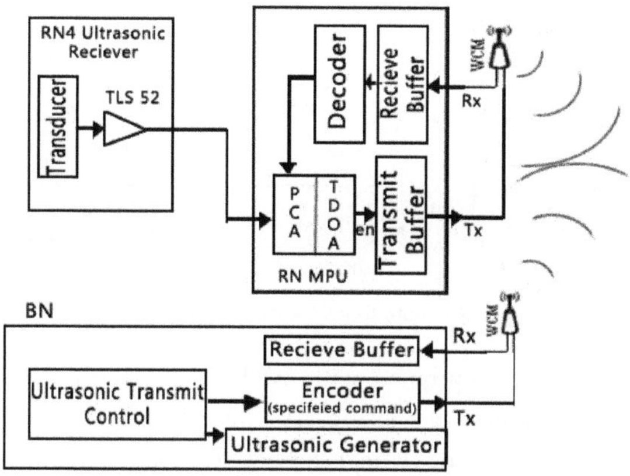

Fig. 2 Communication system.

Map matching algorithm and process

(1) Acquiring position information transmitted by ZigBee/GSM.
(2) Applying vertical projection algorithm in relative distance between reference node and anchor point to calculate accurate 3D location results.
(3) Matching above results to show in 3D electronic map.

3. INS/WSN Integrated Navigation

The integrated navigation model is divided into two parts, training area and adaptive compensation area. In the area equipped with sensor nodes (training area), both the WSN and INS navigation systems work. Firstly, WSN provides relative position information calculated from the measurement of distances to unknown nodes. And the INS navigation technology is applied for absolute position information. Then, the extended Kalman are used for data fusion to get an ideal position data. Meanwhile, WSN and INS error mathematical model are used to establish a new mathematical model of integrated navigation error.

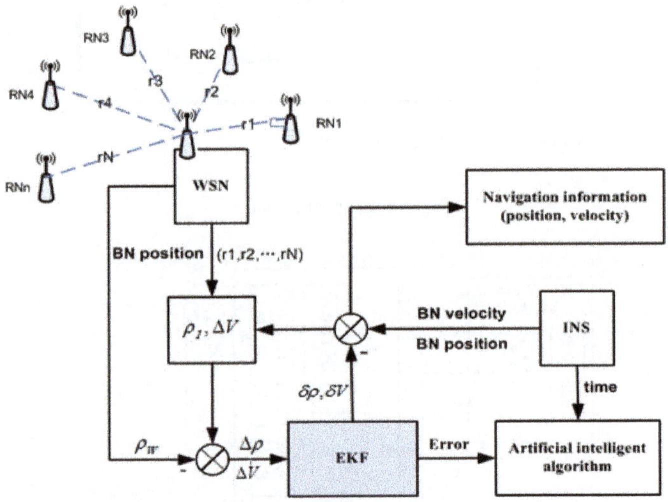

Fig. 3 Construction of integrated navigation system.

When out of the area equipped with WSN, the system will enter into the adaptive compensation area (seen in Fig. 4). Only INS can be depended on. The INS uses training error mathematical model to make compensation for the measurement of absolute positioning information. It avoids precision problems caused by the deficiency of WSN. [7-9]

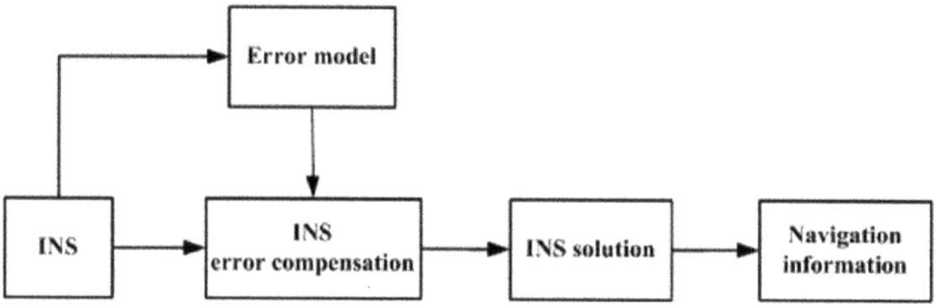

Fig. 4 Navigation in adaptive compensation area.

4. Extended Kalman Filter (EKF)

The ordinary Kalman filter is used when the process and measurement are linear, and the error is in accordance with Gaussian distribution. The introduced navigation system is certainly a non-linearity problem. So extended Kalman filter is used to realize the linearization of nonlinear part. [8-9]

4.1. *Linearization of nonlinear system*

The system model is established on the characteristics of system: [8-10]

$$\dot{x}(t) = f(x(t),t) + g(x(t),t)w(t) \tag{1}$$

$$z(t) = C(x(t),t) + v(t) \tag{2}$$

Among them

$$E(w(t)) = 0, Cov(w(t), w(\tau)) = Q(t)\delta(t-\tau) \tag{3}$$

$$E(v(t)) = 0, Cov(v(t), v(\tau)) = R(t)\delta(t-\tau) \tag{4}$$

$$Cov(w(t), v(\tau)) = 0 \tag{5}$$

Assuming that the filter estimates of system state x have been acquired at time t, the algorithm starts with linearization near the new estimation results, then expand the sum into Taylor series. After that ignore the second order and higher order term to get linear equation: [8-10]

$$\dot{x}(t) = F(t)x(t) + u(t) + G(t)w(t) \tag{6}$$

$$z(t) = H(t)x(t) + y(t) + v(t) \tag{7}$$

Among them

$$F(t) = \frac{\partial f(\hat{x}(t),t)}{\partial \hat{x}(t)} \tag{8}$$

$$H(t) = \frac{\partial C(\hat{x}(t),t)}{\partial \hat{x}(t)} \tag{9}$$

$$G(t) = g(\hat{x}(t),t) \tag{10}$$

$$u(t) = f(\hat{x}(t),t) - \frac{\partial f(\hat{x}(t),t)}{\partial \hat{x}(t)}\hat{x}(t) \tag{11}$$

$$y(t) = h(\hat{x}(t),t) - \frac{\partial C(\hat{x}(t),t)}{\partial \hat{x}(t)}\hat{x}(t) \tag{12}$$

4.2. *Algorithm of extended Kalman filter*

The extended Kalman filter is divided into prediction and correction. The core algorithm can be explained by the following equations. [10]

State estimation equation:

$$\dot{\hat{x}}(t) = F(\hat{x}(t),t) + K(t)[z(t) - C(\hat{x}(t),t)] \tag{13}$$

Gain equation:

$$K(t) = P(t)H^T(\hat{x}(t),t)R^{-1}(t) \tag{14}$$

Error covariance equations:

$$\dot{P}(t) = F(\hat{x}(t),t)P(t) + P(t)F^T(\hat{x}(t),t) + G(t)Q(t)G^T(t) - K(t)R(t)K^T(t) \tag{15}$$

5. Simulations

WSN/INS integrated navigation can keep a high precision through the simulation. The fluctuations at a particular point are in Gaussian distribution. So they are simulated by giving a zero-mean Gaussian random signal to system.

When the changes of real coordinates conform to the constant function ($y=5$, $0<x<10$), it can be seen clearly in Fig. 5 that the errors of two positioning systems are within the scope of 1 cm. But the integrated navigation is more accurate. Though the positioning precision of INS/WSN integrated navigation is kind of low at first, the function is in convergence soon.

When the changes of real coordinates conform to the linear first-order function ($y=x+1$, $0<x<10$), its simulation results can be seen in Fig. 6. The precision of WSN and INS navigation decreases while the integrated navigation still keeps a high positioning precision.

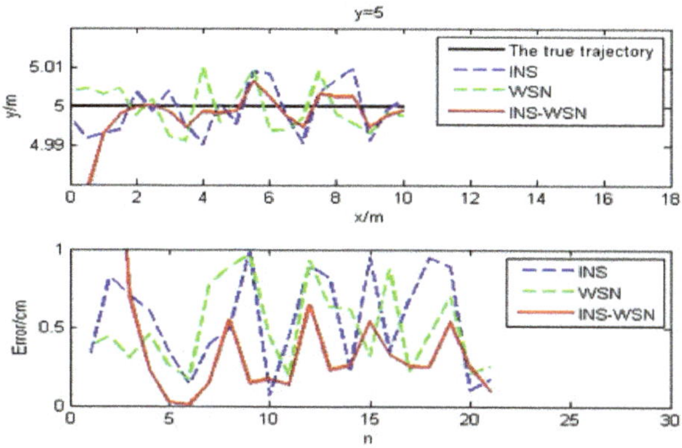

Fig. 5 Result and error of constant function positioning.

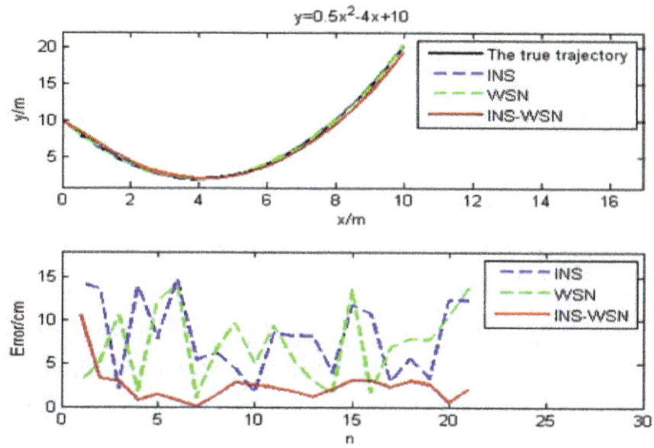

Fig. 6 Result and error of linear first-order function positioning.

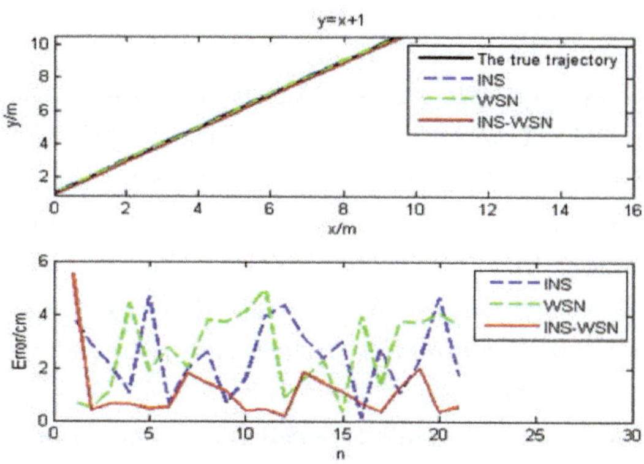

Fig. 7 Result and error of quadratic function positioning.

When the changes of real coordinates conform to the quadratic function ($y = 0.5x^2 - 4x + 10$, $0<x<10$), its simulation results can be seen in Fig 7. The fluctuation of precision is fierce in WSN and INS navigation. But the precision of integrated navigation is still high.

The simulation results above show the random error can be effectively reduced by applying the extended Kalman filter.

References

1. Retscher G and Fu Q. *An intelligent personal navigator integrating GNSS, RFID and INS for continuous position determination*. Boletim de Ciéncias Geodésicas, 2009, 15(5): 707–724.
2. Filyashkin, N.K., Yatskivsky, V.S. *Prediction of inertial navigation system error dynamics in INS/GPS system Actual Problems of Unmanned Air Vehicles Developments Proceedings (APUAVD)*, 2013 IEEE 2nd International Conference, 2013: 206-209.
3. Liu jianwei, HuiSale. *The study of ZigBee networking with wireless sensor*, Consumer Electronics, Communications and Networks (CECNet), 2012 2nd International Conference on 2012,1488-1492.
4. Fang S H and Lin T N. *Cooperative multi-radio localization in heterogeneous wireless networks*. IEEE Transactions on Wireless Communications, 2010, 9(5): 1547–1551.
5. You Ke, Liu Ruiqiang, Zhang Cuixia, *Work mode of ZigBee WSN*. Information Management, Innovation Management and Industrial Engineering, 2008. ICIII'08. International Conference on, 2008, 2: 536-538.
6. Guifen Gu, Guili Peng, *The survey of GSM wireless communication system. Computer and Information Application (ICCIA)*, 2010 International Conference on, 2010, 121-124.
7. Liu H, Darabi H, Baneoee P, et al. *Survey of wireless indoor positioning techniques and systems*. IEEE Transactions on Systems, Man and Cybernetics—Part C: Applications and Reviews, 2007, 37(6): 1067–1080.
8. Xu Y and Chen X Y. *Tightly-coupled model for INS/WSN integrated navigation based on Kalman filter*. Journal of Southeast University (English Edition), 2011, 27(4): 384–387.
9. LI Q H, Chen X Y, and Xu Y. *Distributed $H\infty$ fusion filter design for INS/WSN integrated positioning system*. Journal of Southeast University (English Edition), 2012, 28(2): 164 - 168.
10. KALMAN R. *A new approach to linear filtering and Prediction problems* [J]. Journal of Basic Engineering, 1960, 82(1): 35-40.

Analysis of Dynamic Characteristics of Micro-Gas Turbine Rotor System Based on Three-Dimensional Finite Element Method and Component Mode Synthesis

Zhaoli Zheng
Key Laboratory of Thermal Fluid Science and Engineering, Ministry of Education, School of Energy and Power Engineering, Xi'an Jiaotong University, Shaanxi, Xi'an, China
E-mail: 664311537@qq.com

Zhongyang Shen
School of Energy and Power Engineering, Xi'an Jiaotong University, Shaanxi, Xi'an, China
E-mail: 978215031@qq.com

Di Zhang
Key Laboratory of Thermal Fluid Science and Engineering, Ministry of Education, School of Energy and Power Engineering, Xi'an Jiaotong University, Shaanxi, Xi'an, China
E-mail: zhang_di@mail.xjtu.edu.cn

In this paper, the dynamic characteristics of a Micro-gas Turbine rotor system were studied by the CMS (component mode synthesis). Four types of analytical models were prepared to test the CMS, of which the results valid the accuracy and efficiency of proposed method. Modal analysis of the rotor system indicates that effects of stress stiffening have greater impact on dynamic frequency than spin softening and the frequency corresponding to the blade modes is reduced due to the effect of the shaft. Results indicate that component mode synthesis is more efficient in solving large scale problem.

Keywords: Micro-gas turbine; component mode synthesis; rotor dynamics; prestressed modal analysis.

1. Introduction

As one kind of power propulsion system with high energy density ratio, Micro turbine engine (MTE) plays an increasingly vital role in various types of unmanned aerial vehicles, cruise missiles and other mini-aircrafts [1]. The rotor system is a crucial component of MTE. Its stability and dynamic performance directly affects the working state and service life of the engine, so that it will have significant research values and application prospects in the future. The increasing complexity of rotor systems offers unique challenges for engineers, and fixed-interface component mode synthesis was proposed against that background. The component mode synthesis method, first proposed by Hurty [2], has significant condensation advantages, and it is well suited for modeling and simulation of large and complex systems [3, 4, 5].

2. Component Mode Synthesis

Component mode synthesis is a method adopted in substructure analysis. It reduces the system matrices to a smaller set of interface DOFs between substructures and truncated sets of normal mode generalized coordinates. For a damped system, the matrix equation of motion is:

$$Mu''+Cu'+Ku=F \tag{1}$$

Partitioning the matrix equation into interface and interior DOFs:

$$u=\begin{bmatrix} u_m \\ u_s \end{bmatrix}, M=\begin{bmatrix} M_{mm} & M_{ms} \\ M_{sm} & M_{ss} \end{bmatrix}, C=\begin{bmatrix} C_{mm} & C_{ms} \\ C_{sm} & C_{ss} \end{bmatrix}, K=\begin{bmatrix} K_{mm} & K_{ms} \\ K_{sm} & K_{ss} \end{bmatrix}, F=\begin{bmatrix} F_m \\ F_s \end{bmatrix}$$

where subscripts m refers to master DOFs defined only on interface nodes and s refers to all DOFs that are not master DOFs. The physical displacement vector u may be represented in terms of component generalized coordinates as in Eq. (2) [6].

$$u=\begin{bmatrix} u_m \\ u_s \end{bmatrix}=T\begin{bmatrix} u_m \\ \gamma_\delta \end{bmatrix} \tag{2}$$

where and are truncated set of generalized modal coordinates and transformation matrix of fixed-interface method [7], respectively. After applying the transformation in Eq. (2) into the matrix equation of motion Eq. (1), the equation of motion in the reduced space is obtained. The reduced stiffness, mass, and damping matrices and the reduced force vector of the CMS will be:

$$\bar{K}=T^T KT,\quad \bar{M}=T^T MT,\quad \bar{C}=T^T CT,\quad \bar{F}=T^T F \tag{3}$$

3. Results and Discussion

To test component modal synthesis, four types of analytical models were prepared. These models are all integrated circle blades of second stage compressor, as illustrated in Fig. 1. Model 1-3 are divided into four, ten and twenty components, respectively. For comparison, a calculation by conventional method was carried out.

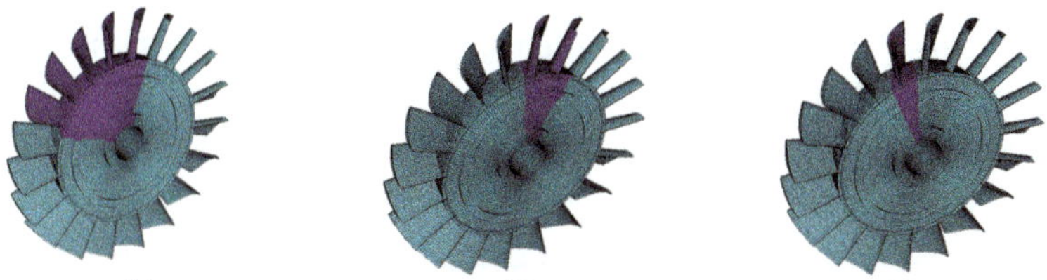

(a) (b) (c)

Fig. 1 Model 1 (a), model 2 (b), model 3 (c).

Table 1 gives the frequencies obtained by the four models indicated previously and the CPU time of computations in solving these problems. As shown in Table 1, results of the first three models agree with the results of comparison very well, which valid the accuracy of CMS. Model 1-3 reduces the CPU time by 44.1%, 72.3%, 67.7% when compared to the conventional method, which confirming the efficiency of CMS.

Table 1 Results for the four different models.

Model	Mode number								CPU time [minute]	CPU time Reduction
	1	2	3	4	5	6	7	8		
Model 1	8644	8817	8817	8887	8887	8976	8976	90 02	66.3	55.9%
Model 2	8644	8817	8817	8887	8887	8976	8976	90 02	32.9	27.7%
Model 3	8644	8817	8817	8887	8887	8976	8976	90 02	38.3	32.3%
Comparison	8644	8817	8817	8887	8887	8976	8976	90 02	118.7	100%

Even for the same model, different numbers of components causes different CPU time. Generally, the CPU time decreased when the number of components increased. But the CPU time will increased when the number of components goes over a specific amount. This is because the number of master DOFs in the interfaces between every tow components increased when the number of components increased. Master DOFs in the interfaces of model 1-3 are 5624, 8780 and 14040, respectively. The number will become larger and larger which can extends CPU time. Thus, it is very necessary to determine an appropriate number of components.

Finite element model of rotor system is divided into four components and is illustrated in Fig. 2. Static and dynamic frequencies of the rotor system obtained by the proposed method are listed in Table 2. Results in Table 2 shows that dynamic frequency under the speed of 6000 rpm is greater than static frequency. It means that effects of stress stiffening have greater impact on dynamic frequency than effects of spin softening. Frequency in Table 2 is smaller than that in Table 1 of the same modal shape, which indicates that the frequency corresponding to the blade modes is reduced due to the effect of the shaft.

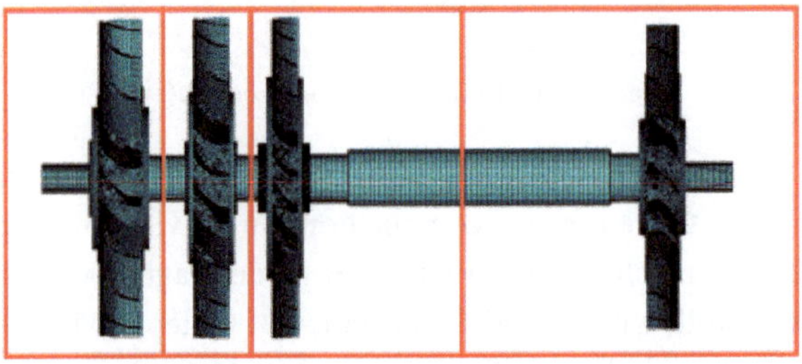

Fig. 2 Finite element model of rotor system.

Table 2 Static and dynamic frequency of rotor system.

Iterms	Mode number							
	1	2	3	4	5	6	7	8
Static frequency	1970	4575	6726	6990	6991	7064	7064	7095
Dynamic frequency	1972	4576	6728	6992	6993	7066	7066	7097

Also for comparison, the CPU time required in solving the whole problem by conventional method and proposed method are listed in Table 3. These results shows that component mode synthesis reduces the CPU time by 68.6% when compared to the conventional method, which means that component mode synthesis is more efficient in solving large scale problem.

Table 3 CPU time in solving problem using the CMS and conventional method.

Model	CPU time [hour]	CPU time Reduction
Conventional method	11.8	100%
CMS	3.7	68.6%

4. Conclusions

In the study of the dynamic characteristics of a Micro-gas Turbine rotor system by the CMS (component mode synthesis) method, major results can be summarized as follows:

(1) The CPU time decreased when the number of components increased unless this number reaches a threshold value.

(2) Modal analysis of the rotor system indicates that effects of stress stiffening have greater impact on dynamic frequency than spin softening.

(3) The frequency corresponding to the blade modes is reduced due to the effect of the shaft.

(4) Component mode synthesis is more efficient in solving large scale problem.

References

1. WENG Yi-wu, SU Ming, WENG Shi-lie. Specific Features of Advanced Micro Gas Turbines and Their Application. Prospects Journal of Engineering for Thermal Energy & Power, 2003, 18(2), 111 - 115.
2. Hurty, W. C., Dynamic Analysis of Structural System by Component Mode Synthesis, AIAA Journal, Vol. 3, No. 4, April 1965, pp. 678-685.
3. Hansteen OE, Bell K. On the accuracy of mode superposition analysis in structural dynamics. Earthquake Engng Struct Dynam 1979; 7: 405.
4. Hurty WC, Collins JD, Hart GC. Dynamic analysis of large structures by modal synthesis techniques. Comput Struct 1971; 1: 535±63.
5. Yuji Aoyama, Genki Yagawa. Component mode synthesis for large-scale structural eigenanalysis [J], Computers and Structures, 2001, 79: 605-615
6. R. R. Craig. A Review of Time Domain and Frequency Domain Component Mode Synthesis Methods. International Journal of Analytical and Experimental Modal Analysis. Vol. 12, No. 2. 59-72. 1987.
7. R. R. Craig and M. D. D. Bampton. Coupling of Substructures for Dynamic Analysis. AIAA Journal. Vol. 12. 1313-1319. 1968.

A New Method of Failure Analysis of the Feed System of CNC Milling Machine Based on Triangular Fuzzy Number

Wang Xian-zhi, Rui Zhi-yuan and Ren Li-na

Engineering Research Center of Nonferrous Metallurgy's New Equipment, Ministry of Education, Lanzhou University of Technology, 730050, China
School of Mechanical and Electronical Engineering, Lanzhou University of Technology, Lanzhou, 730050, China
*E-mail: cagallilan@163.com

In order to solve the problem that classical criticality analysis can't indicate randomness and fuzziness of mechanical failure, a new method of failure analysis is presented based on triangular fuzzy number. Considering influence of fault frequency, maintenance costs, maintenance time, fault effect, decision matrix is established with triangular fuzzy number. In order to reduce subjective influence of determining weights by experts directly, linear programming equations are established to obtain weights by Hausdorff distance. Finally, through establishing possibility degree matrix at different levels of risk attitude, criticality rank of each failure mode is obtained. Taking a case study of XK7132 CNC milling machines, the results show that bearing failure is the most hazardous failure mode. Compared with classical criticality analysis, method in this paper is more scientific and reasonable, and provides a theoretical basis for improving reliability of CNC milling machine.

Keywords: CNC milling machine; feed system; failure analysis; triangular fuzzy number; hausdorff distance.

1. Introduction

With CNC milling machine to develop in the direction of high speed and high precision, people also requires it to have high reliability [1]. According to custom's feedback data, the highest failure rate subsystem of CNC milling machine is feed system. Therefore, improving reliability of CNC milling machine feed system is a inescapable way to improve reliability of CNC milling machine. However, due to diversification of failure modes of feed system, it is unrealistic to treat all failure modes in the same way. Thus, finding out the most important failure mode of feed system cannot be waited.

FMECA (FMECA: Failure Mode, Effect, and Criticality Analysis) is a commonly method to analysis failure mode, effects and criticality. However, the

---

* Email to the Corresponding author.

complexity of mechanical components in feed system, and the randomness and fuzziness of mechanical failure, make the results of classical criticality analysis deviate from the practical [2]. In view of this, many studies combine fuzzy theory with FMECA to indicate the randomness and fuzziness of fault [3-5]. But there are also many defects in these methods. Firstly, due to the influence of subjective intention, and the influence of the low resolution of the Hamming distance and Euclidean distance for fuzzy sets, the weight is not realistic [6]. Secondly, using a certain number to quantify language can not accurately reflect the real situation of feed system in the process of evaluation. Thirdly, all these methods are limited to the influence of fault mode ratio, failure-effect probability and failure rate, ignoring the maintenance costs and other factors. Aiming at these problems, a new method of failure analysis is proposed.

2. Triangular Fuzzy Number

Triangular fuzzy number is a fuzzy number which is used to express uncertain information [7]. The triangular fuzzy number $\tilde{a}=(a^{\mathrm{L}},a^{\mathrm{M}},a^{\mathrm{U}})$ will be taken to mean a uncertain number $\tilde{a}$ between a^{L} and a^{U}, and its most possible value will be a^{M}. When $a^{\mathrm{L}}=a^{\mathrm{M}}=a^{\mathrm{U}}$, the triangular fuzzy number degenerates to a certain number.

Definition [8]: Let $\tilde{a}=(a^{\mathrm{L}},a^{\mathrm{M}},a^{\mathrm{U}})$, $\tilde{b}=(b^{\mathrm{L}},b^{\mathrm{M}},b^{\mathrm{U}})$ be two triangular fuzzy numbers, while $d_h(\tilde{a},\tilde{b})$ is the Hausdorff distance between $\tilde{a}$ and $\tilde{b}$. $d_h(\tilde{a},\tilde{b})$ could be calculated as below:

$$d_h(\tilde{a},\tilde{b})=\max\left\{\left|a^{\mathrm{L}}-b^{\mathrm{L}}\right|,\left|a^{\mathrm{M}}-b^{\mathrm{M}}\right|,\left|a^{\mathrm{U}}-b^{\mathrm{U}}\right|\right\} \tag{1}$$

Definition [8]: Fundamental calculate principles of triangular fuzzy number can be listed as below:

$$\tilde{a}\times\tilde{b}=(a^{\mathrm{L}}b^{\mathrm{L}},a^{\mathrm{M}}b^{\mathrm{M}},a^{\mathrm{U}}b^{\mathrm{U}}) \tag{2}$$

$$\tilde{a}+\tilde{b}=(a^{\mathrm{L}}+b^{\mathrm{L}},a^{\mathrm{M}}+b^{\mathrm{M}},a^{\mathrm{U}}+b^{\mathrm{U}}) \tag{3}$$

Definition [8]: Probability of $\tilde{a}\geq\tilde{b}$ can be indicated as $p(\tilde{a}\geq\tilde{b})$, and can be calculated as following:

$$\begin{aligned}p(\tilde{a}\geq\tilde{b})=\lambda\max\left\{1-\max\left[\frac{b^{\mathrm{M}}-a^{\mathrm{L}}}{a^{\mathrm{M}}-a^{\mathrm{L}}+b^{\mathrm{M}}-b^{\mathrm{L}}},0\right],0\right\}\\+(1-\lambda)\max\left\{1-\max\left[\frac{b^{\mathrm{U}}-a^{\mathrm{M}}}{a^{\mathrm{U}}-a^{\mathrm{M}}+b^{\mathrm{U}}-b^{\mathrm{L}}},0\right],0\right\}\end{aligned} \tag{4}$$

While λ is the risk attitude of decision makers. When $\lambda = 0.5$, the decision makers hold a neutral attitude; when $\lambda > 0.5$, the decision makers pursue risk; when $\lambda < 0.5$, the decision makers hold a cautious attitude.

3. Failure Analysis Based on Triangular Fuzzy Number

The failure analysis for feed system of CNC milling machine can be taken as following steps: first, failure phenomenon should be analyzed. Second, failure cause should be found out. Third, failure frequency statistics should be made. Finally, criticality analysis should be taken. The main steps of calculation for the criticality analysis can be taken as below:

3.1. *Establish the Decision Matrix*

$X = \{x_1, x_2, \ldots, x_n\}^T$ is used to express failure mode of feed system, and $Y = \{y_1, y_2, \ldots, y_m\}$ is used to express each evaluation. The value of y_n to x_n is a_{ij}, then the decision matrix can be expressed as:

$$A = \begin{bmatrix} a_{11} & a_{12} & \cdots & a_{1m} \\ a_{21} & a_{22} & \cdots & a_{2m} \\ \vdots & \vdots & & \vdots \\ a_{n1} & a_{n2} & \cdots & a_{nm} \end{bmatrix} \tag{5}$$

3.2. *Normalize the Decision Matrix*

In order to eliminate the influence of different physical dimension, b_{ij} can be obtained by normalizing a_{ij}. It can be calculated as:

$$b_{ij}^k = \frac{1/a_{ij}^k}{\left\| 1/a_j^k \right\|} \tag{6}$$

That is:

$$\begin{cases} b_{ij}^{L} = \dfrac{1/a_{ij}^{L}}{\sqrt{\sum_{i=1}^{n}(1/a_{ij}^{U})^2}} \\ b_{ij}^{M} = \dfrac{1/a_{ij}^{M}}{\sqrt{\sum_{i=1}^{n}(1/a_{ij}^{M})^2}} \\ b_{ij}^{U} = \dfrac{a_{ij}^{U}}{\sqrt{\sum_{i=1}^{n}(1/a_{ij}^{L})^2}} \end{cases}$$

3.3. *Establish linear programming model*

$\theta = (\theta_1, \theta_2, \cdots \theta_m)$ is used to express the weight sets of $Y = \{y_1, y_2, \ldots, y_m\}$. It is inaccurate when experts give a certain number to indicate weights due to the influence of subjective intention. Thus, establishing a linear programming equation to determine weights by using a weighting interval $0 \le a_i \le \theta_i \le b_i$ which is given by experts, is closer to the practice.

But it is difficult to compare the size of two triangular fuzzy numbers b_{ij} even they are normalized. Thus, the Hausdorff distance of triangular fuzzy number is used to establish linear programming model as below:

$$\max D(\theta) = \sum_{i=1}^{m} C_i \theta_i$$

$$s.t. \begin{cases} 0 \le a_i \le \theta_i \le b_i \\ \sum_{1}^{m} \theta_i = 1 \end{cases} \tag{7}$$

while:

$$C_i = \sum_{j=1}^{n} \sum_{k=1}^{n} d_H(\tilde{b}_{ij}, \tilde{b}_{ik}) \tag{8}$$

i=1, 2, 3, ······, m

3.4. *Determine comprehensive attribute values of failure mode*

After solving $\theta = (\theta_1, \theta_2, \cdots \theta_m)$, the comprehensive attribute value of each failure mode $\widetilde{Z}_j$ should be calculated as below:

$$\widetilde{Z}_j = \left(\sum_{i=1}^{m} L_{ij}^{r}\theta_i, \sum_{i=1}^{m} M_{ij}^{r}\theta_i, \sum_{i=1}^{m} U_{ij}^{r}\theta_i \right) \tag{9}$$

j=1, 2, 3, ……, n

while:

$$\begin{cases} L_{ij}^{r} = \dfrac{\min\{b_{ij}^{\mathrm{L}}\}}{b_{ij}^{\mathrm{U}}} \\ M_{ij}^{r} = \dfrac{\min\{b_{ij}^{\mathrm{M}}\}}{b_{ij}^{\mathrm{M}}} \\ U_{ij}^{r} = \dfrac{\min\{b_{ij}^{\mathrm{U}}\}}{b_{ij}^{\mathrm{L}}} \end{cases}$$

3.5. *Establish possibility degree matrix*

$\widetilde{Z}_j$ is also a triangular fuzzy numbers, and it is still difficult to compare their size. Thus use the Eq. (4) to establish possibility degree matrix as below:

$$P_{ij} = p(\widetilde{Z}_i \geq \widetilde{Z}_j) \tag{10}$$

i=1, 2, 3, ……, m
j=1, 2, 3, ……, n

3.6. *Calculate ordinal number* f_i

In order to compare easily, the possibility degree matrix is transformed into real number f_i

$$f_i = \frac{\sum_{j=1}^{n} P_{ij} + \frac{n}{2} - 1}{n(n-1)} \tag{11}$$

i = 1, 2, 3, ……, m

Through the ordinal number f_i, rank it from big to small. The most hazardous failure mode will be the biggest f_i.

4. A Case Study

The failure data from a machine tool plant production of 73 sets of XK7132 type CNC milling machine is used for analysis in this paper. The failure frequency statistics, failure mode and failure cause are listed in the Table 1. The rank of each failure mode is determined by RPN (RPN: Risk Priority Number)in classical FMECA. That is

$$RPN = \alpha_{ij}\beta_{ij}\gamma_i \tag{12}$$

while: α_{ij} is the failure mode ratio that the component i is failed which caused by failure mode j. β_{ij} is the failure-effect probability that the component i is damaged which caused by failure mode j. It is determined from experience. It is also called the conditional probability of loss function by the national standard draft. γ_i is the failure rate of component i. That is

$$\gamma_i = \frac{N_i}{t} \tag{13}$$

while: N_i is the total failure number of component i in the stipulated time; t is the accumulated working time of component i. It is 46720h in this paper.

Through calculating the RPN, rank it from big to small. The most hazardous failure mode will be the biggest RPN.

Table 1 Failure mode, failure cause and classical FMECA analysis.

	Failure mode	Failure cause	Frequency		α	β	γ	RPN	Rank
X_1	Excessive gap	Excessive gap in X, Y, Z axis	21		0.500	0.5		2.25×10^{-4}	1
X_2	Return to zero inaccurate	Encoder error	2		0.048	0.5		2.14×10^{-5}	4
X_3	Moving parts stuck	The piston is stuck	2		0.048	0.5		2.14×10^{-5}	4
X_4	Loose	Frame loose	3	42	0.071	0.1	9×10^{-4}	6.42×10^{-6}	7
X_5	Damage of components	bearing failure	7		0.167	1		1.50×10^{-4}	2
X_6	Damage of components	screw failure	2		0.048	1		4.28×10^{-5}	3
X_7	Abnormal noises	lock nut loose	5		0.119	0.1		1.07×10^{-5}	6

In method in this paper, X_1~X_7 is used to express above failure modes. Y_1~Y_4 is used to express Failure frequency, Maintenance costs, Maintenance time and Failure Effect. The decision matrix is established as Table 2.

Normalize decision matrix according to Eq. (6). Then establish linear programming equation according to Eq. (7) and Eq. (8). While, weight interval is given by experts as below:

Table 2 Decision matrix.

	Y_1 Frequency			Y_2 Maintenance costs			Y_3 Maintenance time			Y_4 Failure Effect		
				a^L	a^M	a^U	a^L	a^M	a^U	a^L	a^M	a^U
X_1	21	21	21	0.1	1.0	1.0	2	4	5	3	4	5
X_2	2	2	2	2.0	3.0	3.5	1	2	2	1	2	3
X_3	2	2	2	0.1	1.0	3.0	1	2	4	1	2	2
X_4	3	3	3	0.1	0.1	0.1	1	1	2	1	2	2
X_5	7	7	7	1.0	1.5	1.5	1	2	3	2	3	3
X_6	2	2	2	4.0	5.0	6.0	2	4	5	2	4	5
X_7	5	5	5	0.1	0.1	0.1	1	1	2	1	3	4

$$\begin{cases} 0.15 \le \theta_1 \le 0.35 \\ 0.2 \le \theta_2 \le 0.25 \\ 0.2 \le \theta_3 \le 0.35 \\ 0.25 \le \theta_4 \le 0.35 \end{cases}$$

The result is: $\theta =$ (0.3, 0.25, 0.2, 0.25)

$\widetilde{Z}_j$ is calculated as Eq. (9). The result is:

Z_1=(0..0559, 0.3350, 4.5541)

Z_2=(0.0236, 0.2794, 0.7785)

Z_3=(0.0104, 0.1929, 4.6014)

Z_4=(0.1413, 0.6252, 1.1938)

Z_5=(0.0267, 0.2025, 0.5021)

Z_6=(0.0322, 0.3302, 0.7781)

Z_7=(0.1697, 0.8279, 1.8180)

Establish the possibility degree matrix by Eq. (10). Then calculate the ordinal number f_i by Eq. (11). While, the risk attitude of decision makers λ will be 0.3, 0.5, and 0.8 in this paper. The final result is listed as Table 3.

Table 3 Ranking of criticality at different levels of risk attitude.

	0.3		0.5		0.8		Classical
	fi	Rank	*fi*	Rank	*fi*	Rank	
X_1	0.1132	6	0.1222	5	0.1358	5	1
X_2	0.1715	2	0.1676	2	0.1618	2	4
X_3	0.1248	5	0.1396	4	0.1617	3	4
X_4	0.1265	4	0.1206	6	0.1119	6	7
X_5	0.1915	1	0.1860	1	0.1778	1	2
X_6	0.1670	3	0.1618	3	0.1541	4	3
X_7	0.1056	7	0.1021	7	0.0970	7	6

5. Analysis of the Result

As shown in Table 3, the result of method in this paper is different from the result of classical FMECA. In classical FMECA, X_1 is the most hazardous failure mode and also the highest fault frequency failure mode. But, X_5 is the most hazardous failure mode in this paper's method. The reason is that X_1 can be repaired in a short period of time, and machine can still work when the failure happened. But it will result a series effects on the other components when bearing is damaged. And it will seriously affect the processing quality and determine whether the machine can still work. Thus, the result that X_5 is the most hazardous is more reasonable. Some conclusions can be seen though above evidences: the highest fault frequency failure mode is not necessarily the most hazardous failure mode; the higher fault frequency failure mode is not necessarily hazardous than the lower fault frequency failure mode.

X_2 and X_3 tied for the fourth order which is obtained the same RPN value in classic FMECA. But these two failure mode is not parallel in the method in this paper. In engineering practice, although these two failure mode is same in fault frequency, maintenance time, and failure effect, but they are different in maintenance costs. Illustrate shows that this method avoids the same numerical, and effectively distinguish hazardous of these two kinds of failure mode.

Finally, it is concluded that the most hazardous failure mode is X_5, and its failure reason is bearing failure. In order to prolong the service life of bearing, the producer should improve the design in bearing lubrication, sealing and other conditions; users should also timely replace better bearing after failure to avoid this problem happens again.

6. Conclusions

(1) Introducing triangular fuzzy number to the failure analysis for feed system of CNC machine tools, we can indicate the randomness and fuzziness of mechanical failure much better, and can quantify language more accurately. Introducing the linear programming to determine weights, the influence of subjective intention can be reduced. Compared with classical FMECA method, this method is more accurate and scientific.

(2) Different ranking of criticality is showed at different levels of risk attitude.

(3) More attention should be paid on the hazardous failure mode in the design, manufacturing, using and maintenance. It has great significance for improving the reliability of CNC milling machine.

Acknowledgments

This work was financially supported by the National international science and technology cooperation projects (2011DFR70670), the Program for Changjiang Scholars and Innovative Research Team in University of Ministry of Education of China (IRT1140), and the youth science technology foundation of Gansu province, China (No. 145RJYA307).

References

1. Chen W, Jiang B, Jia Z C. Reliability Analysis for CNC Machining Tools during Early Failure Period, J. Material Mechanical & Manufacturing Engineering II, 2014.
2. Jia Z C, Yang Z J, Shen G X. Early Failure Mode Effect and Criticality Analysis for CNC Machining Tools, J. Applied Mechanics & Materials, 2013, 303-306: 1653-1656.
3. Ying-zhi Z, Shan Z, Gui-xiang S, et al. Criticality analysis for CNC turret adopting importance and fuzzy reasoning, J. Journal of Jilin University (Engineering and Technology Edition), 2012, 42(5): 1157-1162.
4. Zhang G B, Zhang L, Ran Y. Reliability and Failure Analysis of CNC Machine Based on Element Action, J. Applied Mechanics and Materials, 2014, 494: 354-357.
5. Yang Z, Xu B, Chen F, et al. A new failure mode and effects analysis model of CNC machine tool using fuzzy theory, J. Information and Automation, IEEE International Conference on, 2010: 582-587.
6. Xiao C. Method of Triangular Fuzzy Number Multiple Attribute Decision Making based on a New Distance Neasure, J. Jilin Normal University Journal, 2014.
7. Yu Z, Qian L, Yong L. Study on Method for Supplier Selection Based on Triangular Fuzzy Number, J. Logistics Technology, 2013.
8. Wei Guiwu. Fuzzy Information Multiple Attribute. Economic Press· CHINA. 2010.

Design of Test Platform for Piezoelectric Stick-Slip Actuator

Shuzhen Liu and Xiaofeng Zhou
Institute of Mechanical Engineering, Ningbo University of Technology,
Ningbo, 315016, China
E-mail: shuzhenl@163.com

Yubao Zhang
[2]*Institute of Information Engineering, Zhejiang Textile and Fashion College,*
Ningbo, 315211, China
E-mail: abao@163.com

Wenjun Zhang
Department of Mechanical Engineering, University of Saskatchewan, Saskatoon,
Saskatchewan, S7N 5A9, Canada
E-mail: chris.zhang@usask.ca

Piezoelectric stick-slip actuator (PSSA) is well-known by its simple configuration, minute step size, high resolution and theoretically unlimited displacement, and has been used in applications where high positioning resolution with large range of movement is required. This project designs an experimental test platform of stick-slip actuator which can be used to investigate the effects of temperature and pressure to the performance of end-effector. Embedded construction is applied for temperature sensor installation, which makes it easy to get more accurate temperature of the friction plate. A non-contact, electromagnet system is introduced in pressure adjustable mechanism. By changing the voltage direction and magnitude of coil, the pressure can be adjusted.

Keywords: Piezoelectric stick-slip actuator; pressure; temperature; test platform.

1. Introduction

Piezoelectric material has been widely used in industry, military, medical care such as micro-motor and ultrasound medical. Piezoelectric stick-slip actuators (PSSA) received a great deal attentions due to their advantages of simple configuration, minute step size, high resolution and theoretically unlimited distance [1-4]. Kang developed a model for the displacement of the end-effecter of the PSSA actuators, in which both the pre-sliding friction and the piezoelectric actuator dynamics are considered. The comparison between the model predicted and the experiment results suggests that the model developed is promising for predicting the displacement of end-effecter [5]. Peng presented a model of the end-effector displacement by taking into account the linear dynamics, hysteretic behavior of the piezoelectric actuator, and the pre-sliding friction on the end-effector [6]. This model is capable to represent the influence of applied voltage and end-effector mass on the dynamics of the end-effector. The model is applicable to the actuators in which the end-effector moves horizontally. C. Edeler etc. introduced the LuGre-model (LGM) and the Elastoplastic model (EPM) to represent the dynamics of the end-effector. Different "causes and effects" linked with friction and stick-slip conditions were discussed. Modifications of the EPM are proposed and the modified model is evaluated by simulations and measurements [7]. Li developed temperature measurement system and investigated the affection of temperature rise to the displacement of the end-effector [8-9]. It found that the temperature rise is due to both the friction at two interacting surface and the operation of the piezoelectric element. To understand the dynamics of end-effector, more efforts should be on close the gap between theoretical ideas and practical approaches. Therefore, factors affecting end-effector dynamics, such as the pressure and temperature between end- effecter and platform, should be investigated. This paper tries to make a contribution for development an experimental test platform which can be used to investigate the effects of temperature and pressure to the performance of end-effector.

2. Principle of Stick-slip Actuator

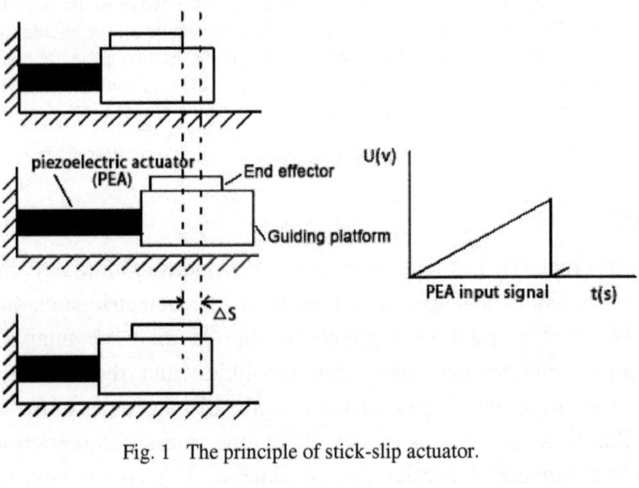

Fig. 1 The principle of stick-slip actuator.

Fig. 1 shows the typical applications of PSSA in micro and nano positioning systems. An inertial mass (end-effector) is supported by a guiding platform, which is driven by a piezoelectric actuator (PEA). During the rise of input signal, the end-effector and the guiding platform move together. However, during the rapid jump of input signal, the PEA and guiding system contract, the end-effector still moves forward due to its inertial. Therefore, the end-effector moves one step (Δs), and this step movement repeats during each cycle of the input signal.

3. Design of Test Platform

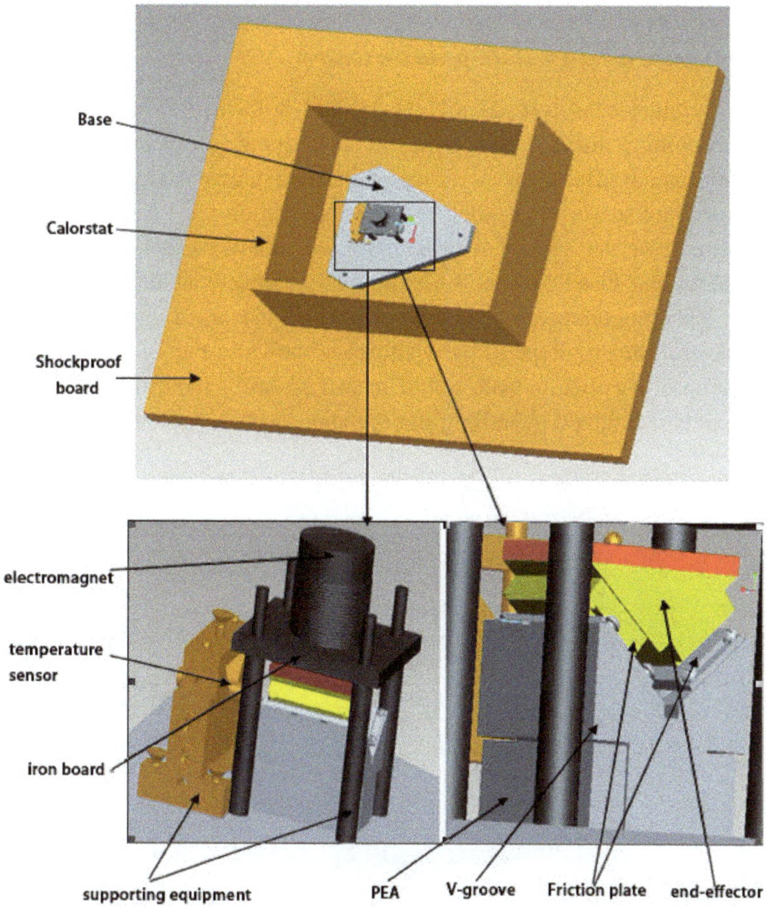

Fig. 2 Three-dimensional model of test platform of piezoelectric stick-slip actuator.

Test platform of the piezoelectric actuator was prototyped as shown in Fig. 2. This test platform was developed based on the actuator in which the end-effector moves horizontally [6]. The whole actuator is placed in a calorstat, under the bottom of which is the shockproof insulating board. The movable platform is driven by the PEA and on the platform is the end-effector, which can slide horizontally via V grooves machined on the platform. Polished silicon wafers are attached to the V grooves as frictional surfaces to ensure the uniformity of the frictional characteristics throughout the traveling range of the end-effector. On the one end of the PEA, a support frame is installed to limit moving direction of it. Arrangement design of temperature sensor and the pressure adjustable equipment will be explained in latter sections.

3.1 *Arrangement design of temperature sensor*

The temperature sensor installed in the blind hole in the end-effector [8-9] makes machining difficult. It is hard to control the depth of the bottom of the blind hole which affects the accuracy of the measurement temperature. When the temperature sensor is installed between the friction plate and the V grooves [9], it is necessary to machine wire holes for temperature sensor in the V groove. Taking into the disadvantages of these two arrangement design, this paper propose installing temperature sensor in the slots machined in the V groove of the platform. The prototype of the platform is shown in Fig. 3. By this method, temperature of the friction plate can be measured easily and drilling holes in the V grooves is substituted by milling slot in them.

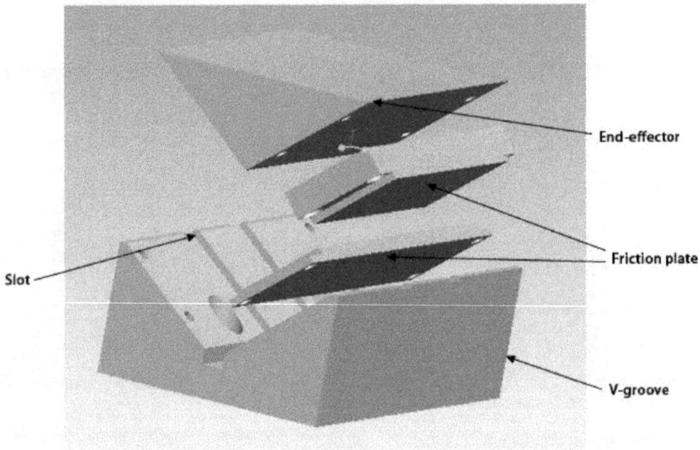

Fig. 3 Prototype of the platform with slots in V-groves.

3.2 *Design of Pressure-adjustable construction*

Electromagnet is applied in this system to adjust the pressure of end-effector actives on the friction plate. The electromagnet is placed on the support plate, which is over the end-effector and supported by four poles installed on the base. On the top of end-effector, an iron plate is sticked on make sure that electromagnet force is active to the end-effect. Changing the direction and magnitude of the voltage on the coil, the pressure acted by the end-effector to the platform can be adjusted. This device has advantages of simple construction and non-contact adjustment, and disadvantage of uneven pressure acted by the end-effector on the platform when the cross-section of electromagnet is not big enough. Therefore, account should be taken to estimate suitable size of electromagnet in this design.

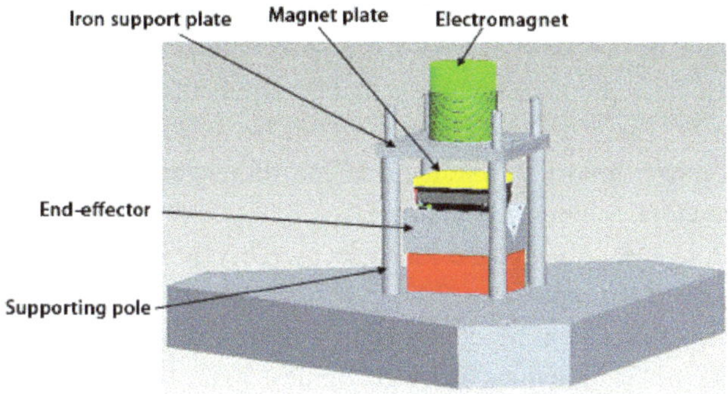

Fig. 4. Electromagnet pressure adjustable mechanism.

4. Conclusion

Piezoelectric stick-slip actuator has been widely applied in nano-positioning. The research dynamics of the end-effector displacement has attracted many research attentions. The temperature and pressure between end- effector and guiding platform are two main factors which affect the performance of the end-effector. It is a challenging task to build theoretical model to predict the practical performance. This study designs a test platform which can measure the temperature of friction plate and adjust the pressure between the end- effector and its guiding platform. The temperature sensor is installed into slots machined in the V grooves in the guiding platform. An electromagnet system is applied in this test platform to adjust the pressure of end-effector active on the friction plate. By changing the direction and magnitude of the voltage on the coil, the pressure can be adjusted. For the uniform pressure distributing along the end-effector, the diameter of electromagnet need to be designed carefully.

Acknowledgment

This work was supported by the grants from Zhejiang Provincial Natural Science Foundation of China (No. LQ13E050005).

References

1. A. Bergander, W. Driesen, T. Varidel, M. Meizoso, and J.M. Breguet, "Mobile cm3-microbots with tools for nanoscale imaging and micromanipulation", Mechatronics and Robotics Conference, pp. 1041-1047, 2004.
2. Micky Rakotondrabe, Yassine Haddab and Philippe Lutz, Voltage/frequency proportional control of stick-slip micropositioning systems, IEEE Transactions on Control Systems Technology, Vol. 16, pp: 1316-132, 2008.
3. Burisch A, Soetebier S, Wrege J, Hesselbach J (2004) Piezoelectric stick-slip-actuator with normal-force-modulation. In: Actuator 2004, 9th international conference on new actuators, Bremen, Germany.
4. Driesen W, Breguet JM, Clavel R (2006) Novel locomotion principles for mobile micro robots. In: Actuator2006, 10th international conference on new actuators, Bremen, Germany.
5. Kang Dong. Modeling of the Piezoelectric-Driven Stick-Slip Actuators [D]. University of Saskatchewan, 2007.
6. J.Y. Peng, X.B. Chen. Modeling and Control of Piezoelectric Actuators [J]. IEEE-ASME Transactions on Mechatronics, 2011, 16(2): 394-399.
7. Christoph Edeler，Ingo Meyer，Sergej Fatikow. Modeling of stick-slip micro-drives，Journal micro-nano mechatronics, Vol. 6, pp: 65-87, 2011.
8. J.W. Li, G.S. Yang, W.J. Zhang, S.D. Tu, X.B. Chen. Thermal effect on piezoelectric stick-slip actuator systems, Review of Scientific Instruments, Vol: 79, pp: 046108-046108-3, 2008.
9. J.W. Li, Experimental Studies on thermal effect on Piezoelectric Stick-slip Actuator Systems [D]. Shanghai: East China University of Science and Technology, 2007.

Vibration Control and Modal Analysis Technology of Scaled Carbody*

Bingrong Miao[a], Ying Zhang, and Xujuan Li
State Key Lab of Traction Power, Southwest Jiaotong University, Chengdu, 610031, China
E-mail: [a]brmiao@163.com
www.swjtu.edu.cn

In order to study the high speed railway vehicle carbody dynamic property and vibration control problems, 1/8 scaled carbody rig has been designed and manufactured. Firstly, the scaled test rig is built and performed an experimental modal test technology. Secondly, finite elements computational modal analysis has been carried out to determine the structural dynamics behavior of the realized model compared the field modal test results. Finally, the achieved results verify the predicted dense lying carbody eigenvalues frequencies between these two kinds of method. The accomplished experimental modal analysis provides a sophisticated basis to improve dynamic property of scaled carbody structure for vibration control. The results are shown that scaled carbody test rig design and modal analysis technology can be effectively used to predict objectively the carbody comfort and bending vibration.

Keywords: Railway; scaled carbody; high speed train; modal analysis; finite element method.

1. Introduction

The lightweight railway vehicle carbody structures require additional control measures to overcome the drawback of increased structural vibrations and fatigue resistance weakens. During the last decade years, many vibration control approaches for suppression of the structure vibration theory were proposed [1, 2]. On the one hand, railway carbody structure vibration control and modal analysis technology were studied during these years. In reference [3] and [4], the 1/10 scaled carbody test rig is built to compare different concepts for suppressing metro carbody structural vibrations. On the other hand, the increasing operational speeds and huge number passenger demands require focusing on the carbody vibration control requirements of railway vehicles. Furthermore, it seems that classical railway vehicles material are being replaced

* This work is supported by National Natural Science Foundation of China (Grant No. 51375405).

by lightweight structure, such as aluminum sandwich panels and composite materials. It is therefore essential to know the different modes of vibration, especially those which, because of their proximity, influence each other. 1/5 scaled carbody dynamic strength test rig was designed for study the problems of vibration fatigue strength problems in reference [5].

For solving carbody structure vibration problems, what is performed by calculations from theoretical models and by experimentation Experimental modal analysis is based on the measurement of the response of the structure submitted to a defined excitation. But the overall carbody structure dynamic strength test and vibration control cost is too large, the scaled carbody test bed can be used to improve the full vehicle test drawbacks and study the smart or adaptive structures. The future development trend of carbody bending vibration control research shows that smart or adaptive structures can be used to overcome the drawback between lightweight and vibration [6]. In this paper, 1/8 scaled carbody test rig which model is adopted from a real high speed railway vehicle carbody concerning the test rig design and structural modes (frequencies, modes shape and etc.) to study the interaction relations between the lightweight structure and structure vibration control problems.

2. Theory Background

The relationship between input (Force excitation) and output (Vibration response) of a linear system structure is expressed as Eq. (1) below:

$$\mathrm{Y}_i=\sum_{i=1}^{n}\sum_{j=1}^{n} H_{\mathrm{ij}} X_{\mathrm{j}} \tag{1}$$

Where $X_j \in R^n$, $Y_j \in R^n$, $H_{ij} \in R^n$. X_j describe the system input loads spectrum at **DOF** (Degree of Freedom) j . X_j describe the system input loads spectrum at **DOF** i . H_{ij} is the frequency function (FRF) between **DOF** i and **DOF** j . The output is the sum of the individual output caused by each of the inputs. The frequencies responses function H_{ij} are estimated from the measured auto and cross-spectra of and between input and output. Only one response **DOF** is needed by one accelerometer position (point and direction) in impact hammer test. Equation (2) is expressed the single-input, single-output test configuration [1] below:

The relationship between input (Force excitation) and output (Vibration response) of a linear system structure is expressed as Eq. (1) below:

$$\begin{Bmatrix} Y_1 \\ Y_2 \\ Y_3 \\ \vdots \\ Y_n \end{Bmatrix} = \begin{Bmatrix} H_{11} & H_{12} & H_{13} & \cdots & H_{1n} \\ H_{21} & H_{22} & H_{23} & \cdots & H_{2n} \\ H_{31} & H_{32} & H_{33} & \cdots & H_{3n} \\ \vdots & \vdots & \vdots & \vdots & \vdots \\ H_{n1} & H_{n2} & H_{n3} & \cdots & H_{nn} \end{Bmatrix} \begin{Bmatrix} X_1 \\ X_2 \\ X_3 \\ \vdots \\ X_n \end{Bmatrix} \tag{1}$$

There are varieties of frequency ranges of interest which are selected based on the deflection pattern of the scaled carbody and the magnitude of natural frequency. Frequency range of interest for Y axis maybe different from X and Z axis. This is to ensure the natural frequency for both methods is closed to each other. The results of natural frequency obtain from the simulation in the frequency range of interest produce a small difference between the two methods. The deflection mode shapes of the scaled carbody depending on the axis selected since the frequency ranges of interest have been set up depending on the axis. For X and Y axis, the pattern of the mode shapes for both methods is almost similar. However, for Z axis, the pattern of the mode shapes is not similar, as in mode 4 for impact test is twisting but for mode 4 by shaker test is bending. The natural frequency obtain for all the three axes is below than 5%, but the pattern of the mode shape for Z axis does not get as desired. This can happens as the tri-axial accelerometer is not accurate compare to the single accelerometer. Tri-axial accelerometer is used on the chassis as the single accelerometer is not suitable for some of the selected DOFs.

3. Numerical Example

3.1. *Test rig design*

In order to get more insight the vibration characteristic of carbody structure, a real carbody model of a railway vehicle is selected for the objective of scaled carbody. In this paper, a dynamics system identification method for a given sensors/actuators configuration can be performed using the identification procedures provided within Matlab or custom programmed algorithms. A scaled test rig and 1: 8 scaled carbody are designed from one real CRH (China Railway High-speed) EMU railway vehicle car body, which have been built to investigate different concepts to suppress structural vibrations by active damping. In contrast to traditional structure modal measurement applications the implementation of closed loop control schemes requires both actuators with suitable amplifiers and a fast and versatile realization of the control unit. A software solution for a short development cycle from design to simulation and finally implementation of a control scheme is therefore necessary. Although different software packages for controller design and even more software solutions for simulation of closed-loop control exist, only few packages provide an integrated solution also covering the implementation of the control unit [3, 4].

To satisfy the vibration control research of the different scaled carbody structure of the different type railway vehicle, the test rig (length is about 4000 mm, width is about 1040 mm, height of is about 2000 mm) has be designed. The scaled carbody vibration test rig is mainly composed: The ends hanger; Middle hangers; The scaled carbody; Soft spring; Exciter; Steel chassis; Wood brackets and other components. The test rig is shown in Fig. 1 (Include the test rig sketch and real test rig).

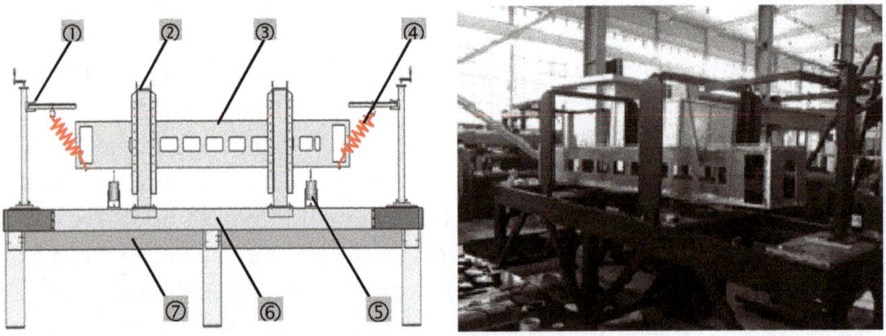

Fig. 1 The multi-objective 1/8 scaled carbody test rig.

3.2. *Experimental modal testing*

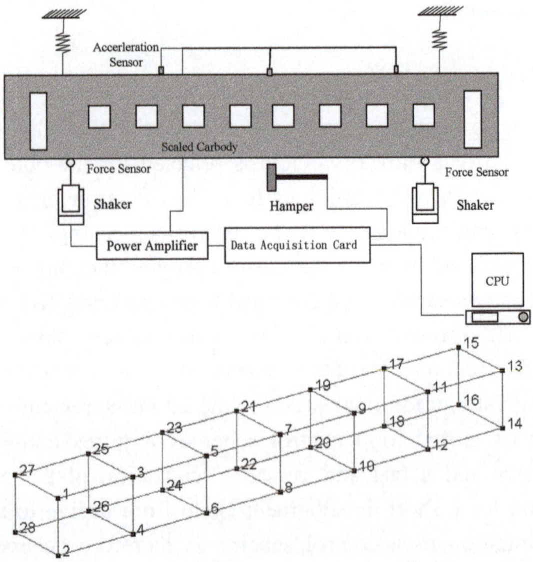

Fig. 2 Experimental modal test principle and measurement points' distribution.

Experimental modal testing is a formalized method for identification of natural frequencies and mode shapes of structures. It utilizes dedicated modal test equipment, and requires a formalized procedure for disturbing, e.g., rapping, the structure into motion, and then recording the distribution of the resulting motions throughout the structure. According to the principle of modal test layout measuring points, hanging modes and measuring points evenly should distribute better [6]. In order to analyze the scaled carbody natural characteristic, the scaled carbody was selected seven different sections, arranged in four vertices of each section of the measuring points, a total of 28 measuring points. The experimental modal test principle and measurement points' distribution are shown in Fig. 2.

3.3. *Modal calculation analysis and compared*

For analysis of force-excited scaled carbody modal measurements systems, two procedure are in use: (1) The response history, in which the modal responses are computed as a function of time and then superposed to obtain the response history of the system; and (2) The response spectrum, in which the peak values of modal responses are determined from the response spectrum or design spectrum that characterizes the excitation, and the peak response of the system is then estimated by appropriately combining the modal peaks. Computational modal analysis is an analytical procedure used to uncouple the structural equations of motion by use of a known transformation, as outlined in the following section. The resulting analysis is then readily achieved by solution of the uncoupled equations. The modal response of the structure is then found through a reverse transformation, followed by a summing of the respective modal responses, in accordance with their degree of participation in the structural motion. Some Eigen-modes calculation results based on FEM are shown in Fig. 3.

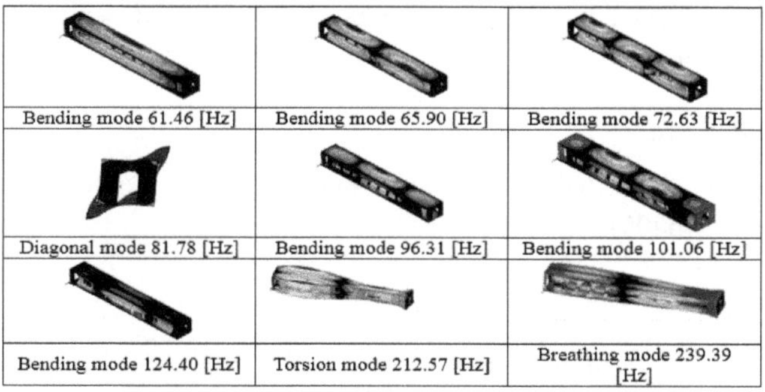

Fig. 3 Some computational modes of carbody structure based on FEM.

In accordance with the test method proposed, respectively, the proportion of body transverse (y direction) and vertical (z direction) to move hammer test method. Since the cause of sensor numbers and distribution, the hammering method using the different reference points should be selected in a different section. The compared results are listed in Table 1.

Table 1 Compared results between the modal test and computational results.

Mode shape	Cal. Modes [Hz]	Exp. Modes [Hz]	Difference [Hz]	Errors
1st Lateral bending	61.46	62.25	0.79	1.27%
2nd Lateral bending	65.90	65.13	0.21	0.34%
3rd Lateral bending	72.63	74.00	0.77	1.18%
Lateral diagonal mode	81.78	83.13	1.35	1.62%
Bending mode	124.40	121.40	3	2.47%

4. Summary and Conclusion

Using 1/8 multi-Objective scaled carbody test rig, it can be used to study the relations between the structure bending vibration characteristics and vibration and control technology. Because of the similarity of the ratio of the carbody structure, respectively, the middle section, the 1/3 section and the 1/6 section are selected as reference points for testing. The results obtained are shown that when the modal sensor is located in the middle position better access to each section of the reference point frequency response function basically the same. The following section focuses on the analysis results for the middle section. The middle section point between 0-130Hz frequency response function and mode shapes in the range are listed and compared with the modal test results. During carbody horizontal and vertical modal test, it can be seen that there are some Eigen-mode frequency dense distribution between 60-80Hz, 80Hz-90Hz, 200Hz-210Hz, and the 230Hz- 245Hz range. Combined with modern structural modal testing and computational theory, the relationship between the lightweight structure vibration mechanism and fatigue resistance of the carbody can be also studied , which greatly reduces the cost and size of the overall vehicle vibration test.

Acknowledgments

This project is supported by National Natural Science Foundation of China (Grant No. 51375405).

References

1. W. Heylen, S. Lammens and P. Sas. Modal Analysis Theory and Testing (Leuven: KU Leuven, Belgium, 1998).

2. J. Hansson, M. Takano and T. Takigami. JSME International Journal Series C. Vol. 47 (2004), pp. 451-456.
3. C. Bilik, C. Benatzky, M. Kozek. Proceedings of the 3rd International Symposium on Remote Engineering and Virtual Instrumentation Cite seer publishing, Maribor, Slovenia, 2006).
4. M. Kozek, C. Bilik and C. Benatzky. http://www.i-joe.org.
5. S.I. Seo, C.S. Park, and K.H. Kim. JSME International Journal Series A. Vol. 48 (2005), pp. 27-34.
6. T. Takigami, T. Tomioka and J. Hansson. Journal of Advanced Mechanical Design systems and Manufacturing, 1 (2007), pp. 649-660.
7. K. Ishiguri, Y. Kobayashi and T. Tomioka. Journal of System Design and Dynamics, 2(1) (2008), pp. 93-104.

CHAPTER 2

Computer Science and Its Application

Location Information Provider Framework Using the Mobius Platform in Mobile Environment

Nanju Kim

Department of Computer Engineering, Hannam University, Daejeon, Republic of Korea
E-mail: 91knj@naver.com

Euiin Choi

Department of Computer Engineering, Hannam University, Daejeon, Republic of Korea
E-mail: eichoi@hnu.kr

Recent various crimes and lost stuff and the like are recognized as a social problem. And users may be the subject of such crimes. To address this, the demand about location information transmission is a situation that is increasing. Therefore various institutions are providing location information service using a mobile device. Also, recently much research has been in progress to provide location-based services using the beacon in the Internet of Things (IoT). In this paper, we investigated definition and technology for Seamless LBS that accuracy is higher than accuracy of GPS in mobile environment. Also, we studied the Mobius platform for interworking with things of IoT. And, we proposed a new location lookup framework that complements traditional location lookup techniques.

Keywords: Seamless LBS; location information; location lookup technique; mobius platform; internet of things.

1. Introduction

Users have been readily exposed with respect to the recent various crimes. So it has emerged as a social issue. Accordingly, the effort is continuing for provide the user location information. So, there is increasing interest in and a need for techniques for providing accurate location. Location Based Service (LBS) are grasp the location of a person or thing based on a mobile network. Then, it is a concept that collectively the application systems and services to take advantage of it. As such LBS have emerged as a major key technology of basis infrastructure for location-based services with the development of wireless communication and Internet. Also ranging from individual, business, and public sector are utilized in a variety of forms. So, recently much research has been in progress to provide location-based services using the beacon in the Internet of Things (IoT). In addition, in case of service of the GPS and Cell-ID mode provided by the mobile phone in the domestic, GPS is impossible to grasp the position of underground or inside buildings. The case of Cell-ID method is result of the grasp the position is larger differences for accuracy requirements level of user. In order to compensate for this problem has emerged Seamless LBS [1]. Provided location information technology is essential to users that not free from crimes. Namely, In order to provide a user location lookup was unthinkable by separating the position-based services such as GPS, LBS. In this paper, we investigated definition and technology for Seamless LBS that accuracy is higher than accuracy of GPS in mobile environment. Also, we studied the Mobius platform for interworking with things of IoT. And, we proposed a new location lookup framework that complements traditional location lookup techniques.

2. Related Works

2.1. *Positioning services*

Now we are living in the one of the great flow of technological change, Internet of Things. These techniques have been developed for identification of objects and its location. And it is being used to remote control and product marketing [1, 2].

2.1.1. *Location Based Service (LBS)*

The definition for the LBS is representing a little differently according each institution. Open GIS Consortium (OGC) is defined as all application software service that acts by the location information or connection and provide of location information.

LBS technology is the same context that developed of mobile communication technology. Namely, LBS technology is track the location of mobile devices in a variety of wired or wireless communication network. And it is collected and processed. Then, it is to service and to making a variety of content using that in the private and public sectors. Thus, location-based service means to create related applications that identify the location of the user using the location detection (check) techniques [3].

2.1.2. *Seamless LBS*

In case of service of the GPS and Cell-ID mode provided by the mobile phone in the domestic, GPS is impossible to grasp the position of underground or inside buildings. The case of Cell-ID method is result of the grasp the position is larger differences for accuracy requirements level of user. In order to compensate for this problem has emerged Seamless LBS.

Seamless LBS mean to LBS technology of the next generation that connected constantly location-based services of the center of the room and Small area.

2.1.3. *Beacon*

Beacon has concept that uses non-audible frequency region machine-to-machine communication. Beacon is a transmitter that uses low energy Bluetooth as a short-range location-aware technology that sends signals to the smart phone [4], tablet pc and smart watches. In particular, the beacon tells all the details of the local area in the indoor or outdoor location as an indoor GPS less than 5cm error. It can automatically forward information required through the application.

2.2. *Location-Based Service Platform*

Location-Based Service Platform is a platform that provides most basic and critical function for LBS and it also provides a common component supporting a variety LBS. In this regard, many platforms have been developed like MPC, GISP, AS, and AP [5].

2.2.1. *Mobile Positioning Center*

Mobile Positioning Center (MPC) is a server acting as elements for the location data retrieval, transmission, storage, and control in the network infrastructure [2, 7]. It uses a Position Determining Entity (PDE) to determine the position using a variety of technologies such as assisted GPS or observed time difference of arrival. MPC and MSC communicate with the emergency services network. The MPC also handles access restrictions to the position information.

2.2.2. *Geographic Information Service Platform*

Geographic Information Service Platform is a platform or content server giving contents as like POI, traffic information and electronic maps for LBS services. GISP uses spatial-temporal location as the key index variable for all other information. Just as a relational database containing text or numbers can relate many different tables using common key index variables, GISP can relate unrelated information by using location as the key index variable. The key is the location and/or extent in space-time [8].

2.2.3. *Application Server and Service Provider*

Application Server and Service Provider are acting like LBS application service provider or client server based on location information from Location-Based Service Platform or Geographic Information Service Platform. [6, 9].

2.3. *Mobius platform*

Mobius platform is an open Internet of Things (IoT) platform, and means interconnecting the things to the network. So it can be to communicate with each other anytime, anywhere between people and things, things and things. First, It is collecting data from the things. Then, provide a service using that data, or provide a control method for the things. Through this, IoT platform can provide personalized, social networks, the smart health, safety such as advanced service.

2.3.1. *Device platform*

Device platform connects the various thing in the IoT infrastructure. Also, it is interworking with the IoT Service Platform. That is, it is software that can provide a IoT service with things. It can provide the communication adapter through the hardware communication module that conversing to the ZigBee communication, mobile communication as 3G/4G, IP communication as Wi-Fi/Ethernet.

2.3.2. *Planet platform*

Planet platform register profile information such as device ID, device name, device location related the IoT device. Planet platform indexes the information. It supports a variety of search based on this information.

2.3.3. *Mashup platform*

The periodic data received and stored about IoT device. Then, the useful information extracts from a IoT device data fusion. So, This platform can provide information to the user. If it is difficult to direct network connection, can directly connect to the device using the Mashup platform.

2.3.4. *Store platform*

The store platform can be registration, upload, and download about IoT device. The platform includes a service application function that provides useful information to the user for interlock with the device application and device.

3. Proposed Framework

The user threat to various crimes is increasing. So, to defend using traditional location provided technology is difficult. As described earlier, the development and research on the user location information is proceeding.

Services for the current position information are provided the GPS, Cell-ID by the way. So it is impossible to grasp a location inside buildings or underground. And the accuracy of the location information is not satisfactory. Indoor and outdoor location measurement using a Seamless LBS order to solve these problems is needed.

Proposed framework provides intelligent services by using the location information to be interoperable Different environments as well as a mobile environment. After that, it will be satisfy a variety of user requirements by connecting with the add-on and location-based services. Developed a framework is configured to interact with the user's needs and user position information that generating in a variety of situations. In addition, since the use of beacon, the framework can be location information transmitting and real-time checking to be based on a beacon. It is possible that according to data processing and integration, various information transfer to users, etc.

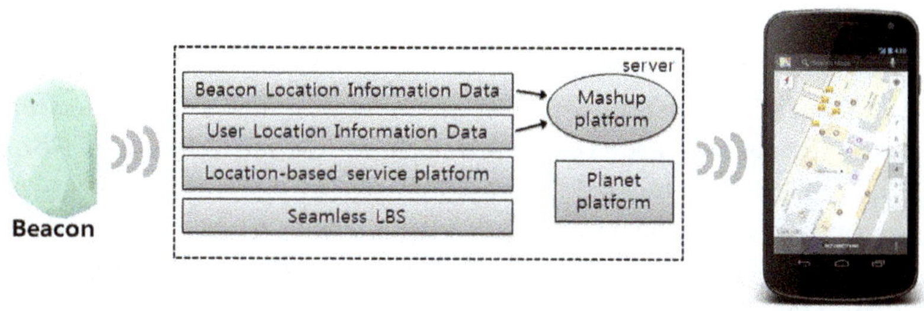

Fig. 1 Proposed framework.

4. Conclusion

Location-based services have been studied and developed in a wide variety application area that has a close connection with our life. But, situation of development for technology or services for precise location information as yet is lacking. Therefore, the study should be continued about Seamless LBS in order to grasp when the user's location information anywhere. So, shall provide a high accuracy about position. Also, it may provide various associated services to meet the user requirements consist the data analysis on the basis of this position information.

Problem with respect to various position information technologies in many fields should analyse. Also, if come true about various service and system research and development, is helping provide highly accurate in position information from a variety of IoT environments.

Acknowledgments

This work (Grants No. C0199617) was supported by business for Cooperative R&D between Industry, Academy, and Research Institute funded Korea Small and Medium Business Administration in 2014.

References

1. H. Choi, LBS, *Location-Based Services trend Computer Software Research*, Korea Electronics and Telecommunications Research Institute, No. 86, 2003.
2. Y. Cho et al, *WARP-P: Wireless signal Acquisition with Reference Point by using simplified PDF* – sys-tem concept and performance assessment, Proc. The ION 2013 Pacific PNT Meeting, Apr, 2013
3. S.H Park, *Location-Based Services (LBS) technology and market trends*, Technical note, Surveying & Mapping Magazine, 3, 2011.
4. D. Tipper el al, *Providing Fault Tolerance in Wireless Access Networks*," IEEE Communication, Mag., Vol. 40, No. 1, Jan. 2002, pp. 58–64.
5. H. Choi, *LBS, Location-Based Services trend Computer Software Research*, Korea Electronics and Telecommunications Research Institute, No. 86, 2003.
6. Application server, *Wikipedia.org/wiki/Application server.*
7. D. Tipper, *Network architecture and protocols for mobile positioning in cellular wireless systems.*
8. Geographic information platform, *Wikipedia.org/wiki/Geographic information platform* .
9. Y. Zhao, *Standardization of mobile phone positioning for 3G systems*, IEEE Communication. Mag, 40(7), pp. 108-116, 2002.

.NET-Based Open Laboratory Management Information System*

Yanyan Wang
College of Urban Rail Transit, Shenzhen University,
Shenzhen, Nanshan District, China
E-mail: wangyanyan@szu.edu.cn

With the continuous expansion of university laboratory scale, the management of laboratory, especially of open laboratory, has become more onerous and complex. Considering the limitations that most laboratories can't meet the requirements of teaching program caused by slow analysis of teaching practice and information updating, this paper proposes an open laboratory management method, which can be used for rapid analysis of teaching task and timely updating of information, by means of which students can make an appointment and conduct experiment installation management independently, etc., to improve the usage rate of laboratory and equipment, and meanwhile reduce laboratory administrative personnel's workload, to increase work efficiency.

Keywords: Open laboratory; experiment reservation; laboratory equipment management; management information system.

1. Introduction

Laboratory is an important place for college teaching and scientific research. Particularly, experiment teaching is more of an important link of college teaching. It plays an irreplaceable role in talent training. However, the significant degree of experiment teaching depends on the constantly developed and perfected experimental contents and management methods [1]. Nowadays, with the expansion of college enrollment scale, the number of students has increased continuously, and the laboratory hardware facilities have also increased in number. Accordingly, the university laboratory scale has expanded constantly. The existing traditional handwork management makes the management work quite tedious, slows down the analysis of the teaching

* This work is supported by Shenzhen University's Fund for the Research of Laboratory and Equipment Management. National Natural Science Foundation of China (11274336), Key Project of Teaching Reform of Guangdong Higher Education in 2013: Research and Practice of the New Urban Rail Transit Talents Training Mode Based on "3+1+X", and Professional Comprehensive Reform Project of Guangdong Higher Schools in 2014: "Transportation Specialty".

practice task ability undertaken by laboratory, and causes information not to be updated timely. As a result, most laboratories can't meet the experimental requirements beyond teaching program, thus reducing the service efficiency of instrument and equipment [2]. To improve the usage rate of laboratory equipment and site, as well as the function of experiment in teaching, this project proposes an open laboratory management method.

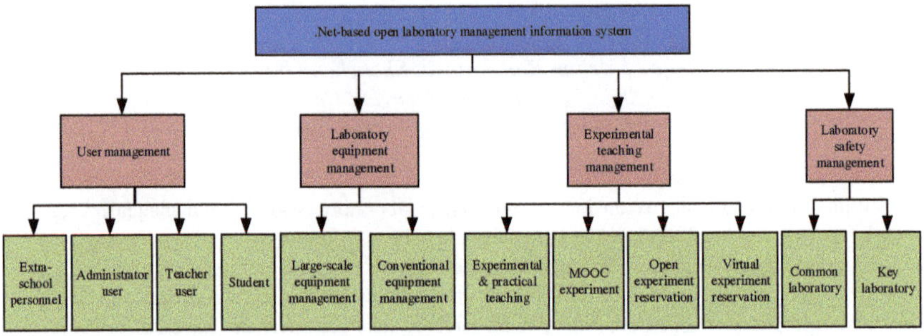

Fig. 1 Functional diagram of laboratory management information system.

2. Main System Functions

Laboratory management information system can fall into four major modules by functions, which are user management, experiment reservation, laboratory equipment management and laboratory safety management.

User management provides a division of user permission for system, by way of which professional administrative personnel can be appointed according to functional modules, with a chief administrator appointed, several device keepers appointed, a few experiment reservation administrators appointed, and a few experiment security administrators appointed. Experimental teaching management module is the most important module in this system. It's mainly used for online reservation experiment, as well as online registration experiment and practical teaching, and the submission of practice report online; it can help teachers submit online experimental plans and review lab reports online. Laboratory equipment management falls into conventional equipment management and large-scale equipment management. Teachers and students can not only examine the using status and detailed parameters of equipment online, but apply for borrowing online. In the process, administrators check and sign borrowing instructions to complete borrowing formalities. For the safety of large-scale equipment, it can't be borrowed unless deposits are paid online in advance. Laboratory safety management includes two parts—hardware and software. Each laboratory is mounted with a hardware system, where experiment can't be carried out unless student or faculty card is swiped. Moreover, cameras are mounted indoors, so that the administrative staff should monitor the indoor situations through the system in time. The figure below is the function block diagram of this system.

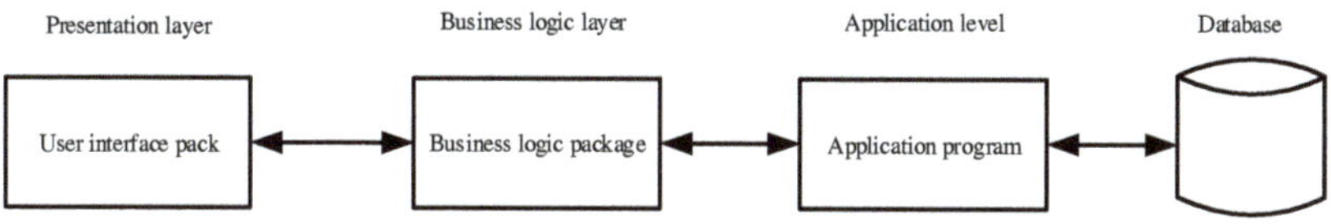

Fig. 2 .NET four-layer structure diagram.

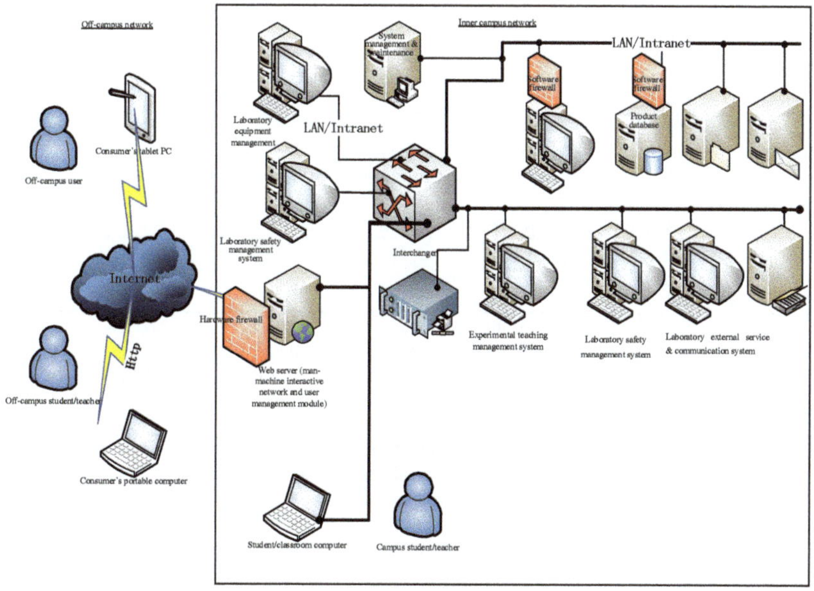

Fig. 3 System software architecture.

3. Software Architecture

This system is equipped with .NET architecture-based B/S four-tier architecture. Four-tier architecture refers to user presentation layer (human-computer interaction interface), business logic layer (the connected logical relationship between human-computer interaction interface and application-level software), application layer (such three major modules as laboratory equipment management system, open laboratory booking system, experiment user management and laboratory safety management), and data access layer (the operation commands set of direct execution to database). The structure is shown in the figure below.

Table 1 User rights.

User	Permission
Chief administrator	1. Manage personal information; 2. Review subordinate administrators (add, delete, suspend, enable and approve); 3. Manage teacher and student account (add, delete, suspend, enable and approve); 4. Have all permissions to subordinate administrators.
Device keeper	1. Manage personal information; 2. Manage teacher's and student's account application (authorize application, refuse application, write a reason for refusal, add user, delete user, suspend and enable user); 3. Manage laboratory (add, delete, edit, suspend and enable); 4. Manage experiment equipment (add, delete, edit, suspend and enable); 5. Manage laboratory reservation (agree, refuse and write a reason for refusal); 6. Manage laboratory equipment reservation (agree, refuse and write a reason for refusal); 7. Manage maintenance application for laboratory equipment; 8. Manage scrapping application for laboratory equipment; 9. Issue notice.
Experiment reservation administrator	1. Manage personal information; 2. Manage experiment (add, suspend and enable); 3. Manage laboratory reservation (approve, mark the completed, mark default and write comments); 4. View experiment reservation and cancel notice.
Laboratory safety administrator	1. Play experimental video; 2. Record laboratory use (add, delete and consult).
Teacher	1. Manage personal information; 2. Manage experiment (add, suspend and enable); 3. Manage laboratory reservation (approve, mark the completed, mark default and write comments); 4. Check laboratory reservation and cancel notice; 5. Reserve laboratory equipment (apply, cancel application, view audit status, and view the using status of all laboratories and all equipment); 6. Apply to repair laboratory equipment; 7. Offer opinions for the management of experiment and equipment; 8. Apply to add laboratory equipment (apply and cancel application).
Student	1. Manage personal information; 2. Reserve experiment (Allow reservation only in 5 days); 3. Cancel laboratory reservation (the ones that have been approved need to be cancelled at least 2 days in advance, and the ones that haven't been approved can be canceled at any time). 4. Submit a lab report and view the comments; 5. Reserve laboratory and equipment (apply, cancel application, view the audit status of application, and view the using status of all laboratories and all equipment); 6. Apply to repair laboratory equipment; 7. Manage scrapping application for laboratory equipment; 8. Offer opinions for the management of experiment and equipment.

Four-layer structure has been developed very maturely and applied extensively. Four-layer structure is stratified very strictly; data is interacted through stratification, and can't be interacted through trans-passing of stratification. For instance, user presentation layer can only interact data with business logic layer. The access request from user presentation layer can only spread to application layer after parsed through business logic layer. Only by then can application layer interact with database access layer for database access and send result to database access layer. Next, database access layer will send it to application layer, and then application layer gives the result to business logic layer to complete relevant rules and logics before business logic layer sends it to user presentation layer [3]. The figure below shows the software architecture of this system.

4. Key Technology

4.1. *User management module*

According to user function, it falls into chief administrator (generally known as experimental center director), device keeper, experiment reservation administrator, laboratory safety administrator, teacher and student.

4.2. *Open experiment reservation module*

Teacher submits experiment application through the system, administrator issues it after approval, and then student makes a reservation according to demand. The figure below shows the detailed flow.

4.3. *Laboratory equipment management module*

Laboratory equipment management falls into conventional equipment management and large-scale equipment management. Teachers and students can not only examine the using status and detailed parameters of equipment online, but apply for borrowing online. In the process, administrators check and sign borrowing instructions to complete borrowing formalities. For the safety of large-scale equipment, it can't be borrowed unless deposits are paid online in advance. The following figure shows the application process for the usage of experimental equipment.

5. Conclusion

.NET-based open laboratory management system offers an effective solution to laboratory personnel (user), experiment reservation and laboratory equipment management. In this way, college teachers and students can conduct experiments more conveniently and flexibly, and laboratory administrators can save plenty of time, to improve the quality of the practical teaching in colleges and universities.

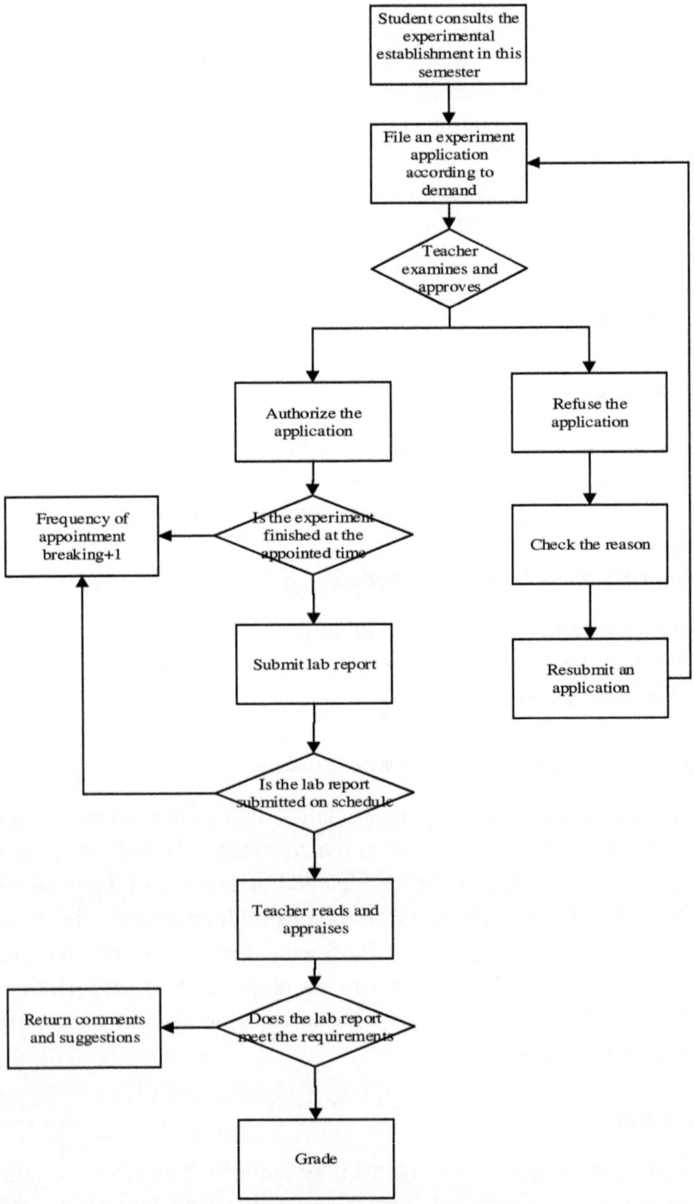

Fig. 4 The flow of Student's experiment reservation.

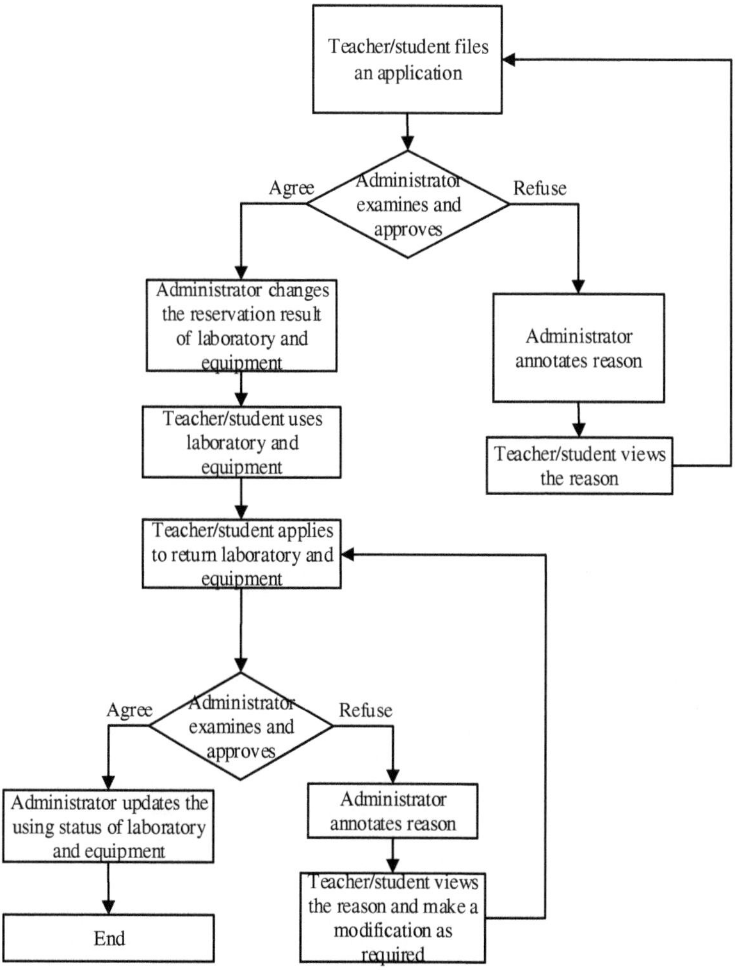

Fig. 5 Application for the usage of experiment equipment.

References

1. Design and Development of Laboratory Teaching Information Management System—a Case of Information Dissemination Experiment Center of Zhejiang Normal University. http://www.docin.com/p-347672440.html.
2. Cai Mingshan. *Research and Design of a Total Management System for University Laboratory* . Hunan University.
3. Min Jiangwei. *Design and Implementation of Bank Office Automation System*. Shanghai Jiaotong University, 2009.

Study on the Key Technology of Measurement Instrument for Mine Spatial Information Integration*

Yu Le-wen[1,2,3†], Zhang Yuan-sheng[1,3] and Zhang Da[1,3]

[1]*Beijing General Research Institute of Mining and Metallurgy, Beijing, China, 102600*
[2]*University of Science and Technology Beijing, Beijing, China, 100083*
[3]*Beijing Key Laboratory of Nonferrous Intelligent Mining Technology, Beijing, China, 102600*
[†]*E-mail: yulewen@bgrimm.com*
www.bgrimm.com

In view of the current situation of measurement system for mining, such as complicated operation, low efficiency, poor portability, poor integrated, a new simple, efficient, hand-held measurement instrument of mine spatial information integration was developed. The instrument can calculate the distance by adopting the phase method and acquire the three-dimensional coordinate data by combining with the dip and the azimuth. The hardware of instrument was developed, with the functions of independent power supply, storage of measurement data, wireless communications and others so as to realize the three-dimensional handheld measurement. The measurement software of the instrument was improved, with the functions of communication interface and measured parameters configuration, real-time display of the survey coordinate, entity modeling and three-dimensional display of the space objects, and analysis and evaluation of the models. When tested in underground mine, the measurement instrument can quickly obtain three-dimensional coordinates of the unknown underground areas and realize the maximum measuring range of the instrument at 83m and maximum measuring error of the instrument at 1cm with the characteristics of simplicity, high efficiency and portability. Its effectiveness and reliability can meet the requirements of the measurement of mine spatial information integration.

Keywords: Mine surveying; three-dimensional coordinate; quickly; three-dimensional construction.

1. Introduction

The traditional measurement instruments of mine spatial information include theodolite, level, total station and three dimensional laser scanner. But there are lots of problems in the actual application. Firstly, it requires professionals to

* This work was supported by the High-tech Research and Development Program of China (2011AA060405) and the National Natural Science Foundation of China (41301436).

mapping. Secondly, it is low efficiency. Finally, the instrument is poor portability, can't meet the needs of the mine complex application [1-4].

In view of the current situation of measurement instrument for mining, a new simple, efficient, hand-held measurement instrument of mine spatial information integration was developed. The instrument can calculate the distance by adopting the phase method and acquire the three-dimensional coordinate data by combining with the dip and the azimuth. It can quickly acquire the three-dimensional shape information of mine.

2. The Measuring Principle

The instrument can calculate the distance by adopting the phase method and acquire the three-dimensional coordinate data by combining with the dip and the azimuth. [5-8]

During the measurement, Firstly, you have to measure the distance, the azimuth and inclination between the instrument and a known coordinate, and calculate the coordinates of the measuring instrument itself. Then measuring the distance and angle between the measuring instrument and any other points. The coordinates of other points can be calculated by the formula 1. The measuring principle is shown in the Figure 1.

Three-dimensional coordinate calculation principle is shown in the Figure 2.

The point $A(x_0, y_0, z_0)$ is known in coordinates, and point $B(x_i, y_i, z_i)$ is any point within the coordinate system. The inclination α and azimuth θ between point A and point B are measured by sensors. That any point coordinates are calculated by formula as follows.

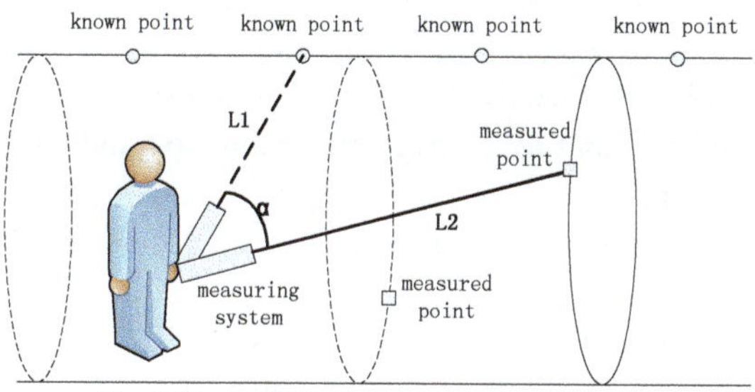

Fig. 1 The method of measurement.

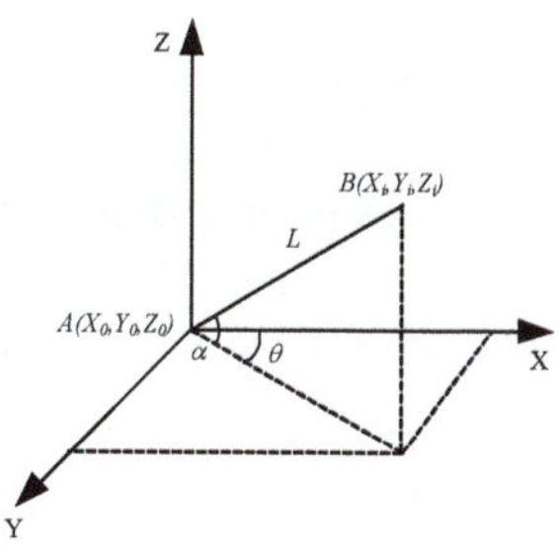

Fig. 2 The principle of measuring.

$$\begin{cases} x_i = x_0 + L \cdot \cos\alpha \cdot \cos\theta \\ y_i = y_0 + L \cdot \cos\alpha \cdot \sin\theta \\ z_i = z_0 + L \cdot \sin\alpha \end{cases} \tag{1}$$

L is the distance between the point A and the point B, (m); α is the inclination between the point B and the point A, (°). θ is the azimuth between the point B and the point A, (°).

The equation of distance is as follow [9-10].

$$L = \frac{\lambda}{4\pi}\phi \tag{2}$$

L is the distance; λ is the wavelength; ϕ is the phase difference.

3. Instrument Development

3.1. *System components*

The instrument consists of hardware system and software platform. The hardware contains sensors, controller, battery, communication cable and PDA. The software platform includes parameter configuration, coordinate real-time display, three-dimensional modeling and display, model analysis and evaluation, and so on.

3.2. *Hardware design*

The instrument acquires the distance by phase-shift of ranging sensor. The azimuth and inclination are measured by electronic compass and tilt sensor. It calculates three-dimensional coordinates by the microcontroller and localized store, or communicating with PDA by wired or wirelessly.

3.3. *Software design*

The software platform is divided into master computer and slave computer. The slave computer software is used for signal acquisition, data processing, data storage, data viewing and transmission. Specific functions as follows:

(1) Parameter settings, including input local magnetic declination and space coordinates of a known point.

(2) Measuring the distance and angle information at the same time for the coordinates calculation.

(3) Data save, save the coordinates of been measured points.

(4) Transferring the data by wired or wireless to master computer.

The master computer has function of coordinates real-time display, three-dimensional modeling, model analysis and evaluation [11-14], specific functions as follows:

(a) Coordinates real-time display, to obtain the coordinates of the measuring point data in real-time communication and display real-time three-dimensional coordinate system;
(b) Three-dimensional modeling, three-dimensional coordinates measuring points were solid modeling
(c) Model analysis and evaluation, to achieve a three-dimensional model of volume, boundary extraction, profile analysis.

4. Experimental

The instrument was tested in a underground mine, which is dust, harsh environment.

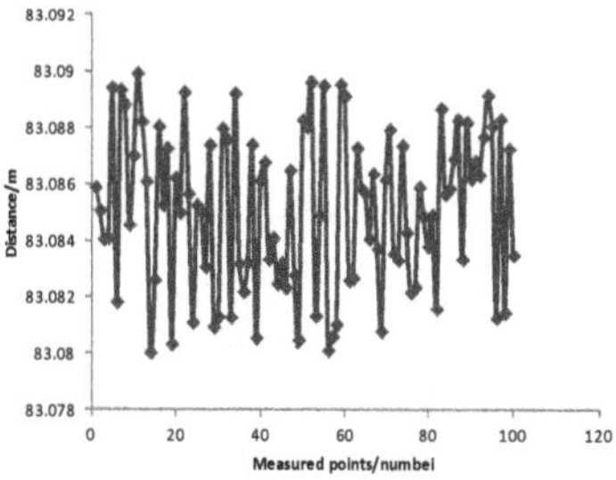

Fig. 3 Rage test.

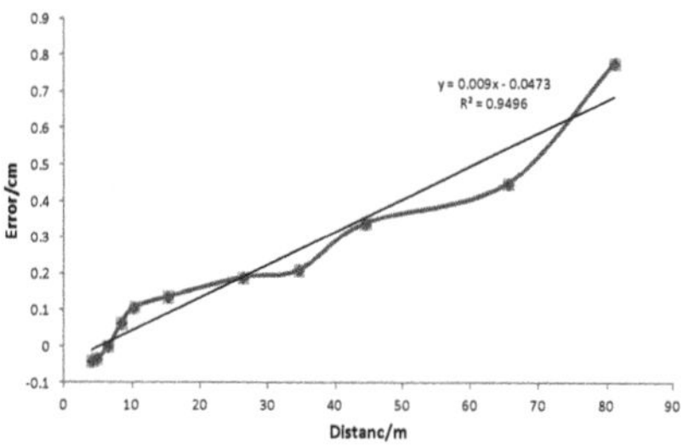

Fig. 4 Accuracy test.

4.1. *Property test*

Putting the instrument on a tripod, testing continuous ranging performance of the instrument by a single point. The measured data is shown in Figure 3.

The intelligent total station range error is less than 1mm, so the test result been accuracy. The data are contrasted between the instrument and the intelligent total station. That is shown in Figure 4.

The furthest ranging of the instrument is 83m in underground, and the measurement error less than 1cm.

4.2. *Measuring test*

Firstly, the instrument measured the distance, the azimuth and inclination between itself and a known coordinate and calculated the coordinate of the instrument itself. Secondly measured the three-dimensional coordinates of any other points in the roadway. The coordinates were displayed real-time in PDA. three-dimensional modeling of the roadway is shown in Figure 5.

The process of roadway measurement is simple. It takes 65 seconds to measure the roadway. The test shows that the instrument can be quickly and accurately to achieve the three-dimensional shape of roadway.

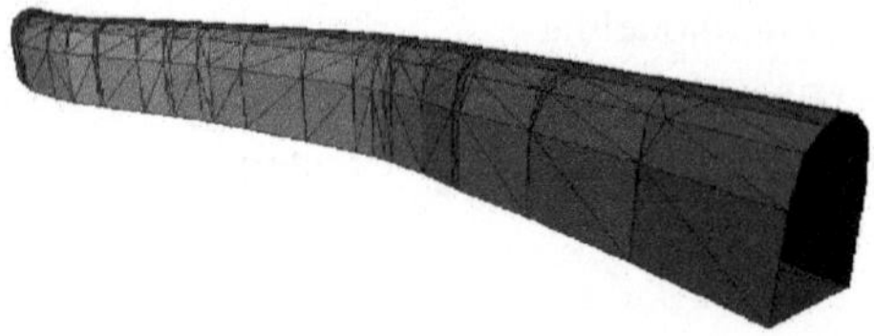

Fig. 5 Three-dimensional model of underground roadway.

5. Conclusion

A new simple, efficient, hand-held measurement instrument of mine spatial information integration was developed, Which can meet the need of mine surveying. It was adapted to harsh environments of mining, ranging capacity of 83m, accuracy of 1cm. The instrument operates simply and quickly measures the three-dimensional shape of roadway to improve measurement efficiency and safety. The instrument can also be applied to high-precision positioning for drilling rig.

Acknowledgments

This work was supported by the High-tech Research and Development Program of China (2011AA060405) and the National Natural Science Foundation of China (41301436).

References

1. Calkins, Joseph Matthew. Quantifying coordinate uncertainty fields in coupled spatial measurement systems [D]. Virginia, USA, Virginia Polytechnic Institute, 2002.
2. Zhang Lingxia, Ma Caiwen, Liu Yi, et al. Method research based on data fusion and simulation analysis of mult-itheodo-lites by intersection [J]. Acta Photonica Sinica, 2002, 31(12): 1528- 1532.
3. Domenico A Maisano, Jafar Jamshidi, Fiorenzo Franceschini, et al. Indoor GPS: System functionality and initial performance evaluation [J]. International Journal of Manufacturing Research, 2008, 3(3): 335- 343.

4. Yu Lewen, Zhang Da, Yu Bin, Yang Xiaocong. Research of three-dimensional Laser Scanning Measurement System for Mining [J]. Metal Mine, (10): 101-103, 107.
5. Ramos P. M., Da Silva F., Cruz Serra V. Improving sine-fitting algorithms for amplitude and phase measurements phase measurements [J]. Proceeding of XVII IMEKO World Congress, Dubrovnik, 2003, pp. 614-619.
6. Wang Tao. Research of the phase laser ranging technology [J]. Laser & Infrared, 2007, 37(1): 29-31.
7. Zhang Yucun, Liu Haibin. A detection method of laser doppler signal based on topological contravariance [J]. Optoelectron Lett, 2009, 5(4): 0295 - 0298.
8. Agrez D. Improving Phase Estimation With Leakage Minimization [J]. IEEE Trans. Instrum. Meas, 2005, 54(4): 1347-1353.
9. Huang Zhen, Liu Bin. New method to measure the time-of-flight in pulse laser ranging [J]. Journal of Optoelectronics·Laser, 2006, 17(9): 1153-1155.
10. Huang Jun-fen, Huang Min-shuang, Sun Ya-ling, et al. High precision time-interval measurement method based on pseudo-nan uniform sampling [J] Journal of Optoelectronics·Laser, 2012, 23(10): 1945-1948.
11. Fiorenzo Franceschini, Maurizio Galetto, Domenico Maisanoa, et al. On-line diagnostics in the mobile spatial coordinate measuring system [J]. Precision Engineering, 2009, 33(4): 408-417.
12. Gai Zhi-gang, Zhao Jie, Yang Li, et al. Development of new laser intelligent water level measuring system [J]. Journal of Optoelectronics·Laser, 2013, 24(3): 569-572.
13. Wu Yonghua, Hu Yihua, Xu Shilong, et al. Design of airport wake vortex monitoring system based on 1.5μm pulsed coherent doppler lidar [J]. Optoelectron Lett, 2011, 7(4): 0298-0303.
14. Zhang Yuansheng. Multi-scal modeling technology for underground mines [J]. Nonferrous Metals(Mining Section), 2012, 64(1): 1-4.

Design of Water Quality Monitoring System Based on STM32 & GPRS Communications and Android

Xiao-lang Sun[a] and De-an Zhao
Electric & Information Engineering School of Jiangsu University, Zhenjiang, China
[a]*E-mail:1067836970@qq.com*

The monitoring system conducts the remote sampling, data processing and mobile phone monitoring analysis on three important parameters of the water samples including the temperature, dissolved oxygen, and PH values. The STM32F103VET6 with ARM Core-M3 as the core processor is used for sampling and the collected data is sent to the remote server through ATK-SIM900A GPRS module with a 12-bit AD converter, the Android mobile phone users can download the data directly from the server. The system can realize the remote monitoring of field water quality through the Android mobile phone, providing a convenient real-time, continuous monitoring of water quality for the users.

Keywords: Monitoring system; STM32; GPRS; android.

1. Introduction

With the rapid development of science and technology, the development of Internet of things has the important practical significance for promoting economic development and social progress, and the Internet of things technology has rapidly penetrated into all areas of daily life. At present, in foreign countries, in the field of agricultural ecological environment monitoring, USA, France and Japan and some other developed countries mainly build advanced agricultural ecological environment monitoring networks mainly through comprehensive use of high-tech means, realizing the automatic monitoring of the agricultural ecological environment and ensuring the sustainable development of agricultural ecological environment by using advanced technologies of sensor perceptual system, data collection, data confusion and the Internet to build the platform of agricultural information that covers the whole country. In the water quality measurement, the automatic monitoring equipment used in foreign countries is higher in measuring accuracy, but the data is transmitted by wires in most cases at a higher cost; while in domestic, water environment monitoring is mainly conducted manually subject to with artificial sampling and chemical analysis, which needs a lot of effort and is also very time-consuming with lower precision and bad real-time performance, as well as some problems in difficult maintenance for a few portable instruments, etc.

2. The Overall Design Scheme

The system is composed of some parts including a water quality monitoring module, a GPRS communication module, a field handheld device, a remote server monitoring system, and an Android mobile phone client. The monitoring module includes a sensor and the circuit of signal adjusting for some water quality parameters such as temperature, PH, and dissolved oxygen, shown as in Figure 1. The field handheld device consists of a LCD and buttons, while the remote server is mainly used for receiving GPRS sent data and establishing communication with the mobile phone client via the wireless network. The Android mobile phone client mainly performs data display, storage and other functions.

3. Design of the System Hardware

The system is used for continuous sampling of the water quality parameters, data processing, remote transmission, the server data storage and data monitoring at the mobile phone terminal. The system hardware frame diagram is as shown in Figure 2. The working principle of the hardware is to calibrate the water samples with the handheld device before amplifying, filtering, computing and storing the sensing signals with the STM32F103VET6 microcontroller, and then send the 3 groups of 32-bit hexadecimal water quality parameters output continuously by the microcontroller to GPRS module through the RS232 serial port, followed by that GPRS module sends the data to the remote server based on the TCP/IP protocol, the remote server first processes the 3 groups of hexadecimal parameters in line with the data protocol, store and display at last. The server sends the data to the Android mobile phone terminal through the wireless network and the set port number, to realize the real-time data monitoring. This system uses the power supply isolation and block coupling relationship in the hardware to reduce crosstalk caused by simultaneous measurement of DO (dissolved oxygen) and PH. GPRS module that is used is the ATK-STM900A industrial-grade double-frequency module produced by SIMCOM, supporting an ultra-wide working range of 5V-24V, and its embedded TCP/IP protocol facilitates the connection to the Internet, meeting the demand of the main control equipment.

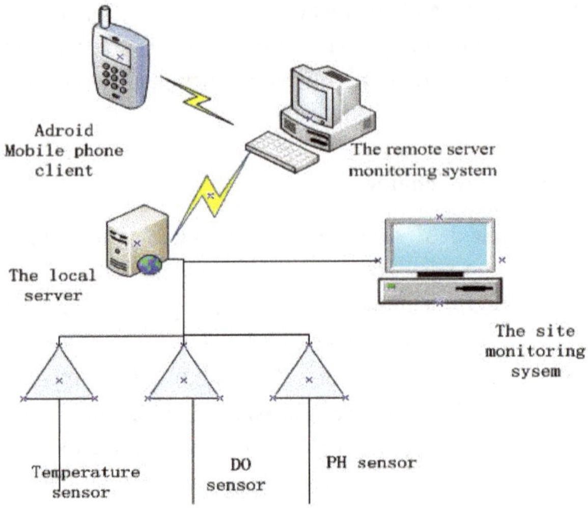

Fig. 1 The system structure diagram.

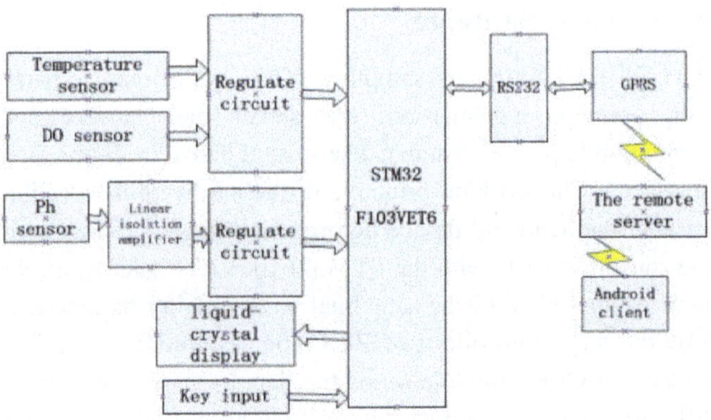

Fig. 2 The overall frame diagram of the system hardware.

4. Design of the System Software

System initialization, data acquisition and transmission. Upon running, the system first completes the initialization of the underlying data sampling part and the communication between GPRS and the upper computer. The underlying data initialization includes conditioning circuit address configuration, initialization of AT24C64 port, LED, USART1, ADC, LCD and the key program, etc. The initialization of the communication between GPRS and the upper computer is achieved by sending the IP address with the mobile phone. After initialization, the system begins to enable applications. The data acquisition application make the time collection of the water quality parameters based on the initialized clock parameters, and the transformed data by AD is sent to the remote upper computer through GPRS wireless network according to the custom protocols. The software design flow chart of the system is as shown in Figure 3.

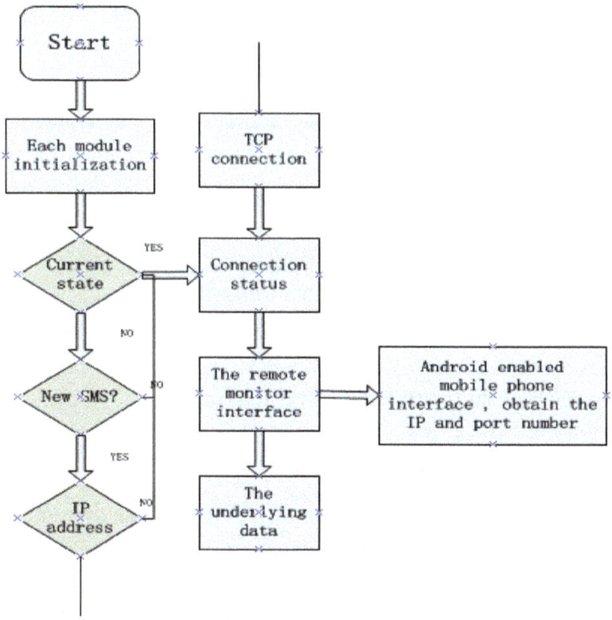

Fig. 3 The software design flow chart.

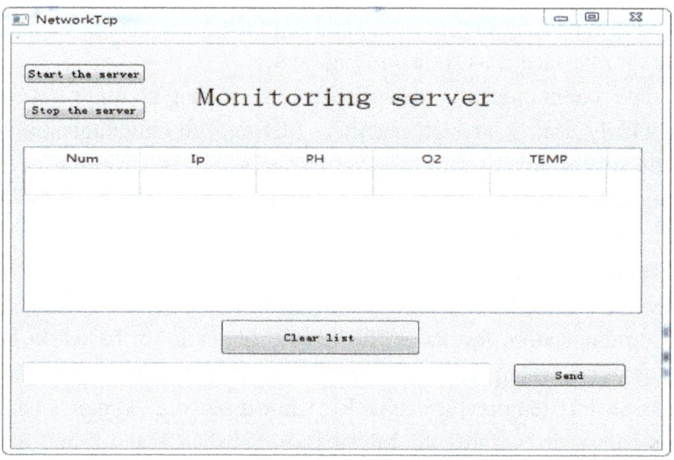

Fig. 4 Interface.

5. GPRS Communication

GPRS module is the key part to connect the underlying part and the upper computer. Before receiving or sending data, the connection between GPRS and the remote monitoring terminal, GPRS and the underlying sampling module must be established first. At first, initialize GPRS wireless module through AI instruction to have it attached to GPRS network, to get GPRS terminal IP address that is dynamically distributed by the network operator, to establish TCP connection to the remote monitoring terminal. And then extend the connection between MAX232 standard serial port and STM3 data acquisition terminal through the serial port 0, easily establishing communication with GPRS communication in accordance with the agreed protocol. The followings are the main AT instructions for establish the TCP connection for GPRS module:

AT+AUTO = NO; //set the module working type

AT+IPR = 9600; //set the baud rate of data transmission

AT+DNS = szzby1127.gicp.net, 19999; //set the domain name and the port of the server

AT+AUTO = YES; // set the module working type

6. Design of the Remote Monitoring Terminal

The remote monitoring terminal is an important part of the system, programmed with QT software in C++ programming language and mainly used for accepting, transmitting, processing, analyzing and displaying data, as well as other functions. The remote monitoring terminal interface contains buttons, a dialog box, a list and other parts. The buttons respond the corresponding performance functions after obtaining button actions through the associated private slots. The remote server interface is as shown in Figure 4.

The data communication design uses the socket communication mode, which is widely used with high stability. At first, the communication pointer, namely, the socket pointer of TCP/IP is instantiated. QT envelops such pointer readily. Socket contains two parts (IP and port number). The IP of the design is that used by the network server under the port number 19999.

```
m_pTcpServer = new QTcpServer();
m_pTcpServer->listen(QHostAddress::Any,19999);
```

The communication format of the remote server is set based on the lower position computer, which sends the upper computer the following format data:

Ip192.168.1.1* temperature value PH value dissolved oxygen value #

The upper computer captures the information between * and # and inputs into data by searching characters.

7. Design of the Android Mobile Phone Terminal

The Android mobile phone client is ZTE Q802T mobile phone, version Android 4.3, kernel 3.4.0, developed in AndroidSDK+JAVA JDK6+Eclipse3.5. The server can communicate with a plurality of mobile phone clients at the same time by distributing 1 port number for each client. After entering the system, the user first acquires the IP address of the server from the database, and then starts the receiving button to obtain the water sample data. As shown in Figure 5.

Table 1 Monitoring data of water quality for 10h.

Time	Temperature(°C)	PH	DO(mg/L)
7:00	16.5	7.1	8.3
8:00	18.3	7.3	8.2
9:00	20.4	7.5	8.5
10:00	23.6	7.4	8.1
11:00	24.3	7.2	8.3
12:00	25.5	7.8	8.1
13:00	26.2	7.2	8.9
14:00	27.4	7.3	8.3
15:00	24.7	7.4	8.2
16:00	23.2	7.2	9.1

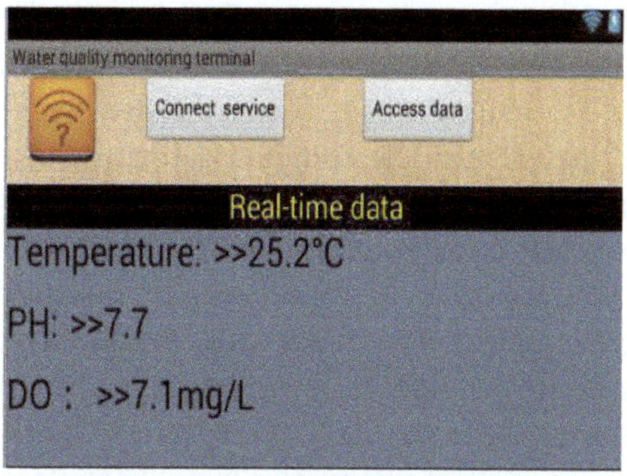

Fig. 5 The actual monitoring interface.

The Android system, whose interface is designed in a scripting language, mainly contains the login interface, the main function interface and a number of main control interfaces of the water quality. In the main function interface, the accepting button can be clicked to download the data that the underlying module sends to the server. The client is designed under the multi-threaded task mode for inter-communication at the server end by connecting to the 19999 port at the server end. After successful handshake, they begin to communicate. The codes to use the socket communication mode are as follows:

```
socketAddress=new
InetSocketAddress(MainActivity._ipText.getText().toString(),
Integer.parseInt("19999"))
```

The client interface is designed by using Scrollview space. ScrollView and HorizontalScrollView are employed to add scroll bars to the control or the layout, set by layout_width and layout_height, with ScrollView used for setting the vertical scroll bar while HorizontalScrollView used for setting the horizontal scroll bar and scroll bars used for setting the direction of scrollbars, in conjunction with the use of TextView control. The communication connection between the mobile phone terminal and the server is under the way to send a connection request to the server through the port number, the connection communication module mainly uses SOCKET communication mode, where the SOCKET (socket) is an abstraction layer, through which the application sends and receives data. At first, it throws exception by using the domain name (IP address) of the server to fail in establishing new SOCKET at the port. Then it is ready to receive the environmental parameters sent from the specified server port after a successful connection to start up the client, before applying Message processing to receive and display the data. The data is sent and received by reading the data flow, the sent or received data must be subject to the character code conversion. To implement a communication program, declare the permissions in the configuration file manifest.xml, otherwise it is impossible to use. The designed communication is by TCP, TCP/IPsocket consists of two parts: 1. input stream and 2. output stream, its basic working principle is: firstly, instantiate how to send the server PrintWriter out information from the client, by doing that, to such an object out is what to be sent. Compared to the server, PrintWriter out is our output stream, if we want to receive the data from the server, we must first instantiate such an object of BufferedReaderbr, also compare to the server, our client is to receive InputStreamReader input stream.

Now, we are conducting an uninterrupted test to a pool behind a school library for 10h. The monitoring data of the upper computer is as in Table 1

It is seen from Table 1 that in the range of 10h, the system can obtain the real-time and accurate water quality parameters on temperature, PH ad dissolved oxygen, with schedule reaching up to 0.1.

8. Conclusion

This system realizes the remote wireless monitoring of real significance based on the Android mobile phone, with a user-friendly operation interface, convenient control, real-time capability, and high performance to price ratio. The system debugging gets good effect, enjoys high control precision, and is quick-witted for remote control output, with great value on the spreading and use.

References

1. SERFASS D; YOSHIGOE K Wireless Sensor Networks using android virtual devices and Near Field Communication peer-to-peer emulation 2012.
2. Liu Fengnan, Dong Xueren, Ma Yuzhen. Mariculture Dynamic Monitoring System Based on 3G Technology [C], 2011.
3. Wang Leda, Xu Lihong, Huang Pei. An Aquaculture Monitoring System Based on Multipoint Data Acquisition, [Journal] -{H}, Fishery Modernization, 2012 (04).
4. Zhang Jun, Shang Min, Chen Jian. Intelligent Agriculture Remote Monitoring and Management System Based on 3G Technology [J], Computer Measurement and Control, 2012, 19(5).
5. PHILLIP G LEE. Process control and artificial intelligence software for aquaculture 2000 (1-3).
6. Zhan Chengguo, Zhu Wei, XuMinji. Design and Development of the Measurement and Control Device Human-Computer Interface Based on Android [J]-{H} Electric Power Automation Equipment, 2012 (01).
7. Lin Cheng. Application and Development Practice of Android 2.3 [J]. China Machine Press, 2011: 17-321.
8. Han Chao. Android Classic Application Development [J]. Human Resource Publishing House, 2011: 5-18.
9. Liu Weiguo, Yao Yuyu. Research and Implementation of Instant Communication between Android and J2ME Platform [J]. School of Information Science & Engineering of Central South University. 2008, No. 12: 118-120.
10. Liu Ping. A Data Interaction Method for the Android Mobile Phone to Access the Server [J]. Network and Modern Education Technology Center of Xi'an Financial Services Institute, 2010-09: 96-102.

A Weighted Round Robin Based Scheduling Method for ARINC653 System

Yue Meng[a] and Likou Zou
Dujiangyan Campus, Sichuan Agricultural University
Dujiangyan, Sichuan, 611830, China
[a]E-mail: mengyuemm@163.com
www.sicau.edu.cn

ARINC653 system is the current mainstream operating system in avionics system. In order to ensure real-time performance in avionics systems, ARINC653 defined two-level scheduling policy. However, the essence of partition level scheduling policy is the off-line static scheduling determined at the early stage of design, which lacks of flexibility and prone to produce idle time. On this basis, an improved method of two-level scheduling based on weighted round robin is proposed in the paper, and an extended scheduling plug-in of OSATE tool is developed and applied for schedulability analysis. Experiment that adopts avionics flight planning system as an example validates the effectiveness of the proposed method in reducing idle time of processors.

Keywords: ARINC653 system; two-level scheduling; weighted round robin; schedulability analysis.

1. Introduction

Avionics system is an important part of the aircraft. Along with the development of technology, avionics architecture continues to evolve from discrete architecture, combined architecture, and highly integrated architecture to integrated modular architecture nowadays. The processor, which is the core model in integrated modular avionics system, supports lots of application-layer software. It effectively brings relatively discrete aviation electronic components onto a standard hardware platform.

With the expansion of avionics software size, integrated modular avionics software is facing unprecedented challenges. Avionics software may gradually reduce reliability. Individual applications may highly rely on or influence by each other, or applications may illegal access memory segments which don't belong to them, resulting in a system crash.

ARINC653 (Avionics Application Standard Software Interface) is a software specification for space and time partitioning in safety-critical avionics real-time operating systems [1]. It allows hosting multiple applications of different software levels on the same hardware in the context of integrated modular avionics architecture.

2. Overview of ARINC653

Partition is a core concept in ARINC653, which divides the avionics system from the function view. ARINC653 use partition as basic unit of scheduling, allocating resources and application protection. Each partition consists of one or more concurrent processes, sharing processor resources. These processes are uniquely identified, and they contain properties which affect scheduling, synchronization, and the entire execution. Partition contains two levels of isolation: time and space. Time isolation of partition means OS (Operating System) periodically scheduling individual partition without taking partition priority into consideration, and OS will schedule the partition only when its corresponding time window comes. Space isolation of partition means the adoption of MMU (Memory Manage Unit) mechanism, which ensures that each partition has an independent virtual memory space to execute [2].

On this basis, ARINC653 standard uses a hierarchical scheduling model, which can be divided into two levels: partition level scheduling and process level scheduling [3]. Partition level scheduling is static and periodical. Process level scheduling means the scheduling inside a partition and is more flexible since the process level scheduling policies can be defined by the system designer [4-5]. Therefore, each partition can use different scheduling policy for scheduling tasks (processes).

3. Partition Level Scheduling based on Weighted Round Robin

In ARINC653 system, each partition gets its own execution time based on partition level round robin scheduling and task scheduling inside a partition relies on process level scheduling algorithms chosen by partition designer. Though ARINC653 has many advantages, there are still some following disadvantages:

(1) Partition design is not included in ARINC653 standard.

(2) Partition level scheduling policy is the off-line static scheduling determined at the early stage of design, which lacks of flexibility and prone to produce idle time.

(3) Idle time might be produced in the main time window and cannot be utilized.

This section presents a partition level scheduling method for ARINC653 based on weighted round robin scheduling, which use idle time sharing mechanism to schedule idle time that occurred in the activation process, to improve the response time of the system as a whole. And we have developed an extended scheduling plug-in of OSATE (Open Source AATL Tool Environment) tool to perform schedulability analysis of proposed scheduling method.

3.1. *Idle partitioning model based on Weighted Round Robin*

Our scheduling method adopts idle partitioning model based on weighted round robin and scheduling algorithm uses partition weight to schedule each partition. The relevant definitions are as follows.

Definition 1: Suppose the system has a partition set $P = (P_1, P_2, ..., P_n)$, where n is the cardinality of set P and $n \geq 1$. Each partition P_i contains a parameter tuple (T, E, W), where T is a set of time periods $\{(s_1, e_1), (s_2, e_2), ..., (s_n, e_n)\}$, and n is the cardinality of set P and $n \geq 1$, satisfy $(0 \leq s_1 < e_1 < s_2 < e_2 < ... < s_n < e_n \leq E)$; s_i represents the starting execution time of partition i; e_i represents the end execution time of partition i. E represents execution cycle, W represents the set of partition weight values and $W = \{w_1, w_2, ..., w_n\}$, each w_i is the weight value of partition i.

Definition 2: a partition performs task group $G = \{task_1, task_2, ..., task_m\}$, where $m \geq 0$, if $m = 0$ means the partition is an idle partition.

Definition 3: a task j has property tuple $task_j = (c_j, p_j, d_j)$, where c_j represents the maximum execution time for the task j, p_j indicates the execution cycle of task j, and d_j represents deadline of task j.

3.2. *Calculating method of weight values*

In above section scheduling model has been given, in which each partition is scheduled according to its weight value. Therefore, the key point is how to calculate the weight value of each partition.

The System assigns tasks of each partition onto the processors to perform. At partition level, partitions with high weight value can perform multiple tasks in one round robin period. Since there has no priority concept in ARINC653, priority of partition will not be taken into consideration. Weight value of partition is calculated by formula 3-1.

$$w_i = \log_2(taskNum_i + 1) \tag{3-1}$$

In this formula, $taskNum_i$ represents the task number of partition i.

3.3. *Scheduling algorithm based on weighted round robin*

In ARINC653 system, the main time window size of entire operation system is fixed. It also leads to idle partition occurs when the ARINC653 system is in operation. For an idle partition, although its weight is 0 (no task is included in the partition), the operating system will still schedule this idle partition to run and this will lead to waste of processor resources.

Therefore, considering the above problems, scheduling policy is given as follows:

1) Partitions can occupy multiple time windows.

2) Partitions are scheduled based on weighted round robin.

3) All partitions at ready state share idle partition. Idle partition sharing principle is defined as follows: the scheduler will always assign idle time to the maximum weight partition, or randomly pick one if there are multiple partitions with the same maximum weight.

In the application, partition switching consumes time, therefore, partition switching time need to be considered. If the time length of idle partition is smaller than or equal to the partition switch time, scheduler will continue to retain the idle partition. Besides, how to identify greater weight partition in all partitions at ready state is important when an idle partition is detected. A bitmap algorithm is used to manage partitions in order to improve search efficiency.

Based on the above consideration, execution flow in one round robin cycle of the proposed partition level scheduling algorithm is depicted in Figure 1.

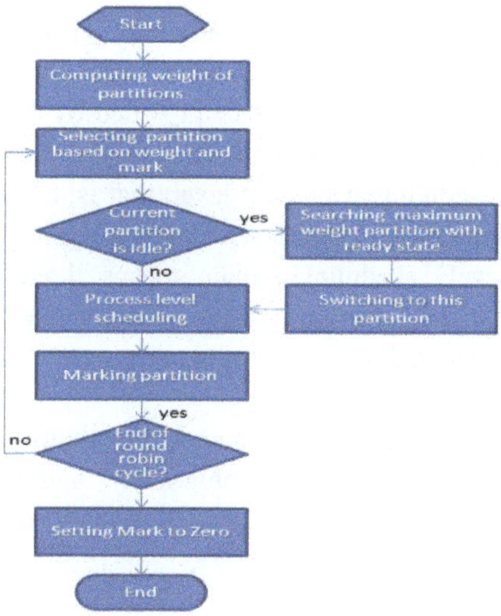

Fig. 1 Execution Flow of the proposed.

4. Schedulability Analysis

If all tasks in the system can be completed before its deadline, then it says the system is schedulable. Meanwhile verifying that the system is schedulable or not is called schedulability analysis. Schedulability analysis is an effective approach to verify system and it can predict the time behavior of the target system [6].

We use OSATE (Open Source AADL Tool Environment) tool for schedulability analysis of partition scheduling based on weighted round robin. OSATE is an AADL [7] (Architecture Analysis & Design Language) open source integrated development environment developed by Carnegie Mellon University [8]. It can be used for AADL modeling, compilation, and analysis. OSATE developed a variety of analyses plug-ins. Scheduling plug-in is one of those plug-ins, which can execute schedulability analysis and return the processor load as the result. Currently, two-level scheduling simulation is not supported by OSATE. Therefore, extended development is needed for OSATE scheduling plug-in in order to apply two-level scheduling simulation. Extend development steps are described as follows:

First of all, process component and thread component has its own properties in OSATE, but the original scheduling plug-in of OSATE only uses properties of thread component and doesn't take properties of process component into consideration. Since process component impersonate the concept of partition, the process component's properties represents the partition's property information. Therefore, by parsing XML documents that store model information, process component's properties can be accessed.

Secondly, to achieve two-level scheduling, partition scheduling algorithm described in section 3 and process component's properties must be imported into the plug-in by using scheduling interface provided by the plug-in, thus partition level scheduling simulation can be performed.

Then, when scheduling at process level, that is, a certain partition is being executed, the original scheduler of scheduling plug-in need to be invoked to realize process level scheduling, which means thread components will be scheduled. When the deadline of the current partition reaches, actions of partition switching will be executed. And scheduling at process level of the new selected partition will be performed.

Finally, load percentage of processors will be returned as the final result.

Based on the original scheduling plug-in, we added scheduling of process components so that the partition level scheduling can be simulated. The difference is shown in Figure 2.

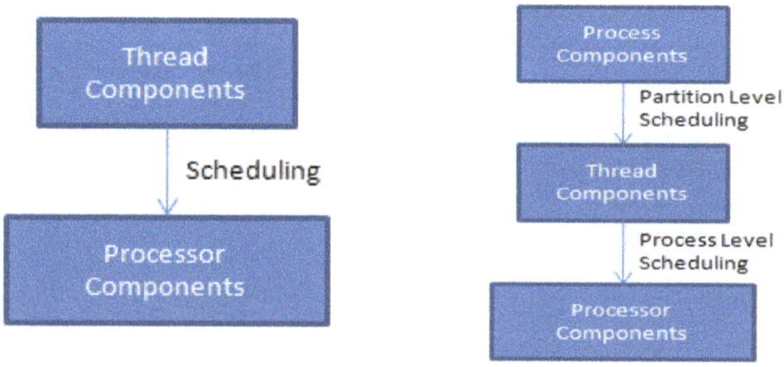

a

b

Fig. 2 a) Original plug-in scheduling diagram. b) Extended plug-in scheduling diagram.

5. Case Study

In this section, an avionics flight planning system is used for demonstration. The AADL model of flight planning system is shown in Figure 3, which includes six processes: Navigation Process, IntegrateNavigation Process, Flight Perfor Process, Guidance Process, Flight Plane Process and Data Display Process. The hardware components include Device (Sensor), FMProcessor (Processor), MeM (Memory) and Processor_Mem_Bus (Bus). Data is transferred between different processes (partition) is via bus, and partition use RMS to schedule. RMS (Rate Monotonic Scheduling) is adopted inside process (partition). Tasks attributes and corresponding attribute values of each process (partition) are given in Table 1.

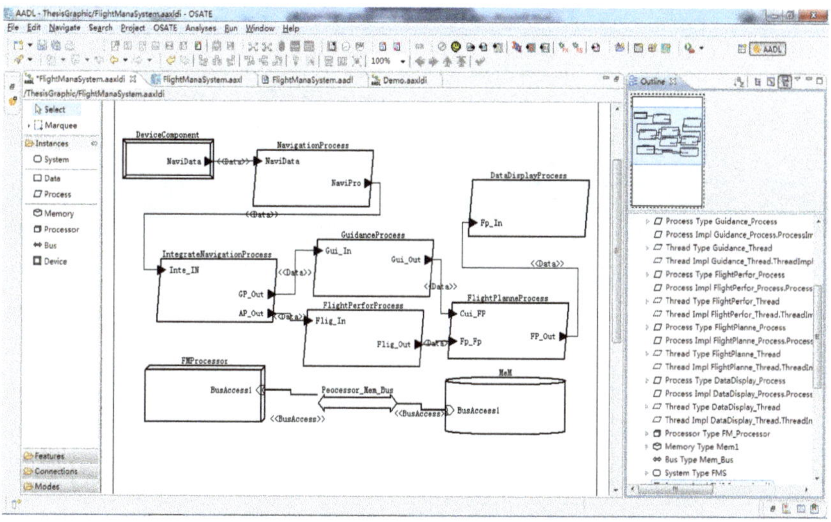

Fig. 3 Flight planning system architecture diagram.

Table 1 Tasks attributes and corresponding attribute values.

Task Title	**Period (ms)**	**Execution Time (ms)**	**Deadline (ms)**
Navigation_thread	20	3~6	20
IntegrateNavigation_thread	20	4~8	20
FlightPerfor_thread	20	2~4	20
Guidance_thread	20	5~10	20
FlightPlane_thread	20	6~12	20
DataDisplay_thread	20	8~14	20

Applying the extended scheduling plug-in, the simulation results of off-line static scheduling and weighted round robin scheduling are shown in Figure 4a and Figure 4b, respectively. As Figure 4a shows, when using off-line static scheduling, the processor load is 75% and the processor idle rate is 25%. While in Figure 4b, when using a scheduling based on weighted round robin, the processor load is 90% and the processor idle rate is 10%. Therefore, the processor idle rate of scheduling based on weighted round robin is less than that of off-line static scheduling.

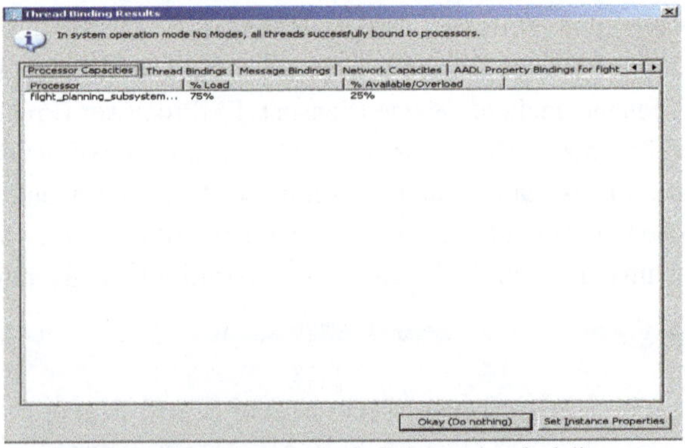

Fig. 4 a) Simulation result of off-line static scheduling.

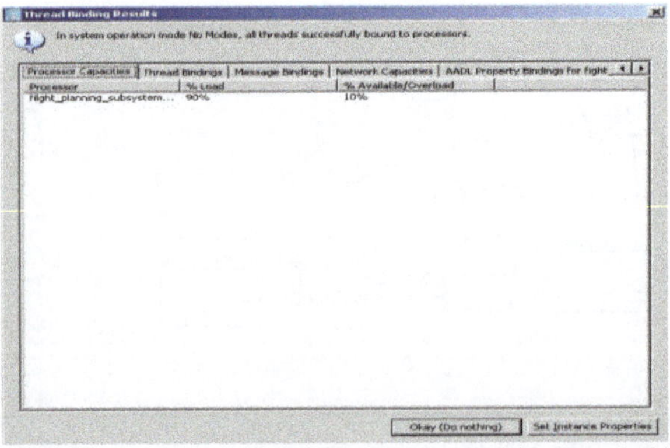

Fig. 4 b) Simulation result of scheduling based on weighted round robin.

6. Conclusion

This paper presents a partition level scheduling method based on weighted round robin, which provides an improved solution for the ARINC653 partition scheduling. Using weight to schedule partition can effectively reduce idle time of processors. An extended scheduling plug-in of OSATE tool is developed and applied for schedulability analysis. Based on the result of schedulability analysis, application designers can make a better choice in the early design stage.

References

1. A. Dubey, G. Karsai, R. Kereskenyi, et al. A Real-time Component Framework: Experience with CCM and ARINC-653 [C]. Proceedings of 13th IEEE International Symposium on Object/Component/Service-Oriented Real-Time Distributed Computing (ISORC'2010), IEEE, 2010, 143-150.
2. Li X. Y., Gu J., He F., et al. Two-level Partition Scheduling in Hard Real-time system under Strong Partition Constraints [J]. Chinese Journal of Computers, 2010, 33(6): 1032-1039.
3. Easwaran A, Lee I, Sokolsky O, et al. A Compositional Scheduling Framework for Digital Avionics systems [C]. Proceedings of 15th IEEE International Conference on Embedded and Real-Time Computing Systems and Applications (RTCSA'2009), IEEE, 2009, 371-380.
4. Cao G. X., Jiang Z. J., Wang L. F., et al. Study of Real-time Scheduling Algorithm under Strong partition constraints [J]. Microelectronics and Computer, 2012, 29(5): 108-112.
5. Qiao N. Q., Xu T., & Gu Q. F. Research and improvement of ARINC653 partition schedule algorithm [J]. Computer Engineering, 2011, 37(20): 249-251.
6. Zhang Y.Y., Sun Y., Li Y., et al. Research and Implementation of Schedulability Determination Tools in Complex Real-time System [J]. Computer Engineering, 2013, 39(1): 270-274.
7. P. H. Feiler, D. P. Gluch, and J. J. Hudak. The Architecture Analysis & Design Language (AADL): An Introduction [R]. Technical Report, 2006, CMU/SEI-2006-TN-011.
8. The SEI AADL Team. An Extensible Open Source AADL Tool Environment (OSATE) [R]. Software Engineering Institute, Carnegie Mellon University, 2006.

Automatic Vehicle Identification in Coating Production Line Based on Computer Vision

Li Xiang[a] and Dean Zhao[b]
Jiangsu University School of Electrical and Information Engineering, Zhenjiang, China
[a]270897695@qq.com, [b]zhaodean228@126.com

Kunming Yu
Jiangsu Puma Intelligent Equipment Co., Ltd., Changzhou, China
ykm198603083610@163.com

This thesis introduces a computer vision system which is applied to coating production line to automatically identify the vehicle model. This system controls camera to collect pictures by receiving signals of field sensor and processes these pictures by using grey level histogram similarity comparison technique and digital template matching technique, thus obtains the fittings' model of car body loaded by the lever body and the lever body number, and finds all corresponding information entering in advance into IPC (Industrial Personal Computer). When it needs the information of vehicle body in a link of production line, IPC will input corresponding information according to the lever body number through experimental tests, both image identification methods have good effects on identification of vehicle model and lever body number.

Keywords: Coating production line; computer vision; vehicle model identification; identification of lever body number.

1. Introduction

Along with the rapid development of automobile manufacturing and related industries, the competition among these industries has become very intense. And it is the most major problem being faced by all manufacturers how to improve efficiency and product quality in production. Automatic Vehicle Identification System (AVI system) may improve the intelligent level and information management level of vehicle coating production line, and play an important role to improve production efficiency and product quality. But it is the key problem for AVI system how to collect information. With the scientific and technological development, and the improved requirements of intelligence, safety and eligibility of coating production line, the constituent parts of AVI have changed, especially the information collection of AVI, which has changed from traditional bar code scheme to current universal RFID scheme.

Because the bar code identification system has gradually been obsoleted due to limitation of its own technology and low accuracy, and current primary RFID system is with high cost and its environmental factors make the carrier labels easy to be covered and damaged and affect reading, so new AVI system data collection schemes are proposed, mainly including infrared electric switch scheme, open type metal bar code scheme, image identification scheme and software reasoning scheme. And there are various methods of information collection in image identification scheme, such as obtaining information by identifying the home-made information sign for lever body. As for the computer vision scheme in this thesis, it mainly identifies vehicle models and lever body number.

2. Introduction of Principle of Computer Vision System

The main vehicle body identification system in production line at present is RFID system. Its principle is that the workers input the information of RFID tag of lever body when loading the vehicle body on the lever body, including vehicle model, production requirement (color), lever body number and so on. When the information of vehicle body is needed in a link of production line like spraying robot and automatic wiping, the tag of lever body will be read. During the process of production, several kinds of problems as below may come up:

1 Due to the special environment of coating production line, the tags may be covered by oil paint or damaged in the heat, and thus result the failure of information reading.

2 It is unable to be detected if workers input wrong information of vehicle body (vehicle model, color and so on) when loading the vehicle.

The principle of computer vision system is: enter the work plan into the IPC in advance, next the workers load the vehicle body by lever body according to the information provided by the computer, then IPC collect and identify the vehicle model and lever body number on the lever body by camera and signals provided by sensor in existing production line, finally compare them with the information in IPC. If there is an error about loaded vehicle model, this system will raise the alarm to make manual adjustment and modification. The loaded vehicle body by lever body moves along the production line, and when it arrives at a link which needs the information of vehicle body, the system will identify the lever body number by camera, then find out all corresponding information in the work plan from IPC and IPC transmits the information to field equipments (such as spraying robot).

The differences between the computer vision system and RFID system lie in:

1 The computer vision system enters the production schedule into IPC in advance, so that the workers need not to make information input of loaded vehicle model every time. As long as they load vehicle body according to the information provided by IPC, the mistakes during the vehicle loading could be found and adjusted timely. In this way, the production efficiency and accuracy get improved.

2 The lever body in RFID system has no fixed lever body number, so the workers need to define the lever body number when loading the vehicles. And every lever body number is fixed in computer vision system and must be embodied on the lever body for ease of computer identification and artificial identification.

3 All information of vehicle body in RFID system moves along with lever body in the production line, and is read when required. All information in computer vision system is stored in IPC and provided by IPC when required.

3. Principle of Computer Identifying Information

During the computer vision processing, OpenCV software is mainly used to process the image information collected in the field, grey level histogram similarity comparison is used to identify the vehicle model, and template matching digital identification technique is used to identify the lever body number.

4. Setting of ROI

ROI (Region of Interest) refers to a stated rectangular region in the picture. If ROI has been set, the program will process the stated region, while if ROI has not been set, the program will process the whole picture. It is very necessary to set ROI, because it not only can process the tiny difference between two similar pictures, but also can improve the processing efficiency.

5. Grey Level Histogram Similarity Comparison

After the camera collects the pictures conditionally in the collection point, the system confirms the vehicle model by comparing the collected pictures with the vehicle models in the database of IPC in sequence. In this process, it involves the issue of comparing two pictures. There are a variety of methods in OpenCV to compare two pictures, such as corner-point feature match and histogram similarity comparison. At this point, histogram similarity comparison is adopted in consideration of the fittings, colors, shapes and other conditions of car body.

Histogram is one of the most classical tools in computer vision. In brief, histogram is carrying on the data statistics and organizing the statistical values into a series of pre-defined bins, whose value is the statistical magnitude of features calculated by the data. And these data may be characteristic of gradient, direction and color, so histogram obtains the statistical chart of data distribution. Actually, histogram is a method which can display the image features conveniently.

Grey level histogram is the function of gray level, and it indicates the number of pixels with every kind of grayscale in an image and reflects the occurrence frequency of each grayscale in an image. An image may be expressed in a matrix, in which each figure corresponds to the grayscale value of points in the image. The gray level histograms of different pictures are different. It is able to confirm the information of vehicle model by comparing the gray level histograms of the collected pictures with the pictures in the database in sequence. The gray level histograms of pictures are shown as the Figures 1 and 2: The test results are in Fig. 3 and Fig. 4:

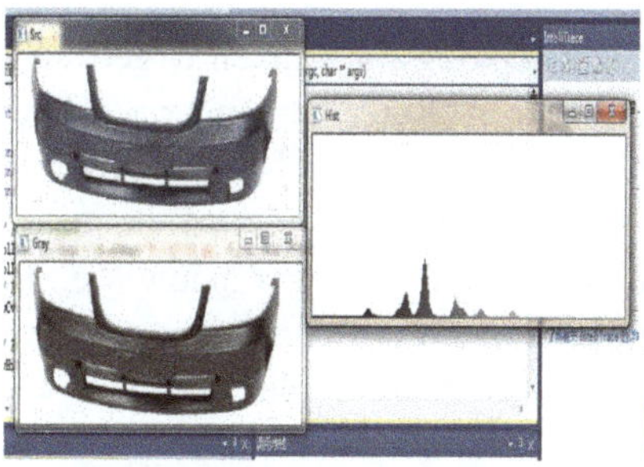

Fig. 1 Gray and gray level histogram of model 1.

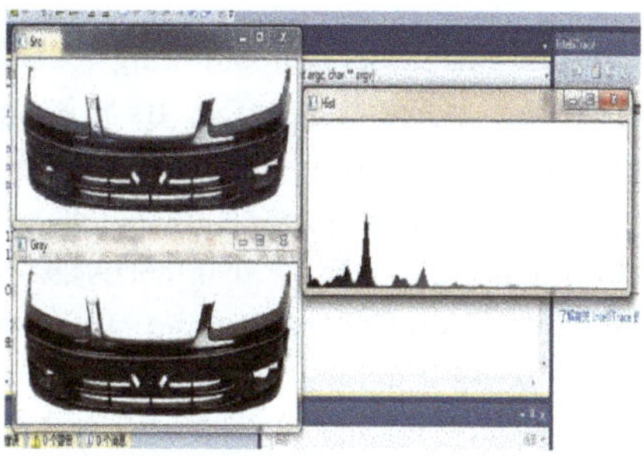

Fig. 2 Gray and gray level histogram of model 2.

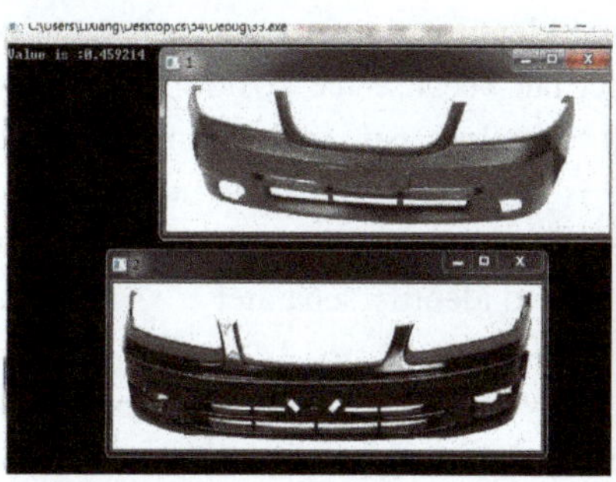

Fig. 3 Comparison of gray level histogram between model 1 and model 2.

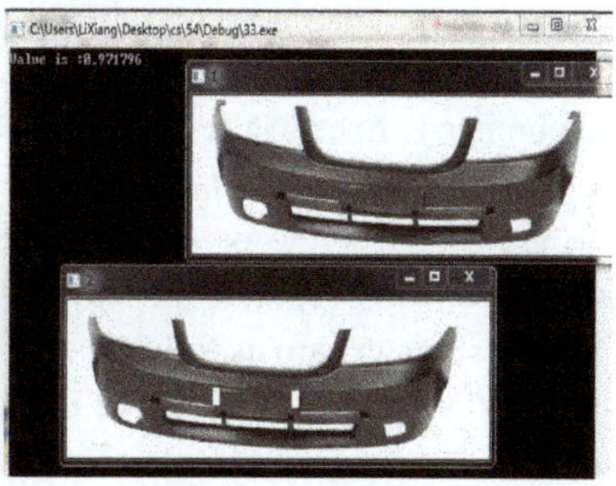

Fig. 4 Comparison of gray level histogram between model 1 and similar model.

Seen from above Figure 3, the score is very low obtained by comparing similarity of different fittings. And in Figure 4, the similarity comparison value is very high when there are only tiny differences between two pictures. If two pictures are same, the value is 1.

Because the result of image identification to identify the vehicle body is similarity, it may be misjudged when identifying two very similar car parts in shape and color due to high similarity and setting of threshold value. So it is necessary to perform secondary identification for two similar car parts. For example, vehicle a and b are quite similar on a whole and only have differences at a certain part. When the picture of fittings of vehicle a in the production line is collected and processed by IPC, the similarity values obtained by comparing with a and b in the database are very close and cause the error. But when we set the different regions of a and b as ROI in advance, and the IPC judges that the vehicle in the production line may be a, it is able to obtain an accurate judgment on vehicle body by making a histogram similarity comparison between the ROI of the collected vehicle model in the field and the ROI of a and b.

6. Template Matching

Template matching is positioning technology looking for a given target image (T) in the source image (S). Its principle is to measure the similarity of two image blocks through some criteria of similarity. This method is usually used for some plane image processing, such as the recognition of printed characters. While matching T in S, it is necessary to slide the matching window (i.e., the size of the template image) and calculate the similarity of corresponding image area between template image and the window. After the whole S image is slid, several match results will be obtained, and the best match results within all the match results will be obtained (the minimum or maximum value depends on the calculation way of similarity).

In computer vision system, the digital identification can use the recognition technology of license plate for reference, but because the position of the lever body number is fixed while shooting, all the colors and sizes of numbers are the same and shooting angle of the camera is consistent, thus it is unnecessary to rotate the digital angle or segment the characters or other steps. Setting ROI region can directly separate the single figure to identify separately.

The test results are as follows:

Firstly, assume No. 47 of the lever body number is collected to be handled by IPC, and the whole picture is treated as the source image (S), successively scan the target images (T) 0-9 in the source image (S) which are collected ahead of time from the IPC bank. Search the best matching region with the correlation coefficient matching method. Set the threshold value for the best matching value so as to exclude the pictures which are not matched successfully, to see whether the template matching is feasible. As shown in Figures 5 and 7, target images 4 and 7 have found matching areas, but in Figure 6, the target image 8 is excluded for its maximum of best matching result in the source image (S) is smaller than the threshold value.

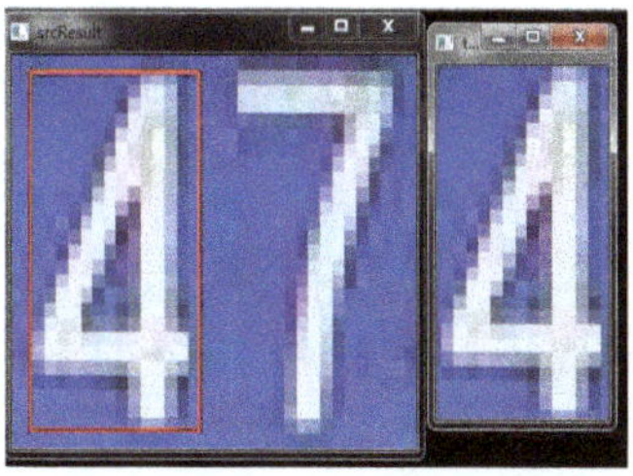

Fig. 5 The template 4 most similar template matching region in the source graph.

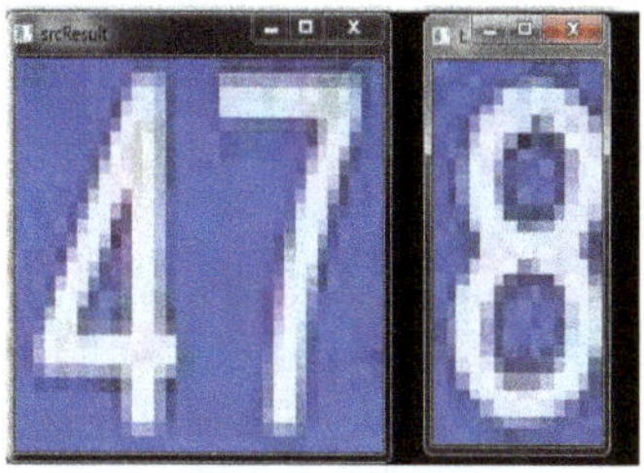

Fig. 6 Template 8 most similar matching region is not found in the source region graph.

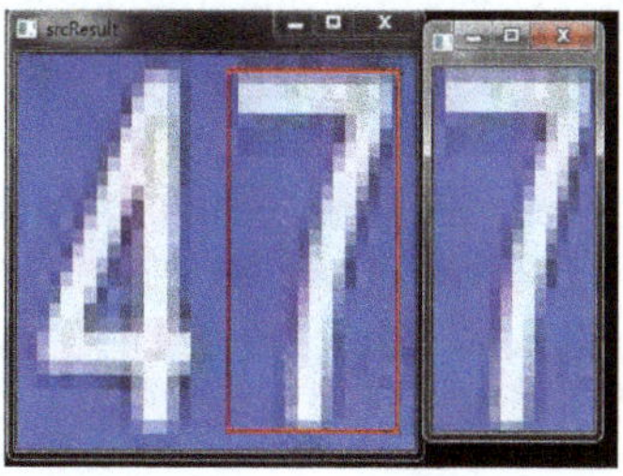

Fig. 7 The template 4 most similar template matching region in the source graph.

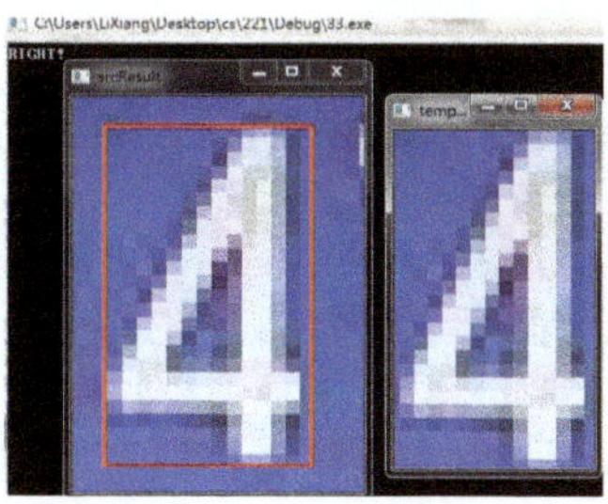

Fig. 8 The template 4 most similar template matching region in the splitted graph.

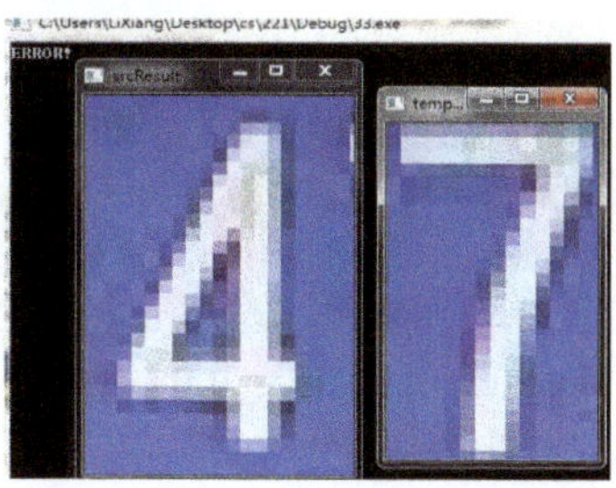

Fig. 9 The template 7 most similar template matching region not found in the region splitted graph.

After determining that the template matching can be used to identify the numbers, segment the character 4 and 7 through setting ROI region on the collected pictures. Respectively match in proper orders as the source image (S) so as to confirm the lever body number As shown in Figure 8, after the target image 4 matches with the first matching template, the best matching result is greater than the set threshold value; and in Figure 9, the target Figure 7 is excluded as its best matching result is smaller than the threshold value after the first matching.

7. Conclusion

Compared with the present REID system, the computer vision system not only reduces hardware costs, but also improves the level of coating production line intelligence, but the simplification of hardware makes the system software more complicated.

In the computer vision system, it is feasible to confirm the vehicle model with the contrast method of histogram similarity. However, in order to ensure the correctness of recognition, it is necessary to further recognize the ROI region of secondary identification for similar models. Segment the lever body number into separate characters through ROI, and then recognize it with the method of template matching, which is effective seeing from the test result.

Acknowledgments

Transformation project of scientific and technological achievements in Jiangsu Province, “A research and development on energy-efficient, environmentally friendly, flexible and intelligent coating production line for high-and-mid-end passenger vehicles” (BA2014079).

References

1. Zhang Chengli, Pang Luoming. The Application of Vehicle Automatic Identification Technology in the Automotive Coating Production Line, J. Automobile Technology and Materials, 2010, 04: 23-28.
2. Shen Ming, Yu Heqing. The Application of Radio Frequency Identification Technology in the Automotive Coating Production Line, J. Computer and Telecommunication, 2008, 07: 72-74. In Chinese.
3. Liu Jun, Xueming, Li Guili. The Application of RFID Vehicle Recognition and Information Processing in Automotive Production, J. Manufacturing Automation, 2006, 11 (28): 84-88. In Chinese.
4. Wang Qiwei. The Study of Image Histogram Feature and its Application, D. University of Science and Technology of China, 2014, 29-36. In Chinese.

5. Wei Wu, Zhang Qisen, Wang Mingjun, Huang Zhongxiang. A License Plate Identification Method Based on Template Matching and Neural Networks, J. Chinese Journal of Highway and Transport, 2001, 14 (1): 104-106. In Chinese.

GPU Accelerated DC Power Flow Analysis

Xu Zhang[a], Gan Zhou[b], Yanjun Feng[c] and Bingru Li[d]
School of Electrical Engineering, Southeast University, Nanjing, 210096, China
E-mail: [a]xuzhang@seu.edu.cn, [b]zhougan2002@seu.edu.cn, [c]fengyanjun@seu.edu.cn, [d]libingru1991@gmail.com
www.seu.edu.cn

Yupei Jia
China Electric Power Research Institute, Beijing, 100192, China
E-mail: jiapy@epri.sgcc.com.cn

Jinghuai Lin
Fujian Electric Power Dispatching and Control Center, Fuzhou, 350003, China
E-mail: linjinghuai@163.com

Graphics processing unit (GPU) has broad prospects in computation and memory intensive realms due to its superior performances in calculation capability, memory bandwidth and power consumption, and has natural applications in computational intensive power system analyses. Direct current power flow (DCPF) is often used in power system analysis, such as power flow analysis, security analysis and contingency screening. DCPF is a problem of solving sparse linear systems. This paper uses Jacobi iteration method to solve DCPF. Numeric studies on a 900-bus system have shown that the GPU-accelerated algorithm, in compared with its counterpart CPU version, can achieve about 2.3 times speedup. This highly promising performance has demonstrated that carefully designed performance tuning in conjunction with GPU programing architecture is imperative for a GPU-accelerated application.

Keywords: Graphics processing unit (GPU); Direct current power flow (DCPF); Jacobi iteration.

1. Introduction

In recent years, the graphics processing unit (GPU) has been used to accelerate the calculation in computation and memory intensive realms, such as petroleum survey, and computational fluid dynamics. Compared with same generation CPU, GPU has some unique advantages[1]. Therefore, applications of GPU technology in power systems have drawn increasingly more attention. Direct current power flow (DCPF) is a problem of solving a sparse linear system. So, GPU can be used to accelerate the calculation.

LU factorization is commonly used to solve linear system in power system. However, LU factorization is a serial algorithm and difficult to parallelize due to the tight data dependency during factorization. Meanwhile, LU factorization will be effective for smaller systems while its performance is limited for larger systems[2]. So, Jacobi iteration method have been adapted to solve DCPF accelerated by GPU.

2. DC Power Flow

The DCPF model, which is widely used in power system realm, is a linear model simplified from nonlinear alternative current power flow[3]. DCPF can be expressed as follows.

$$\boldsymbol{B}_{n\times n}\boldsymbol{\theta} = \boldsymbol{P} \tag{1}$$

where $\boldsymbol{B}$ is the bus reactance matrix (excluding the slack bus); the subscript $n\times n$ represents the dimension of matrix (n is the total number of buses in power network excluding slack bus); $\boldsymbol{P}$ is a $n\times 1$ vector of nodal active power injection; $\boldsymbol{\theta}$ is the $n\times 1$ vector of nodal voltage angle. $\boldsymbol{B}$ and $\boldsymbol{P}$ are known parameters and $\boldsymbol{\theta}$ is unknown.

Because of the characteristics of power system, $\boldsymbol{B}$ is a highly sparse matrix. DCPF is essentially solving the sparse linear system.

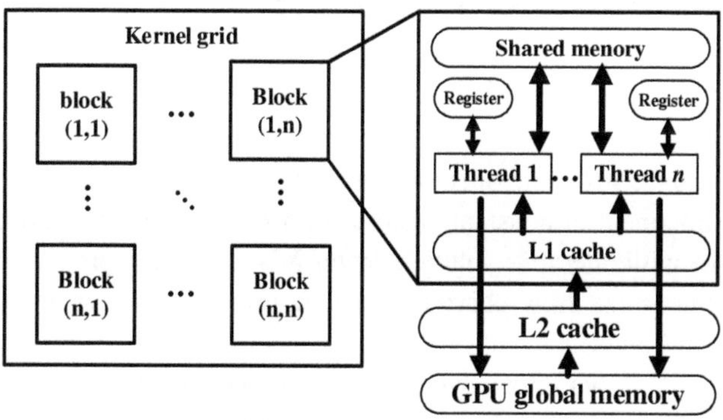

Fig. 1 GPU architecture.

3. GPU Architecture and CUDA Runtime Model

The NVIDIA GPU architecture is shown in Fig. 1. A GPU consists of some streaming multiprocessors (SM), and each SM is composed of many CUDA cores, L1 cache, shared memory, and some special functional units. In Kepler architecture, each SM has 192 CUDA cores. The global memory has much more storage capacity and longer access latency than other storages[4].

NVIDIA GPUs execute programs in a single-instruction multiple-thread (SIMT) manner. SMs execute threads in groups of 32 concurrent threads called a warp. Several warps are grouped into a thread block. One thread block is executed on one SM, and one SM can hold several concurrent thread blocks. Data can be easily shared within a thread block through the shared memory.

4. Implementation of Jacobi Iteration on GPU

Iterative methods are suitable for large scale linear equations. There are three commonly used iterative methods: Jacobi's iterative method, Gauss-Seidel iterative method and SOR iterative method. The last two iterative methods' convergence speed is faster than Jacobi's iterative method but lack of parallelism. They have advantages to Jacobi method only when implemented in sequential fashion. On the contrary, Jacobi iteration has inherent parallelism. It's suitable to be implemented on GPU to run concurrently on many cores. Linear equations in matrix form is

$$\boldsymbol{AX}=\boldsymbol{b} \tag{2}$$

$\boldsymbol{X}$ is the iterative solution vector. Vector $\boldsymbol{b}$ is constant vector. Coefficient matrix $\boldsymbol{A}$ is a sparse matrix stored in CSR format.

The solving process of Jacobi's iterative method is as follows:

$$X_i^{(k+1)} = \frac{1}{a_{ii}}\left(b_i - \sum_{j\neq i} a_{ij} X_j^{(k)}\right) \tag{3}$$

Where $X_i^{(k+1)}$ is the i-th component of the (k+1) times iterative solution vector; b_i is the i-th component of constant vector $\boldsymbol{b}$ in $\boldsymbol{AX}=\boldsymbol{b}$; a_{ij} is element of $\boldsymbol{A}$ in row i, column j. The initial iterative solution vector $\boldsymbol{X}$ is a zero vector.

Fig. 2 shows the flow chart Jacobi iteration implementation on GPU. Its details are as follows:

(1) There is no global thread synchronization mechanism on CUDA. But each time iteration need to be synchronized. Just one block is launched and each thread is in charge of calculating one X_i.

(2) In order to avoid frequently reading convergence mark *flag* in global memory by each thread. The convergence mark *flag* is stored in shared memory.

(3) In the calculation, because of the (k+1) times iterative solution vector $\boldsymbol{X}^{(k+1)}$

and the (k) times iterative solution vector $\boldsymbol{X}^{(k)}$ are shared in a block and used in every iteration, $\boldsymbol{X}^{(k+1)}$ and $\boldsymbol{X}^{(k)}$ are also stored in shared memory.

(4) Vector $\boldsymbol{b}$ is a constant vector in the iteration, which is stored in constant memory.

(5) In convergence judgment, each thread will write convergence mark *flag*. This process is in serial and time-consuming. So, before judgment in each thread, the mark flag will be checked firstly. If flag has be changed, the write operation will not be executed.

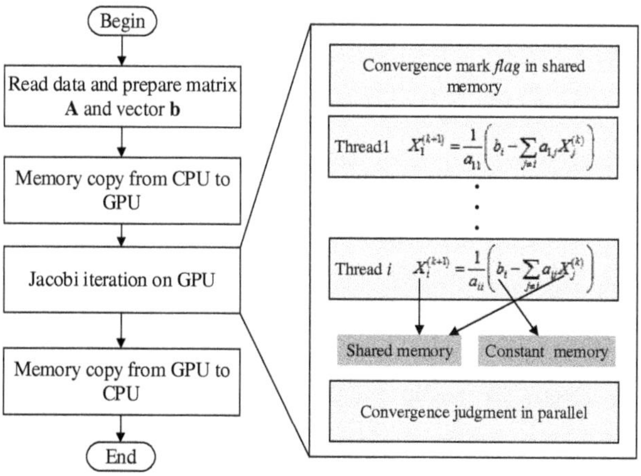

Fig. 2 Flow chart of Jacobi iteration implementation on GPU.

5. Experimental Results

We implement Jacobi iteration method both in traditional fashion that runs on CPU and parallel fashion on NVIDIA GPU. The convergence accuracy is 1e-7.

The test platform is a computer equipped with a NVIDIA NVS5400M GPU and an Intel Core i7-3520M 2.90 GHz CPU. The CUDA driver version is 6.0. Operation system is Windows 7. Our sequential program runs only on one CPU core.

All tested sparse linear systems are from DCPF model in matpower[5].

The above figures shows the CPU and GPU calculation time and the speedup. It can be seen that the speedup increases with the growth of matrix order. When the matrix order is over 200, the speedup increases very slowly and run into the bottleneck. The speedup reach the peak of 2.3 when the matrix order is 900. The reason is, this GPU is based on Femi architecture, on which computing resources are used 100% when one block contains more than 192 threads.

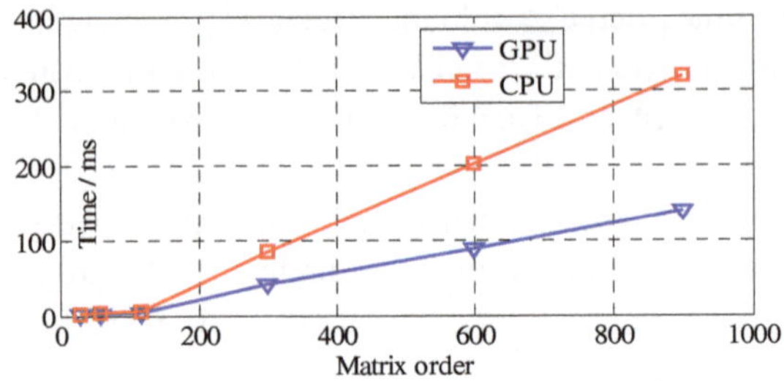

Fig. 3 Calculation time of CPU and GPU algorithm.

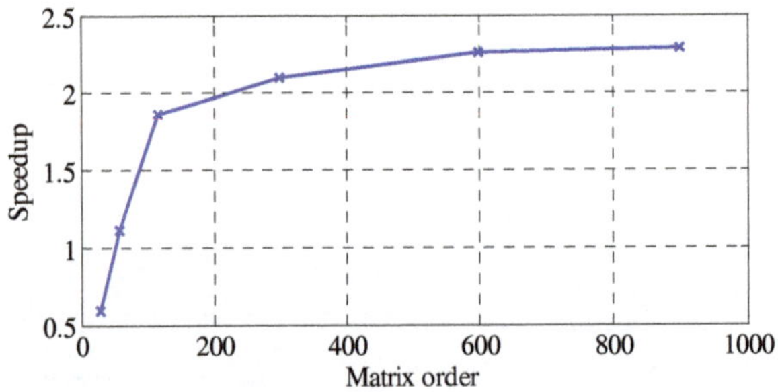

Fig. 4 The speedup of GPU-accelerated Jacobi iteration.

6. Conclusion

Taking advantages of NVIDIA's CUDA technology, Jacobi iteration are implemented on GPU for sparse linear systems. The maximum 2.3 times speedup has be achieved comparing with traditional sequential program on CPU. Because of the characteristics of GPU and Jacobi iteration algorithm, the speedup is not obvious and the matrix order is limited. Further, we will explore other methods of solving sparse linear system to improve computing efficiency.

Acknowledgments

This study was supported by the National Natural Science Foundation of China (51207020) and the Science and Technology Foundation of State Grid Corporation of China (DZ71-14-040).

References

1. E. Lindholm, J. Nickolls, S. Oberman, J. Monyrym, NVIDIA Tesla: A unified graphics and computing architecture, *IEEE Micro* **28**, 39-55 (2008).

2. X. Li, F. Li, GPU-based power flow analysis with Chebyshev preconditioner and conjugate gradient method, *Electric Power Systems Research* **116**, 87-93 (2014).
3. B. Stott, J. Jardim, O. Alsac, DC power flow revisited, *IEEE Trans. Power Systems* **24**, 1290-1300 (2009).
4. J. Nickolls, I. Buck, M. Garland, S. Kevin, Scalable parallel programming with CUDA, *ACM Queue* **6**, 40-53 (2008).
5. R. D. Zimmerman, C. E. Murillo-Sánchez, D. Gan, MatPower – A Matlab Power System Simulation Package (2015), `http://www.pserc.cornell.edu/matpower/`.

Lunar Image Enhancement Algorithm Using Dark Channel Prior and Histogram Equalization*

Ip Ka Meng
Faculty of Information Technology, Macau University of Science and Technology, Macau, China
E-mail: ipzxve2678@gmail.com
http://www.must.edu.mo

Xiaolin Tian
Faculty of Information Technology, Lunar and Planetary Science Laboratory/Space Science Institute, Macau University of Science and Technology, Macau, China
E-mail: xltian@must.edu.mo

A new Enhancement Algorithm of Lunar CCD Images based on the Dark Channel Prior & Histogram technology has been proposed in the paper. The Dark Channel parts of Lunar CCD Images have been detected through the Dark Channel Prior Algorithm first, and then only Dark Channel parts of images have been enhanced by Histogram Equalization technique. After combined enhanced Dark Channel parts with the other non-Dark Channel parts, a new Histogram modification technique has been designed and implemented to reduce the blocking effect in combined images. The new algorithm has been tested and results have been compared with other enhancement algorithms based on the histogram technology on Lunar CCD Images. The testing results have shown that Lunar CCD Images enhanced by the new algorithm proposed could become clearer, and the topography in the Lunar CCD Images becomes more prominent, color softer compared with results by other tested algorithms.

Keywords: Lunar CCD image; dark channel prior; histogram equalization; histogram modification.

1. Introduction

One of the most obvious characteristics in the lunar CCD images is that the image looks dim and dark. It would be harder to do any further research if those lunar CCD images could not be enhanced. There are many different algorithms for lunar CCD images enhancement which have been published recently. Such as Image Sharpen [2], Bi-histogram Equalization [3], Photometric correction [4]

* This work is supported by the Science and Technology Development Fund of Macao, Macao SAR, China (No.059/2013/A2).

and Fast Matching [5].

A new enhancement algorithm of lunar CCD images based on Dark Channel Prior & histogram technology has been proposed in the paper. The new algorithm has been implemented and tested on lunar CCD images. Enhancement results based on histogram technology only have been tested too, which have shown that the new algorithm proposed using Dark Channel Prior & Histogram technology has better performance on promoting image clarity, due to the multiple dependencies of lunar CCD Images and Dark Channel Prior enhanced images, which has laid a solid foundation for subsequent research of Moon.

2. New Enhancement Algorithm of Lunar CCD Images

First of all, the new algorithm proposed will detect sub-images to be enhanced by introducing the Dark Channel Prior info to distinguish which area should be enhanced in the lunar CCD images. Then those sub-images detected will be enhanced by Histogram Equalization. Enhanced sub-images will replace or be merged back to the original image. Finally, a new histogram modification technique has been designed and implemented to reduce the blocking effect in combined images. The flow chart of the new enhancement algorithm proposed has been shown in the Figure 1. Details of the new algorithm proposed will be given step by step.

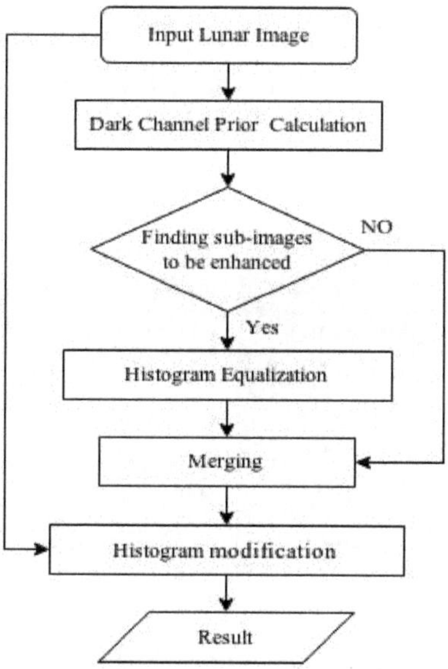

Fig. 1 Flow chart of new enhancement algorithm for the lunar CCD images proposed.

2.1. *Dark channel prior calculation*

In most of non-astronomical images, at least one color channel has very low intensity at some pixels. In the other words, the minimum intensity in such channel should have a very low value. Formally, for an image *J*, define

$$J^{dark}(x) = \min_{y\in\Omega(x)}(\min_{c\in\{r,g,b\}} J^c(y)) \quad (1)$$

$\boldsymbol{J}^c$ is a color channel of $\boldsymbol{J}$ and $\boldsymbol{\Omega(x)}$ is a local patch centered at $\mathbf{x}$.

The new enhancement algorithm for the lunar CCD images proposed will use dark channel prior algorithm to process the original image. It is more effectively to find out the terrain feature which needs to focus on strengthening through Dark channel processing. And analysis different Dark Channel image is helpful to analysis Lunar Surface.

After calculating the Dark Channel Prior from the original image, the Dark Channel result image will be divided into 100 pieces of the same size sub-images, then calculate the average grey value of each image to decide which sub-images should be enhanced.

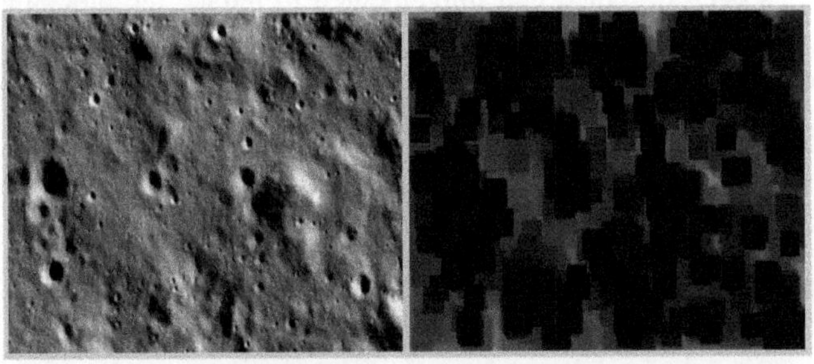

Fig. 2 Lunar image and its dark channel.

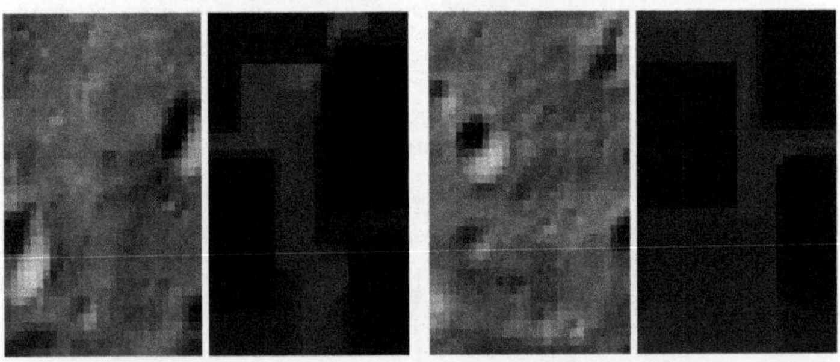

Fig. 3 Divided sub-image with its dark channel image.

2.2. *Dark channel block enhancement by histogram equalization*

Histogram equalization is a technique for adjusting image intensities to enhance contrast. This method usually increases the global contrast of many images, especially when the usable data of the image is represented by close contrast values. Through this adjustment, the intensities can be better distributed on the histogram. This allows for areas of lower local contrast to gain a higher contrast. Based on chunked dark channel images, histogram equalization will be implemented to every dark channel block, when the average gray value of the block is smaller than a fixed value (0.16 was used in the testing).

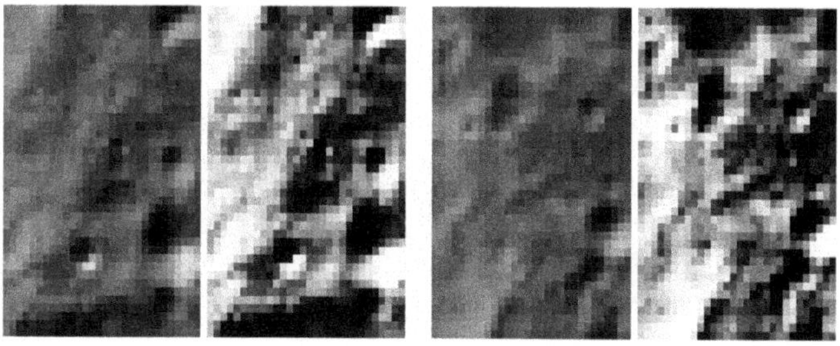

Fig. 4 Sub-image and its equalization result.

2.3. *Merging sub-images*

In this step, enhanced sub-images will be merged back with those not-enhanced sub-images to form a whole result image. And then the histogram modification will be implemented to avoid potential block effects, because merged images may have some block effects in the result. The histogram will be modified according to the histogram of the result image. Fig. 5. has showed the merged result image with its corresponding histogram, which will offer the reference value for the histogram modification.

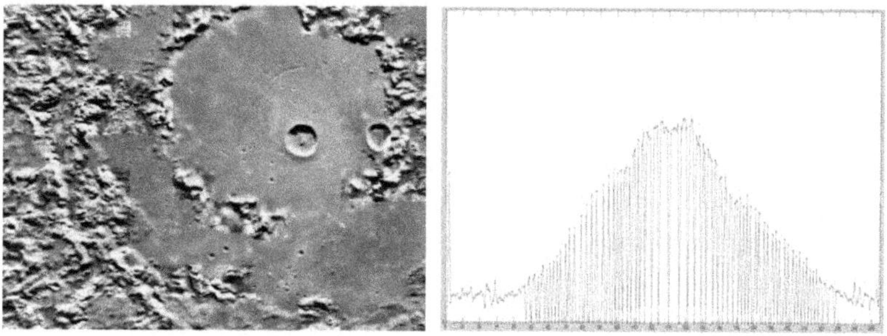

Fig. 5 Merged result image with its corresponding histogram.

2.4. *Histogram modification*

Histogram modification is a method to modify image histogram to a required shape. It is possible to use histogram matching to balance detector responses as a relative detector calibration technique. It can be used to normalize two images, when the images were acquired at the same local illumination over the same location, but by different sensors, atmospheric conditions or global illumination. Utilizing reference value graph combined image as new parameters into the original image histogram modification process. It can avoid the images to be not unified, balanced color tone.

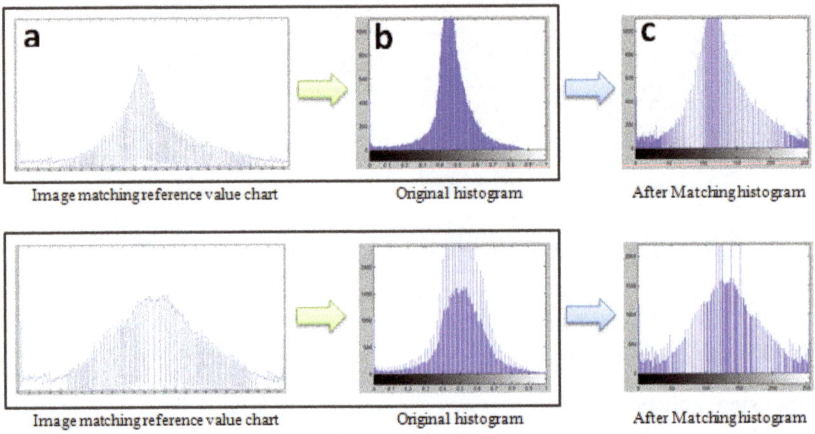

Fig. 6 Histogram modification processing.

3. Testing Results

To evaluate the new algorithm proposed, the other two Histogram technology related enhancement methods have been tested too for comparison purpose. They are Method1: Full histogram equalization; Method2: Chunked histogram equalization; and the Method3: The method proposed in this paper.

One of the testing result images have been shown in the Fig. 7 for better explaining the results.

From the Figure 7 we could see that Fig. 7a Histogram distribution focus, colors dim, terrain features are not clear. Fig. 7b Histogram distribution dispersion, color imbalance, after enhancing local topography appears dim; the whole is not uniform unfavorable observation. Fig. 7c Histogram distribution of scattered, not unified tone image appears uneven terrain features are not clear. Fig. 7d Histogram distribution average, lunar terrain features more obvious, the overall tone of the average image clearer, favorable observation.

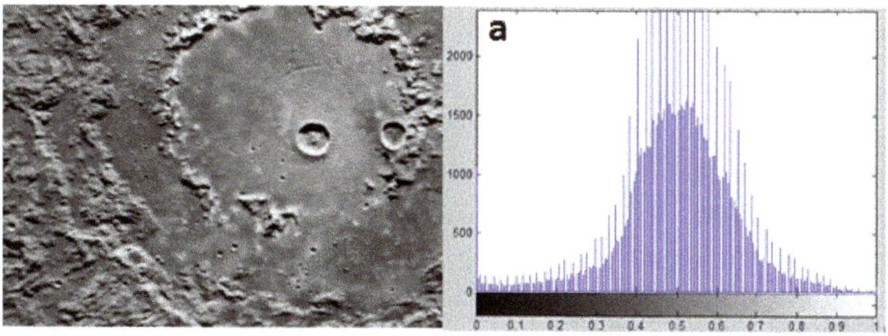

(7a) The original image with it's histogram

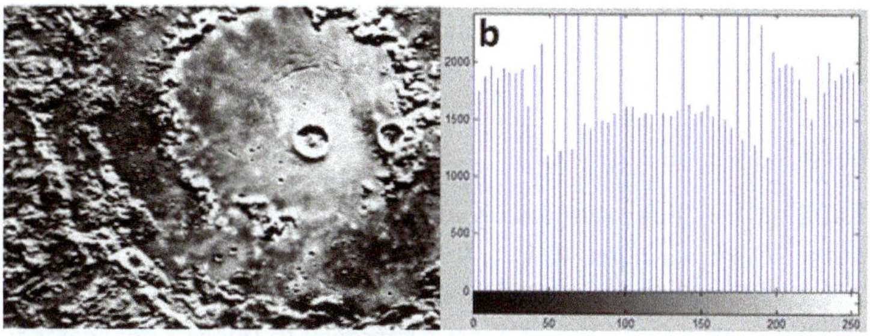

(7b) The result image by whole image equalization

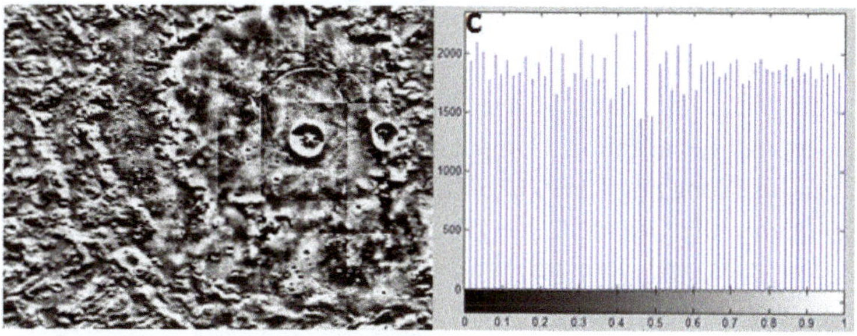

(7c) The result image by chunked equalization

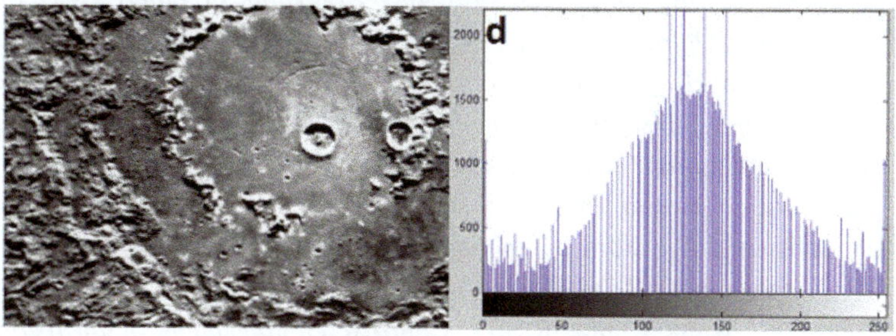

(7d) The result image by the new algorithm proposed

Fig.7 Experimental Results by different enhancement algorithms.

4. Conclusion

A new algorithm of lunar CCD image enhancement based on Dark Channel Prior & histogram technology has been proposed in the paper. Testing results have shown that the new enhancement algorithm proposed is suitable for enhancing the lunar CCD images, and it is more effective to highlight the topography of the lunar surface using relevant characteristics as a parameter. According to the experimental results, It is easier to see that the new algorithm proposed could offer better enhancement results than other histogram equalization methods. The new algorithm proposed could solve the tone uneven terrain dim and other issues, and it could be a reliable basis of further research in the future.

References

1. Kaiming He, Jian Sun, and Xiaoou Tang, *Single Image Haze Removal Using Dark Channel Prior.* IEEE TRANSACTIONS ON PATTERN ANALYSIS AND MACHINE INTELLIGENCE, (2011).
2. Negi, S.S, Bhandari, Y.S, A hybrid approach to Image Enhancement using Contrast Stretching on Image Sharpening and the analysis of various cases arising using histogram, Recent Advances and Innovations in Engineering (ICRAIE), (2014).
3. WU Ying, Adaptive Image Enhancement Algorithm Based on Bi-histogram Equalization, Computer Engineering, P244-245, (2011).
4. Yan Lu, Yongqing Chen, Chao Chen, Xiao Zhou, *Photometric correction of lunar image from CCD stereo camera on Chang'E-1 satellite of China,* Geoscience and Remote Sensing Symposium (IGARSS), 2013 IEEE International.
5. Wang Junduo, Wang Riwei, Wen Xianbin, Zou Yongliao, Zheng Yongchun, Wang Ling, *Fast Matching Algorithm of Lunar CCD Image [J]. Laser & Optoelectronics Progress,* 2012, 49(1): 011102.
6. Park, D., Ko, H., *Fog-degraded image restoration using characteristics of RGB channel in single monocular image.* Consumer Electronics, 2012 IEEE International Conference on, pp. 139--140, IEEE Press (2012).
7. Aedla Raju, Dwarakish G.S, Reddy D. Venkat, Satellite image contrast enhancement algorithm based on plateau histogram equalization, Region 10 Symposium, (2014) IEEE.
8. Santhi K, WahidaBanu, R.S.D, *Contrast enhancement of bi-histogram equalization with neighborhood metrics, Computing*, Communications and Networking Technologies (ICCCNT), (2013).

9. JIANG Ju-lang, ZHANG You-sheng, XUE Feng, HU Min1, *Local Histogram Equalization with Brightness Preservation*, ACTA ELECTRONICA SINICA, (May 2006).
10. CHEN Wei tao, YAN Bo kun, ZHANG Zhi, THE IDENTIFICATION OF SPECIAL TARGETS BASED ON SPATIAL FEATURES OF CHANG'E CCD DATA, REMOTE SENSING FOR LAND & RESOURCES, (2009).
11. LI Guo, GONG Zhi-hui, LEI Yang, HE Yu, Genetic Algorithm Optimization Enhancement on Fourier Frequency Domain of Degraded Image Achieved by Chang'E-1 Orbiter, Opto-Electronic Engineering, (2012).
12. LI Chunlai. Photogrammetric Processing and Lunar Global Topographic Map form the Chang'E-1 3 Line-array CCD Data. Acta Geodaetica et Cartographica Sinica, (2013).
13. PAN Zhiqiang, GU Xingfa, LIU Guodong, MIN Xiangjun, *Relative Radiometric Correction of CBERS-01 CCD Data Based on Detector Histogram Matching*, GEOMATICS AND INFORMATION SCIENCE OF WUHAN UNIVERSITY, (2005).
14. Mostafa Fakhar, Peyman Moalem, Mohamad Ali Badri. *Lunar Crescent Detection Based on Image Processing Algorithms*. Earth, Moon, and Planets, (2014).
15. Cai Shidong, Yang Fang, *Image Enhancement Based on Histogram Modification*, OPTOELECTONIC TECHNOLOGY, (2012-9), pp.155-159.
16. LI Chun-hui, LIU Hui, ZHONG Cheng, *Histogram Equalization in Image Enhancement Application*, JOURNAL OF HUBEI UNIVERSITY OF TECHNOLOGY, 2011, 26(2).

Performance Evaluation Method of Image Registration in Diffusion-Tensor Imaging Based on Gray Level Co-Occurrence Matrix

Yang Chen, Min Lu, Xiaojie Zhang and Weibei Dou[a]

Department of Electronic Engineering, Tsinghua University, Beijing, 100084, China
[a]E-mail: douwb@tsinghua.edu.cn

Medical image registration is the key technique of multimodal medical image processing, because it directly influences the results of information fusion of multimodal signals. It is one of the most important technique in Diffusion-Tensor Imaging (DTI), since the tensor calculation depends on the registration of Diffusion-Weighted Imaging (DWI) of different gradient direction. Therefore, the evaluation of the registration performance is a very important step for evaluating the result of information fusion. But traditional subjective evaluation method varies from person to person, while some objective evaluation methods are related to different registration algorithm or software. To solve this problem, an automatic evaluation method of DWI registration is proposed in this paper. The evaluation criteria used in this method include entropy, contrast, and correlation calculated by gray level co-occurrence matrix of Fractional Anisotropy (FA) image. Two registration results obtained by rigid and affine methods, and non-registered data are used in our testing experiment. The experiment results of 5 subjects data showed that the proposed evaluation method not only can integrate whole-brain information automatically, but also can reflect the performance of different registration methods accurately.

Keywords: Diffusion-tensor imaging; image registration; evaluation.

1. Introduction

Diffusion tensor imaging [1], is a magnetic resonance imaging technology by measuring water molecule diffusion direction and degree in the brain. In the process of diffusion tensor image acquisition, the head motion of subjects and eddy current effect caused by changed gradient magnetic field would lead to image shift and distortion. Therefore, in order to reduce the influence of image spatial relationship, registration is needed before using DWI and b0 image.

At present, 7-parameter rigid registration, 12-parameter affine registration and a few non-linear registration algorithms are commonly applied in DTI registration. In order to compare the performance of different algorithms on the clinical application, evaluation method is needed. Medical image registration evaluation, usually has no real gold standard. Researches on the image registration evaluation methods are disperse. Hence this paper proposes a novel rapid registration evaluation method which has a positive theoretical support.

2. Related Work

The current registration evaluation methods can be divided into subjective evaluation and objective evaluation. Subjective evaluation method is based on human visual system. Malinsky [2] introduced checkerboard image method by observing the reference image and target image directly. K. Choil [3] proposed a method by means of observing the fiber bundles based on FA image. But all these methods require priori knowledge. Objective quantitative evaluation methods become a popular trend. Kinoshita *et al.* [4] proposed using inverse consistency error as a criterion. Similar criteria are proposed by Non-rigid Image Registration Evaluation Project [5]. Malinsky [2] takes the mean of FA value in white matter as a criterion, while Oubel E [6] uses the mean FA value of cerebrospinal fluid. However, these evaluation methods rely on other software's segment result. Therefore, this paper presents a novel evaluation method based on gray level co-occurrence matrix. This method evaluates registration results by directly calculating characteristic parameters based on co-occurrence matrix, meanwhile it doesn't need other software and consider the whole information.

3. Evaluation Method Based on Gray Level Co-Occurrence Matrix

Since the brain has distinct textural features, the texture of the FA image which was generated from registered image can be used to evaluate the registration results. Gray level co-occurrence matrix is the most commonly used analysis method in texture analysis, and this matrix reflects different gray levels' distribution in the space [7]. Hence this study uses gray level co-occurrence matrix to evaluate the textural features.

In order to describe the image textures intuitively, complicated gray level co-occurrence matrix is replaced by its secondary statistic parameters. This paper uses three main parameters.

(1) Entropy

$$E = -\sum_{i=0}^{N-1}\sum_{j=0}^{N-1} P_{d,\theta}(i, j)\log P_{d,\theta}(i, j) \tag{1}$$

Entropy is a measure of the information. The element of gray level co-occurrence matrix is more random, the entropy is higher. If the texture is fuzzy, it means the intensity distribution is close to random and the noise is big, and the entropy is high. In theory, the image processed by better registration algorithm has sharper textures and has a higher non-uniformity, so the entropy is smaller.

(2) Contrast

$$CN = \sum_{n=0}^{N-1} n^2 \left\{ \sum_{|i-j=n|} P_{d,\theta}(i,j) \right\} (i,j = 0,\cdots,N-1) \quad (2)$$

Contrast reflects image's clarity and the level of texture grooves. The deeper texture grooves will be visually clearer, and the contrast is higher. In theory, the image processed by better registration algorithm has higher contrast.

(3) Correlation

$$CR = \frac{\sum_{i=0}^{N-1}\sum_{j=0}^{N-1} ijP_{d,\theta}(i,j) - \mu_1\mu_2}{\sigma_1^2\sigma_2^2} \quad (3)$$

Where μ_1, μ_2 are mean, σ_1, σ_2 are variance.

Correlation is used to measure the similarity of gray level co-occurrence matrix elements in the direction of row and column, and reflects the gray correlation of image. The image processed by better registration algorithm has sharper textures, so the correlation is smaller.

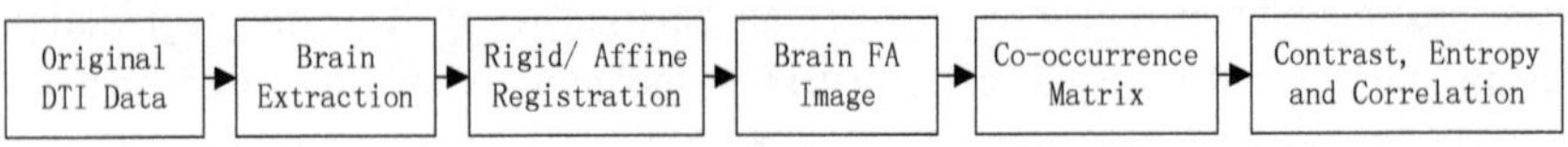

Fig. 1 DTI registration evaluation framework.

4. Experiments and Results

DTI data acquisition: 5 subjects were from Beijing Tian Tan Hospital. They are scanned by using EPI sequence performed on a 3.0T Siemens MRI. Specific parameters are as follows, 20 non-collinear diffusion gradient directions with b value of 1000 s/mm2, the image size is 128x128x25, voxel size is 1.8x1.8x5.2mm.

Figure 1 shows the proposed DTI registration evaluation framework. Entropy, contrast and correlation of gray level co-occurrence matrix generated by different registration methods are calculated, verifying the reliability of the evaluation criterion.

Because of useless skull tissue and background noise, the skull and background noise need to be removed before image registration. This paper uses the brain extraction tool BET in the FSL (FMRIB Software Library) software to remove the skull and background noise, and get the accurate brain FA image.

The steps of DTI registration evaluation framework are as follows.

(1) Use BET on b0 image, and get the corresponding binary image.

(2) Use rigid registration and affine registration on DTI data separately. In the registration process, b0 image is used as the reference image and each different direction DWI is target image.

(3) Get abrain FA image without background.

(4) Compute the four main directions' gray level co-occurrence matrix based on the FA image from different registration methods.

(5) Compute the entropy, contrast and correlation in each slice and the mean value of all the parameters in all four main directions.

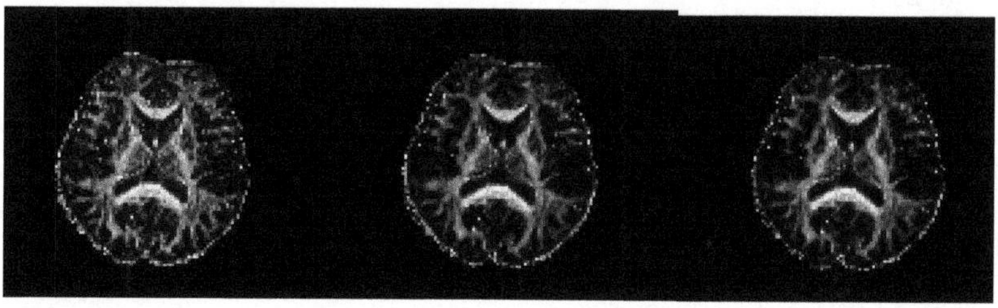

(a) (b) (c)

Fig. 2 (a) original FA image, (b) rigid registered FA image, (c) affine registered FA image.

The registration algorithms were implemented by using Automated Image Registration (http://bishopw.loni.ucla.edu/AIR5/). The tensor and FA were calculated by DtiStudio (http://www.mristudio.org/).

The clearer images have less noise and lower entropy, so the lower entropy means better registration. Experiment result shows that, as shown in Figure 3(a), the entropy of affine registration is the lowest, followed by the rigid registration, and the images without registration have the highest entropy. The result confirms the reliability of entropy as an evaluation criterion.

The clearer images have deeper texture grooves and less noise, so the contrast is greater. Experiment result shows that, as shown in Figure 3(b), the contrast of affine registration is highest, followed by the rigid registration, and the images without registration have lowest contrast. The result confirms the reliability of contrast as an evaluation criterion.

Similarly, the clearer image has lower correlation, as shown in Figure 3(c). Experiment result show that correlation is a reliable evaluation criterion because the affine registration performs best in all subjects.

Therefore, it is feasible to use entropy, contrast and correlation based on gray level co-occurrence matrix as registration evaluation criteria. In addition, in order to compare with the traditional method, the mean FA value of cerebrospinal fluid (CSF) [6] has also been calculated. Table 1 presents the two criteria in 5 subjects.

All experiment results show that three new evaluation criteria have an excellent performance. However the traditional criterion was failed in 2 subjects. Thus one of the three new criteria can be chosen to evaluate registration algorithm, especially, the contrast can significantly distinguish performance. Furthermore, in order to be more persuasive, all three criteria can be chosen and then using majority voting method to estimate the performance of the different algorithms.

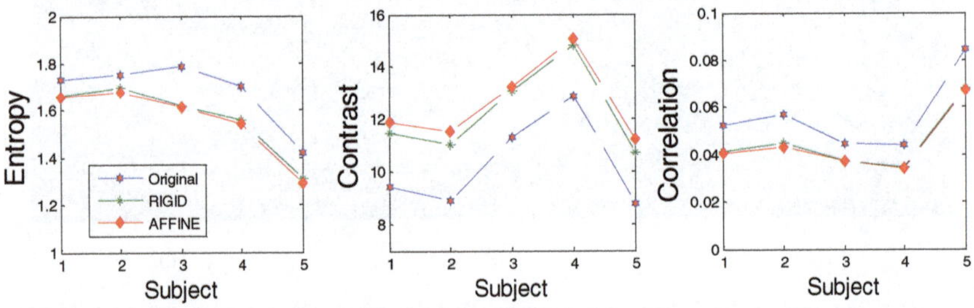

Fig. 3 Entropy, Contrast, Correlation distribution of 5 subjects processed by different registration algorithms.

Table 1 The evaluation criteria on the five subjects. CN=Contrast(the new criterion), A=mean of FA in CSF(the traditional criterion). For each criterion of a subject, the better values are underlined.

Method	subject 1		subject 2		subject 3		subject 4		subject 5	
	CN	FA	CN	FA	CN	FA	CN	FA	CN	FA
AFFINE	<u>11.87</u>	<u>0.10</u>	<u>11.53</u>	<u>0.15</u>	<u>13.23</u>	0.09	<u>15.05</u>	<u>0.08</u>	<u>11.20</u>	<u>0.08</u>
RIGID	11.50	<u>0.10</u>	11.03	0.18	13.08	<u>0.08</u>	14.82	0.09	10.72	0.09
Original	9.41	0.13	8.89	0.22	11.31	0.12	12.85	0.11	8.75	0.12

5. Discussion

The evaluation criteria of entropy, contrast and correlation based on gray level co-occurrence matrix can integrate full brain information, so it is more accurate than other no global-brain parameters. It has more superiority and convenience than the methods relying on the software. In the experiment, 12-parameter affine registration, using more transform parameters, shows a better result compared with 7-parameter rigid registration and non-registration.

In the registration process, skull and background are usually removed in preprocessing, which can reduce the influence of background noise. In order to rule out the influence of different slices and different matrix generated directions, the averages of entropy, contrast and correlation in each slice and each direction is calculated.

6. Conclusions

This paper presents a novel registration evaluation method of DWIbased on gray level co-occurrence matrix. The result shows that the three criteria can distinguish registration algorithms effectively. Combining three criteria and using majority voting can guarantee the validity of evaluation.

Acknowledgment

This work was supported by the projects of NSFC-61171002, NSFC-60372023 and Tsinghua University Initiative Scientific Research Program 20131089382.

References

1. Mori S. *Introduction to diffusion tensor imaging* [M]. Elsevier, 2007.
2. Malinsky, M., Peter, R., Hodneland, E., Lundervold, A. J., Lundervold, A., & Jan, J. (2013). Registration of FA and T1-weighted MRI data of healthy human brain based on template matching and normalized cross-correlation. Journal of digital imaging, 26(4), 774-785.
3. K. CHOI, A. R. Franco, P. E. Holtzheimer, H. S. Mayberg, and X. P. Hu. Diffusion tensor imaging distortion correction with T1. Proc. Intl. Soc. Mag. Reson. Med. 19 (2011), 1946-1947.
4. Kinoshita, M., Hashimoto, N., Goto, T., Kagawa, N., Kishima, H., Izumoto, S., & Yoshimine, T. (2008). Fractional anisotropy and tumor cell density of the tumor core show positive correlation in diffusion tensor magnetic resonance imaging of malignant brain tumors. Neuroimage, 43(1), 29-35.

5. Christensen, G. E., Geng, X., Kuhl, J. G., Bruss, J., Grabowski, T. J., Pirwani, I. A., & Damasio, H. (2006). Introduction to the non-rigid image registration evaluation project (NIREP). In Biomedical image registration (pp. 128-135). Springer Berlin Heidelberg.
6. Oubel, E., Rousseau, F., Noblet, V., Koob, M., Armspach, J. P., & Dietemann, J. L. (2009). Evaluation of Different Strategies for Distortion Correction in Fetal Diffusion-Weighted Imaging.
7. Arvis, V., Debain, C., Berducat, M., & Benassi, A. (2011). Generalization of the cooccurrence matrix for colour images: application to colour texture classification. Image Analysis & Stereology, 23(1), 63-72.

Design of Extended 'Digital Communication Theory' Hardware Implementation Platform*

Lu Jihua[a], Zhou Ronghua and Luo Shixun
School of Information and electronics, Beijing Institute of Technology, Beijing, 100081, China
[a]*E-mail: lujihua@bit.edu.cn*

Conventional 'Digital Communication Principles' experiment platform consists of discrete components, which are lack of extensibility and flexibility. Meanwhile, software platform exhibits waveforms and functions of different communication modules. However, Due to the absence of practical coherent signals, the software platform cannot satisfy the future practical needs of profound "digital communication principle" related courses. Hence, a novel "digital communication experiment" platform bearing high expansibility and flexibility compared with traditional hardware and software experiment platform is proposed, which is useful for both experimental teaching and stimulating students' interests and awareness toward digital communication. Moreover, the extended platform allows students to design extra components, which will further improve their abilities of manipulation and innovation.

Keywords: Digital communication; hardware platform; expansibility; practice and innovation.

1. Introduction

With the rapid development of information theory and increasing enrollment of undergraduates, 'Digital Communication Principles' course is getting more and more important and it has become one of the main courses for undergraduate communication and engineering major students. Also, the teaching effects of this course has significant influence on the students' professional abilities [1-2]. The course of 'Digital Communication Principles' is carried out after courses of Digital Signal Processing, Signal and System, Analog Circuit, Digital Circuit, et. al., which bears characteristics of many abstract theories. Therefore, congruity of theory and practice should be emphasized. Moreover, the basic

* The work has been supported by the National Science Fund (61002014, 6097201 and 60972018), Foundation for Distinguished Young Talents in Beijing Institute of Technology (X01011), National Major Scientific and Technological Special Project for Next-generation broadband wireless mobile communication network (2010ZX03002-003-03).

experiment skills and practical abilities should also be grasped and enhanced through teaching practices [3-4].

As the rapid growing developing pace of wireless communication and software simulations, teaching of 'Digital Communication Principles' should combine software and hardware experiments together, which also is popular recently, and the joint teaching mode of such courses has been widely applied and accepted [4-6].

Most of the digital communication experimental platforms are based on hardware modules, which only contain several parts of an integrated digital communication system, like sampling theorem, modulation/demodulations and channel coding. Such experiment platforms could hardly satisfy the increasing requirements of experiment teaching to catch up the technology trend. Full-featured, flexible and extended digital communication experimental platform can supplement the existing experiments, which can carry out various teaching activities and achieve good teaching effects. The main features of the proposed hardware platform is that all the algorithms can be simulated and verified through matlab programs. Moreover, the verifications can be realized based on software and hardware simultaneously, which help students to acquire profound knowledge. The proposed extended experimental platform designed can be used as hardware platform for teaching practice, which can realize functional modules as modulation, channel coding, filter and complete communication system in both hardware and software. Also, it has advantages of visualization, verification and large operational capacity.

Teaching practices show that the extended experimental platform can enhance students' mastering of the digital communication principles, harden their experimental and self-design capabilities through the combination of actual hardware measures and software program process. Moreover, the students' interests in learning and motivation can be improved by independent design, debugger the program, and comparisons with measures of the hardware platform.

2. The Conventional Hardware Platform of Digital Communication

2.1. *Overview of conventional hardware platform*

Previous experiments of digital communication are based on "digital communication experiment hardware platform", which can be grouped as follows:

(1) Sampling theorem

This set consists four experiments of PAM (Pulse Amplitude Modulation), PCM (Pulse Code Modulation), ADPCM (Adaptive Differential Pulse Code Modulation), and CVSD (Continuous Variable Slope Delta Modulation).

(2) Modulations

This set consists modulations and demodulations of AM (Amplitude Modulation), FM (Frequency Modulation), BPSK (Binary Phase Shift Keying), DBPSK (Differential Binary Phase Shift Keying), FSK (Frequency Shift Keying), MSK (Minimum Shift Keying), GMSK (Gaussian Minimum Shift Keying), QPSK (Quadrature Phase Shift Keying), OQPSK (Offset Quadra phase Shift Keying), QAM (Quadrature Amplitude Modulation) and etc.

(3) Source and channel codes

Including of Hamming, Scrambling codes, AMI (Alternative Mark Inversion), HDB3 (3rd Order High Density Bipolar), and CMI (Coded Mark Inversion).

(4) Interface experiments

Including Subscriber Loop, DTMF (Dual Tone Multi-Frequency), RS442 and RS232 transmissions.

(5) Systematic experiments

Including IS95 transmission, Walsh codes, CDMA/DS, and fading channels.

The aforementioned hardware experimental platform covers the major modules of the digital communication principle, which reflects the combination of the basis theory, engineering practice, and some of the latest technology methods [4].

2.2. *Constraints of conventional experimental hardware platform*

The conventional digital communication experimental platform has been used for years without being updated. There exists some major problems in practical experiments such as inflexible parameter settings, fewer manipulated operations and larger gaps between software simulations and hardware measurements. The basic functional modules consisted in the experimental box such as sampling and analog phase-locked loop modules employ specific analog chips, which is easily to be damaged, less flexibility and almost unchangeable on the few parameters.

The experiments of digital modulation in the traditional experimental platform are lack of transparency on each parts of digital processing, parameters cannot be modified to some extent. Conventional "digital communication experimental hardware platform" is restricted by the chip sizes and processing capacities, which causes by limited expanding spaces, less flexibility and leads to less interests and less teaching effects. Students cannot achieve full and independent design on these existing modules. Moreover, the existing analog segments in traditional "Hardware platform of digital communication principle" is damageable, which also leads to the high cost of repairs.

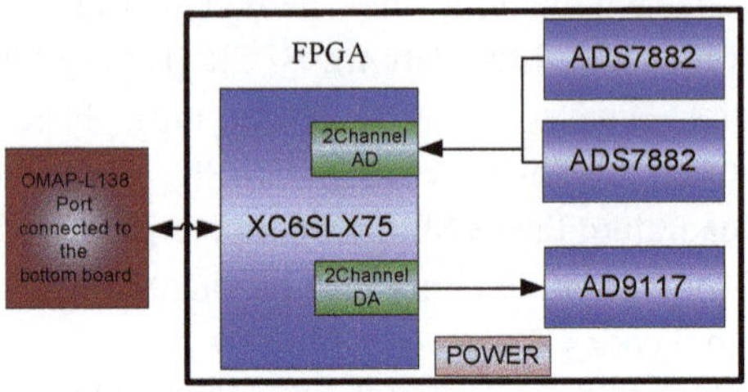

Fig. 1 Block diagram of extended digital communication experiment platform.

3. Extended Digital Communication Experimental Platform

3.1. *Architecture of extended digital communication experimental platform*

The block diagram of proposed experiment platform is shown in Figure 1.

The main design ideas are as follows:

Experiment board, adopting sub-board plus bottom board mode, consists three parts: one bottom board and two sub-boards (FPGA sub-board and OMAP sub-board). Among them, FPGA sub-board contains main chips of SPARTAN6 FPGA, ADC and DAC. The EMIF in FPGA board is interface to bottom board through Board to Board Connector. OMAP sub-board contains a minimal system which is named OMAP-L138. All the interface of OMAP connect with bottom board through standard DIMM-200. The bottom board provides various peripheral interface: network interface, USB, UART, SD card and so on, used to be connected to OMAP and FPGA board.

3.2. *FPGA sub-board of extended platform and available experiments*

3.2.1. *Design criteria of FPGA sub-board*

The FPGA board is designed to implement digital modulation, digital demodulation and bidirectional data transfer with OMAP board, which contains one FPGA chip, two single channel A/D converter, one double-channel D/A converter and the power supply. Moreover, the FPGA sub-board is connected to the baseboard by a board-board connector.

Assume the baseband bandwidth is less than 50KHz, the intermediate frequency (IF) is 500KHz and the sampling rate is 2MHz. When the information rate of QPSK is 5M bps, then a simple QPSK modem consumes about 8% hardware resource of 4vlx60ff1148 (600K Gates' FPGA). Since, other information rates in this platform is designed to less than 300K bps, then, the hardware resource consumed of such system is predicted to be 10K logic gates. Thus, we choose XC6SLX75 (the main characteristic of which is shown in Table 1) bearing 70K logic gates, which is redundant to implement other high complexity algorithms, i.e. guarantee the expansibility of the extended experiment platform.

Also, AM/FM and some other modulation method can be realized based on the DSP chip in OMAP board, and the expansibility of platform can be further enhanced. The ADC and DAC chips are selected as A/D: ADS7882 (TI), single channel, 12bit, 3MSPS; D/A: AD9117 (ADI), double channel, 14bit, 125MSPS.

Table 1 Characteristics of resources using in XC6SLX75*.

Device	Logic Cells(1)	Configurable Logic Blocks (CLBs)			DSP48A1 Slices(3)	Block RAM Blocks		CMTs(5)	Memory Controller Blocks (Max)(6)	Endpoint Blocks for PCI Express	Maximum GTP Transceivers	Total I/O Banks	Max User I/O
		Slices(2)	Flip-Flops	Max Distributed RAM (Kb)		18 Kb(4)	Max (Kb)						
XC6SLX45	43,661	6,822	54,576	401	58	116	2,088	4	2	0	0	4	358
XC6SLX75	74,637	11,662	93,296	692	132	172	3,096	6	4	0	0	6	408
XC6SLX150	147,443	23,038	184,304	1,355	180	268	4,824	6	4	0	0	6	576

*Chip selected for FPGA board is highlighted in table.

3.2.2. *Experiments Available on FPGA Sub-board*

The experiments available on FPGA sub-board include modulations and demodulations (BPSK, QPSK, MSK, FM, AM and etc); filter designs and equalizations, which aim to help the students using HDL (Hardware Description Language) and gain the abilities of system design.

3.3. *OMAP sub-board of proposed experimental platform*

3.3.1. *Design criteria of OMAP sub-board*

OMAP is mainly used for flexible expansion algorithms, which is relative independent and can be fitted into the backplane via DIMM-200. From the perspective of experience board simplification, the number of this module can be configured flexibly. This module, with powerful function of control and algorithm, is the main platform for development, which can provide students flexible and ample space to design. The chip of this sub-board uses OMAP-L138, whose configure system block diagram is shown in Fig. 2.

OMAP sub-board has some main advantages as follows:

(1) Multi-core structure, ARM926EJ and C6748 float DSP with 300MHz clock;

(2) ARM module can realize the system transplantation, including Linux and Wince and DSP in data transmission;

(3) Design system in modules, connect to the system board by DIMM-200, with flexibly and friendly maintenance interface.

The OMAP sub-board contains audio, LAN, serial port, SD card, SATA, video, touch screen interfaces, and EMIF connected to FPGA.

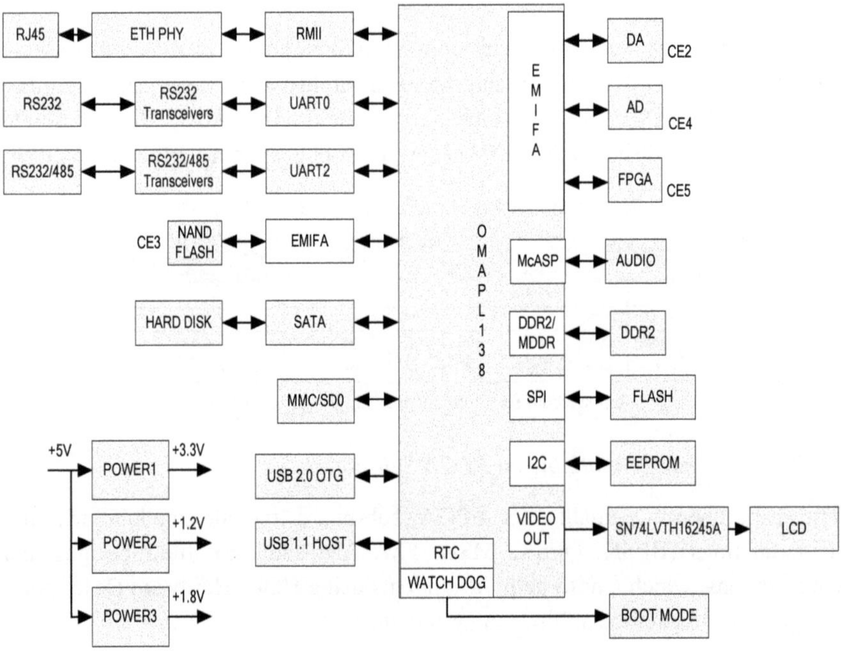

Fig. 2 Block diagram of OMAP sub-board.

3.3.2. *Available experiments in OMAP sub-board*

There are the following groups of experiments available in OMAP sub-board:

1) Audio processing: recording and playing; 2) Video processing: image acquisition and LCD display; 3) Transplantation of peripheral drivers: LAN, serial port, SD card and SATA; 4) Design of modulations, digital filters et. al. through DSP programming; 5) OS Transplantation: Linux, Wince, aiming to cultivate the students' abilities of grasping C, OS and etc.

3.3.3. *Other available experiments*

(1) Flash R/W(read/write): Light the lamps on the circuit board orderly, write the program in Flash, load in OMAP, run and testify the program;
(2) Digital-analog Conversion (DAC): Input triangle or sine wave data into DAC through EMIFA interface, and test the output signal from the output interface with an oscilloscope;
(3) Analog-digital Conversion (ADC): Send ADC samples to the input interfaces of DAC; or using signal source in CCS to input signal, sample and write data into OAMP via EMIFA. Finally, analyze the precision of ADC through the FFT algorithms;
(4) McASP transmission: Sample the external audio signal through McASP;
(5) DDR2 R/W(read/write): R/W data in specific format through programming;
(6) LCD display: Output graphic data from OMAP to buffers through the LCD control interface, and display it on LCD. The transmitted graphs shall continuously show up;
(7) R/W(read/write) via Serial Peripheral Interface (SPI);
(8) R/W(read/write) via Inter-Integrated Circuit (I2C);
(9) RS232 transmission: First, read data from DDR2 OR Flash; Then, communicate with PC via RS232 and SPI interfaces. Finally, verify the transmitted and received data;
(10) RJ45 interface: First, connect PC via RMII, Eth physical layer by RJ45;
(11) SATA R/W(read/write) via SATA interface;
(12) SD card R/W(read/write) via SDIO interface;
(13) USB 2.0 and 1.1 transmission(2.0 master/slave modes; 1.1 master mode);
(14) RTC read and RTC setting;
(15) Linux experiments of NFS boot and RAM DISK boot.

4. Matlab Verifications of the Digital Communication Experiments

The block diagram of verification matlab platform is shown in Fig. 3. The same software functions related to the verifiable hardware modules are illustrated in the dashed box, and those at the receiving end are vice versa. Coding and modulation modules contain common channel code and modulation scheme, respectively.

Fig. 4 shows the verification of BPSK eye diagram generated from hardware (right) by the similar one generated from matlab (left).

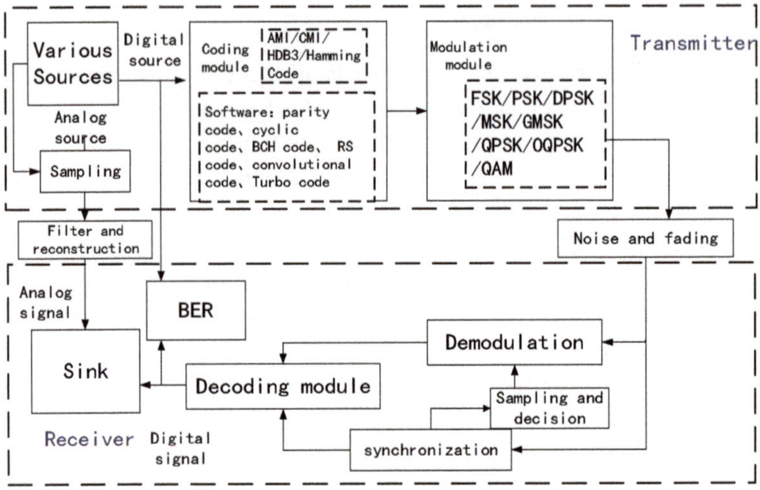

Fig. 3 Block diagram of the matlab verification platform.

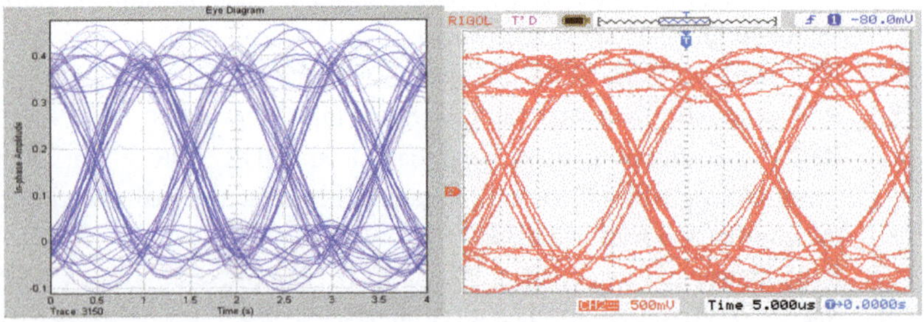

Fig. 4 Comparisons of the Eye diagrams generated by matlab and hardware platform.

5. Conclusion

The extended hardware platform of "digital communication principles" is designed and implemented, of which, two main sub-boards and their corresponding experiments are elaborated, including the chips' selection, block diagrams and experiments. Besides the hardware design, the experimental platform contains software verification part. The software simulation and hardware implementations can be carried out simultaneously. Also, the experimental results and measurements can be verified through comparing software simulation and hardware implementation. Moreover, an example of verification the hardware eye diagram by matlab simulation is illustrated. The extended hardware platform of "digital communication principles" can not only help students to grasp the information theory learned in class, but also can stimulate their enthusiasm and enhance their practical manipulation ability.

References

1. Fan changxin, Cao lina. Communication Principles [M]. Bei jing, National defence of Industry Press, 2011.
2. Jiang hong, Mo xiulin, Kang jian, etc. Research of the teaching model of "Digital mobile communication principles" [J]. Journal of electrical and electronic education, 2011, 33(4): 23-24.
3. Zhou youbin. The design of the teaching and research model of communication principles [D]. Jiang su, Suzhou University, 2006.
4. Li shaosong, Yin dong, Mu dejun, Dai guanzhong. The design and implementation of extended Mapreduce based on FPGA [J]. Computer technology and development. 2012, 2, 103-106.
5. Ling lin, Su yinjie, Jin chun. The application of software simulation in teaching of communication principles [J]. Experimental technology and management, 2013, (5).
6. Wen huafeng, Hu qianmiao, Yang yan. Visualization of digital communication system design based on MATLAB [J]. Journal of Ningbo University, 2006, 19(3): 302-205.
7. Nanjing zhehua. Technology Co., Ltd., Research on communication technology of the Jiangsu Liyang Hua Yang. ZH5001A Instruction experiment of comprehensive experiment system for communication principle [M].
8. Nanjing zhehua. Technology Co., Ltd. ZH7001 Instruction experiment of comprehensive experiment system of modern communication theory [M]. 46-115.
9. Liao yunya. The design and implementation of virtual experiment platform for digital communication based on Java and Matlab [D]. Hu nan, Central South University, 2007.
10. Jiang wei. Design and implementation of simulation platform for communication signals [D]. Chang sha, National University of Defense Technology, 2006.
11. Zhong lihui, Lv danjv. The reform of experiment teaching of communication principle based on MATLAB [J]. Electronic design engineering, 2012, 20(6): 76-78.
12. Zhang haitao, Wang fuchang. Design and implementation of experimental teaching software channel coding based on MATLAB [J]. Research and Exploration in Laboratory, 2005, 24(1): 46-49.

CHAPTER 3

Medical Science and Biological Engineering

A Coordination Speed Control Method Between Patient and Treadmill in the Rehabilitation Training*

Shen Linyong, Gao Shunxin[a], Zhang Yanan and Yang Lvjian
Precision Machinery Department, Shanghai University,
Shanghai Zhabei District Yanchang Road No. 149, China
[a]E-mail: GSX_SHU@163.com

In order to make patients have a better experience and better rehabilitation effect in rehabilitation training, designed a coordination speed control method and apparatus between patient and treadmill. The system adopt acceleration sensor to detect human movement trend and figure out the expected speed of the human body. Designed a PI controller with anti-windup algorithm to adjust the speed of the treadmill, so that the treadmill can follow the speed of human to change. The experimental results show that this control method can meet the running machine speed with adaptive requirements.

Keywords: Rehabilitation training; treadmill; speed coordination; control method.

1. Introduction

In medical science, the patients usually through repetitive and task-specific training to conduct enough repetitive activity so that the cerebral cortex which is in reorganization can through a profound experience to learn and store the correct movement patterns [1]. Treatment of weight loss gait training is based on this principle to proceed the patient training, and achieved good clinical effect which become the main method of lower limb rehabilitation therapy [2].

Treadmill-assisted rehabilitation for patients with lower limb motor dysfunction is a very effective training methods. In treadmill training process, change the speed of the treadmill play a crucial role in the lower limb rehabilitation process [3]. When the practical speed of the patient training is changed, the speed of treadmill is required to be changed automatically. Both speed must be coordinated well. If coordination is not good, the patient will not follow the normal gait rehabilitation, and could even lead to accidents during training patients. So that patients will suffer secondary damage and worsen the

---

* This work is supported and grant by the Chinese National Natural Science Foundation (No: 51275282) and the Chinese Ministry of Higher Education Doctoral Foundation (No: 2012310 8110009).

state of illness [4,5].

However, in practical rehabilitation system, the treadmill speed is usually set to a constant or only given by therapists which is based on rehabilitation of patients. So it can not be achieved on the basis of the patient's intention to proceed the automatic acceleration and deceleration, which is not consistent with the natural walking speed changing law so that the rehabilitation is not very obvious. Therefore, the study of treadmill speed adaptation controlling method is extremely necessary [6-8]. Manchester Metropolitan University has through the ultrasonic sensor to detect the displacement of people, and constantly calculate and control the speed of the treadmill so that the location of people is held in a predetermined position [9], we propose a speed coordination control method of the treadmill which is based on the body's gravity acceleration.

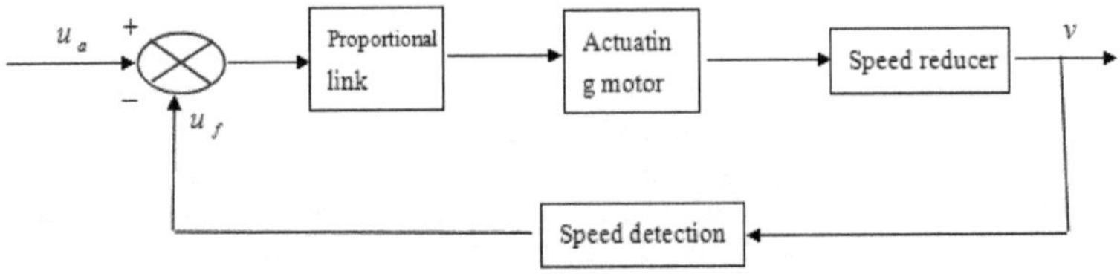

Fig. 1 Treadmill systems modeling block diagram.

2. The Modeling of Treadmill System

The treadmill system modeling block diagram shown in Figure 1. The servo motor control voltage is u_a, and the velocity output signal of the speed reducer become the feedback signal to the controller after speed detection device, which forming a speed feedback signal u_f. The u_a and u_f together to control the motor running after a proportional link, and the motor drives the reducer to produce the corresponding displacement, so that the treadmill output a corresponding speed.

The actuator of the system is based on the structure of belt drive transmission, and the rotation of the servo motor eventually turn into the movement of running belt by gear drive and belt drive.

Because the treadmill system is a typical electric actuators, after linearization, the mechanical properties of the servo motor can be directly expressed as:

$$M_m = -C_\omega \omega + M_S \tag{1}$$

Where M_m is the output torque of the motor, ω_m is the angular velocity of the motor (rad/s); $C_\omega = dM_m / d\omega_m$ is the damping coefficient, which is the slope of the mechanical characteristic curve after linearization.

The mathematical model of the treadmill system is shown in Figure 2.

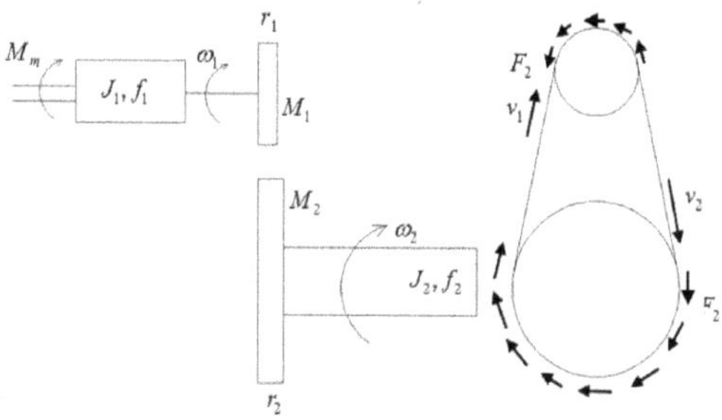

Fig. 2 The mathematical model of the treadmill system.

After theoretical analysis and simplified calculation, the form of the transfer function of the treadmill system is:

$$G(s) = \frac{V(s)}{U_a(s)} = \frac{k}{s+a} \tag{2}$$

In actual experiments, the friction coefficient and the damping coefficient of the treadmill is different with the theoretical value. In order to determine the actual model of system we need to cooperate with system identification experiment to determine the transmission function of the system. In the experiment, the experimental data obtained by the system step response experiments, then using Matlab System Identification Toolbox to process the data, and a total of 10 groups of experiments have been done. After Matlab identification and calculation, the transfer function model as shown in equation (3), and the match results of the model is 94.07%.

$$G(s) = \frac{0.9977}{1+0.0806s} \tag{3}$$

3. The Speed Coordination Control between Human and Treadmill Based on Acceleration Sensor

3.1. *The relationship between walking speed and acceleration of body center of gravity*

In order to identify the specific relationship between walking speed and acceleration of body center of gravity when walking, it is necessary to do some preliminary experimental data acquisition and analysis. In this study, built the data acquisition experiment platform of people walking on the treadmill. Experiment collected a total of 20 individual experimental data, and everyone was repeated experiments, then processed each set of data with off-line analysis techniques. The specific method is: First, remove the DC component of all the center of gravity acceleration, and get the volume of the amplitude of acceleration information which is cyclical changes over time. Then moving average process the data, and get the changes of gravity acceleration amplitude over a certain period of time. Because the body center of gravity acceleration amplitude is varied within a specific range even if the person's walking speed is constant, the experimental mainly extracted three characteristic quantities in the acceleration information, they are the minimum, average and maximum values of the acceleration amplitude at a constant speed.

This is the result of a person, the data processed by MATLAB, and after two function fitting, the results are shown in Figure 3. There are three fitting curves, representing three fitting function, they are maximum fitting function $f_{\max}(v)$, average fitting function $f_{avg}(v)$, Minimum fitting function $f_{\min}(v)$.

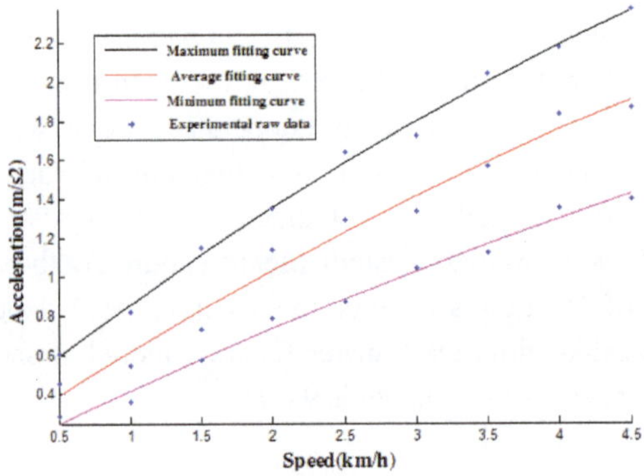

Fig. 3 Correlation between gravity acceleration and walking speed.

Through the existing experimental data amply demonstrated that people walk faster, the greater his acceleration, the two variables are linearly related. So take the average fitting function $a = f_{avg}(v)$ as the current speed reference. If we assume that the human change factor is K_m, K_m is vary from individual height, weight and walking habits, it can be adjusted according to actual, The speed (V_t) can be show as:

$$V(t) = K_m(a(t)+b)^2 + p \tag{4}$$

Where b, p are the constants, they are adjustable parameters of the human change factor which can be obtained through the early experimental data.

The coordination speed control algorithm of the treadmill is shown in equation (5):

$$E(t) = V_c(t) - V_t(t) = K_n^{-1} \bullet K_p\{k(t) \bullet a(t)\} \quad (5)$$

Where $E(t)$ is the speed adjustment errors of the treadmill. V_t is the current speed of the treadmill. V_c is the desired speed of the treadmill. K_n is the rate adjustment factor, the greater the K_n, the longer adaptive time the system take, and the shorter the accelerated process of the experiment. $k(t)$ is a nonlinear gain function, nonlinear gain function has many representations, in this article, using the equation (6) and (7) to describe $k(t)$ [14,15]:

$$k(t) = \frac{e^{k_0 a(t)} + e^{-k_0 a(t)}}{2} \quad (6)$$

$$f(t) = \begin{cases} a(t), & a_{\min} < a(t) < k_1 f_{\min}(v), k_2 f_{\max}(v) < a(t) < a_{\max} \\ a_{\max}\,\mathrm{sgn}(a(t)), & |a(t)| > a_{\max} \\ 0 & k_1 f_{\min}(v) < a(t) < k_2 f_{\max}(v) \end{cases} \quad (7)$$

Where k_0, k_1, k_2 are user defined constants. The value of k_0 determines the range of $k(t)$, k_1 and k_2 are response coefficients of $k(t)$, they determine the change of system response interval. $a_{\max}$ and $a_{\min}$ are the maximum and minimum response acceleration sensor response value, which are designed to prevent the speed adjustment of the treadmill too fast. When people in uniform motion, $f_{\max}(v)$ and $f_{\min}(v)$ are the boundary function of the fluctuation range of the acceleration, and if the sensor detects a value within this range, the control system will not respond.

After trier wear the experimental apparatus and adapt to walking on the treadmill, trier uniform walking on treadmill for a while, and according to the experimental data to fit out the three key functions ($f_{\max}(v)$, $f_{avg}(v)$, $f_{\min}(v)$) of trier, and then deduce the human variation factor (K_m) of the trier as well as the fixed constant (b, p). In this experiment, set the parameters $K_p = 0.302$, $k_0 = 0.136$, $k_1 = k_2 = 0.1$.

The acceleration sensor data curve and the corresponding treadmill speed curve during the experiment are shown in Figure 4. In the Figure 4(a), the top curve is the response upper limit curve of acceleration value; the middle curve is the actual measurement value of acceleration sensor; he bottom curve is the response lower limit curve of acceleration value. In the experiment, the experimenter adjust his walking speed gradually. When the experimenter are trying to accelerate, the acceleration sensor detects the acceleration amplitude greater than the response interval, then the treadmill followed the experimenter to accelerate; When the experimenter are trying to decelerate, the acceleration sensor detects the acceleration amplitude less than the response interval, then the treadmill followed the experimenter to decelerate. The experimental results show that this algorithm can meet the requirements that the speed of the treadmill follow the speed of experimenter to change.

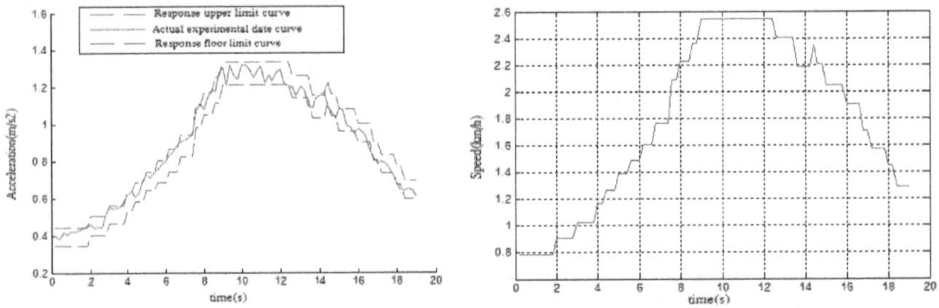

(a) (b)

Fig. 4 Acceleration curves and treadmill speed curves.

3.2. *Controller design*

The design principle of the treadmill speed coordinated controller is as follows: firstly, considering the tracking performance of the control system, In order to make the treadmill can quickly follow the input desired speed. In this paper, the common used PI control algorithm is used to design the speed following controller of the treadmill; secondly, in order to suppress the acceleration of the treadmill, and avoid the injury to patients caused by too large acceleration, anti-integral saturation suppression module is added to the designed treadmill speed tracking controller. The PI controller designed can be shown in Figure 5.

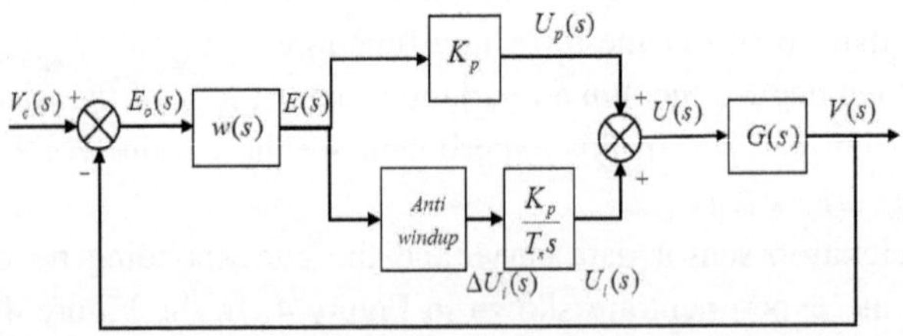

Fig. 5 The design principle diagram of the speed following control system of treadmill.

In Figure 5, $w(s)$ represents the transfer function of the low-pass filter. represents the transfer function of treadmill. Through simulation and experiment, figure out the parameters of the controller system, the result is: $K_p = 40$, $T_i = 0.5$. The Anti windup module is anti-integral saturation suppression module, the specific algorithm is as follows:

$$\Delta u_i = \begin{cases} 0 & |u_p + u_i| > u_m, \text{and} \quad e \cdot u_i \geq 0 \\ e & \text{else} \end{cases} \tag{8}$$

Where is saturation voltage of the servo motor amplifier, and in the simulation, $u_m = 1\text{v}$.

4. Simulation and Results

To simulate changes in acceleration of patient during their movement, and verify that the speed tracking performance and acceleration inhibition effect of the designed controller, firstly, it is assumed that the desired speed is a step signal which amplitude is 0.3, with anti-integral saturation suppression module, the output speed of the treadmill as shown in Figure 6. It can be seen from the figure, not only the actual speed can quickly track the desired speed in the acceleration uninhibited stage, but also the acceleration of treadmill also obtained the expected effective inhibition.

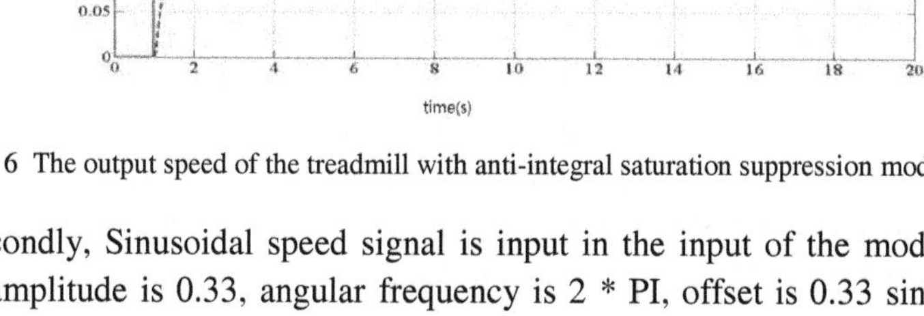

Fig. 6 The output speed of the treadmill with anti-integral saturation suppression module.

Secondly, Sinusoidal speed signal is input in the input of the model, with which amplitude is 0.33, angular frequency is 2 * PI, offset is 0.33 sine speed signal, the output speed of the treadmill as shown in Figure 7. Conversely, the dotted line represents the desired speed of the treadmill, solid line shows the actual speed of the treadmill. With restraining acceleration model, the actual speed of the treadmill can well track the desired speed.

From the above simulation results, Treadmill speed coordinated controller is designed to ensure the stability of the whole control system, and when the patient's acceleration is too large, the designed PI controller with restraining acceleration can effectively suppress the acceleration of the treadmill, so as to ensure patient's safety in the training process, to avoid treadmill sudden acceleration or deceleration caused by muscle spasm of patients which can cause the secondary damage. In addition, it also ensures that the speed of treadmill can track the desired speed of the patients in the acceleration uninhibited stage, and achieve the coordinated movement of mechanical leg system and treadmill. The simulation results prove that the designed treadmill speed of coordinated controller which is based on the coordination between man and treadmill mutual force detection, can be used to control the feasibility of coordination between the trainer and treadmill.

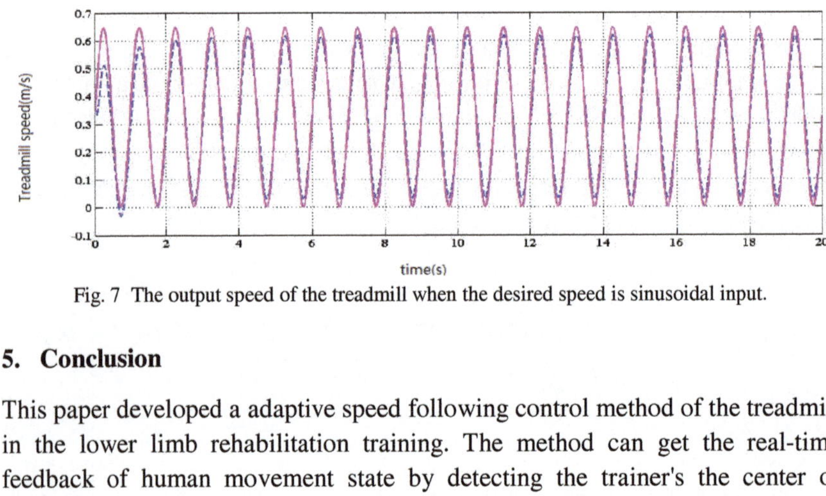

Fig. 7 The output speed of the treadmill when the desired speed is sinusoidal input.

5. Conclusion

This paper developed a adaptive speed following control method of the treadmill in the lower limb rehabilitation training. The method can get the real-time feedback of human movement state by detecting the trainer's the center of gravity acceleration when he walks. Besides, PI controller with anti-integral saturation suppression is designed to achieve speed coordination control between people and the treadmill in the rehabilitation training. The experiment results show that this control method can achieve Coordinated movement between robot system of the lower limb rehabilitation training and the treadmill, and the feasibility of the designed controller.

References

1. Sterr A, Freivogel S. Motor-improvement Following Intensive Training in Low-functioning Chronic Hemiparesis, Neurology, Vol. 61 (2003), pp. 842 - 844.
2. Hesse S, Konrad M, Uhlenbrock D. Treadmill Walking With Partial Body Weight Support Versus Floor Walking in Hemiparetic Subjects, Arch Phys Med Rehabil, Vol. 80 (1999), pp. 421-427.
3. A Wernig, S Muller, Laufband Locomotion With Body Weight Support Improved Walking in Persons With Severe Spinal Cord Injuries, Paraplegia, Vol. 30, (1992), pp. 229-238.
4. A.E. Minetti, L. Boldrini, L. Brusamolin, et. al. A feedback-controlled treadmill (treadmill-on-demand) and the spontaneous speed of walking and running in humans [J]. Journal of Applied Physiology, 2003, 95(2): 838-843.
5. L. Lichtenstein, J. Barabas, R. L. Woods, et. al. A feedback control instrument for treadmill locomotion in virtual environments [J]. ACM Transactions on Applied Perception, 2007, 4(1): 1-17.
6. Souman J.L, Giordano P.R, Frissen I, De Luca A, Ernst M.O, Making Virtual Reality Real: Perceptual Evaluation of a New Treadmill Control Algorithm, ACM Trans. Applied Perception, Vol. 7 (2010).
7. L. Lichtenstein, J. Barabas, R. L. Woods, et. al. A feedback control instrument for treadmill locomotion in virtual environments [J]. ACM Transactions on Applied Perception, 2007, 4(1): 1-17.
8. Z. V. Zitzewitz, M. Bernhardt, R. Riener. A novel methods for automatic treadmill locomotion in virtual environments [J]. IEEE Transactions on Neural Systems and Rehabilitation, 2007, 4(1): 401-409.
9. Minetti A, Boldrini L, Brusamolin L, Zamparo P, McKee T, A Feedback-controlled Treadmill (Treadmill-on-demand) and the Spontaneous Speed of Walking and Running in Humans, J. Appl. Physiol., Vol. 95 (2003), pp. 838-843.
10. Seraji H. A New Class of Nonlinear PID Controllers with Robotic Applications. J Robot Syst, Vol. 15 (1998), pp. 161-81.
11. Koenig A, Voluntary Gait Speed Adaptation for Robot-assisted Treadmill Training, IEEE Int. Conf. on Rehabilitation Robotics. JPN, (2009) pp. 419-424.

Brain Neurocognitive Processing of Morphologically Complex Uyghur Words: Evidence from Event-Related Potentials*

Abudoukelimu Abulizi[a], Minghu Jiang[b], DengfengYao
Lab of Computational Linguistics, Center for Psychology and Cognitive Science, School of Humanities, Tsinghua University, Beijing 10084, China
Email: [a]keram1106@163.com, [b]jiang.mh@mail.tsinghua.edu.cn

Halidanmu Abudoukelimu
Department of Computer Science and Technology, Tsinghua University, Beijing 10084, China

We used event-related potentials (ERPs) to investigate electrophysiological correlates of Uyghur morphological word processing in lexical decision paradigm. We found N400 effects for bimorphemic complex words and pseudowords in the 350-550 time windows demonstrated that subjects failed to lexical search when they processing bimorphemic pseudowords and probably reflected access and possible interaction of the stem and suffix. We also found the neurocognitive underpinning that support monomorphemic word, bimorphemic word and both pseudoword processing is also different.

Keywords: Morphological complex words, Uyghur; ERPs, pseudowords.

1. Introduction

The description of morphological processes, the principles by which complex words are formed, has always been a challenge to theoretical linguistics as well as to psycholinguistics. Lexical access to polymorphemic word like "Work+s", "house+s" are represented and processed in the brain has stirred considerable interest in the field of psycholinguistics.

To answer this question, some scholars have suggested that the recognition of all morphologically complex words occur through decomposing the stem and affix during recognition [1]. While others have assumed that all complex word forms are stored as whole units in the mental lexicon.

There is lot of scholars used Event-related brain potentials investigated inflectional word processing. Most of their experiment violation of the regular

* This work was supported by the National Natural Science Fund (61171114) and Key Fund (61433015), and National Social Science Major Fund (14ZDB154) of China.

inflection elicit a left anterior negativity (LAN). This LAN effect has been interpreted morphological structure building process to the inflectional words. Several studies also found N400 effects elicit for violation of inflectional words. This N400 effects has been reported when an irregular suffix was applied to regular stem as well as in stem violation (change one or two letters in the stem). This N400 effects also observed in the single regular and irregular word decision experiment.

2. The Aim of Present Study

As we see, previous electrophysiological brain studies of morphological word processing have mostly been conducted with Indo-European languages, and in their experiment they have mainly addressed the distinction between regular and irregular inflection. There is reason to expect that the morphological typology of a speaker's language effect the way representations are accessed and stored.

As Uyghur belong to the Karluk branch of Turkic language, we expect that morphological complex word processing in Uyghur different from other Indo-European language, and expect observe some brain cognitive components that is different from the other language. We think it is very important to demonstrate neurocognitive components that be found in the other language and universality of the components in other language that has different morphological structures.

3. Materials

We selected high frequency Uyghur nouns in four condition: monomorphemic nouns, monomorphemic pseudowords, bimorphemic complex nouns and bimorphemic complex pseudowords, for each condition 160 words. Monomorphemic nouns don't contain any suffixes. Bimorphemic complex nouns in our experiment include four Uyghur noun case suffixes (possessive case, locative case, dative case and ablative case). For example " دۆلەت+تىن " (from country, دۆلەت country+تىن from). The real words and pseudoword were matched by length (all of the words in our experiment consist of six letters).

3.1. *Participants*

We recruited 19 Uyghur subject (9 female and 10 male) from Minzu university of China. They are all native and born in the Xinjiang Uyghur autonomous region of China. All participants has normal or correct normal vision and none of them reported any visual defects, linguistic dysfunction or neurological disorders.

3.2. *Procedure*

Participants were tested individually in a sound attenuated room and gave informed consent before the experiment start. The participants was instructed to look at the computer screen placed in front of him/her (distance 1.9m) and to avoid unnecessary movements. When experiment start red fixation point (+) appeared middle of the screen 800ms, Following the fixation point, there was a stimulus remained for 400ms, and then double question marks (??) presented middle of the screen 1500ms, require to subjects respond as quickly and accurately as possible. To avoid extra eye blinks in experiment, end of a trial there would be present empty screen in grey for 1000ms, for subject's eye blinks.

4. EEG Data Recording and Analyses

EEG data were collected from 64Ag/AgC1 electrodes (sampled at 500Hz, band-pass filtering=0.1-100Hz, notch filtering=50Hz) in a BP (Brain Product GmbH, Munich, Germany) head-cap on the scalp, according to the international 10/20 system. The electrode FCz was used as reference. Electrode impedances were below 10KΩ for all channels.

4.1. *Data analyses*

EEG data were analyzed by Brain Vision Analyzer software BP (Brain Product GmbH, Munich, Germany), and eye blinks were removed from further analyses. One subjects' data were rejected from analysis due to high eye blinks. Filter high-pass 0.01Hz/24 and low-pass 30Hz/24 were applied.

4.2. *ERP results*

The grand averaged ERPs for 9 electrodes (frontal, central an posterior region of brain) for the visually presented monomorphemic and biomorphemic complex words and pseudowords are presented in Fig. 1.

350-550ms time window the main effect for lexicality was statistically significant [$F(1,19)=15.17$, $P=0.004$]. Due to the fact that the main amplitudes for the pseudowords were more negative than those for the real words. The main effect for morphology was significant [$F(1,19)=11.66$, $p=0.008$], mean amplitude were more negative for the bimorphemic word stimuli than for the monomorphemic word stimuli.

The morphology × hemisphere interaction was significant [$F(2,18)=9.97$, $p=0.002$], as the main amplitudes for the bimorphemic words were more negative in the right hemisphere electrodes. Separate ANOVAs for the words and pseudowords confirmed that the increased negativity for the bimorphemic words most prominent in the right hemisphere electrodes [$F(2,18)=12.88$, $p=.0.006$].

There in significant interaction between lexicality and region [$F(2,18)=8.98$, $p=0.003$], with the negativity effect for the pseudowords at the centroposterior electrode. The negativity effect for the pseudoword was stronger over right hemisphere as compared to the left hemisphere. Subsequent ANOVAs for each electrode site revealed that the increased negativity for the bimorphemic pseudowords was most prominent at the right central and right parietal electrodes.

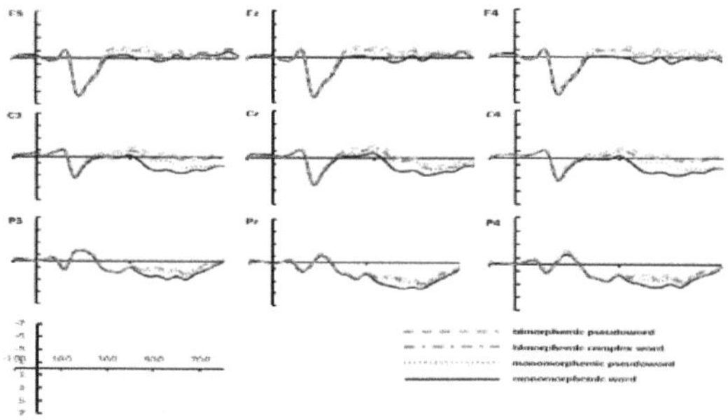

Fig. 1 Grand average ERPs from 9 scalp sites (F3, Fz, F4, C3, Cz, C4, P3, Pz, P4) to the monomorphemic word (black solid line), monomorphemic pseudowords (blue dotted line) bimorphemic complex word (red dash line), bimorphemic pseudoword (green dash line), after baseline correction in the 100ms prestimulus interval. Negative polarity is plotted upward.

5. Conclusions

This conclusion supported by two findings. Frist both monomorphemic word and bimorphemic words elicited their distinct characteristic ERP effects. We found strong N400 effects for the bimorphemic pseudowords, the N400 effects was elicit when we compared the processing of the morphological real words with pseudowords. This effect demonstrated that subjects failed to lexical search when they parsing morphologically complex words. Bimorphemic words also elicited an N400 effect. The N400 effect for the bimorphemic words most probably reflected access and integration of the stem and suffix. Second, the neurocognitive underpinning that support monomorphemic word, bimorphemic word and both pseudoword processing is also different. Mean amplitudes for the bimorphemic word were more negative in the right hemisphere electrodes than for the monomorphemic words. Negative effect for the pseudowords was stronger over the right hemisphere as compared to the left hemisphere.

References

1. Taft and Forster, Lexical Storage Retrieval of Prefixed Words. Jou of verbal and verbal behavior. 14, 638-646 (1975).

Study on the Factors Affecting Indigenous Microbial Bioaugmentation Remediation of Oil-Polluted Soil*

Xiaolou Li
Architecture and Environmental Engineering Department,
Sichuan Vocational and Technological College, Suining, Sichuan, China
lixiaolou677@126.com

Bioaugmentation technology is a promising and low-cost method of bioremediation. There are many factors affecting the efficiency of microbial bioaugmentation remediation including composition and molecular weight of oil, the physical condition and concentration of oil, and the composition, temperature, nutrient and pH of the soil. Combined with the actual research work, this study made a comprehensive analysis of the impact of the indigenous microbial concentration, soil temperature, soil humidity, and soil pH on the petroleum hydrocarbon degradation efficiency by supplying $(NH_4)_2SO_4$ and KH_2PO_4 as the N and P sources, respectively. This study took advantage of indoor pots simulation experiment to analyze the factors such as indigenous microbial bioaugmentation remediation. The results showed that by adding an appropriate proportion of N, P and sawdust, and at temperature of 30°C, humidity of 20%, pH of 7.0, the efficiency of petroleum hydrocarbon degradation by strengthening indigenous microbial is the best.

Keywords: Microbial remediation; oil-polluted soil; autochthonous bioaugmentation.

1. Introduction

With increasing utilization of oil, the problems of environmental pollution are worsening. Taking advantage of indigenous microbial to remediate petroleum contaminated soil has great potential as it has the advantages of safety and no secondary pollution, etc., thus it has been used more and more widely. But in the actual research and application process, there are problems of low efficiency, poor stability and other issues. Combined with the actual research work, this study made a comprehensive analysis of the factors affecting indigenous microbial remediation of petroleum contaminated soil, using indoor pots simulation test which provide references for the indigenous microbial bioaugmentation remediation of oil-polluted soil.

* This work is supported by key projects of Sichuan Provincial Education Department under Grant No. 13ZA0036.

The factors affecting the indigenous microbial bioaugmentation remediation of oil-polluted soil mainly include three aspects. The first factor is the feature of the oil pollutants including the composition and molecular weight of the oil. Petroleum accumulated in the contaminated soil, the composition and molecular weight are important factors affecting the indigenous microbial degradation of the oil [1]. Biodegradable of oil is very different according to its molecular weight and composition. Oil component is more simple and the molecular weight is smaller, the more susceptible it can be degraded by indigenous microbial. In the component of oil, aromatic saturated hydrocarbon is relatively easily be degraded by indigenous microorganisms. Resins and asphaltenes are extremely difficult to be degraded by indigenous microorganisms [2]. Only with full contact between the components of oil and the indigenous microbes, the petroleum is likely to be degraded by indigenous microorganisms, and concentrations of petroleum pollutant can also affect indigenous microbial activity.

The second factor is feature of indigenous microbial which including the groups, number and identity of indigenous microorganisms, co-metabolism of indigenous microbial and indigenous microorganisms biofortification. The constitution of indigenous microbial in soil is the most direct factor affecting the efficiency of oil biodegradation. Because crude oil has complex components, it is difficult to completely be degraded by a single bacterium. In the soil ecosystem, it widely spread microorganisms which can degrade petroleum hydrocarbons. Different microbial species have nutritional types and different physical and chemical tolerance properties of petroleum contaminants. Thus, constitution of indigenous microbial directly affects the degradation of oil pollutants. Co-metabolism of indigenous microbial refers to that as a non-growth substrate; the pollutants can be degraded or oxidized when the microbes grow on the substrate. Co-metabolism of indigenous microbial plays an important role for the decomposing of pollutants in the contaminated soil. Indigenous microbial bioaugmentation technology is a promising bio-remediation method with low-cost. It mainly used microorganisms composed of one strain or some strains with degradation ability to enhance degrade ability of soil pollutants. Autochthonous bioaugmentation technology was developed by Japanese scientists Ueno et al in 2007 [3]. It mainly refers to that separation and enrichment local petroleum-degrading microorganisms from the oil-contaminated soil and reputing the enhanced microorganisms into the oil-contaminated soil to degrade the oil. Many studies have shown that bioaugmentation technology can significantly improve the efficiency of petroleum hydrocarbon degradation.

The third factor is the soil environment which includes soil structure, soil tillage and crop species, soil temperature, types of nutrients, and the pH and humidity of the soil [4]. The entire soil environment plays important roles in affecting the microbial metabolic activity and thus affects the indigenous microbial bioaugmentation remediation of oil-polluted soil. And this study analyzed the role of factors including concentration of indigenous microbial, soil temperature, types of nutrients, and the pH and humidity of the soil played in the efficiency of petroleum hydrocarbon degradation.

2. Materials and Methods

2.1. *Sampling and the physical and chemical properties of the sample soil*

Sample soil was taken from the abandoned oil-well in Shehong, Sichuan province. When sample the soil, the 5 cm of the surface was thrown, and the sample soil was taken between 5~10 cm soils using diagonal cross 5 point sampling method. Then, sieve to remove impurities, mixing the soil for spare. We detect that in the soil, the petroleum hydrocarbons content was 5.3%, organic carbon was 23g/kg, nitrate was 0.164g/kg, ammonia nitrogen was 0.38g/kg, the dissolution of phosphorus is 0.042g/kg, and moisture is 16.14%.

2.2. *Indigenous microbial bioaugmentation*

The microbial in the sample soil is taken as bacteria source. Taking 2g contaminated soil inoculated in the indigenous microbial enrichment medium to enrich the microbial [5]. Then, cultivate the indigenous microbial under 30°C with 180r/min shaking for 5 days. Then, taking 1ml liquid from the enrichment culture to inoculate into fresh enrichment medium to enrich and acclimatize the indigenous microbial, and then cultured it under identical conditions 5 days, repeated this process three times to obtained domesticated and enriched indigenous microorganisms, stored them for use.

2.3. *Basin simulation experiment research*

Put sample soil collected into spare pots with the same specifications, and the pots should have holes at the bottom of packing. Every pot was loaded with 1 kg sample volume; then put the pots of soil samples in under different conditions culture 30d, stir them once every day. The sample of 0, 10, 20, 30 days were taken for testing analysis.

2.4. *Activator treatment*

In the study we used sawdust as the activator to detect whether it affect the efficiency of petroleum hydrocarbon degradation by strengthening indigenous microbial. We added the sawdust as the ratio of 1:10 of the weight of soil. Other conditions are the same as the experiment before [6].

3. Results

3.1. *The effects of microbial concentration on the efficiency of petroleum hydrocarbon degradation*

In the experiment, we added 10, 20, 30 ml indigenous microorganisms prepared before into the pots of soil; as the control, we also added the same volume bacilli which have been sterilized. And all the samples were cultured at 25°C with 25% humidity. Then, we tested the sample every 10 days to analyze the degradation of petroleum hydrocarbon in the contaminated soil. The result is shown in Figure 1. It can be seen that at 30 days, the degradation efficiency of petroleum hydrocarbon showed no significantly differences among the samples with different bacilli concentrations added.

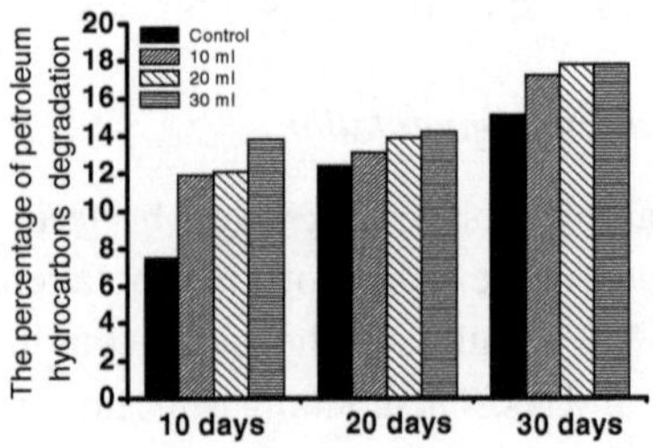

Fig. 1 The effects of microbial concentration on the efficiency of petroleum hydrocarbon degradation.

3.2. *The effects of soil humidity, temperature and PH on the efficiency of petroleum hydrocarbon degradation*

To detect the effects of soil environment on the efficiency of petroleum hydrocarbon degradation, we tested the degradation efficiency under different humidity, temperature and pH. The results were shown in Figure 2. It can be seen that when the humidity is at the range of 10% to 25%, the degradation efficiency increased as the humidity increased; however, when the humidity is over 25%, the degradation efficiency decreased as the as the humidity increased

(Fig. 2A), which may because that the high humidity can decrease the oxygen concentration in the soil and thus inhibit the growth of the microbial. At the temperature range from 10°C to 25°C, the degradation efficiency increased as the temperature increased; when the temperature is over 25°C, the degradation efficiency decreased as the temperature increased (Figure 2B). The pH of soil also affects the degradation efficiency. As shown in Figure 2C, when the pH is 7.0, the degradation efficiency is about 2 times of that in pH 4.5 or pH 8.5. Thus, the most suitable condition is the temperature of 25°C, humidity of 25% and pH of 7.0.

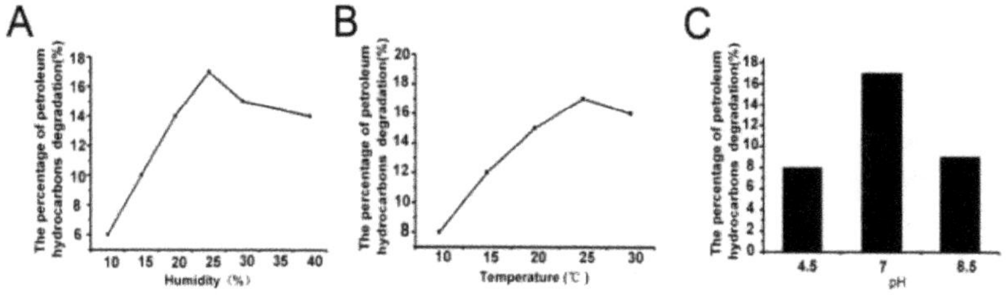

Fig. 2 The effects of soil environment on the efficiency of petroleum hydrocarbon degradation.

3.3. *The effects of nutrients of microbial concentration on the efficiency of petroleum hydrocarbon degradation*

In our study, we supplied $(NH_4)_2SO_4$ and KH_2PO_4 as the N and P sources, respectively. Thus, we added $(NH_4)_2SO_4$ or KH_2PO_4 and both of them into the pots of soil to detect the efficiency of petroleum hydrocarbon degradation. And the culture condition is the temperature of 25°C, humidity of 25% and pH of 7.0, and the volume bacilli is 20 ml. The tested soil samples are added with N source according to C/P=25, and added P source of C/P=150, added N+P of C: N: P=150:6:1. We also added the same volume bacilli which have been sterilized as the control. It can be found that only add strengthening of bacteria without N and P nutrients, there is little effect on the degradation efficiency of petroleum hydrocarbons. As shown in Figure 3, the nutrients of N and P greatly affect the rate of degradation of petroleum hydrocarbons in soil. When appropriate proportion of N source and P source are added to the soil, the degradation rate of the oil has been greatly improved up to 73.4%; when added strengthen bacteria, the degradation rate of the highest up to 77.8% compared with the control group which is 62.4%.

3.4. *The effects of activator on the efficiency of petroleum hydrocarbon degradation*

To detect whether other activator play a role in the efficiency of petroleum hydrocarbon degradation, we added sawdust (1/10 of the weight of soil), and then dected the degradation percentage as before. The result is shown as Figure 4. The experiment used bacilli which have been sterilized and strengthen bacteria as control; it can be seem that the application of activator can significantly increase the degradation efficiency. Thus, we further added both activator and N and P, it can be found that when added activator to the N and P applied soil, the degradation efficiency was 85%, which was increased compared with application N and P (77.5%), and activator (75.6%). As sawdust can not only supply as nutrient substance, but also can make the soil become loose which can increase the oxygen concentration in the soil, and thus to increase the degradation efficiency [7]. Thus, the activator (sawdust) can also improve the degradation efficiency of petroleum hydrocarbons.

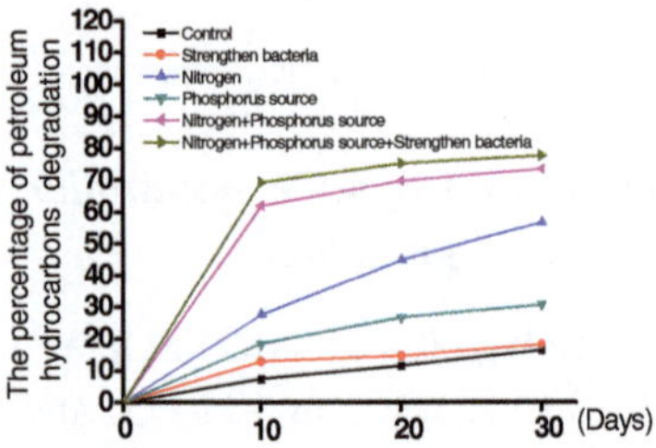

Fig. 3 The effects of nutrients of microbial concentration on the efficiency of petroleum hydrocarbon degradation.

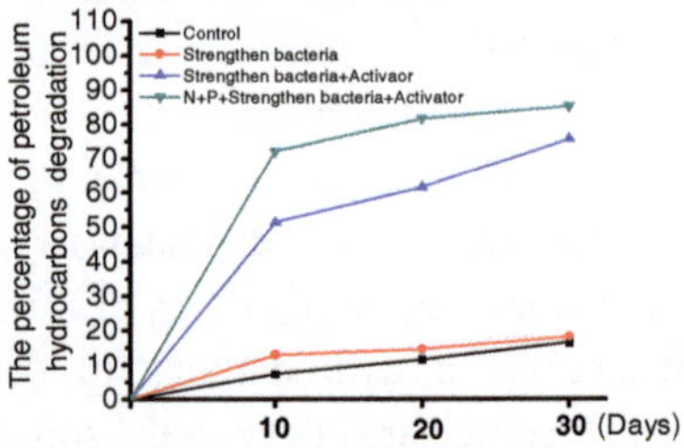

Fig. 4 The effects of sawdust on the efficiency of petroleum hydrocarbon degradation.

4. Conclusions

Factors affecting the indigenous microbial remediation of petroleum contaminated soil contaminants include the concentration of indigenous microorganisms, composition and molecular weight of oil, and the composition, temperature, nutrient and pH of the soil [8]. Our results showed that condition of t 25°C, 25% humidity and pH 7.0 is the most suitable for the efficiency of petroleum hydrocarbon degradation, and the concentration of strengthen indigenous microorganisms did not has significantly affect on the efficiency of petroleum hydrocarbon degradation. However, nutrients of N and P greatly affect the rate of degradation of petroleum hydrocarbons in soil. And added sawdust as the activator can also increase the degradation efficiency of petroleum hydrocarbons. Appropriate proportion of N and P source and sawdust are added to the soil, the degradation rate of hydrocarbon degradation has been greatly improved, up to 85%.

References

1. Xiuxia Zhang, Zhi Teng, Jiadong Wu, et. al. The optimization of the condition for microbial bioaugmentation remediation of oil-polluted soil by the treatment of activated agent. *Journal of petroleum.* 29(2), pp. 353-357, 2013.
2. Lihua Mao, Hua Lu, Zijun Li. Mechanism and Methods of Bioaugmentation Remediation of Petroleum Hydrocarbon contaminated Soil. *Journal of nonferrous metals.* 58(1), pp. 92-95, 2006.
3. Ueno A, Ito Y, Yamamoto I, et al. Isolation and characterization of bacteria from soil contaminated with diesel oil and the possible use of these in autochthonous bioaugmentation. *World J Microbiol Biotech.* 23(l), pp. 1739-1745, 2007.
4. Liu Hong, Yu-hang Wu, Zhiping Li. Remediation of Petroleum Hydrocarbons Contaminated Soil by Stimulating in Digenous Microorganisms. *Journal of Jilin Institute of Chemical Technology.* 29(7), pp. 60-63, 2012.
5. Fenglan Xu, Guiyin Feng, Wen Ma et. al. Screening bacteria of efficient oil degradation ability. *Biotechnology Bulletin.* 7, pp. 221-226, 2010.
6. Hui Y. Research progress in microbial degradation of petroleum hydrocarbons. *Shanxi Chemical Industry.* 29 (4), pp. 25-28, 2009.
7. Xiang He, Hai Wu, Wei Wei. Bactert-Based Bioremediation Technique for Oil Polluted Soi. *Soil.* 37 (3), pp. 338-340, 2005.
8. Lin Li, Huifang Yang, Jia Shengfen. Study on bioremediation of petroleum polluted soil. *Shanghai Environmental Sciences.* 7, pp. 325-329, 2000.

DNA Motifs and Transcription Factor Binding Sites Analysis of Regulatory Regions of MicroRNAs Relating to Psoriasis Disease*

Lina Wang[1], Yuxiao Jing[1], Jianqiang Du[1], Xiaoming Wu[1,a], Jiaqi Guo[1,2] and Yan Zheng[1,2,b]

[1]The Key Laboratory of Biomedical Information Engineering of Ministry of Education, School of Life Science and Technology, Xi'an Jiaotong University, Xi'an 710049, China
[2]Department of Dermatology, Second Affiliated Hospital, Xi'an Jiaotong University Xi'an, 710061, China
E-mail: [a]wxm@mail.xjtu.edu.cn, [b]zenyan66@126.com

Psoriasis is a complex disease, in which microRNAs played an important role in regulating target genes, and thus affecting gene expression and conducting cell proliferation. To analysis the regulation of microRNAs, and to illustrate the interaction of microRNAs with psoriasis related genes, we analyzed the upstream regions of the differentially expressed microRNAs relating to psoriasis. The polymerase binding site motifs were discovered by MAST using profiles of 13 polymerases in the upstream region for each microRNA, and a SVM (Support Vector Machine) was used to identify the motifs mostly related to microRNA expression level. Result shows that motif 3 and motif 6 are key to the gene expression type of psoriasis related microRNAs.

Keywords: Gene expression regulation; microRNAs; psoriasis; transcription factors.

1. Introduction

The etiology of psoriasis is multifactorial, involving complex interactions between the skin and the immune system, in addition to genetic alterations and environmental factors [1]. It is characterized by epidermal hyper-proliferation, vascular remodeling and inflammation. Some observations suggest T cells, dendritic cells and inflammatory cytokines are key to the pathogenesis of psoriasis, and microRNA is probably one reason for the regulation of these cells. MicroRNAs take an important role in target genes regulation, they can bind to part of mRNA target genes, and inhibit their translation and cause accelerated turnover or transcript degradation. However, the underlying principle of gene expression for microRNA still needs to be clarified, since it is also a reason for disease development. In this study, we focused on the regulatory regions of the

* This work was supported by the National Natural Science Foundation of China (81102085, 81371732, 81201231), and the Fundamental Research Funds for the Central Universities (2012jdhz47, xjj2013117).

differently expressed microRNA genes to characterize their sequence feature and to illustrate the regulatory function of each part of them.

2. Materials and Methods

2.1. *MicroRNA gene selection*

Joyce et. al. have conducted a deep sequencing experiment to discover the difference of microRNA profiles in psoriasis patients and health individuals [2]. Their research identified 98 differentially expressed novel and known microRNAs. In the dataset, 73 microRNA genes are up-regulated and 27 microRNA genes are down-expressed. Those microRNAs were served as source for researching the expression mechanism in this study.

2.2. *Polymerase binding sites identification*

2000bp long upstream region relating to each microRNA was extracted from genome sequences, according to the annotation data of each microRNA in mirBase. Perl script and Samtools were used to make the sequences data preparation. MAST web service was used to find sub-sequences matching a predefined profiles. In this case, we uses profiles of 13 curated polymerase binding sites obtained from TRANSFAC database [3].

2.3. *Discriminative binding site discovery*

A procedure of SVM (Support Vector Machine) selection was used to find the best motif combination that can discriminate the up-regulated and down-regulated microRNAs. The approach was first introduced by Wu et. al. [4]. Briefly, each gene was classified as up-regulated or down-regulated according to its expression, and then it was represented by a set of motif features which was the existence number in the upstream region of each microRNA. A SVM was constructed and trained according to the genes attributes. If the gene expression type is related to some motifs, the algorithm can find out the motif sets having the best discriminate result for the gene expression type, which is up-regulated or down-regulated.

3. Results

3.1. *Motif existences in upstream for each microRNA*

Motif 1, motif 3, motif 4, motif 6 and motif 11 have occurred in the upstream region of these genes, while other 8 polymerase binding sites don't appear. It can be seen that different microRNA gene would prefer different kind of motifs with different number of instances; the distribution of transcription binding site in each gene is uneven.

3.2. *Motifs related to microRNA gene expression*

We used a SVM to search the motif combination that account for gene expression type. For a single motif, motif 6 has the best ability to discriminate the gene type, which is up-regulated or down-regulated. The precision is 0.75. When two motifs combination were considered, motif 3, together with motif 6 can get a discriminative value of 0.63. The profile of motif 3 and motif 6 are showed in Table 2.

3.3. *Transcription factor binding site in regulatory area of microRNA*

By using ChIP-Seq technology, many transcription binding site have been discovered in a genomic scale. Transcription factor distribution in a genomic scale can be downloaded from website (https://genome.ucsc.edu/ENCODE/). The merged track data were served as the source for true protein binding sites. In down-regulated microRNA, has-mir-2110 and has-mir-375 contain most protein binding evidence, showing the importance of these two microRNAs. In up-regulated microRNA, hsa-mir-142 and hsa-mir-200c contain most protein binding evidence.

4. Discussion

Gene expression is determined by many factors, and the transcription factors binding site in the upstream region is the primary one. In this study, motifs related to microRNA gene expression in psoriasis disease were identified. motif 3 and motif 6 were reported to have the main effect to arouse the microRNA gene expressions. When the two motifs are considered together, the synergy effect to arouse gene expression would decrease, which means the two motifs have an opposite effect to arouse the same microRNA gene expression in psoriasis lesion.

5. Tables

Table 1 Motif occurrence count in the upstream of microRNA genes.

Name	Total count	Polymerase name	Minimum count in sequence	maximum count i sequence
Motif 1	129	POL001	0	2
Motif 3	260	POL003	1	11
Motif 4	100	POL004	0	2
Motif 6	108	POL006	0	2
Motif 11	195	POL011	1	9

Table 2 Motif profiles and their function.

Name	Consensus sequence logo	Function
Motif 3	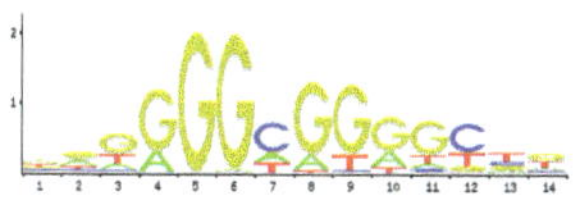	Motif 3 binds to GC-box-binding protein such as transcription factor SP1, which is RNA polymerase II promoter elements.
Motif 6	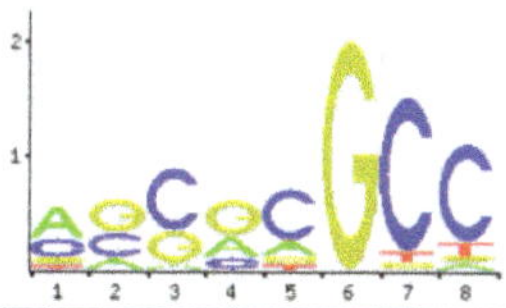	Motif 6 is transcription factor IIB recognition element, affecting the ability of transcription factor IIB to enter transcription complexes and supporting transcription initiation.

Note: The profiles and sequences logo are derived from Transfect database.

References

1. E. Sonkoly, M. Stahle and A. Pivarcsi: MicroRNAs: novel regulators in skin inflammation *Clinical and experimental dermatology.* **33**(3), 312 (2008).
2. C.E. Joyce, X. Zhou, J. Xia, C. Ryan, B. Thrash, A. Menter, W. Zhang and A.M. Bowcock: Deep sequencing of small RNAs from human skin reveals major alterations in the psoriasis miRNAome. *Human molecular genetics.* **20**, 4025 (2011).
3. V. Matys, O. Kel-Margoulis, E. Fricke and E. Wingender: TRANSFAC and its module TRANSCompel: transcriptional gene regulation in eukaryotes *Nucleic acids research.* **34**(Database issue), 10 (2006).
4. X. Wu, L. Wang, X. Wang, H. Zhang and J. Du: Conserved DNA Sequences Discovered From Atrial Fibrillation Related Genes *International Heart Journal.* (52), 295 (2011).

Discriminant Analysis of Bean Curd with Blood From Duck, Pig or Cattle Based on Real-Time PCR

Wang Jianming[a] and Geng Yongran
College of Food Engineering and Biotechnology, Tianjin University of Science & Technology, Tianjin, 300457, China
[a]E-mail: wjm-1115@126.com

Wei Wei and Lu Fei[b]
Beijing Supervision & Testing Center I for Foods and Alcoholic Products, Beijing, 100075, China
[b]E-mail: lufei@bitri.cn

Based on the real-time quantitative polymerase chain reaction technology and Fisher discriminant analysis method, a new approach is established to rapidly discern the bean curd with blood from duck blood, pig or cattle. Through the primer design and specificity validation of duck, pig and cattle, the real-time quantitative polymerase chain reaction technology is used to identify the components of 81 samples of blood curd. The discriminant analysis model of species identification of bean curd with blood of duck, pig or cattle is established on the basis of taking two indicators, the content of iron and that of protein, as discriminant factors and using SPSS 19.0 to calculate the discriminant coefficient. The result shows that, in the case of Fisher linear discriminant analysis model, the accuracy of identifying the authenticity of bean curd with duck blood, pig blood or cattle blood is respectively 83.0%, 82.7%, 75.3%. Through the combination of iron and protein content with Fisher discriminant analysis method, the bean curd with duck blood, pig blood, or cattle blood can be identified relatively easily. This is a new and simple way of distinguishing bean curd with blood.

Keywords: Bean curd with blood; iron; protein; discriminant analysis.

1. Introduction

The blood curd is the solidified product similar to bean curd on the basis of taking animal blood as raw material [1]. The blood curd is smooth, tender and soft, which is favored by people because of abundant nutrients. It enjoys the reputation of "liquid meat" [2]. As the duck blood has higher nutritional value and better edible effect [3], its price is significantly higher than that of pig blood. So, some merchants may adulterate the duck blood with pig blood and even cattle blood for more profits, greatly harming the interests of consumers.

Therefore, it is particularly important to establish a simple and quick method to identify the authenticity of blood curd and control its quality.

Currently, the meat adulteration detection mainly relies on the gene detection technology of PCR (polymerase chain reaction) expansion in vitro of nucleic acids [4-6]. The real-time fluorescent quantitative PCR technology has become an important tool in the molecular biology study [7-8] because of its advantages: strong specificity, high sensitivity and totally closed reaction. However, this method is complicated and tedious in operation; moreover, it has relatively high requirements on laboratory and operators. However, the discriminant analysis is different. First, a discriminant function is established on the basis of determining the quantitative relationship between the variable of describing individual characteristics and its category according the variable value and the known information of its category. On this basis, those individuals which are not known or classified are grouped through discrimination; that is, this classification method is based on the prediction of those whose categories are not known [9-11]. Discriminant analysis is a kind of multivariate statistical analysis method with strong application [12], which has penetrated into all areas. But it has not been found that this method is applied in the identification of adulterated bean curd with duck blood in combination with PCR technology. In this paper, 81 samples are taken randomly, which are used for the identification of three kinds of genes: duck, pig and cattle. In addition, taking iron and protein as indicators and following the Fisher linear discriminant criterion, a discriminant model of identified bean curd with blood is established. Thus, a simple and quick way of distinguishing true and false bean curd with duck blood is expected to obtain.

2. Material and Methods

2.1. *Preparation of samples*

The fresh blood of ducks, pigs, hens/cocks, oxen and sheep were taken from Beijing Anding Slaughterhouse.

81 blood curd samples were taken randomly, including 44 in bulk and 37 in box. The boxed samples concerned fifteen popular brands in Beijing markets, which were taken from ten districts in Beijing, such as Fengtai, Changping, Shunyi.

2.2. *Identification of components of the sample*

2.2.1. *Preparation of genomic template*

A small amount of sample was weighed and placed in the centrifuge tube of 2.0mL, and then the steps were followed according to Magnetic Genomic DNA Kit DNA Extraction Kit Instructions provided by Tiangen Biotech. The extracted OD_{260}/OD_{280} ratio was animal tissue DNA of 1.6 to 2.0.

2.2.2. *Primer probe design synthesis*

The replication was made according to the mitochondrial cytochrome b (Cyt b) gene sequences of duck, pig and cattle obtained from the database of NCBI. Then the results were fully contrasted. According to the primer probe design principle, Primer Express 3.0 software was used to design primer and probe with specificity. Oligo7 was used to score the design primer sequence, and the final results were good. The specific species sequences were as Table 1.

Table 1 Sequences of the oligonucleotide primers and probes.

Primer/probe	Sequence 5'-3'
Duck-F	GCAACTGCCTTCGTAGGTTATGTC
Duck-R	GGAGGGCTGA AAATAAGTTGGTAA
Duck-probe	FAM- ATGAGGACAAATATCGTTCTGAGGAGCTACCGTA-TAMRA
Pig-F	TTTGTGCATGACTGCGTCAAC
Pig-R	CTTGGTGGTCGTGG TCACTGT
Pig- probe	FAM- CACCGTCAAGCAGC-(NFQ)(MGB)
Cattle-F	CAACAGGAATCTCCTCAGACGTAGA
Cattle-R	GCTAGAATT AGTAAG AGGGCCCCTAA
Cattle-probe	FAM-CCCATTCCACCCCTACTATACCATTAAGGACA-TAMRA

2.2.3. *Real-time fluorescent PCR reaction system and reaction cycle parameters*

The volume of reaction system was 20μL: Buffer of 10μL; upstream primer of 1μL; downstream primer of 1μL; fluorescently labeled probes of 1μL; template DNA of 2μL; the insufficient rest was filled with sterile double distilled water. The reaction cycle parameters: 95℃, 30s; 95℃, 5s; 60℃, 35s, and 40 cycles.

2.2.4. *Primer specificity validation*

DNA extracted from pure blood of oxen, pigs and ducks has the concentration of approximately 50ng/μL, which was respectively taken in the amount of 2μL for real-time PCR reaction to verify the specificity of designed primers and probes.

2.2.5. *Sample measurement*

In order to lay a foundation for rapid detection model of adulterated bean curd with duck blood, DNA was extracted from the taken sampled. In addition, the adulteration was identified through the cycle threshold value (Ct) red by the real-time fluorescent quantitative PCR in combination with amplification curve.

2.3. *Measurement of content of iron in the sample*

2.3.1. *Conditions of iron measurement*

The wavelength was 248.3nm; the slit width (or the spectral passband) was 0.2nm; the lamp current was 6.0mA; the flame was C2H2/air; the gas flow was 65L/h; the combustion head was 100mm in type; the combustion head height was 6mm; the atomizer's lift amount was 5.0mL/min.

2.4. *Measurement of content of protein in the sample*

2.4.1. *Preparation of standard series*

The Kjeldahl method was used to measure the content of protein in the blood curd.

3. Results and Analysis

3.1. *Specificity experiment*

The upstream and downstream primer genes and probe sequences of different species were the total gene synthesis provided by BGI Gene Synthesis Technology Co., Ltd. Under the optimized fluorescent PCR reaction system and reaction conditions, for DNA of the extracted duck blood, pig blood and cattle blood, the fluorescent quantitative PCR specificity inspection was made respectively to verify the specificity of primers and probes. The amplified PCR curve is shown below.

The results show that only the targeted detection object has an amplification curve and other appropriate control and blank control have no amplification curve. This indicates that the designed primer and probe have higher homology with the target detection object and corresponding species. According to the result, the designed primer and probe are good, which have stronger specificity. Thus, they can be used to identify the authenticity of blood curd sampled from the market.

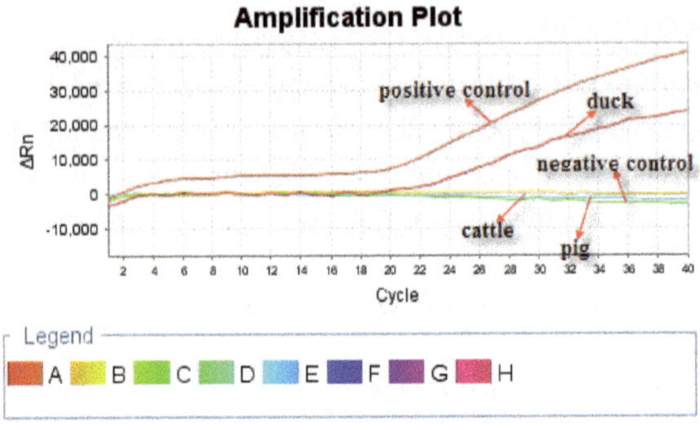

Fig. 1 Real time PCR result of specificity test of the duck.

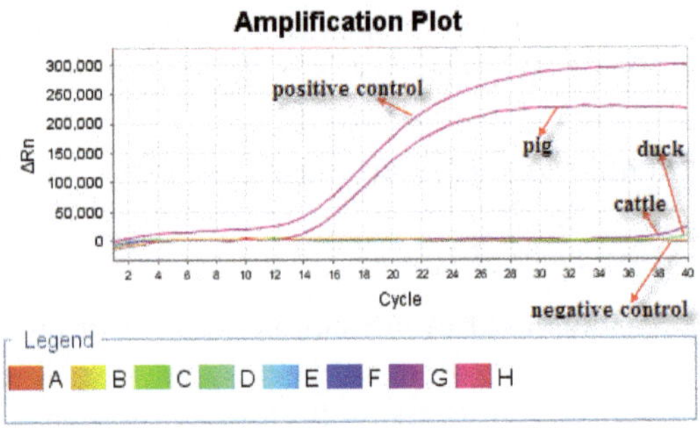

Fig. 2 Real time PCR result of specificity test of the pig.

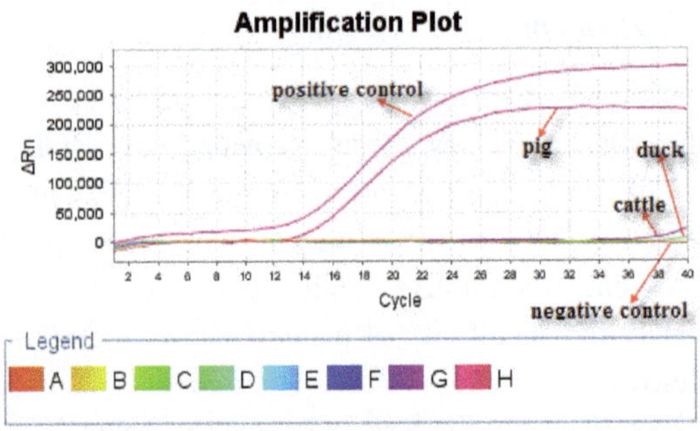

Fig. 3 Real time PCR result of specificity test of the cattle.

3.2. *Measurement results of specie components and iron and protein content*

Based on the optimized conditions, the real-time fluorescent quantitative PCR technology was used to identify the genetic components of extracted 81 samples. The Ct value red through the PCR instrument was used to identify whether there exist the source components of duck, pig and cattle. In addition, the content of iron and protein in the appropriate samples was measured. The results are shown in Table 2.

Table 2 Result of genetic identification and concentrations of DNA of the samples.

No.	Ct of duck	Ct of pig	Ct of cattle	Fe (mg/kg)	Protein (g/100g)
1	23.6	40	40	125.40	6.98
2	29.5	40	39.3	130.95	9.94
3	33	39	40	133.55	8.00
4	22.1	40	40	81.73	6.46
5	25.1	40	40	178.25	8.02
6	27.5	40	40	138.80	6.15
7	23.3	40	40	175.50	6.88
8	25.1	39.6	40	227.05	8.78
9	22.8	40	40	309.75	8.32
10	32.1	38.3	40	229.60	7.83
11	25.9	40	40	231.55	8.30
12	37.6	30.6	40	193.95	7.98
13	40	36.6	40	200.25	4.54
14	31.7	35.5	40	199.90	8.62
15	29.3	39.3	40	174.00	6.82
16	26.7	40	40	269.20	6.37
17	40	31.1	40	166.45	4.36
18	26.3	40	40	269.10	7.00
19	27	40	28.7	180.70	6.23
20	25.5	40	40	219.10	9.27
21	40	28.3	40	202.45	8.02
22	29	40	40	208.90	7.00
23	29	38.9	40	210.85	7.98
24	40	40	40	224.60	3.41
25	40	40	40	123.75	4.50
26	30.6	40	40	294.40	6.38
27	30	39.8	40	177.05	8.62
28	40	40	40	174.90	4.06
29	30.1	40	40	157.25	9.13
30	29.5	40	40	180.90	7.05
31	19.3	40	40	121.50	6.15
32	23.7	40	40	140.25	8.15
33	40	29.2	40	256.85	11.40
34	40	25.6	40	289.75	11.30
35	29.1	30	40	281.35	8.53
36	39.2	26.9	40	207.10	10.80
37	37.9	28.4	40	170.15	11.50
38	40	36.3	25.8	140.60	6.00
39	40	40	24.1	103.20	5.19
40	40	36	26.1	203.15	6.18
41	40	35.9	26	147.20	7.33
42	40	36.6	26.6	156.10	5.13
43	40	36.8	25.8	172.30	6.55
44	40	36.1	25.1	140.70	5.09
45	40	36.5	24.2	188.25	8.75
46	40	35.9	24.3	138.20	5.79
47	40	29	40	114.60	9.44

48	40	37	22.1	263.45	7.39
49	40	35.7	24.9	229.60	8.23
50	40	36.5	24.3	230.55	6.75
51	40	37	24.2	331.90	7.90
52	40	37.2	24.4	195.10	5.73
53	40	38.5	26.4	330.15	6.55
54	40	36.8	27.5	282.50	5.54
55	40	37.7	26.5	173.00	7.33
56	40	38	24.7	189.75	5.83
57	40	36.6	25	252.95	7.25
58	40	40	24.4	157.30	6.62
59	40	40	24.8	190.65	6.63
60	40	40	24.7	196.00	6.17
61	40	36.9	23.9	205.65	6.81
62	40	40	24.7	300.15	6.67
63	40	40	24.2	209.10	7.94
64	40	37.9	25.1	99.00	5.35
65	40	40	24.2	145.60	4.35
66	40	31.8	40	253.50	10.50
67	40	31.7	40	272.00	10.40
68	40	36.7	23.3	130.65	4.82
69	40	40	26	120.35	4.39
70	40	29.1	40	267.80	11.50
71	40	25.9	40	389.40	10.00
72	40	40	26.2	115.50	5.07
73	40	40	26.5	212.85	4.53
74	40	36.7	40	196.55	5.07
75	40	25.5	40	389.50	10.30
76	40	28.2	40	237.40	9.68
77	40	28.3	40	181.20	9.83
78	40	40	23.2	229.30	5.15
79	40	40	23.4	257.35	5.89
80	40	40	23.8	254.45	5.08
81	40	38.5	25.8	220.30	4.58

The number of 1 to 37 is blood curd in bulk and the number of 38 to 81 is blood curd in box.

The gene components of samples taken from the market were identified. It can be seen from Table 2 that the adulteration of blood curd is seriously; the source blood curd components of duck, pig and cattle. Therefore, in the Fisher discriminant analysis, the quick method to identify the authenticity of blood curd would be established.

3.3. *Establishment of discriminant analysis model*

3.3.1. *Establishment of discriminant analysis model of duck component*

It can be seen from Table 3 that one discriminant function is extracted in this analysis. Obviously, the cumulative percentage indicates 100% that this discriminant function completely extracts the information of samples. The significant test result is Sig value=0.000<0.05, which shows that this discriminant function expression is of great significance.

Table 3 Eigenvalue and function test of discriminant analysis of the duck.

Eigenvalue	Variance %	Cumulative %	Positive correlation	Wilks' Lambda	Chi-square	Df	Sig.
0.058[a]	100.0	100.0	0.234	0.945	4.389	2	0.000

Table 4 Functional determine of discriminant analysis of the duck.

	Canonical discriminant function coefficients			Centroid function	
Function	Protein coefficient	Iron element coefficient	Constant	Not detected	Detected
1	0.498	-0.012	-1.086	-0.163	0.346

Table 4 shows the non-standardized canonical discriminant function coefficients, which are considerably important in the discriminant function. The standardized coefficient table is not convenient for the subsequent verification through using the observation value. For the mean vector of discriminant scores of each group, under the premise that the above table for category gravity is given and the discriminant function expressions in the table are combined, it can be first put in the formula for calculation as long as the data of measured protein and Fe are grasped in the subsequent operation. Finally, an X value is obtained. If this X value is approaching one value in two items (undetected and detected), it means that it belongs to this category. Therefore, the non-standardized coefficient table is the main reference. It can be inferred from the above table that the discriminant function equation is $D = -1.086 + 0.498 \times \text{protein} - 0.012 \times \text{Fe}$.

The discriminant model of duck component is verified, and the results are shown that the accuracy of the discrimination of all cases, cross-validation and discriminant validation is 83% and 80.7% respectively. Obviously, the discriminant effect of duck discriminant function is better.

3.3.2. *Establishment of discriminant analysis model of pig component*

Table 5 Eigenvalue and function test of discriminant analysis of the pig.

Eigenvalue	Variance %	Cumulative %	Positive correlation	Wilks' Lambda	Chi-square	df	Sig.
0.707[a]	100.0	100.0	0.644	0.586	41.716	2	0.000

It can be seen from Table 5 that one discriminant function is extracted in this analysis. The cumulative percentage indicates 100% that this discriminant function completely extracts the information of samples. The significant test result is Sig value=0.000<0.05, which shows that this discriminant function expression is significant.

Table 6 Functional determine of discriminant analysis of the pig.

	Canonical discriminant function coefficients			Centroid function	
Function	Protein coefficient	Iron element coefficient	Constant	Not detected	Detected
1	0.618	0.003	-5.004	-0.412	1.674

Table 6 shows the non-standardized canonical discriminant function coefficients. It can be inferred from the above table that the discriminant function equation is $D = -5.004 + 0.618 \times$ protein+$0.003 \times$ Fe. For the mean vector of discriminant scores of each group, under the premise that the above table for category gravity is given and the discriminant function expressions in the table are combined, it can be first put in the formula for calculation as long as the data of measured protein and Fe are grasped in the subsequent operation. It can be seen from analysis that the accuracy of the discrimination of all cases, cross-validation and discriminant validation is 82.7% and 82.7% respectively. Obviously, this discriminant function has a certain practical significance.

3.3.3. *Establishment of discriminant analysis model of cattle component*

Table 7 Eigenvalue and function test of discriminant analysis of the cattle.

Eigenvalue	Variance %	Cumulative %	Positive correlation	Wilks' Lambda	Chi-square	df	Sig.
0.309[a]	100.0	100.0	0.486	0.764	21.012	2	0.000

It can be seen from Table 7 that one discriminant function is extracted in this analysis. The cumulative percentage indicates 100% that this discriminant function completely extracts the information of samples. The significant test result is Sig value=0.000<0.05, which shows that this discriminant function expression is of great significance.

Table 8 Functional determine of discriminant analysis of the cattle.

	Canonical discriminant function coefficients			Centroid function	
Function	Protein coefficient	Iron element coefficient	Constant	Not detected	Detected
1	0.603	-0.003	-3.651	0.491	-0.614

Table 8 shows the non-standardized canonical discriminant function coefficients. It can be inferred from the above table that the discriminant function equation is $D = -3.651 + 0.603 \times$ protein $-0.003 \times$ Fe. It can be seen from analysis that the accuracy of the discrimination of all cases, cross-validation and discriminant validation is 75.3% and 72.8% respectively.

4. Conclusions

Through the duck, pig and cattle primer design and specificity validation, the real-time fluorescent quantitative PCR technology is used to analyze five gene components of 81 samples. Through using the discriminant analysis model of statistical analysis software SPSS 19.0 and taking iron and protein as the discriminant factors, the discriminant analysis model is established based on the Fisher linear discriminant analysis model principles. The discriminant function formula of duck component is: $D = -1.086+0.498\times\text{protein} -0.012\times\text{Fe}$; for the group mass center function, −0.163 is for "not detected", 0.346 is for "detected". The discriminant function formula of pig component is: $D = -5.004 + 0.618 \times \text{protein} + 0.003 \times \text{Fe}$; for the group mass center function, −0.412 is for "not detected", 1.674 is for "detected". The discriminant function formula of ox component is: $D = -3.651 + 0.603 \times \text{protein} -0.003 \times \text{Fe}$; for the group mass center function, 0.491 is for "not detected", −0.614 is for "detected". The results show that the accuracy rates of discriminant function formula in the identification of adulterated bean curd with duck blood and pig blood and cattle blood are 83%, 82.7% and 75.3%. Through sampling validation, the results show that sheep blood is not the source of adulterated duck blood and that the adulteration of chicken blood is not obvious. Thus, this method can be effectively applied to practice, that is, it is a new way of identifying the adulteration of the bean curd with duck blood. However, although many samples are used in this study, all the samples are taken from Beijing. Thus, for the identification of adulterated duck blood in other regions, this method needs further research.

References

1. Xin Cheng, Weiling He, Feng Huang, Ming Huang, Guanghong Zhou. Multiplex real-time PCR for the identification and quantification of DNA from duck, pig and chicken in Chinese blood curds. Food Research International, 2014, 60(6): 30-37.
2. Sen Li. Study of key technology of boxed pig blood processing. Meat Industry, 2009, 35(11): 17-19.
3. Fei Chen, Yingdao Wang, Yongzhi Zhu, *et al.* Effect of Different Heating Time on Quality of Duck Blood Curd. Southwest China Journal of Agricultural Sciences, 2011, 24(4): 1515-1518.

4. Nicolai Z. Ballin, Finn K. Vogensen, Anders H. Karlsson. Species determination-Can we detect and quantify meat adulteration. Meat Science, 2009, 83(2): 165-147.
5. Sónia Soares, Joana S. Amaral, Isabel Mafra, M. Beatriz P.P. Oliveira. Quantitative detection of poultry meat adulteration with pork by a duplex PCR assay [J]. Meat Science, 2010, 85(3): 531-536.
6. Zülal Kesmen, Yasemin Celebi, Ayten Güllüce, Hasan Yetim. Detection of seagull meat in meat mixtures using real-time PCR analysis. Food Control, 2013, 34(1): 47-49.
7. John J. Dooley, Kelly E. Paine, Stephen D. Garrett, Helen M. Brown. Detection of meat species using TaqMan real-time PCR assays. Meat Science, 2004, 68(3): 431-438.
8. Muhammad Safdar, Yasmeen Junejo. Development and validation of fast duplex real-time PCR assays based on SYBER Green florescence for detection of bovine and poultry origins in feedstuffs. Food Chemistry, 2015, 173(8): 660-664.
9. Hyejin Shin. An extension of Fisher's discriminant analysis for stochastic processes. Journal of Multivariate Analysis, 2008, 99(6): 1191-1216.
10. E. Colman, W. Waegeman, B. De Baets, V. Fievez. Prediction of subacuteruminal acidosis based on milk fatty acids: A comparison of linear discriminant and support vector machine approaches for model development. Computers and Electronics in Agriculture, 2015, 111(2): 179-185.
11. Angelo Pavesi. Prediction of the determinants of thermal stability by linear discriminant analysis: The case of the glutamate dehydrogenase protein family. Journal of Theoretical Biology, 2014, 357(18): 160-168.
12. G. Kouvoutsakis, C. Mitsi, P.A. Tarantilis, M.G. Polissiou, C.S. Pappas. Geographical differentiation of dried lentil seed (Lens culinaris) samples using Diffuse Reflectance Fourier Transform Infrared Spectroscopy (DRIFTS) and discriminant analysis. Food Chemistry, 2014, 145: 1011-1014.

Effects of Treadmill Speed on Joint Angles of Human Lower Limbs During Walking*

Jianfeng Li†, Sa Wang and Qihuan Zhang
College of Mechanical Engineering and Applied Electronics Technology,
Beijing University of Technology, Beijing, 100124, China
†E-mail: lijianfeng@bjut.edu.cn
www.bjut.edu.cn

Chunjing Tao and Run Ji
National Research Center for Rehabilitation Technical Aids
Beijing, 100176, China

In order to study the influence of different walking speeds on locomotive information of healthy human lower limbs in the sagittal plane, frontal plane and transversal plane, VICON three dimensional motion capturing system was adopted to measure the movement information of seven healthy human pelvis, hip, knee and ankle, when human was walking on the treadmill at 1km/h, 2km/h, 3km/h. The pelvic, hip, knee and ankle kinematics and the relationship of joint angles of lower limbs in the sagittal plane, frontal plane and transversal plane were analyzed. The results show that for three joints of lower limb, increasing of the treadmill velocity increases the maximum angle of the flexion and variation range of joint in the sagittal plane while increasing velocity has little impact on the shapes of the curves except curves of hip joint in the transversal plane; regarding pelvic movement, increasing velocity has small effects on amplitude and shape of curves of pelvis motion; with velocity increasing, the modes of joint movement kept invariant, knee movement is stabilized and ankle movement is complicated. The results provide kinematics information for designing and controlling lower extremity rehabilitative robot.

Keywords: Human lower limbs; VICON; treadmill velocity; kinematics analysis.

1. Introduction

In recent years, more and more people are suffering from mobility problems caused by lower limbs damage or nervous system damage. People are increasingly concerned about their rehabilitation training. Treadmills are frequently used as training device. The user can improve motor coordinative skills and increase their muscular strength and endurance [1]. One important

* This work is supported by the National Natural Science Foundation of China under Grant No. 61273342, the Beijing Natural Science Foundation under Grant No. 3132005.

rehabilitation technique, so-called treadmill training, was created in 90's [2]. Different types of lower limb rehabilitation robots have been developed for the patient's lower limb rehabilitation. Such as Lokomat [3]. In treadmill training, the patient is standing on a treadmill and his body weight is reduced by a special suspension system [2]. The movement of patient's leg are assisted by two physiotherapists. Walking on a treadmill is more safety for elderly people and patient.

For designing and controlling lower extremity rehabilitation robot, it is essential to define normative kinematic data. Usually, kinematic data is extracted from experiment result of unimpaired people walking on the ground or treadmill, such as, clinicians collect data from healthy subjects who walk on the ground at their normal self-selected speed [4] or slow self-selected speed or walk on the treadmill at their slow self-selected speed. However, walking speed of patient is less than able-bodied person. a neurological or neuromuscular condition can often reduce an individual's gait speed more than 50% [3]. It is difficult for older population and individuals with disabilities to adapt the individual treadmill-based gait in natural walking [5]. Several studies have investigated the influence of velocity on human lower limbs. Some researchers have studied the effects of treadmill velocity on spatio-temporal, kinematic with young healthy subjects [4, 5] and older adults [6]. And Ya li Han et al. [7] have studied the effects treadmill velocity on kinematic and kinetic with young healthy subjects, Ilaria C et al. [8] found the difference of spatio-temporal and kinematic between overground walking and treadmill walking. However, previous work almost did not involve the effects of treadmill velocity on hip, knee and ankle kinematics data in the frontal plane and transversal plane.

This paper will offer pelvic kinematics data, hip, knee and ankle kinematics data in the sagittal plane, frontal plane and transversal plane at different treadmill speeds and the relationship of joint angles of lower limbs in the sagittal plane, frontal plane and transversal plane.

2. Materials and Methods

The measurements were realized in Human Biomechanics laboratory of National Research Center for Rehabilitation Technical Aids using VICON three-dimensional motion capturing system.

Seven young healthy volunteer (7 male, aged: 23-26, weight: 58-90kg, height: 1.70-1.82m, average leg length: 964.35mm, average knee width: 86.46mm, average ankle width: 73.56mm) with no reported orthopedic disorders performed gait on the treadmill at different speeds (1km/h, 2km/h, 3km/h) without using the treadmill handrails. Leg length is the distance from anterior superior iliac spine to sole, knee width is the distance from medial point on tibial plateau to lateral point on tibial plateau, ankle width is the distance from tip of the medial malleolus on ankle to tip of the lateral malleolus on ankle. The description and location of the Markers are presented in Figure 1 and Table 1.

Before the start of collection, every volunteer was performed to walk on the treadmill at each velocity for adapting his walking pattern to the measuring conditions. For each selected velocity five trials were performed, each trial having duration of approximately 5 seconds.

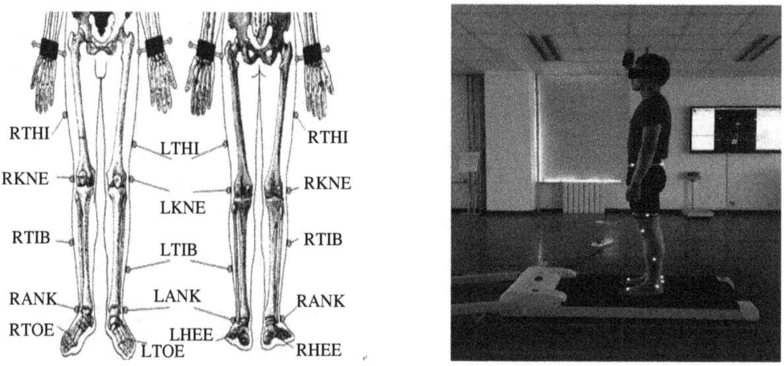

Fig. 1. Location of the marker.

Table 1 The description and location of markers.

Makers name	Description and location
R/LASI	Right/left anterior superior iliac spine
R/LPSI	Right/left posterior superior iliac spine
R/LTHI	Right/left thigh. Placed over the lower lateral 1/3 surface of the thigh
R/LKNE	lateral epicondyle of the right/left knee
R/LTIB	Right/left tibial wand marker. Placed over the lower 1/3 of the shank
R/LANK	Right/left ankle. Placed on the lateral malleolus
R/LTOE	Right/left toe. Placed over the second metatarsal head
R/LHEE	Right/left heel. Placed on the calcaneous

3. Results and Discussion

Three dimensional motion data was obtained for pelvis, hip, knee and ankle joints of both lower limbs. The raw data were exported from the system software and each velocity one gait cycle was selected. For pelvic (Fig. 2), the rotation movements are pelvic rotation (rotation about Z axis), pelvic tilt (rotation about Y axis) and pelvic obliquity (rotation about X axis). Positive direction of curves of pelvic movement is counterclockwise.

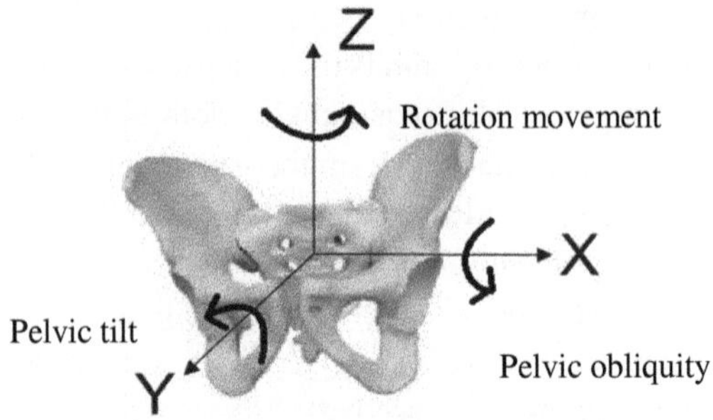

Fig. 2 Definition of axial composition and motion of pelvic.

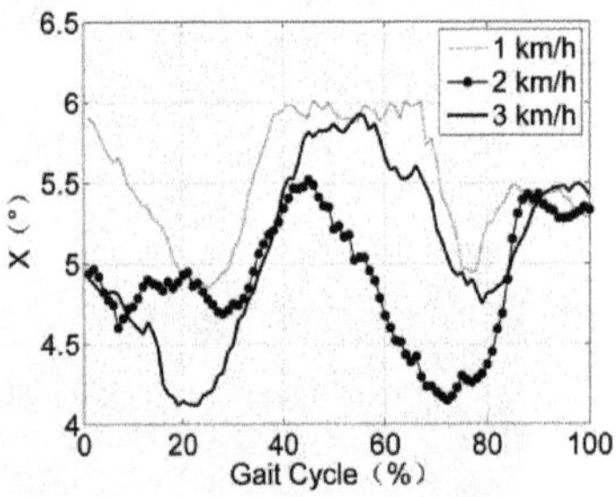

(a) pelvic obliquity

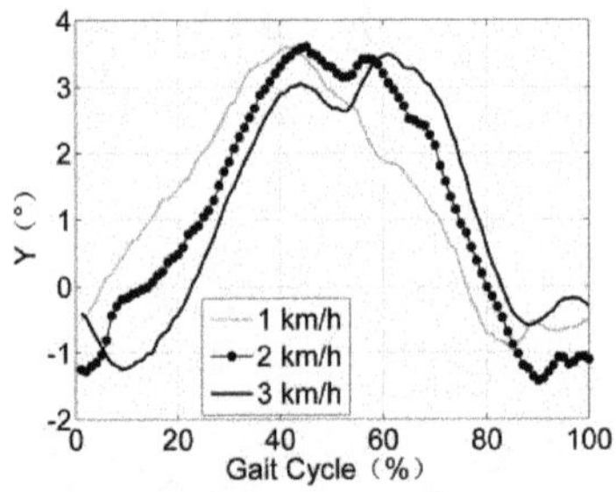

(b) pelvic tilt

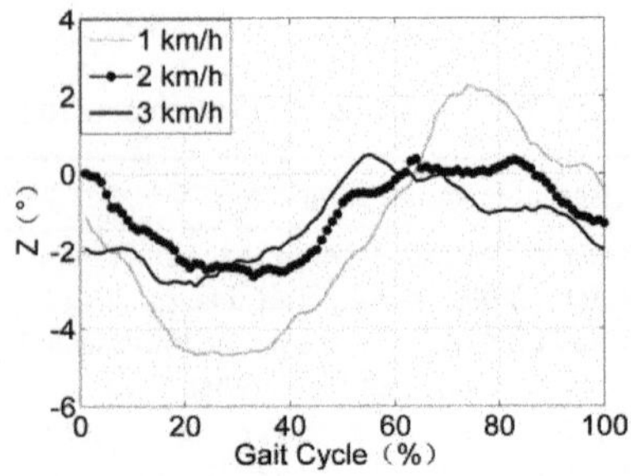

(c) pelvic rotation

Fig. 3 Curves of pelvic movement.

The X, Y, Z in diagram and Table 2 and Table 3 indicates sagittal, frontal and transversal plane respectively and positive value of angles of hip (Fig. 4), knee (Fig. 5) joints indicates flexion, adduction and internal rotation. For ankle joint (Fig. 6), positive value of angles indicates dorsiflexion, adduction and internal rotation. Positive/negative value of curves indicates direction. Due to the periodicity of human gait, the curve of hip, knee and ankle are presented for left lower limb only.

Angle graphs of pelvic movement are presented in Fig. 3(a-c). The amplitudes of rotation movements are small and shape of curves almost remind same at different velocity. Curves of pelvic rotation are similar to cosine wave. Curves of pelvic obliquity and pelvic tilt have two ups and downs in one gait phase by enhancing velocity and the maximum angle appear in the swing phases. In Fig. 3(a). Variation range of pelvic obliquity (1km/h: 1.18°; 2km/h: 1.38°; 3km/h: 1.82°) increase with velocity increasing. When velocity is 1km/h, curve of pelvic obliquity remains almost unchanged. In Fig. 3(b), when the velocity increases, the arising time of maximum angle lags and curves have valleys in approximately 55% gait phases. There is a reversal in fluctuation of curves of pelvic rotation with velocity increasing (see Fig. 3(c)).

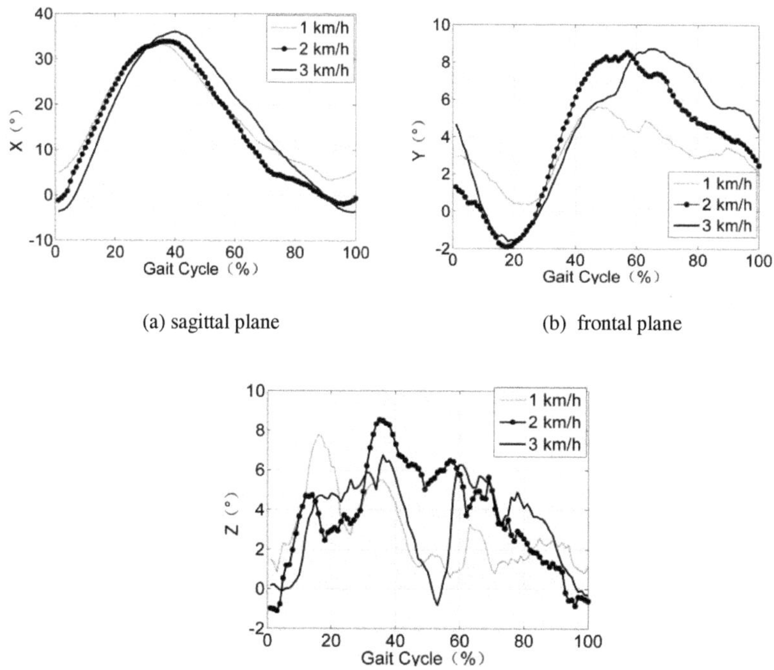

(a) sagittal plane

(b) frontal plane

(c) transversal plane

Fig. 4 Curves of hip angles in the sagittal plane, frontal plane and transversal plane.

Fig. 4(a-c) illustrates the variation of average angle in hip joint for one gait cycle. The value of hip joint curves are almost above the zero line. The maximum flexion angle (1km/h: 33.36°; 2km/h: 33.89°; 3km/h: 36.06°) and variation range of hip joint (1km/h: 29.95°; 2km/h: 35.7°; 3km/h: 39.74°, see Table 3) increase with velocity increasing in Fig. 4(a).

In Fig. 4(b), curves of hip joint are similar to sine wave. The maximum adduction angle (1km/h: 5.6°; 2km/h: 8.54°; 3km/h: 8.72°) increases and the arising time of maximum adduction angles lags gradually with velocity increasing (see Fig. 4(b)).

In Fig. 4(c), with velocity increasing, angle of hip joint in transversal plane have no regular variations. But the trends of the curves at different velocity are increased in the early stage of the gait phases then decreased in the late stage of the gait phases. When velocity is 3km/h, the curves of hip joint has more clear wave trough in the nearly 55% gait phases than velocity is 1km/h and 2km/h.

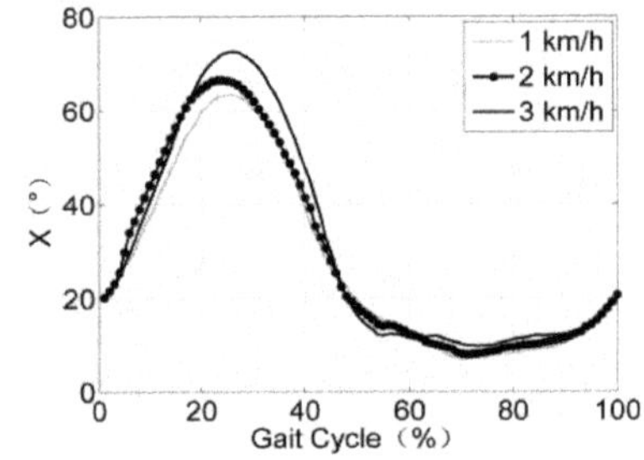

(a) sagittal plane

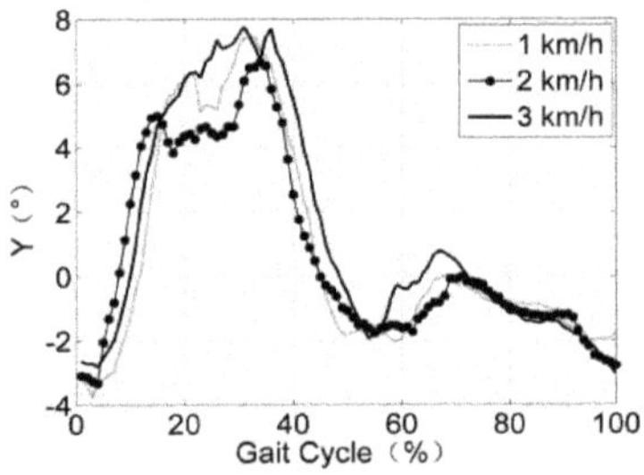

(b) frontal plane

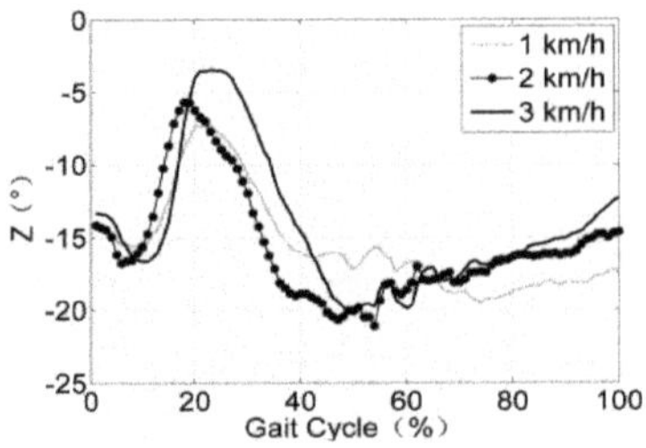

(c) transversal plane

Fig. 5 Curves of knee angles in the sagittal plane, frontal plane and transversal plane.

The variation of average knee joint angle for one gait cycle is presented in Fig. 5(a-c). The maximum flexion angle (1km/h: 63.47°; 2km/h: 66.57°; 3km/h: 72.64°) and variation range of knee joint (1km/h: 56.49°; 2km/h: 58.67°; 3km/h: 62.89°, see Table 3) increases with velocity increasing in Fig. 5(a).

According to Fig. 5(b), the three knee joint curves have similar shapes (difference of the maximum angle nearly 1°, see Table 3). And curves of knee joint have one up and down in support phases and swing phases respectively, but don't have regular variations with velocity increasing.

In Fig. 5(c), curves of knee joint in transversal plane were under the zero line. With velocity increasing, the peak value of curves (1km/h: -7.26°; 2km/h: -5.71°; 3km/h: -3.47°) and variation range of knee joint (1km/h: 12.24°; 2km/h: 15.4°; 3km/h: 16.79°) increases. And the trends of the curves are increased firstly, then decreased, in the late stage of the gait phases increased again.

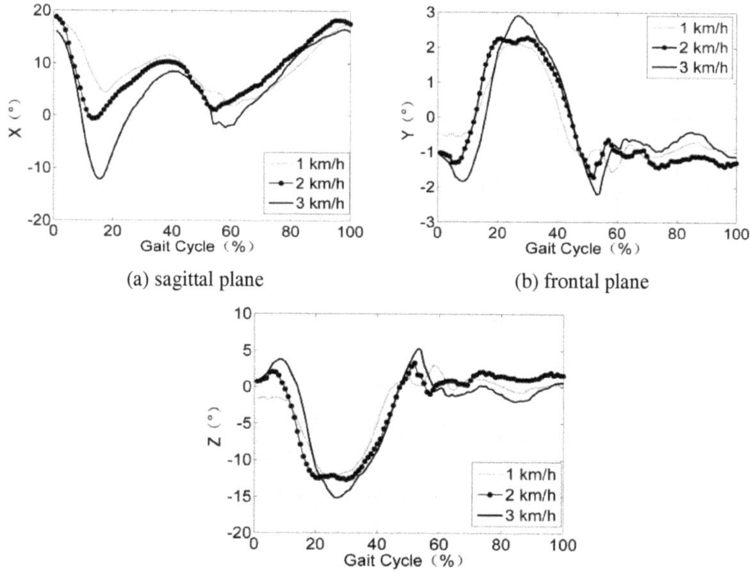

(a) sagittal plane

(b) frontal plane

(c) transversal plane

Fig. 6 Curves of ankle angles in the sagittal plane, frontal plane and transversal plane.

The variation of average ankle joint angle for one gait cycle is presented in Fig. 6(a-c). According to Fig. 6(a), there are two valleys and one peak in one gait cycle. The two valleys value of ankle curves increased with velocity increasing. On the contrary, the peak value of ankle curves is decreased with velocity increasing. The peak value (see Fig. 6(b)) and valley value (see Fig. 6(c)) that occurs around swing phases of ankle curves. The variation range of ankle joint curves in Fig. 6(b) (1km/h: 3.67°; 2km/h: 3.99°; 3km/h: 5.1°) and Fig. 6(c) (1km/h: 15.17°; 2km/h: 16.03°; 3km/h: 20.99°) are increased with velocity increasing. Coincidentally, the curves of ankle joint in the frontal plane and transversal plane have opposite variation. This phenomenon is characteristics of lower limbs motion and the variation correspond with previous work [10].

Angular phase diagrams are used to show the relationship and tendencies of angles in the sagittal plane, frontal plane and transversal plane with the same time variable. It is very convenient to compare the variation of joint angle in different states. Arrows in each figure indicate the direction of joint rotation, and swing phase is the start phase [6, 9].

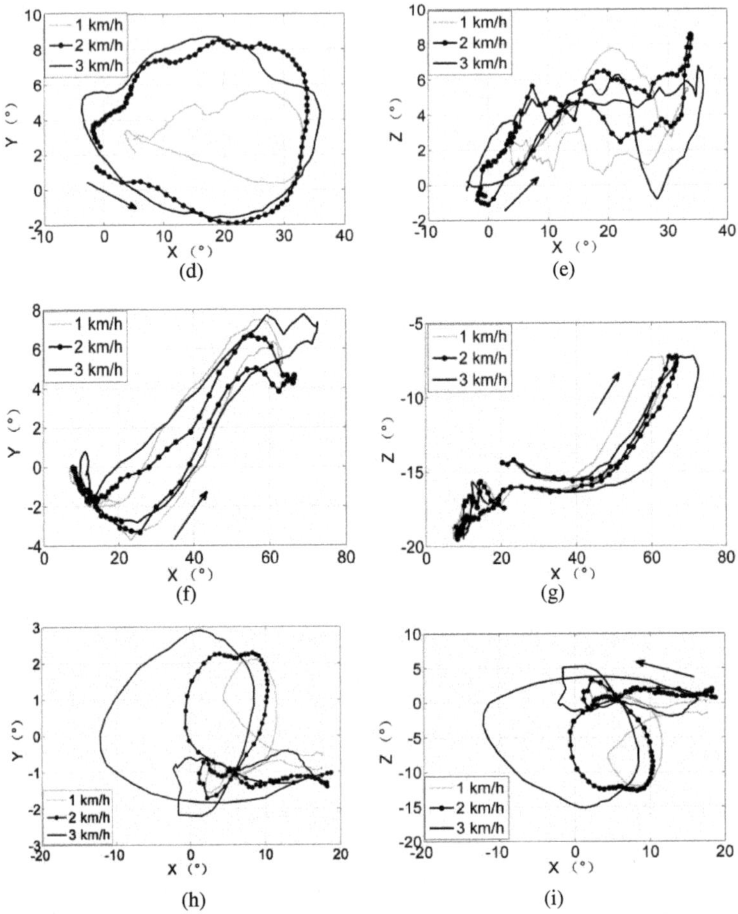

Fig. 7 Diagrams of sagittal plane- frontal plane angles and sagittal plane- transversal plane angles of joints at different speeds: (d-e) Hip (f-g) Knee (h-i) Ankle.

The hip, knee and ankle kinematics and the relationship of joint angles of lower limbs in the sagittal plane, frontal plane and transversal plane are shown in Fig. 7 (d-i). With velocity increasing, the shapes of angular phase diagrams at different speed almost keep unchanged, which indicates that the modes of joint movement keep invariant with speeds increasing. And the closed area in three joints, changing extent of joint angles, gradually increase with speeds increasing.

while the closed area of knee joint (see Fig. 7(f-g)) almost remain the same at different velocity, which shows that knee movement is stabilized. In Fig. 7 (h-i), closed loops appear in one gait phase, which indicates the complexity of ankle movement.

Table 2 The angular value of pelvis motion at different speeds.

	pelvic obliquity		pelvic tilt		rotation movement	
	Max(°)	Min(°)	Max(°)	Min(°)	Max(°)	Min(°)
1km/h	6.02	4.84	3.60	-0.92	2.28	-4.69
2km/h	5.52	4.15	3.60	-1.42	0.38	-2.65
3km/h	5.92	4.12	3.49	-1.25	0.48	-2.9

Table 3 The angular value of hip, knee and ankle at different speeds.

		Hip		Knee		Ankle	
		Max(°)	Min(°)	Max(°)	Min(°)	Max(°)	Min(°)
Sagittal plane	1km/h	33.36	3.41	63.47	6.98	17.74	1.91
	2km/h	33.89	-1.81	66.57	7.90	18.74	-0.63
	3km/h	36.06	-3.68	72.64	9.75	16.51	-12.16
Frontal plane	1km/h	5.60	0.35	7.47	-3.73	2.11	-1.56
	2km/h	8.54	-1.90	6.67	-3.33	2.28	-1.71
	3km/h	8.72	-1.62	7.76	-3.03	2.90	-2.20
Transversal plane	1km/h	7.77	0.58	-7.26	-19.50	3.08	-12.09
	2km/h	8.54	-1.11	-5.71	-21.11	3.34	-12.69
	3km/h	6.76	-0.82	-3.47	-20.26	5.30	-15.69

4. Conclusions

This paper presents some kinematic particulars about pelvic movement, hip, knee and ankle joint in the sagittal plane, frontal plane and transversal plane at different treadmill velocity, which provides kinematic data for designing and controlling lower extremity rehabilitation robot.

For hip, knee and ankle joint, increasing of the treadmill velocity increases the maximum angle of the flexion and variation range of joint in the sagittal plane. Increasing velocity has little impact on the shapes of the curves except curves of hip joint in the transversal plane.

For pelvic movement, there are a little change on amplitude and shape of curves with velocity increasing, which exhibits the stability of rotation movement with treadmill velocity increasing.

The joint angle and variation range of ankle joint in the frontal plane and transversal plane increases with velocity increasing while the same regular variations of knee joint appear only in the transversal plane and only in the frontal plane the changes of angles arise for hip joint, which indicates increasing velocity has greater effects on ankle joint activities than hip joint and knee joint.

With velocity increasing, the modes of joint movement kept invariant and the changing extent of knee joint angles remind not much changed, which explains knee movement is stabilized and knee joint can act as a cushion in support phases.

The results of this paper are presents above; some revelations have come to us. The reference trajectories are selected by consideration of influence of treadmill velocity. For patents, adaptable reference trajectory should be applied by a strict regulation because there are different in kinematic data of lower limbs with different velocity. Treadmill velocity should correspond to reference trajectory extract by same velocity.

References

1. J. von Zitzewitz, M. Bernhardt and R. Riener, A Novel Method for Automatic Treadmill Speed Adaptation, *IEEE Transactions on Neural Systems and Rehabilitation Engineering*. **15**, 401 (2007).
2. S. Jezernik, G. Colombo and M. Morari, Automatic Gait-Pattern Adaptation Algorithms for Rehabilitation with a 4-DOF Robotic Orthosis, *IEEE* Transactions on Robotics and Automation. **20**, 574 (2004).
3. Colombo G, Joerq M, Schreier R, et al. Treadmill training of paraplegic patients with a robotic orthosis. *J Rehabil Res Dev*. 37, 693 (2000).
4. D. I. Stoia, M. Toth-Tascau, Influence of treadmill velocity on joint angles of lower limbs during human gait, in *Proc. E-Health and Bioengineering Conference (EHB),* (Iasi, Romania, 2011).
5. Weijun Tian, Qian Cong, Zhen Yan, Yi Ma and Yurong Liu, Spatio-temporal Characteristics of Human Gaits based on Joint Angle Analysis, in 3rd *Proc. Conference on Computer Science and Information Technology* (ICCSIT), (Cheng Du, China, 2010).
6. Kang, H G, Dingwell, J B, Separating the effects of age and walking speed on gait variability, *Gait Posture*, **27**, 572 (2008).
7. Yali Han, Xingsong Wang, The biomechanical study of lower limb during human walking. *Sci China Tech Sci*. **41**, 592 (2011).
8. I. Carpinella, P. Crenna, M. Rabuffetti and M. Ferrarin, Coordination between upper-and lower-limb movements is different during overground and treadmill walking, *Eur Journal Appl Physio*. **108**, 71(2008).
9. K. D'Août, P. Aerts, D. De Clercq, K. De Meester and L. V. Elsacker, segment and joint Angles of Hind Limb During Bipedal and Quadrupedal

walking of the Bonobo (PanPaniscus), *Am J phys Anthropol.* **119**, 37 (2002).

10. S. M. Kidder, Jr. F. S. Abuzzahab, G. F. Harris and J. E. Johnson. A system for the analysis of foot and ankle kinematics during gait, *IEEE Transactions on Rehabilitation Engineering*. **4**, 25 (1996).

On Global Stability Analysis for SEIR Models in Epidemiology with Nonlinear Incidence Rate Function*

Xiuxiang Yang
College of Mathematics, Weinan Normal University,
Weinan, Shaan'xi 714000, P.R.China
E-mail: yangxiuxiang2000@aliyun.com

Lifei Zheng†
Department of Applied Mathematics, Northwest A&F University,
Yangling, Shaan'xi 712100, P.R.China
E-mail: zhenglifei@nwsuaf.edu.cn

We study an SEIRS epidemic model with an isolation and nonlinear incidence rate function. We have obtained a threshold value R_0 and shown that there is only a disease free equilibrium point when $R_0 < 1$ and an endemic equilibrium point if $R_0 > 1$. We have shown that both disease free- and endemic equilibrium point are globally stable.

Keywords: Nonlinear infectious rate; threshold; equilibrium point; global stability.

1. Introduction

The global stability of SEIR models with nonlinear incidence rate has been conjectured [1] and has been stated as an outstanding open question for the classical bilinear models [2-6]. By applying the Poincare-Bendixson property of dynamical system in space, authors [3-8] have proven the conjecture for the bilinear model with enough long average immunity period, and all authors have shown the case with enough long average infection period [9-10].

In this paper, we solve the open problem for the bilinear case completely and relax the constraint on general nonlinear transmission function for the global stability. As usual, we let *S(t), E(t), I(t)* and *R(t)* be the fraction of susceptible, exposed, infected and recovered at time t, respectively. Moreover, we assume

---

* Supported by Weinan Normal University (No. 13YKF003), National Higher-education Institution General Research and Development Project (No. 2014YB023) and the National Natural Science Foundation of China (No. 11461024).

† Corresponding author.

that all new-born individuals are susceptible, no death due to disease and having constant birth rate ν as well as constant natural death rate d, thus the total population is constant, $S + E + I + R = 1$.

The corresponding system of differential equations of the model is:

$$\begin{cases} S'(t) = \nu - \beta S g(I) - dS + \delta R \\ E'(t) = \beta S g(I) - (d+\varepsilon)E \\ I'(t) = \varepsilon E - (\gamma + d)I \\ R'(t) = \gamma I - (\delta + d)R \end{cases} \tag{1.1}$$

Where the nonlinear transmission rate $g(I)$ is C^1 on (0, 1] and $g(0)=0$, $g(I)>0,\ I\in(0,1]$. The parameter $\varepsilon>0$ is the constant rate of exposed becoming infectious, $\gamma>0$ is the rate of infectious becoming recovered, $\delta>0$ is the rate of recovered lost the immunity. Physically, $\frac{1}{\varepsilon}$ is understood as the average of the latent period, $\frac{1}{\gamma}$ as the average of infectious period, $\frac{1}{\delta}$ as the average of loss of immunity. In [2], the author have considered the SEIR model with general transmission rate where the constraint $|Ig'(I)|\le|Ig(I)|$ first appeared, and also used assumption (H) If $c = \lim_{t\to 0^+}\frac{g(I)}{I} < \infty$, $g(I)\ge cI$ for sufficiently small $I>0$.

2. Steady States and Local Stability

There is always a disease free equilibrium $P_0(1,0,0,0)$. To find an endemic equilibrium point $P_*(S_*,E_*,I_*,R_*)$, where $I_*\ne 0$, Denote

$$k_1 = \frac{(\varepsilon+d)(\gamma+d)(\delta+d)-\delta\gamma\varepsilon}{\varepsilon d(\delta+d)}(>1),\ k_2 = \frac{(\varepsilon+d)(\gamma+d)}{\varepsilon\beta},\ k_3 = \frac{\gamma+d}{\varepsilon},$$

$$k_4 = \frac{\gamma}{\delta+d},\ R_0 = \frac{\varepsilon\beta g'(0)}{(\varepsilon+d)(\gamma+d)},$$

By the mean value theorem for continuous functions, there is always an endemic equilibrium $P_*(S_*,E_*,I_*,R_*)$, $I_* < \frac{1}{k_1}$, whenever $R_0>1$, and following relations hold

$$E_* = k_3 I_*, R_* = k_4 I_*, S_* = 1 - k_1 I_*, \beta S_* g(I_*) = k_2 I_* \tag{2.1}$$

(H1) $I\,|\,g'(I)|\le(1+\tau)g(I), \tau = \dfrac{d}{d+\min\{\gamma,\varepsilon\}}$;

(H2) $k_1 + k_2(\frac{I}{g(I)})' \geq 0, 0 < I < 1$.

We begin with some qualitative properties of the solutions. Since we have assumed that the population is of constant size, we can also easily verify that the simplex $\Gamma = \{(S,E,I,R); 0 \leq S,E,I,R, S+E+I+R=1\}$ is positively invariant. Furthermore, we have

Theorem 1 *Suppose that* $R_0 > 1$, *then the endemic equilibrium* $P_*(S_*,E_*,I_*,R_*)$ *of (1.1) is locally asymptotically stable and the disease free steady state* $P_0(1,0,0,0)$ *is unstable: for any initial value* $(S_0,E_0,I_0,R_0), E_0 + I_0 > 0$ *the associated solution will leave* P_0. *If* $R_0 \leq 1$ *and moreover suppose that* $Ig'(I) \leq g(I), 0 < I < 1$ *holds, then there is no endemic equilibrium and the disease dies out.*

According to Hurwitz criteria, the $P_*(S_*,E_*,I_*,R_*)$ is proved locally asymptotically stable (prove a brief).

3. Global Stability Principle

In this section, we make a very brief review of geometrical global stability principle [2-6]. Consider the system of differential equations

$$x' = f(x), x(0) = x_0 \in D \subset R^n \tag{3.1}$$

where D is an open, simply connected domain is locally Lipschitz in D and is the only equilibrium of (3.1). The unique solution to the initial value problem of (3.1) will be denoted by $x(t,x_0)$. We have the global stability principle

Theorem 2 *Let* $\tau_1 = \frac{d}{d+\varepsilon}$, *suppose that* $(H1)$ *and* $(H2)$ *holds, then the unique endemic equilibrium* $P_*(S_*,E_*,I_*,R_*)$ *of (1.1) is globally asymptotically stable.*

Proof Using the Jacobian of (1.1), We can get the third additive compound matrix of J_3 (see appendix) and the associated linear system $z'(t) = [dI + J_3]z(t)$ of (1.1) at any periodic orbit is

$$\begin{cases} X'(t) = -(2d+\gamma+\varepsilon+\beta g)X + \delta W \\ Y'(t) = \gamma X - (2d+\delta+\varepsilon+\beta)Y + \beta S g'[Z+W] \\ Z'(t) = \varepsilon Y - (2d+\delta+\gamma+\beta g)Z \\ W'(t) = \beta g Z - (2d+\delta+\gamma+\varepsilon)W \end{cases} \tag{3.2}$$

To show the equi-uniformly asymptotical stability of (3.2), we consider similarly as in [3] the Lyapunov function $V = \max\{V_1, V_2\}$, where

$$V_1 = |X| + |Y| + \frac{\delta}{\varepsilon}(|Z| + |W|), V_2 = \frac{E}{I}(|Z| + |W|) .$$

We see that there are constants C_1, C_2 independent of any solution (*S,E,I,R*) such that

$$C_1(|X| + |Y| + |Z| + |W|) \le V(X,Y,Z,W) \le C_2(|X| + |Y| + |Z| + |W|) .$$

In order to estimate the Dini derivative of *V*, we start with

$$\begin{cases} D_+X \le -(2d+\gamma+\varepsilon+\beta g)|X| + \delta|W| \\ D_+Y \le \gamma|X| - (2d+\delta+\varepsilon+\beta)|Y| + \beta Sg'(|Z|+|W|) \\ D_+Z \le \varepsilon|Y| - (2d+\delta+\gamma+\beta g)|Z| \\ D_+W \le \beta g|Z| - (2d+\delta+\gamma+\varepsilon)|W| \end{cases} \tag{3.3}$$

And thus

$$\begin{cases} D_+(|X|+|Y|) \le -(2d+\varepsilon+\beta g)(|X|+|Y|) - \\ \delta|Y| + \delta|W| + \beta S|g'|(|Z|+|W|) \\ D_+(|Z|+|W|) \le -(2d+\gamma+\delta)(|Z|+|W|) + \varepsilon(|Y|-|W|) \end{cases}$$

If $I|g'(I)| \le (1+\tau_1)g(I), \varepsilon < \gamma$, then we deduce this form

$$\begin{cases} D_+(|X|+|Y|) \le -(2d+\varepsilon+\beta g)(|X|+|Y|) \\ -\delta|Y| + \delta|W| + (1+\tau_1)\beta Sg'(|Z|+|W|) \\ D_+(|Z|+|W|) \le -(2d+\gamma+\delta)(|Z|+|W|) + \varepsilon(|Y|-|W|) \end{cases} \tag{3.4}$$

By the persistence conclusions in [2], we may choose small $\eta > 0$ such that $\beta g,\ \delta > \eta$, and derive from (3.4)

$$D_+V_1 \le -(2d+\varepsilon+\eta)V_1 + \frac{(1+\tau_1)\beta SgV_2}{E} \tag{3.5}$$

$$D_+V_2 \le (\frac{E'}{E} - \frac{I'}{I})V_2 - (2d+\varepsilon+\eta)V_1 + \frac{(1+\tau_1)\beta SgV_2}{E} \tag{3.6}$$

Using the relationships $\frac{(1+\tau_1)\beta Sg_2}{E} = \frac{(1+\tau_1)E'}{E} + 2d + \varepsilon, -\frac{I'}{I} + \frac{\varepsilon E}{I} = d + \varepsilon$ we deduce where after from (3.5) in the case

$$\begin{cases} V = V_1 \ge V_2 \\ D_+V = D_+V_1 \le -(2d+\varepsilon+\eta)V_1 + \frac{(1+\tau_1)\beta SgV_2}{E} = (\frac{(1+\tau_1)E'}{E} - \eta)V_1 := h(t)V \end{cases}$$

In similar way, if $V = V_2 \ge V_1$, using the idea of rewriting.

$$\frac{E'}{E}=\frac{(1+\tau_1)E'}{E}+d-\frac{\tau_1\beta Sg}{E}<\frac{(1+\tau_1)E'}{E}+d\ ,$$

we obtain

$$D_+V=D_+V_2\le(\frac{E'}{E}-\frac{I'}{I}-2d-\varepsilon-\eta+\frac{\varepsilon E}{I})V_2\le(\frac{(1+\tau_1)E'}{E}-\eta)V_2=h(t)V,\quad (3.7)$$

Finally, estimates (3.6) and (3.7) lead to $D_+V_2\le h(t)V$. Because for any

$$0\le s\le t,\int_s^t h(x)dx=(1+\tau_1)\ln(\frac{E(t)}{E(s)})-\eta(t-s)\,,$$

then it follows from $D_+V_2\le h(t)V$ and persistence conclusion in [2], that $c\le E(s)$ and whence for large t,s,

$$V(t)\le V(s)(\frac{E(t)}{E(s)})^{(1+\tau_1)e^{-\eta(t-s)}}\le V(s)Me^{-\eta(t-s)},M=\frac{1}{c^{(1+q)}}\,,$$

thus the system (3.2) is equi-uniformly asymptotically stable, and the proof is complete. According to stability theory of [2], then the unique endemic equilibrium of (1.1) is globally asymptotically stable.

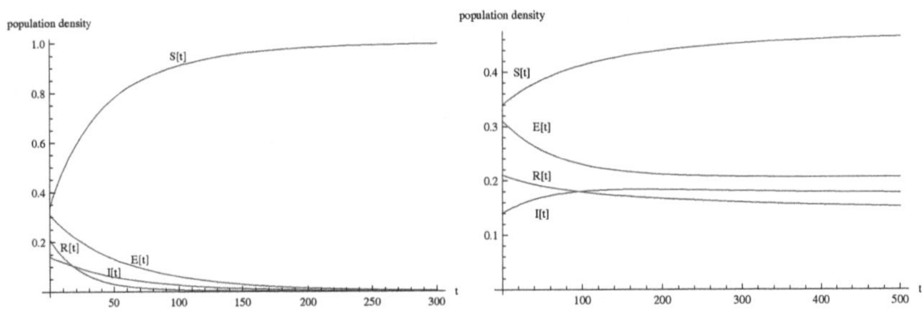

a. b.

Fig. 1(a). Numerical simulation with parameters $\beta=0.02;\nu=0.02;\delta=0.024;$ $\varepsilon=0.003;\gamma=0.004;S(0)=0.34;E(0)=0.31;I(0)=0.14;R(0)=0.21$
b. Numerical simulation with parameters $\beta=0.02;\nu=0.002;\delta=0.004;$ $\varepsilon=0.006;\gamma=0.005;S(0)=0.34;E(0)=0.31;I(0)=0.14;R(0)=0.21$

4. Example

In this section, we gave an example for above results. Some values of all parameters were given and showed that the disease free steady state and the endemic equilibrium are global asymptotically stable respectively. Let $g(t)=\frac{t}{1+0.004t}$, and according to Theorem 1, we can give parameter value satisfying, $Ig'(I)\le g(I), 0<I<1$ and $R_0 \le 1$, then P_0 is Global asymptotically stable, which shows in Figure 1(a).

By theorem 2, we can give parameters' value satisfying (*H1*)-(*H2*) and $R_0 > 1$, then the equilibrium point P_* is Global asymptotically stable, which shows in Figure 1(b).

5. Conclusion and Discussion

In this paper we have presented an SEIRs epidemic mathematical model with an isolation and nonlinear incidence rate function. We determined the system's equilibria and performed the stability analysis of them. The analytical and unmerical investigations show when the function $g(I)$ satisfied the conditions (*H1*) and (*H2*), the unique endemic equilibria is globally asymptotically stable. So we solved the open problem for the bilinear case completely and relax the constraint on general nonlinear transmission function for the global stability.

Of course there still have some problems to solve. For example, when the function *g*(*I*) does not satisfy the conditions (*H1*) and (*H2*), we need to know how to solve the open problem for the bilinear general nonlinear transmission function for the global stability. These problems will be further work in the future time.

References

1. W. M. Liu, H. W. Hethcote and S. A. Levin, Dynamical behavior of epidemiological models with nonlinear incidence rates. J. Math. Biol. 25 (1987), 359-380.
2. M. Y. Li, J. S. Muldowney and P. Van den Dreissche, Global stability of the SEIRS model in epidemiology, Canadian Appl. Math. Quarterly, 7 (1999), 409-425.
3. M. Y. Li, J. S. Muldowney, Geometric approach to global stability problems, SIAM J. Math. Annal. 27 (1996), 1070-1083.
4. H. W. Hethcote and P. van den Driessche, Some epidemiological models with nonlinear incidence rate. J. Math. Biol. 29 (1991), 271-287.
5. M. Y. Li, J. R. Graef, L. Wang and J. Kasari, Global dynamics of a SEIR model with varying total population size. Math. Biosci. 160 (1999), 191-213.
6. M. W. Hirsch and H. Smith, Monotone dynamical systems. Handbook of

differential equations: ordinary differential equations. Elsevier, Amsterdam, Vol. 2 (2005), 239-357.

7. M. Y. Li, Dulac critieria for a autonomous system having an invariant affine manifold. J. Math. Anal. Appl. 199 (1996), 374-390.

   A. Margheri and C. Rebelo, Some examples of persistence in epidemilogical models. J. Math. Biol. 46 (2003), 564-570.

8. M. Y. Li, J. S. Muldowney, Dynamics of differential equations on invariant manifolds, J. Diff. Equa. 168 (2000), 295-320.

9. D. Xiao and S. Ruan, Global analysis of an epidemic model with nonmonotone incidence rate. Math. Biosci. 208 (2007), 419-429.

10. Yang Xiu-xiang, Cheng Yuan-ji, Xue Chun-rong, Global stability analysis of isolation epidemic model with nonlinear incidence rate. J. of Biomathematics 27(4) (2012), pp. 1-12.

A Simple Pre-Culture Treatment Significantly Enhances the Colchicine Induced Chromosome Doubling Effects in Purple Coneflower (*Echinacea purpurea* L.)

Rong Chen

The Key Laboratory of High Quality Crops Cultivation and Safety Control, Honghe University, Mengzi, Yunnan 661100, China
E-mail: chentianyigl@126.com

Weizhen Jiang, Xinglian Li, Xiaolu Chen, QingLing Li, Yuesheng Yang* and HongWu

Guangdong Technology Research Centre for Traditional Chinese Veterinary Medicine and Natural Medicine, South China Agricultural University, Guangzhou 510642, China
**E-mail: ysyang@scau.edu.cn*

A haploid clone recovered from anther cultures and 10 diploid clones prepared from seedlings of purple coneflower (*Echinacea purpurea* L.) were used to compare chromosome doubling colchicine treatments. It was found that, although routine methods of culturing explants directly on colchicine containing medium could induce chromosome doubling, the efficiencies were generally low. However, by first culturing explants on a colchicine-free medium, followed by culturing the explants on a colchicine medium, the number of chromosome doubled plantlets could be significantly increased. Two pre-culture treatments lasting two and four days, and two treatments cultured in 240 mg colchicine l^{-1} for four and eight days, were tested for haploid cells with similar results that a step of pre-culture was conducive to the obtaining of regenerated tetraploid plants. Experiments on diploid clones comparing the durations of pre-culture and the duration of 120 mg colchicine l^{-1} treatments indicated that pre-culture for four days was more effective than eight days, and treating with colchicine for 12 days was more effective than 24 days. In addition, the mechanism of pre-culture for enhancing the chromosome doubling efficiency is discussed and a potential application of the present method for more plant species is proposed.

Keywords: Chromosome doubling; colchicine; haploid; *in vitro* culture; purple coneflower; tetraploid.

1. Introduction

Purple coneflower (*Echinacea purpurea* L.), known for its medicinal properties, [1, 2] has been cultivated in many countries outside of its natural range in North America. [3, 4] Natural purple coneflower plants are diploid with 22 chromosomes in a somatic cell (2n=2×=22), [5] but haploid and tetraploid karyotype plants have already been created. [6, 7] Polyploidization has been shown to be an efficient strategy in crop breeding, [8-11] and recent investigations confirmed that tetraploid purple coneflower plants have higher production and accumulation of functional secondary metabolites than diploid plants, [12, 13] suggesting a higher cultivation value for tetraploid plants. However, the doubling of haploid individuals results in homogenous diploid and tetraploid individuals, which are fundamentally different from diploid and tetraploid plants developed from natural plants with heterogeneous chromosomes that result from entomophilous pollination. [5]

Offspring produced by crossing between homogeneous parents are heterotic, and crosses between homogeneous diploid and tetraploid individuals may result in triploid seeds, which benefit from being both heterotic and polyploid. It has also been observed that variation in performance among plants that grow from seeds in the field [14] and explants taken from different seedlings *in vitro* [15] was large. This suggests inducing more genotype tetraploids from diploids for selection might be a practical way for breeding more advantageous varieties. In the present paper, a simple and effective *in vitro* method for obtaining homogeneous and heterogeneous tetraploid plants through the adoption of a pre-culture step before colchicine treatment is described.

2. Materials and Methods

2.1. *Preparation of plant materials*

Haploid plants were obtained from anther cultures, [6] and a haploid clone was procured by inducing axillary bud proliferation [14] from one haploid plantlet. Diploid plantlets of 10 genotypes were grown from seeds *in vitro* by conventional disinfection and aseptic culture methods, and then ten clones of the same diploid genotypes were established by the same method used for the haploid clones. [14] A half–strength, hormone-free Murashige and Skoog (MS) medium was used for the culture of these plantlets. Explants were prepared by isolating and cutting the petioles of the plantlets into approximately 5 mm segments.

2.2. *Induction of chromosome doubling and the regeneration of adventitious buds*

The explants were cultured on medium containing 120 and 240 mg colchicine l^{-1} for two, four and eight days for the induction of chromosome doubling by the method described before. [7] After treatment with colchicine, the explants were transferred to a medium containing 0.4 mg benzyladenine (BA) l^{-1} and 0.01 mg naphthalene acetic acid (NAA) l^{-1} for induction of the regeneration of adventitious buds.

2.3. *Growing the regenerated buds and the identification of the ploidy levels*

Buds regenerated from the colchicine treated explants were isolated and cultured on a half–strength MS medium with 0.05 mg NAAl^{-1} to initiate root growth and become intact plantlets. Root tips were cut from the plantlets and root tip cells were observed under a microscope (Leica DLMB2) in order to assess the chromosome numbers following a serial preparation by the method reported in Zhao et al. (2006). [6]

2.4. *Preparation of medium*

To prepare the medium, approximately 200 ml glass bottles were filled with about 40 ml of medium. The medium contained MS basal elements (macro-elements were reduced by half), 3% sucrose, and was adjusted with 0.1 N NaOH to a pH value of 5.8. The medium was then gelled using 0.5% agar powder and autoclaved 20 minutes at 121°C. When the colchicine containing medium was prepared, colchicine was added using a 0.22 micrometer pore size (diameter) sterile membrane filter.

2.5. *Maintenance of the cultures*

The cultures were stored at 25-27°C. Cultures used for seed germination were first kept in darkness for ten days, then under a photoperiod of 12-h light (about 50 μ mol $m^{-2}s^{-1}$)/12 h darkness; pre-cultures of the explants were kept under a photoperiod of 12-h light/12 h darkness; cultures for the treatment of colchicine were not exposed to light; cultures for the regeneration of adventitious buds and for rooting of the isolated buds were kept under a photoperiod of 12-h light/12 h darkness.

2.6. *Data record and analysis*

Each treatment consisted of four bottles inoculated with eight explants each. Data for adventitious bud formation were recorded 80 days later through a single subculture to fresh medium of the same composition. Buds of at least one cm in height, without hyperhydricity and at least two visual leaves were considered as valid buds. Data were statistically analyzed using the Student Newman-Keuls means separation test using SAS (SAS Institute, Cary, NC, 1995). Significant differences among means were determined by Duncan's multiple range tests at $P \leq 0.05$.

3. Results

3.1. *Regeneration of adventitious buds and the identification of ploidy levels*

Adventitious buds were regenerated from haploid and diploid explants on medium containing 0.4 mg BA l^{-1} and 0.01 mg NAA l^{-1} (Fig. 1A) after various colchicine treatments. When these buds were isolated from the mother tissues and inoculated to a medium containing 0.05 mg NAA l^{-1}, intact plantlets were obtained and could be classified into three groups based on root morphology (Fig. 1B-D). Although ploidy chimeras were detected, most plantlets in Fig. 1B were identified as haploid, in Fig. 1C as diploid and in Fig. 1D as tetraploid (Fig. 2).

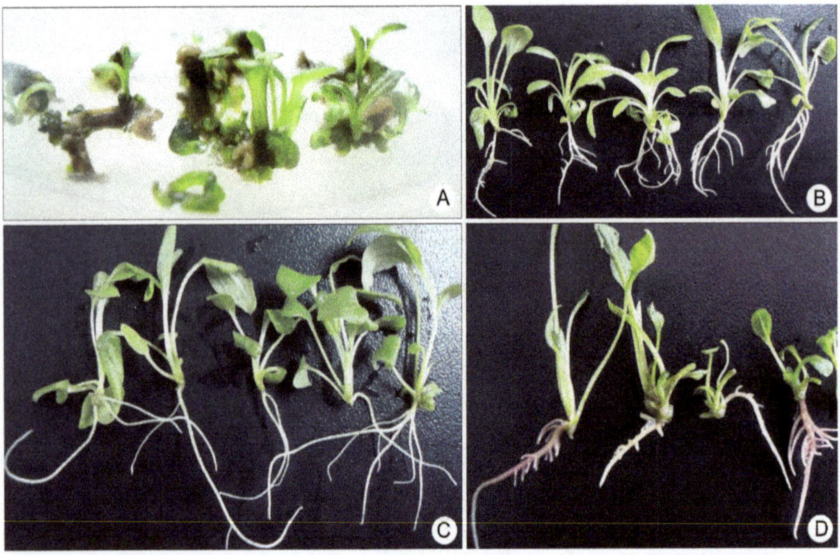

Fig. 1 Regenerated buds and plantlets. (A) Buds regenerated from explants following colchicine treatment. (B) Regenerated plantlets with thin, highly branched roots. (C) Regenerated plantlets with thick roots and minimal branching. (D) Regenerated plantlets with thick, shortly branched roots.

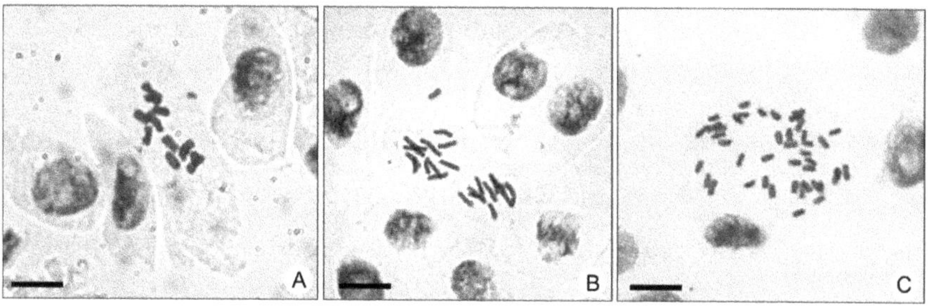

Fig. 2 Chromosomes in root tip cells of the regenerated plantlets. (A) haploid (2n = 1× = 11). (B) diploid (2n = 2×= 22). (C) tetraploid (2n = 4× = 44). Bar =15μm.

3.2. *Treatments of haploid explants with 240 mg colchicine l^{-1}*

3.2.1. *For four days*

Before being treated with 240 mg colchicine l^{-1} for four days, the explants were pre-cultured on medium containing 0.4 mg BA l^{-1} and 0.01 mg NAA l^{-1} for two and four days. The effects of the duration of pre-culture were summarized in Table 1. Pre-culture could largely or even significantly enhance the regeneration of adventitious bud formation with more valid buds being regenerated. Although both the pre-culture treatments could not increase the percentage of the regenerated tetraploid buds, the numbers of tetraploid buds per bottle were increased by 37.5% for two days pre-culture and 75% for four days pre-culture.

Table 1 Influence of pre-culture duration on the effects of 240 mg colchicine l^{-1} treatment for four days in haploid purple coneflower *in vitro* cultures.

Duration of pre-culture (day)	% adventitious bud formation	No. valid bud per bottle	% tetraploid bud	No. tetraploid bud per bottle
0 (control)	37.5 ± 10.2 b	7.5 ± 2.1 c	51.8 ± 8.9 a	4.0 ± 1.6 b
2	53.1 ± 15.7 ab	11.3 ± 2.2 b	48.2 ± 7.9 a	5.5 ± 1.7 ab
4	68.8 ± 16.1 a	15.5 ± 1.7 a	45.2 ± 5.4 a	7.0 ± 1.2 a

*Data in the same column followed by different letters are significantly different by Duncan's test at ≤ 5% level.

3.2.2. *For eight days*

Before being treated with 240 mg colchicine l^{-1} for eight days, the explants were pre-cultured on medium containing 0.4 mg BA l^{-1} and 0.01 mg NAA l^{-1} for two and four days. The effects of the duration of pre-culture were summarized in Table 2. Pre-cultures could largely or even significantly enhance the regeneration of adventitious bud formation based on the duration of the pre-culture. Although both the pre-culture treatments could not increase the percentage of the regenerated tetraploid buds, the numbers of tetraploid buds per bottle were increased significantly.

Table 2 Influence of pre-culture duration on the effects of 240mg colchicine l^{-1} treatment for eight days in haploid purple coneflower *in vitro* cultures.

Duration of pre-culture (day)	% adventitious bud formation	No. valid bud per bottle	% tetraploid bud	No. tetraploid bud per bottle
0 (control)	21.9 ± 12.0 b	2.8 ± 1.5 b	68.8 ± 23.9 a	1.8 ± 1.0 b
2	37.5 ± 10.2 ab	8.0 ± 1.8 a	56.3 ± 10.0 a	4.5 ± 1.3 a
4	46.9 ± 12.0 a	11.8 ± 2.8 a	49.0 ± 7.1 a	5.8 ± 1.5 a

*Data in the same column followed by different letters are significantly different by Duncan's test at ≤5% level.

3.3. *Treatments of diploid explants with 120 mg colchicine l^{-1}*

3.3.1. *For 12 days*

Before being treated with 120 mg colchicine l^{-1} for 12 days, the explants were pre-cultured on medium for four and eight days. The effects of the duration of pre-culture were summarized in Table 3. Our results found that these pre-culture methods can significantly enhance the regeneration of adventitious buds. Although four days pre-culture treatment was not as effective as eight days for the percentage of adventitious bud formation and number of valid buds per bottle, a greater number of tetraploid buds per bottle and tetraploid genotypes were obtained in the four day pre-culture treatment.

Table 3 Influence of pre-culture duration on the effects of 120 mg colchicine l^{-1} treatment for 12 days in diploid purple coneflower *in vitro* cultures.

Duration of pre-culture (day)	% adventitious bud formation	No. valid bud per bottle	No. tetraploid bud per bottle	No. genotypes obtaining 4 X plantlets
0 (control)	55.9 ± 1.6 c	28.6 ± 6.4 c	0.0 c	0
4	73.1 ± 1.5 b	40.4 ± 3.6 b	6.0 ± 1.4 a	5
8	86.1 ± 3.8 a	62.3 ± 6.3 a	0.6 ± 0.2 b	1

*Data in the same column followed by different letters are significantly different by Duncan's test at ≤5% level.

3.3.2. *For 24 days*

Before being treated with 120 mg/l colchicine for 24 days, the explants were pre-cultured on medium for four and eight days. The effects of the duration of pre-culture were summarized in Table 4. Pre-culture could significantly enhance the regeneration of adventitious bud formation and increase the number of valid buds per bottle significantly. In comparison with the pre-culture treatment for eight days, the pre-culturc treatment for four days was more effective for obtaining more tetraploid buds and tetraploid plantlets of more genotypes.

Table 4 Influence of pre-culture duration on the effects of 120 mg colchicine l^{-1} treatment for 24 days in diploid purple coneflower *in vitro* cultures.

Duration of pre-culture (day)	% adventitious bud formation	No. valid bud per bottle	No. tetraploid bud per bottle	No. genotypes obtaining 4 X plantlets
0 (control)	20.8 ± 3.3 c	12.4 ± 1.4 c	0.3 ± 0.2 b	1
4	44.3 ± 2.5 b	20.9 ± 2.6 b	2.7 ± 0.6 a	3
8	62.7 ± 4.0 a	34.6 ± 2.2 a	1.8 ± 0.3 a	2

*Data in the same column followed by different letters are significantly different by Duncan's test at ≤5% level.

4. Discussion and Conclusion

Chromosome doubling of diploid purple coneflowers occurred through the direct culture of explants on a colchicine containing medium. [7] However, conventional *in vivo* methods have been used in the induction of chromosome doubling by colchicine in purple coneflower, [12, 16] suggesting low efficiency of *in vitro* treatment used in the experiments reported by Nilanthi et al. [7] On the other hand, pre-cultures are short in duration, generally aiming to modify the physiological status of the explants [17-20] in order to increase plant response in the main culture Results of the present experiments indicated that, by applying a pre-culture step before colchicine treatment, the chromosome doubling efficiency in purple coneflower by means of *in vitro* culture could be greatly improved.

There were three reasons which would account for the results of the present experiments. First, when petiole explants were prepared, the cells were not undergoing mitosis because petioles are made up of differentiated cells. After the explants were cultured, some of the cells began to divide and de-differentiate in response to the composition, mainly the hormones, of the medium. However, before the initiation of cell division, a period is required to physiologically and biochemically prepare the cell to activate this process. Secondly, at certain concentrations, colchicine is toxic to plant cells. [21, 22] It is probable that the cells of freshly prepared explants were more sensitive to the toxicity of the compound because the tissues have not yet recovered from the injury during explant preparation, as well as not yet getting used to the culture conditions.

Finally, the accepted mechanism of chromosome doubling by colchicine is by blocking the formation of spindle fibres, and can therefore only occur when the cells are actively dividing. [22-24] From this, we are able to conclude that the pre-culture period allows the explant cells to initiate division in the absence of the toxic colchicine. Further, pre-cultured cells undergo more effective chromosome doubling in response to colchicine treatmentsbecause cells that were in the course of division following the pre-culture were more susceptible to the influence of colchicine.

Obtaining of tetraploid from haploid explants by one-step colchicine treatment has been previously reported. [25] The results of this study may be explained in two ways. First, the haploid state is not as stable as the diploid state. In a range of anther cultures diploid, [26-28] triploid [29] and mixoploid [30] plants have been obtained without colchicine treatment for the induction of chromosome doubling. Second, the colchicine treatment in the present experiments continued for four to eight days. The prolonged exposure of cells to colchicine may increase the likelihood for the chromosome number to be twice doubled. Our results support that the efficiency could be increased significantly by adopting a pre-culture stage before colchicine treatment.

In conclusion, adopting a pre-culture period before colchicine treatment was a simple and effective method for increasing the *in vitro* chromosome doubling efficiencies in haploid and diploid purple coneflower. This method may possibly be applied to other plant species given that the chromosome doubling mechanism may be the same in all plants.

Acknowledgments

This research was funded by a grant (2011B031700026) of Science and Technology Planning Project from the government of Guangdong Province, China.

References

1. Barnes J, Anderson LA, Gibbons S, Phillipson JD. *Echinacea* species (*Echinacea angustifolia* (DC.) Hell., *Echinacea pallida* (Nutt.) Nutt., *Echinacea purpurea* (L.) Moench): a review of their chemistry, pharmacology and clinical properties. J Pharm Pharmacol. 2005; 57: 929-54.
2. Barrett B. Medicinal properties of *Echinacea*: a critical review. Phytomedicine. 2003; 10: 66–86.
3. Landy N, Ghalamkari GH, Toghyani M, Moattar F. The effects of

Echinacea purpurea L. (purple coneflower) as an antibiotic growth promoter substitution on performance, carcass characteristics and humoral immune response in broiler chickens. J Med Plants Res. 2011; 5: 2332-2338.

4. Hudson JB. Applications of the phytomedicine *Echinacea purpurea* (Purple Coneflower) in infectious diseases. JBiomed Biotech. 2012; doi: 10.1155/2012/769896 PMCID: PMC3205674.
5. Sejdler LK, Dabrowska J. Studies on the biology of flowering and fruiting of purple coneflower (*Echinacea purpurea* Moench). Part 1. Biology of flowering and fruiting. Herba Polonica. 1996; 42: 83-87.
6. Zhao F, Nilanthi D, Yang Y, Wu H. Anther culture and haploid plant regeneration in purple coneflower (*Echinacea purpurea* L.). Plant Cell Tiss Organ Cult. 2006; 86: 55-62.
7. Nilanthi D, Chen X, Zhao F, Yang Y, Wu H. Induction of tetraploids from petiole explants through colchicine treatments in *Echinacea purpurea* L. J Biomed Biotech. 2009; doi:10.1155/2009/343485.
8. Luckett DJ. Colchicine mutagenesis is associated with substantial heritable variation in cotton. Euphytica. 1989; 42: 177–182.
9. Dhawan OP, Lavania UC. Enhancing the productivity of secondary metabolites via induced polyploidy: a review. Euphytica. 1996; 87: 81–89.
10. Majdi M, Karimzadeh G, Malboobi MA, Omidbaigi R, Mirzaghaderi G. Induction of tetraploidy to feverfew (*Tanacetum parthenium* Schulz-Bip.): morphological, physiological, cytological, and phytochemical changes. HortSci. 2010; 45: 16–21.
11. Lavania UC, Srivastava S, Lavania S, Basu S, Misra NK, MukaiY. Autopolyploidy differentially influences body size in plants, but facilitates enhanced accumulation of secondary metabolites, causing increased cytosine methylation. Plant J. 2012; 71: 539–549.
12. Mohammad A, Moieni A, Badi HN. Morphological, physiological, cytological and phytochemical studies in diploid and colchicine-induced tetraploid plants of *Echinacea purpurea* (L.). Acta Physiol. Plant. 2013; 35: 2075-2083.
13. Xu C, Tang T, Chen R, Liang C, Liu X, Wu C, Yang Y, Yang D, Wu H. A comparative study of bioactive secondary metabolite production in diploid and tetraploid *Echinacea purpurea* (L.) Moench. Plant Cell Tiss Organ Cult. 2013; doi: 10.1007/s11240-013-0406-z.
14. Chen R, Chen X, Li Q, Yang Y, Wu H. Micropropagation by repeatedly inducing axillary bud formation of different gene dosage purple coneflower plants. In: Proceedings of the 2012 International Conference

on Biomedical Engineering and Biotechnology; 28-30 May 2012; Macau.

15. Li Q, Chen R, Chen X, Yang Y, Wu H. Estimation of the cloning potential in six selected genotypes of purple coneflower (*Echinacea purpurea* L.). Biotechnol Biotech Eq. 2013; 27: 3911-3917.
16. Koul S, Sambyal M, Kitchlu SK, Bakshi SK, Kaul MK. Development, micropropagation and characterization of colchiploid of *Echinacea purpurea* (L.) Moench. Indian J. Biotech. 2010; 9: 221-224.
17. Sorvari S, Ulvinen S, Hietaranta T, Hiirsalmi H. Preculture medium promotes direct shoot regeneration from micropropagated strawberry leaf disks. HortScience. 1993; 28: 55-57.
18. Ozawa S, Yasutani I, Fukuda H, Komamine A. Sugiyama M. Organogenic responses in tissue culture of *srd* mutants of *Arabidopsis thaliana*. Development. 1998; 125: 135-142.
19. Melo CG, Barbosa MHP. Motoike SY, Sabino MV, Ventrella MC, Peternelli LA, Oliveira MAR. Preculture sugarcane tissue in sucrose-supplemented culture medium to induce desiccation tolerance. Crop Breed Applied Biotech. 2011;11: 320-329.
20. Rai GK, Rai NP, Kumar S, Yadav A, Rathaur S, Singh M. Effects of explant age, germination medium, pre-culture parameters, inoculation medium, pH, washing medium, and selection regime on Agrobacterium-mediated transformation of tomato. In Vitro Cell Dev Biol-Plant. 2012; doi:10. 1007/s11627-012-9442-3.
21. Hansen NJP, Andersen SB. In vitro chromosome doubling potential of colchicine, oryzalin, trifluralin, and APM in *Brassica napus* microspore culture. Euphytica. 1996; 88: 159-164.
22. Ade R, Rai MK. Review: colchicine, current advances and future prospects. Bioscience. 2010; 2: 90-96.
23. Hansen A, Gertz A, Joersbo M, Andersen S. Antimicrotubule herbicides for *in vitro* chromosome doubling in *Beta vulgaris* L. ovule culture. Euphytica.1998;101: 231–237.
24. Morejohn LC, Bureau TE, Tocchi LP, Fosket DE. Resistance of *Rosa* microtubule polymerization to colchicine results from a low affinity interaction of colchicine and tubulin. Planta. 1987; 170: 230–241.
25. Nilanthi D, Chen X, Zhao F, Yang Y, Wu H. One-step in vitro induction of diploids and tetraploids from haploid purple coneflower (*Echinacea purpurea* L.) by colchicine treatment. In: Proceedings of the 6th International Conference on Bioinformatics and Biomedical Engineering (iCBBE 2012); 17-20 May 2012; Shanghai (China).
26. Antoine-Michard S, Beckert M. Spontaneous versus colchicine-induced

chromosome doubling in maize anther culture. Plant Cell Tissue Organ Cult.1997; 48: 203–207.

27. El-Hennawy MA, Abdalla AF, Shafey SA, Al-Ashkar IM. Production of doubled haploid wheat lines (*Triticum aestivum* L.) using anther culture technique. Annals Agri Sci. 2011; 56: 63–72.
28. Olszewska D, Kisiala A, Niklas-Nowak A, Nowaczyk P. Study of in vitro anther culture in selected genotypes of genus *Capsicum.* Turkish J Biology. 2014; 38: 118-124.
29. Geng X, Wei Z, Yao X, Zhao Y. Anther culture of *Medicago sativa* L. and ploidy detection. Acta Agrestia Sinica. 2010; 18: 714-718.
30. Kudirka DT, Schaeffer GP, Aenziger S. Stability of ploidy in meristems of plants regenerated from anther calli of wheat (*Triticum aestivum* L. em. Thell.). Genome. 1989; 32: 1068-1073.

A Simple Loading Model for Stress Analysis of Lumbar Intervertebral Discs in Basic Body Positions*

Han Zhang and Weiping Zhu†
Shanghai Institute of Applied Mathematics and Mechanics, Shanghai University, Shanghai 200072, 149 Yanchang Road, China
†E-mail: wpzhu@shu.edu.cn
www.shu.edu.cn

The load acting on human spine is complex and varying in different positions of a body, and direct measurement to obtain the complete load information is not yet possible. The objective of this study was to use a simple model to deliver the realistic load for the stress analysis of the lumbar intervertebral discs in several basic body positions, including standing, sitting, and lying in a supine, prone and lateral position. The validated finite element model of lumbar spine L1-L5 was adapted. And combined with proper constraints, characterized axial force for each body position was applied to the top end of the model according to the normal standing load and the occupied percentage on the experimental data. The stresses and strains in all lumbar intervertebral discs were calculated and their variation tendency was analyzed. The results show that stress distributions in intervertebral discs were similar between standing and sitting, and stress concentration occurred at the anteroinferior and posterior part of annulus fibrosus (AF). Slightly lower stress was found in sitting than in standing. Stress level in each lumbar intervertebral disc was significantly lower in all lying positions than that in standing and sitting. Stress concentration at the AF posterior part partly disappeared for lying. Only a small difference in stress level existed between various lying positions. Moreover, stress level in nucleus pulposus and at the AF anterior part was relatively low, and stress values in intervertebral discs generally increased from L1-2 to L4-5, while stress peak and strain peak were always located at L4-5 intervertebral disc. These features are consistent with those in previous studies mostly. It suggests that our loading model is efficient, the high strain in L4-5 AF may be a reason for leading to high incidence of disk herniation, and more lying supine should be recommended to whom suffering from back problems as a physiotherapy.

Keywords: Lumbar intervertebral disc; stress analysis; body position.

1. Introduction

Spine as the central pillar of human body is composed of intervertebral disc, vertebrae, ligament, etc. Support, buffering and protection are its main

---

*This work is supported by the National Natural Science Foundation of China (31370940).

functions. Lumbar has a large movement range and is the most loaded part of the spinal column [1]. Nowadays half of the people in the global endure spinal pain indifferent degrees, most of them are lumbar disease.

The load on intervertebral disc is obviously different in various body positions. Many efforts [2,3] have been made to obtain the information about the intradiscal load, but direct measurement of complete loading is not yet possible.

In this paper, a finite element model for lumbar spine L1-L5 was constructed, validated, and employed to analysis and compare the stress and strain of lumbar intervertebral discs in several basic body positions. Based on experimental data, a set of axial forces was characterized by a normal standing load and the occupied percentage in each body position. These axial forces combined with proper boundary conditions were respectively applied to the top end of the model for each body position. The stress and strain in all lumbar intervertebral discs were calculated and shown in detail.

2. Material and Methods

2.1. *Spinal load in basic body positions*

Different postures of a body generate different loads acting on the spine. Here the basic body positions mean the standing, sitting, lying in a supine, prone, and lateral position. Loadings on lumbar spine are composed of weight of the trunk, the muscle strength and others [4].

In an upright body position, the spine is loaded with the upper body weight, and the centre of gravity of upper body is in front of the spine, which leads to a forward bending moment acting on the lumbar, but it can be balanced by the muscle contraction from the dorsal side. Thus, the lumbar spine has to bear a higher axial load (see Fig.1, P) caused by almost entire trunk weight and the muscle balancing strength [5].

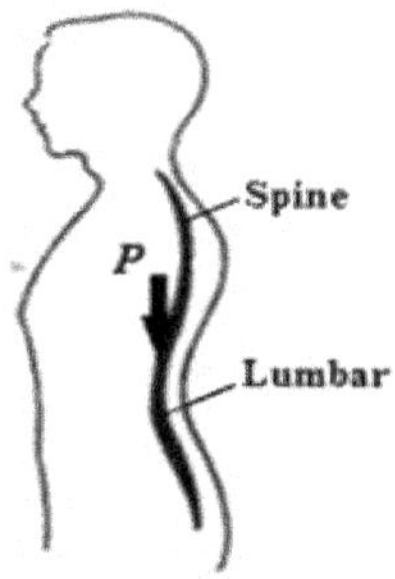

Fig. 1 Resultant loading on lumbar spine (axial load) is the most important load component caused by the weight of the trunk and muscle strength.

As for the lying body positions, the lumbar spine does not have to carry most of the weight of the trunk. So the axial load acting on lumbar spine should be significantly lower in lying than in upright body positions. For quantification, we may define the axial load for each body position according to the following experiments.

Rohlmann et al. [6] equipped internal spinal fixators with load sensors in 10 spinal instability patients through surgery. These measurements indicated that the (flexion) bending moments acting on the implanted fixators in sagittal plane (Mb, sag.) were the most important load component. The bending moments bended the pedicle screws and compressed the longitudinal rods of the fixators [7]. Thus the bending moments in the implants actually reflected the spinal axial compression load [8]. In order to reduce the individual differences, Rohlmann et al. [9] normalized the bending moments in the implants with respect to the bending moment when the same patient was in a standing position, then averaged them over the total number of samples. Let M, M_1, M_2, M_3, and M_4 represent for average bending moments on fixators in standing, sitting, and lying in a supine, prone and lateral position, respectively. The ratios of average bending moments of M_1, M_2, M_3, and M_4 to M will be equal to 0.89, 0.26, 0.32, and 0.34, respectively. These ratios can also be expressed as

$$\frac{M_1}{M} = \frac{P_1 e}{Pe} = \frac{P_1}{P} = 0.89\,,\quad \frac{M_2}{M} = \frac{P_2}{P} = 0.26\,,$$

$$\frac{M_3}{M} = \frac{P_3}{P} = 0.32\,,\ \text{and}\quad \frac{M_4}{M} = \frac{P_4}{P} = 0.34. \tag{1}$$

where e represents the equivalent length between the pedicle screws and longitudinal rods of the fixators, while P, P_1, P_2, P_3, and P_4 represent for average axial loadings on spine in standing, sitting, and lyingin a supine, prone and lateral position, respectively.

2.2. *Finite element modeling*

A three-dimensional finite element model for whole lumbar spine L1-L5 was established by dealing with the CT images in Mimics 10.01 software, Geomagic Studio12.0 and Hypermesh11.0. Totally, there were five vertebrae bodies, four intervertebral discs and six kinds of ligaments, with 64710 nodes and 227644 elements (Fig. 2) in the FEM. Contact at the facet joint was modeled using a zero friction surface-to-surface penalty method. Discs and the adjacent vertebral bodies were connected using tied contacts to ensure the connectivity between the discs and the vertebral bodies. Material properties and element types were assigned to different parts as in references [10-11], given in Table 1.

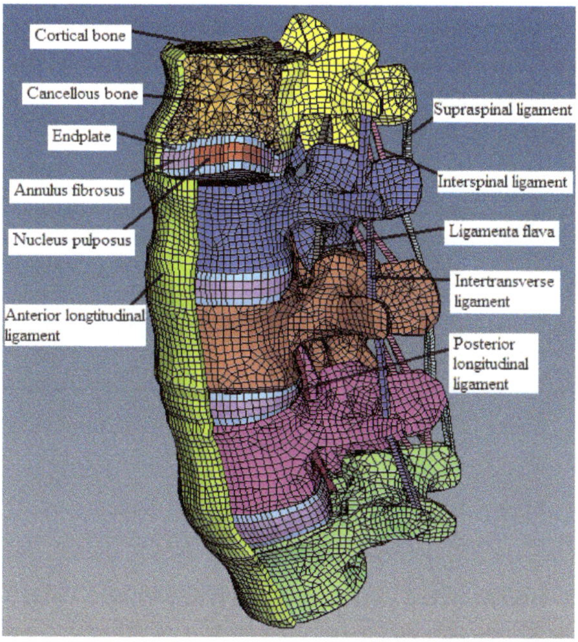

Fig. 2 Finite element model of lumbar spine L1-5.

Table 1 Element type and material properties of the FE model.

Structure	Type of Element	Elasticity Modulus (MPa)	Poisson's Ratio
Cortical bone	Tetrahedral solid elements	12000	0.3
Cancellous bone	Tetrahedral solid elements	100	0.25
Annulus fibrosus	Hexahedral solid elements	4.2	0.45
Nucleus pulposus	Hexahedral solid elements	1	0.4999
Endplate	Hexahedral solid elements	600	0.3
Ligamenta flava	Hexahedral solid elements	5	0.35
Interspinal ligament	Hexahedral solid elements	5	0.35
Supraspinal ligament	Hexahedral solid elements	5	0.3
Anterior longitudinal ligament	Hexahedral solid elements	30	0.3
Posterior longitudinal ligament	Hexahedral solid elements	20	0.3
Intertransverse ligament	Hexahedral solid elements	5	0.3

2.3. *Loadings and boundary conditions*

It has been pointed out in section 2.1 that the axial compressive force is the most important load component acting on lumbar spine in basic body positions.

According to equations (1), we took P=500N as the normal standing load acted on the lumbar spine model [12,13]. When lying down, the displacements of lumbar spine in sagittal plane would be limited by bed. So in the cases of lying body positions, the lateral displacements at the upper surface of L1were constrained in our simulations, while in all cases, the lower surface of L5 were fully fixed. The loading values and boundary conditions are listed in Table 2.

Table 2 Loading and boundary conditions in different positions.

Body position	Standing	Sitting relaxed	Supine lying	Prone lying	Lateral lying
Axial compression force (N)	500	445	130	160	170
Boundary conditions	Six degrees of freedom of the lower surface of L5 were constrained, and lateral displacements at the upper surface of L1 were constrained for lying positions.				

3. Results

3.1. *Stresses of lumbar intervertebral disc in basic body positions*

The stress distributions of intervertebral discs (discs) for standing show that stress concentration occurred at the posterolateral part of annulus fibrosus (AF) in L1-2 disc, posterior part and posterolateral part of AF in L2-3 disc, posterior part of AF in L3-4 disc, anteroinferior part and posterior part of AF in L4-5 disc, respectively. The maximum stress occurred at the anteroinferior part of AF in L4-5 disc, while maximum strain was located at the posterior part of AF in L4-5 disc. The stress in nucleus pulposus and the AF anterosuperior part was relatively low. Maximum stress in each disc from L1-2 to L4-5 was 0.657, 0.580, 0.596, and 1.075MPa, respectively. However, considerable higher stress were found in L4-5 disc than in other discs.

For sitting relaxed, the stress distributions in discs were similar to those in standing state. Our simulations in this study obtained a slightly lower stress for sitting than for standing. The maximum stress in each disc from L1-2 to L4-5 in sitting relaxed was 0.589, 0.520, 0.535, and 0.962MPa, respectively.

When lying in a supine position, the region of high stress are located at the posteroinferior part of AF in L1-2, and L2-3 discs, posterolateral part of AF in L3-4 disc, anteroinferior part, and posterosuperior part of AF in L4-5 disc. The maximum stress occurred at the anteroinferior part of AF in L4-5 disc, while the maximum strain appeared at the posterior part of AF in L4-5 disc. The stress in nucleus pulposus and at the anterior part of AF were relatively low. The stress in L1-2 disc was slightly higher than the stress in L2-3 disc. The maximum stress in each disc from L1-2 to L4-5 first decreased then increased, and the values were 0.131, 0.128, 0.134, and 0.136MPa, respectively.

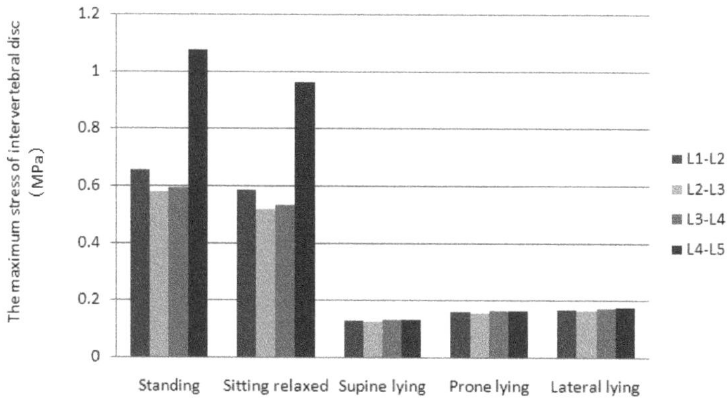

Fig. 3 The maximum stress in intervertebral discs for five different body positions.

No significant differences in stress distributions were found among lying in a supine, prone and lateral position. And stress peak in each disc from L1-2 to L4-5 first decreased then increased, the values for lying prone were 0.161, 0.158, 0.166 and 0.167 MPa, respectively, and for lying lateral were 0.171, 0.168, 0.176 and 0.177 MPa, respectively. However, the stress peak values in all discs were almost same. Fig. 3 shows the maximum stress in each disc for five basic body positions.

Loadings on discs were significantly lower in lying than in upright body positions, but slightly lower in sitting than in standing. Stress concentration located at the anteroinferior part and posterior part of AF partly disappeared in lying. We normalized the maximum stress in each disc with respect to the maximum stress in standing. These relative values are presented in Table 3.

Table 3 Average of relative maximum stress in intervertebral discs for different body positions.

	Standing	Sitting relaxed	Supine lying	Prone lying	Lateral lying
L1-2	1	0.90	0.20	0.25	0.26
L2-3	1	0.90	0.22	0.27	0.29
L3-4	1	0.89	0.23	0.28	0.30
L4-5	1	0.91	0.13	0.16	0.17
Average value	1	0.90	0.20	0.24	0.26

3.2. *Intradiscal pressure in basic body positions*

Wilke et al. (1999) [3] in vivo measured intradiscal pressure in L4-5 disc to several body positions as well as to daily activities. which indicated 0.5MPa for standing, 0.46MPa for sitting relaxed, 0.10MPa for lying spine, 0.11MPa for lying prone and 0.12MPa for lying lateral. These pressures likely represented the hydrostatic pressure in nucleus pulposus.

In our simulations, the average hydrostatic pressures in nucleus pulposus of L4-5 were 0.6MPa for standing, 0.54MPa for sitting relaxed, 0.14MPa for lying spine, 0.17MPa for lying prone, and 0.18MPa for lying lateral. The normalized value of the average hydrostatic pressure in L4-5 nucleus pulposus for sitting, and each lying with respect to standing are given in Table 4. It can be seen that the relative hydrostatic pressures in L4-5 nucleus pulposus in our simulations were consistent with those in vivo experiments [3].

Table 4 Relative hydrostatic pressure in L4-5 nucleus pulposus for each body position.

	Standing	Sitting relaxed	Supine lying	Prone lying	Lateral lying
Wilke [3]	1	0.92	0.20	0.22	0.24
This paper	1	0.90	0.23	0.28	0.30

4. Discussion

The loads acing on spine is very complex and remains unclear, and more investigations are needed. In this study, we introduce a simple loading model for stress analysis of lumbar intervertebral disc in basic body positions

Theoretical analysis shows that the axial compressive force is the most important load component acting on lumbar spine in basic body positions. According to normalized experimental results, we obtained the relative values of axial compressive force for basic body positions with respect to standing. Therefore, we can simulate different basic body postures by applying different loading on lumbar spine.

No matter what kind of body positions there were some common findings, the stress in nucleus pulposus and at anterior part of AF were relatively low. The stress in each disc generally increased from L1-2 to L4-5, while stress and strain in L4-5 disc was always the highest. The high stress and strain in L4-5 disc may be a factor leading to high incidence of lumbar disc herniation [14].

No distinct differences in stress information were found for lying in a supine, prone and lateral positions. However, load for lying in a supine were the lowest in various lying positions. Minor differences in various lying positions were probably resulting from different individual curvature of spine. Incorrect sleeping postures may not only cause viscera and nerve compression, but also have a passive effect on breathing. Thus, lying supine were recommended to those who suffering from low back problem as the basis of physiotherapy.

References

1. Dai, Some basic issues of human lumbar spine biomechanics, *Advances in Mechanics*, 20 (1980), pp. 352-366.
2. A. Nachemson, The load on lumbar disks in different positions of the body, *Clinical Orthopaedics and Related Research*, 45 (1966), pp. 107-122.
3. H.J. Wilke, P. Neef, M. Caimi, T. Hoogland and L.E.Claes, New in vivo measurements of pressures in the intervertebral disc in daily life, *Spine*, 24 (1999), pp. 755-762.
4. V.H. Frankel, M. Nordin, Basic Biomechanics of the Skeletal System. *Lea & Febiger*, Philadelphia (1980).
5. D.K. Damkot et al., *Spine*, 9 (1984), pp. 395.
6. A. Rohlmann, G. Bergmann and F. Graichen, Loads on internal spinal fixators measured in different body positions, *European Spine Journal*, 8 (1999), pp. 354-359.
7. A. Rohlmann, G. Bergmann, et al. Influence of load carrying on loads ininternal spinal fixators, *Journal of Biomechanics*, 33 (2000), pp. 1099-1104.
8. A. Rohlmann, G. Bergmann and F. Graichen and U. Weber, Monitoring *in vivo* implant loads with a telemeterized internal spinal fixation device, *Spine*, 25 (2000), pp. 2981-2986.
9. A. Rohlmann, L.E. Claes, G. Bergmann, F. Graichen, P. Neef, H.J. Wilke, Comparison of intradiscal pressures and spinal fixator loads for different body positions and exercises, *Ergonomics*, 44, 8 (2001), pp.781-794.
10. M. Kurutz, L. Oroszvary, Finite element analysis of weight bath hydrotr action treatment of degenerated lumbar spine segments in elastic phase, *J Biomech*, 43, 3 (2010), pp. 433-441.
11. M. Kasra, A. Shirazi-Adl, Dynamics of human lumbar intervertebral joints: Experimental and finite-element investigations, *Spine*, 17 (1992), pp. 93-102.
12. A.L. Nachemson. Disc pressure measurements. *Spine* (Phila Pa 1976), 6, 1 (1981), pp. 93-97.
13. M. Dreischarf, A. Rohlmann, Rui Zhu, H. Schmidt and Thomas Zander, Is it possible to estimate the compressive force in the lumbar spine from intradiscal pressure measurements? A finite element evaluation, *Medical Engineering & Physics,* 35 (2013), pp. 1385-1390.
14. Jisheng Qin, Yu Wang, et al. Three-dimensional finite element modeling of whole lumbar spine and its biomechanical analysis, *Journal of Medical Biomechanics*, 28 (2013), pp. 321-325.

Transcriptome Analysis Identified Feature Genes and Enriched Gene Functions Relating to Psoriasis

Jiaqi Guo and Yan Zheng[a]
Department of Dermatology, Second Affiliated Hospital, Xi'an Jiaotong University, Xi'an, 710061, China
E-mail: [a]zenyan66@126.com

Lina Wang, Yuxiao Jing, Jianqiang Du and Xiaoming Wu[b]
The Key Laboratory of Biomedical Information Engineering of Ministry of Education, School of Life Science and Technology, Xi'an Jiaotong University
Xi'an, 710049, China
E-mail: [b]wxm@mail.xjtu.edu.cn

Psoriasis is an inflammatory chronic disorder mediated by cells of immune systems. To know more about the pathogenesis underlying differentially expressed genes (DEGs) of psoriasis, we used all the 64102 annotated genes to assay the transcriptome of psoriatic and normal skin based upon public available RNA-Seq data. We identified 2906 DEGs (p.adj<0.05), of which 1365 were down-regulated and 1541 were up-regulated in psoriasis. Transcription-factor binding sites (TFBS) of NFKBRELA, IRF1, STAT1 showed significantly enriched among the up-regulated DEGs. We also confirmed that cytokines in immune system play an important role in psoriasis.

Keywords: Psoriasis; RNA-Seq; transcriptome; inflammation; cytokine.

1. Introduction

Psoriasis is considered as a cutaneous immune disease which NK cells, macrophages and neutrophils are all present in psoriatic lesions. It can reinforce inflammatory cascades by releasing cytokines while activating other inflammatory cell types [1, 2]. Although psoriasis has long been studied, and a wealth of new findings based on whole-transcriptome data have been performed and identified [3-4], the pathogenesis is still not completely clear.

Recently, with the development of high-throughput sequencing, RNA-Seq has emerged as a better alternative that has more power of accuracy and precision than microarrays to identify DEGs or alternative splicing [1]. The analysis of gene expression alone is not sufficient to resolve complex problems such as gene regulation and gene network, using quantitative RNA-Seq data can get more insights.

2. Materials And Methods

2.1. *Data sources*

All the data we used here has been deposited into the NCBI with accession ID: GSE54456 [1]. We downloaded 11 samples from the SRA database (Psoriatic skin: GSM1315778, GSM1315771, GSM1315764, GSM1315765, GSM1315623, GSM1315617 and Normal skin: GSM1315734, GSM1315732 GSM1315663, GSM1315635, GSM1315621). The reference genome (GRCH37.75.fasta) and gene annotation data (GRCH37.75.gtf) were downloaded from Ensemble.

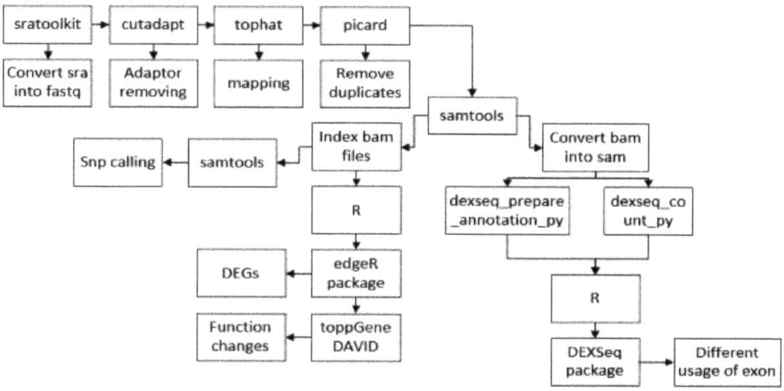

Fig. 1 Analysis strategy. edgeR implements exact statistical methods for multigroup experiments. A particular feature of edgeR functionality is empirical Bayes methods that permit the estimation of gene-specific biological variation.

2.2. *Data processing*

The strategy of raw data processing and data analyzing were showed in Figure 1, together with the tools and workflow.

3. Results

3.1. *Analysis of differentially expressed genes (DEGs)*

Out of all the 64102 annotated genes, we identified 2906 DEGs (FDR<0.05) using R v3.0.1, of which 1365 were down-regulated and 1541 were up-regulated in psoriasis. The 10 most significant DEGs were shown in Table 1.

Table 1 The 10 most significant DEGs.

Gene Name	logFC	LogCPM	PValue	FDR
ENSG00000134827	5.982105	4.969829	1.55E-60	9.91E-56
ENSG00000163221	5.146794	2.701467	3.87E-49	1.24E-44
ENSG00000138642	2.832388	5.542233	6.73E-45	1.44E-40
ENSG00000188373	3.605821	4.667591	3.67E-44	5.88E-40
ENSG00000153802	3.952092	4.621003	2.59E-42	3.32E-38
ENSG00000111335	3.396453	5.679669	1.24E-41	1.32E-37
ENSG00000181333	4.144039	6.276463	1.18E-39	1.08E-35
ENSG00000205413	2.875073	5.169822	1.09E-37	8.71E-34
ENSG00000196805	4.71964	11.23023	7.79E-35	5.55E-31
ENSG00000136688	3.196381	5.224348	9.66E-35	6.19E-31

Gene name means the gene identification according to ensemble database. logFC represent the differences of gene expression value.

3.2. *Enrichment analysis of biological functions/pathways*

We performed gene set enrichment analysis to identify changed-biological functions, and transcription factor binding sites (TFBS) among the DEGs. By using toppGene, the most significantly enriched functions from the up-regulated genes were showed in Table 2.

The most significantly enriched functions in the down-regulated genes included "cell adhesion", "fatty acid metabolic process", "cellular calcium ion homeostasis", "cell-cell signaling". By using DAVID to analyze TFBS, it revealed 41 TFBS, of which 11 are enriched among increased DEGs, 30 are enriched among the decreased DEGs. In the enriched TFBS, NFKBRELA (NF-κB), IRF1 and STAT1 are all involved to flammation and immune responses in various ways.

Table 2 Some changed functions relating to DEG genes.

Name	p-Value	FDR B&H	Genes overlap
immune response	2.923E-48	1.635E-44	189
inflammatory response	8.831E-29	8.234E-26	94
innate immune response	4.078E-27	2.535E-24	114
regulation of cytokine production	1.797E-24	1.005E-21	81
response to bacterium	1.177E-20	4.388E-18	69
response to virus	1.136E-19	3.973E-17	55
cytokine-mediated signaling pathway	7.764E-19	2.413E-16	62
leukocyte activation	3.327E-17	8.091E-15	82
NF-kappa B signaling pathway	1.050E-3	2.080E-2	12
Toll-like receptor signaling pathway	3.067E-3	4.512E-2	12

Note: Function changes (FDR B&H<0.05) among the increased DEGs.

4. Conclusion

We identified 12 increased DEGs that are associated with Toll-like receptor signaling pathway, including MYD88, TLR7, IL1B, IL8, IRF7, STAT1, IKBKE, CCL3, CCL4, CXCL10, CXCL11, and CXCL9. We confirm that immune cells and KCs are associated with psoriasis. Cytokines such as IL-23, IL-27, IL-17, TNF, IFN, chemokine are abnormally produced and released. Toll like signaling pathway are involved in the development of psoriasis.

Acknowledgment

This work was supported by the National Natural Science Foundation of China (81102085, 81371732, 81201231), and the Fundamental Research Funds for the Central Universities (2012jdhz47, xjj2013117).

References

1. T. Terui, M. Ozawa and H. Tagami: Role of neutrophils in induction of acute inflammation in T-cell-mediated immune dermatosis, psoriasis: a neutrophil-associated inflammation-boosting loop *Experimental dermatology.* **9**(1), 1 (2000).
2. J. Fuentes-Duculan, et al. and M.A. Lowes: A subpopulation of CD163-positive macrophages is classically activated in psoriasis *The Journal of investigative dermatology.* **130**(10), 2412 (2010).
3. B. Li, et al. and J.T. Elder: Transcriptome analysis of psoriasis in a large case-control sample: RNA-seq provides insights into disease mechanisms *The Journal of investigative dermatology.* **134**(7), 1828 (2014).
4. J.E. Gudjonsson, et al. and J.T. Elder: Assessment of the psoriatic transcriptome in a large sample: additional regulated genes and comparisons within vitro models *The Journal of investigative dermatology.* **130**(7), 1829 (2010).
5. T. Terui, M. Ozawa and H. Tagami: Role of neutrophils in induction of acute inflammation in T-cell-mediated immune dermatosis, psoriasis: a neutrophil-associated inflammation-boosting loop *Experimental derma-tology.* **9**(1), 1 (2000).

Experimental Study of Bipolarpulsed Magnetic Field on Its Anti-Scaling Effect

Hu Guohui and Zhao Yi
Chongqing Academy of Metrology and Quality Inspection, Chongqing, 400020, China

Li Junwei [a], Xiong Lan, Yang Zikang and He Wei
State Key Laboratory of Power Transmission Equipment & System Security and New Technology, Chongqing University, Chongqing 400030, China
Email: [a]971062034@qq.com

The scaling problem in industrial circulating cooling water is paid more and more attention. In order to obtain bipolar alternating magnetic field, this paper presents a new device model. Moreover, aiming at the air gap flux density as high as 0.1T, we study the possibility of combining permanent magnet and rotating electric machine, then compare it with the electromagnetic generator. In addition, we study on the relationship between the magnetic induction intensity with distance and properties of two permanent magnets by using ANSYS software for magnetic field analysis. In order to realize the stepless rotation speed regulation of the single-phase asynchronous motor, an electronic speed switch was adopted, thus the alternating magnetic field frequency can also be adjusted smoothly. Through three experiments under the same conditions, we found the experimental system had experimental repeatability. Then, we carried out the experiments under alternating magnetic field with different frequencies. Experimental results showed that the alternating magnetic field had stronger inhibition effect than constant magnetic field for groups with pulse frequency as 90Hz respectively, and the highest inhibition rate reaches 33%. The scale inhibition effect of 80Hz group was the same as that of the constant magnetic field group, which indicates that not all frequencies of the alternating magnetic field have high scale inhibition effect.

Keywords: Bipolar; pulsed magnetic fields; ANSYS; frequency; magnetic flux density; scale inhibition.

1. Introduction

Industrial circulating cooling water system is widely used in a variety of heat transfer equipments, the common one is the steam condenser of thermal power plant. However, due to the water system contains scaling ions, it can form crystallization scale on the surface of the steam condenser after long-term use. Crystallization scale is constitutive of carbonates, sulfates, silicates, and their mixture substances, which attaches to the surfaces of cold side steam condenser. Then, it will reduce the heat transfer efficiency of the equipment. According to the calculation of correlation study, crystallization scale can reduce the thermal conductivity of the metal from 70 to 1,000 times. On one hand, it will inevitably result in a waste of energy. On the other hand, it shortens the life of the steam condenser or cause malfunction [1-4].

Bipolar pulse technique is regarded as an effective water treatment method. The research group reported that self-made bipolar high frequency electromagnetic generator shown effective anti-scaling effect in the processing chamber of solenoid. Moreover, they put forward and designed a bipolar magnetic pulse generator based on the permanent magnet, which not only had strong magnetic flux density, but also could output the bipolar pulse waveform of magnetic field. By using the generator for anti-scaling experiments, and measured periodically parameters such as the calcium ion, electrical conductivity and pH in the artificial hard water, and compared and analyzed those experimental data. The final comprehensive evaluation proved the competent anti-scaling effect.

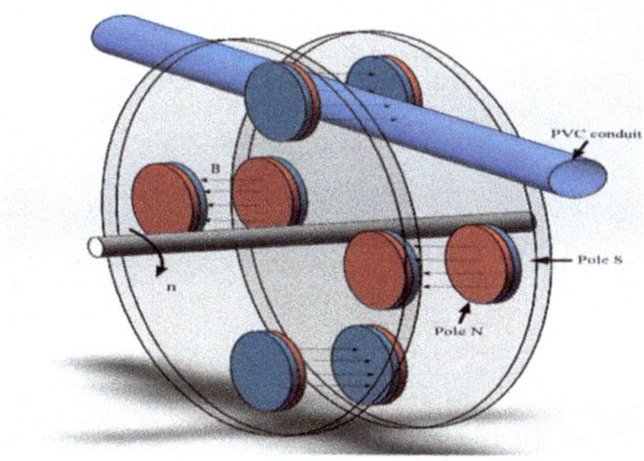

Fig.1 Symmetrical arrangement of four pairs of alien polarities of the permanent magnets on the two discs respectively.

2. Magnetic Pulse Generator

2.1. *The layout of magnetic pulse generator*

In this paper, the requirement for the pulsed magnetic field is that the magnetic flux density is no less than 0.1T, and magnetic field is series of bipolar pulses [5-8].

In Figure 1, four pairs of alien polarities of the permanent magnets are symmetrically fixed along the same circle of two aluminum alloy discs respectively. The waterpipe is fixed between the upper position of the two discs, namely between the magnet air gap of one pair of alien polarities, the diameter of the water pipe is 2 cm. In Figure 2, the single-phase asynchronous motor drives two discs and also four pairs of magnetic poles to rotate altogether. Then the water inside the waterpipe is processed by the bipolar pulsed magnetic field.

Compared to the common electromagnetic generator, the magnetic generator above is simpler, more reliable with low cost. The rotating speed is controlled by SCR stepless speed regulation. A tachometer is used to measure the speed of this single-phase induction motor, the speed range is 1200r/min ~ 2800r/min. Meanwhile, Guass Meter is used to measure the magnetic induction intensity (MII) at the center axis of one pair of alien permanent magnets, the value is 113mT which is the lowest one, while the MII near the permanent magnet is 166mT. The equation 1 shows the relationship among the motor rotational speed (n, r/min), number of pole pairs (p) and frequency (f, Hz). Consequently, the magnetic field frequency ranges from 40Hz to 95Hz.

$$f = \frac{n}{60} \times \frac{p}{2} \tag{1}$$

Therefore, the MII inside the airgap of each pair of magnets ranges from 0.113T to 0.16T, which meets the requirement of pulsed magnetic field.

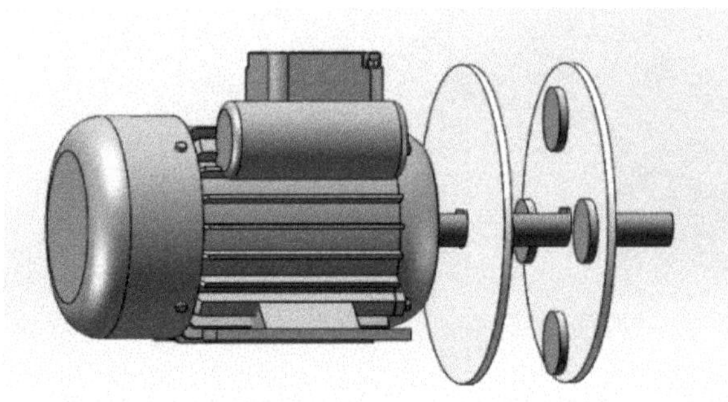

Fig. 2 The single-phase asynchronous motor drives two discs.

2.2. *The ANSYS simulation for the magnetic field intensity inside the air-gap of permanent magnets*

For the magnetic field analysis, we must set the parameters of magnetic permeability, coercivity and conductivity of three materials namely the permanent magnet (NdFeB N35), the aluminum alloy disc, and air. Physical parameters of N35 are shown in Table 1.

The permanent magnet is a cylinder whose diameter is 4cm and thickness is

0.5cm. The aluminum disc is also a cylinder whose diameter is 20cm and thickness is 0.5cm. The distance between two permanent magnets is 3cm. Then, finite element model is shown in Figure 3.

Table 1 Parameters of N35.

Type	N35
Remanence Br (T)	1.14-1.17
Coercivity Hc (KA/m)	860-915
Maximum magnetic Energy Product (kJ/m^3)	263-279
Operating Temperature (°C)	<80

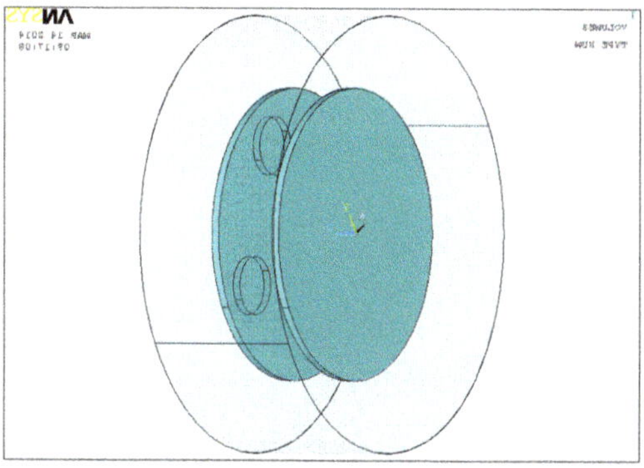

Fig. 3 Structure model of rotating magnets for ANSYS simulation.

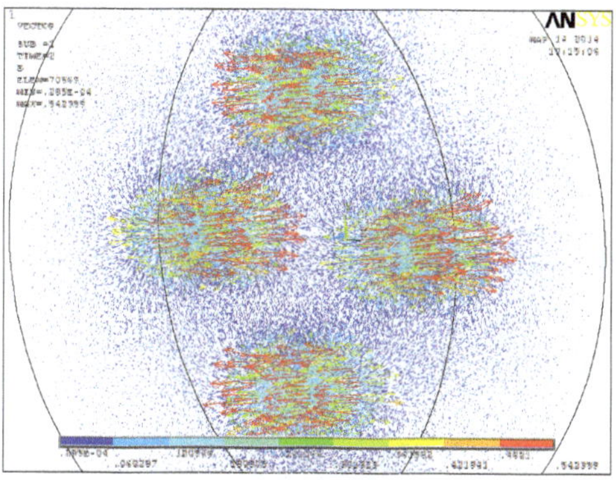

Fig. 4 MII of four pair of alien magnets.

2.3. *Simulation analysis*

After simulation, the MII distribution of four pairs altogether is shown in Figure 4.

MII along the air gap of onepair of alien magnets is shown in Figure 5. The axis of the permanent magnet is the Z axis which is vertical to the surface of magnets.

On condition that the distance between a pair of permanent magnets keeps 3cm or so with the use of N35-type NdFeB magnets, the MII inside the air gap has following characteristics, MII distribution is centrosymmetric, the value in the center of air gap reaches 0.13T, the closer the alien magnets are, the higher MII is. The MII close to the permanent magnets can reach 0.16T. With the rotation of the motor, the MII of the fixed position (water pipe) along the center of air gap will change within ±0.13T alternately and form a periodic bipolar pulsed magnetic field shown in Figure 6.

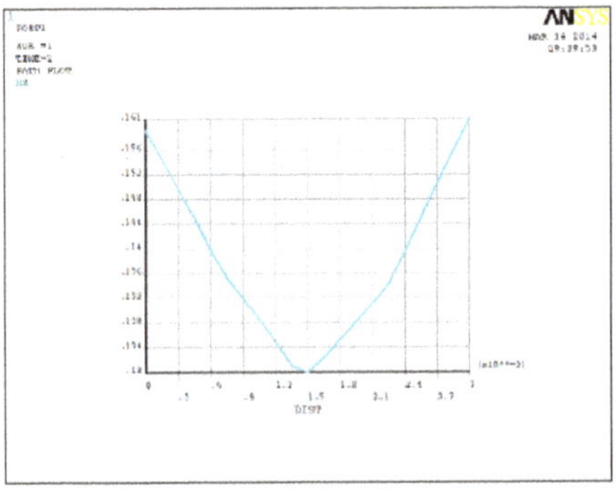

Fig. 5 Curve of MII along air gap as Z coordinates.

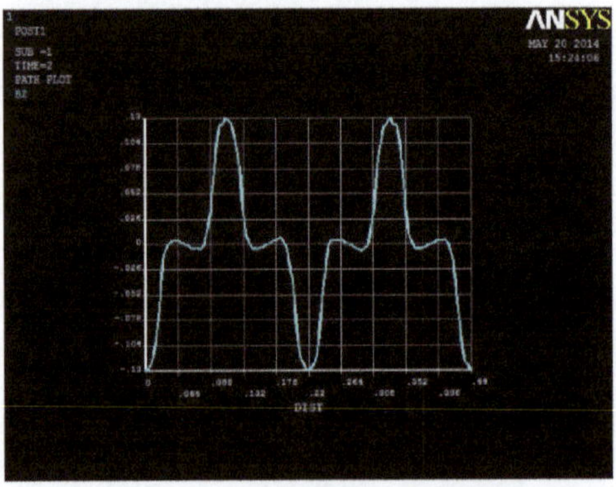

Fig. 6 The waveform of periodicpulsedmagnetic field on treated water.

3. The Anti-scaling Experiments and Data Analysis

We applied this Bipolar Magnetic Pulse Generator to do the anti-scaling experiments. Firstly, the blank experiments were done three times to prove that the experiments data has enough repeatability or not. A non-parametric test of multiple independent systems was chosen, and the significance levels of three groups were all lower than 0.05, which proved the repeatable experiment layout. On this basis, we started the six groups of anti-scaling experiments.

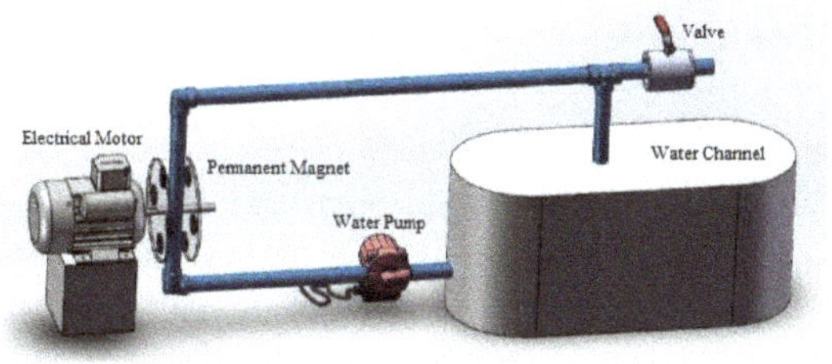

Fig. 7 The experimental platform for water treatment under pulsed magnetic field.

3.1. *Experimental devices and preparation*

Experimental devices included pulsed magnetic generator and the water circulation system shown in Figure 7. Water circulation system included water pumps, pipes, tanks and valves. The values of pH and conductivity were measured with the pH/conductivity meter of Seven Multl series, and the output for measurement results is consistent with GLP norms.

Experimental preparation followed these steps:

We set hard water's hardness to 500ppm (as CaCO3) so that the solubility of Ca2+ was 5mmol/L. The molar ratio Ca2+ and HCO3- is 1:2. As a solvent, they are formulated to 14L of deionized water, the quality of the CaC13 and NaHCO3is 7.77g and 11.76g respectively. EDTA titration was applied for the solubility measurement part of Ca2+. Then, 465mg of ethylenediamine-tetraacetic acid disodium salt was weighed to put into the 250ml flask. In addition, EDTA titration is measured by observing the color alteration, and calcium-acid indicator must color under alkaline conditions, so that it must be equipped with a sodium hydroxide solution. Then, we put 10g of NaOHinto the 250ml volumetric flask each time.

② After the water pump worked, we regulated the valve for appropriate flow rate and also ensured it was constant. After that, we started the motor and adjusted the speed to output the set frequency of pulse magnetic field. Then the whole system ran for experiments.

③ During the experiments, the solubility of Ca2+, conductivity and pH value were measured every half an hour with EDTA titration method and appropriate instruments respectively.

3.2. *The results and analysis*

According to the recorded data, we drew time-dependent curves including pH, conductivity, calcium solubility of three group namely blank group, static magnet groups and rotating magnet group (with four frequencies). The curves are shown in Figure 8, 9, 10 respectively. Therein the data of blank group is the average value of three blank groups.

Calcium solubility can directly reflect the hardness of water. In these experiments, the solubility of Ca2+ all decline gradually. The differences among three different groups are the rate of decline and the final stable value of the curve. Among them, there are overlaps, and the final stable values are different from each other.

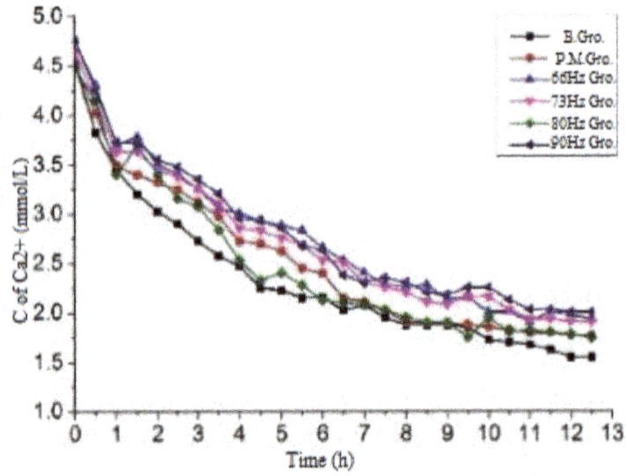

Fig. 8 The curves of calcium ion solubility.

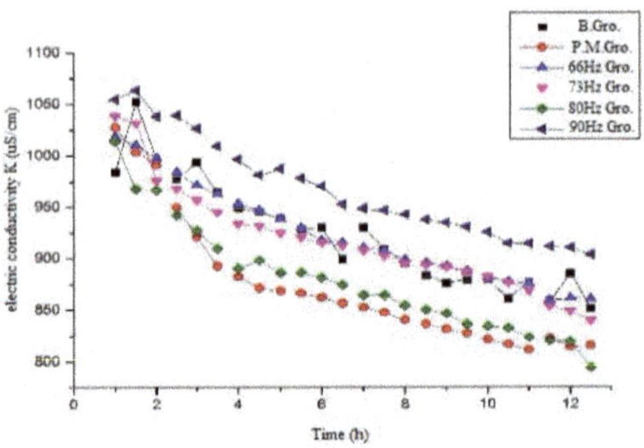

Fig. 9 Conductivity versus time.

Conductivity is a macroscopic manifestation of the number of ions which can move freely within the solution. The ions comprise a large number of Cl-, Ca2+, HCO3-, Na+. Therein the Cl- and Na+ are kept constant quantity so that their influence on the conductivity is negligible. Therefore, the Ca2+ and HCO3- are very important factors for conductivity. Conductivity can reflect the alteration of number of Ca2+ in water. In Figure 10, conductivity curves of the constant magnetic group is closer to that of the 80Hz group and the blank group, whereas conductivity curves of the 73Hz and 66Hz group curves almost coincide together, the 90Hz group curve is on the top of all groups.

Analyze comprehensively the curves of calcium solubility and conductivity, we can conclude that 80Hz group and blank group have not obvious anti-scaling effects, while 66Hz and 73Hz group's do have anti-scaling effects with the same level, and 90Hz group has the strongest anti-scaling effect.

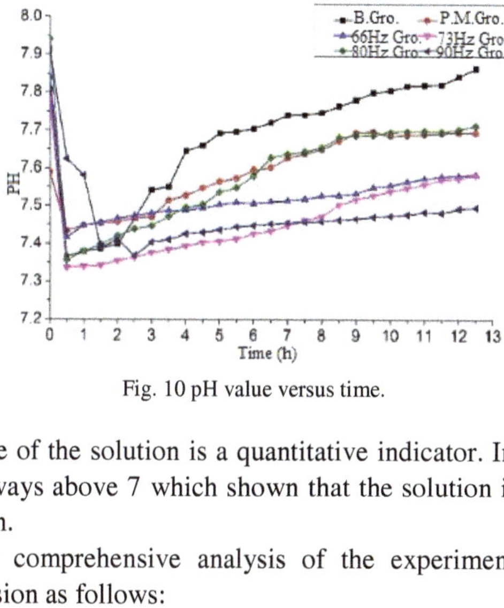

Fig. 10 pH value versus time.

The pH value of the solution is a quantitative indicator. In this experiment, pH value was always above 7 which shown that the solution is a weak alkaline or neutral solution.

Through the comprehensive analysis of the experimental data, we got following conclusion as follows:

1) Not all the anti-scaling effect of pulsed magnetic fields is absolutely better than that of constant magnetic field. It is true for some frequency.

2) Both static and pulsed magnetic field have the anti-scaling effect. However, which kind of parameters of static magnetic field or pulsed magnetic fields have the significant anti-scaling effect is the focus of future research.

4. Conclusion

1) After the reasonable arrangement of magnets, this paper designed a bipolar magnetic pulsed generator which is driven by the motor. The MII inside the center of the air gap flux density ranges from 0.13T to 0.16T and the frequency ranges from 40Hz to95Hz. The generator generates magnetic field nearly one hundred times as common pulsed electromagnetic field.

2) According to the anti-scaling experiment, the best frequency of bipolar pulsed magnetic field for anti-scaling effects is 90Hz, and the anti-scaling rate is 33.3%. 66Hz's anti-scaling effect is similar to 73Hz's, which is slightly lower than 90Hz's. While anti-scaling effect of static magnetic group is close to that of the 80Hz's, which is the lowest one.

Acknowledgment

Project supported by the National Natural Science Foundation of China (No. 51077139); China Scholarship Council; cstc2011pt-gc70009.

References

1. XI Zhaohui. Anti-scaling effect of high frequency electromagnetic field on circulating cooling water in power plant [D]. Chongqing, China: Chongqing University, 2011.
2. LI Guofang. Research on optimized control of power plant high-frequency eletromagnetic water treatment [D]. Shanghai China: Shanghai Jiao Tong University, 2011.
3. WU Yimei. Electromagnetic field analysis and experimental research of high frequency electromagnetic water treatment [D]. Chongqing, China: Chongqing University, 2012.
4. Lipus L C. Dobersek D. Influence of magnetic field on the aragonite precipitation [J]. Chemical Engineering Science, 62 (2007): 2089-2095.
5. Lipus L C. Acko D. Hamler A. Electromagnets for high-flow water processing [J]. Chemical Engineering and Processing: Process Intensification, 50 (2001): 952-958.
6. Fathi Alimi, Mohamed Tlili, Mohamed Ben Amor, Claude Gabrielli, George Maurin. Influence of magnetic field on calcium carbonate precipitation [J]. Desalination, 206 (2007): 163-168.
7. Alimi Fathi, Tlili Mohamed, Gabrielli Claude, Georges Maurin, Ben Amor Mohamed. Effect of a magnetic water treatment on homogeneous and heterogeneous precipitation of calcium carbonate [J]. Water Research, 40 (2006): 1941-1950.
8. F. Alimi, M.M. Tlili, M. Ben Amor, G. Maurin, C. Gabrielli. Effect of magnetic water treatment on calcium carbonate precipitation: Influence of the pipe material [J]. Chemical Engineering and Processing, 8 (2009): 1327-1332.

Connection between Hyaluronic Acid and Toll-Like Receptor in Signal Transduction

Cheng Fan
Department of Geriatrics, Union Hospital, Tongji Medical College, Huazhong University of Science and Technology, Wuhan, Hubei, China
E-mail: fancheng236@126.com

Hui Wang
Department of Genetics, Tongji Medical College, Huazhong University of Science and Technology, Wuhan, Hubei, China
E-mail: huiwang1977@yahoo.com.cn

Toll-like receptor (TLRs) is cell surface receptor family discovered in recent years, which belongs to the first line weapon for immune system to rapidly fight against microbial infection and plays an important role in triggering natural immunity and affecting acquired immunity. High molecular weight hyaluronic acid (HMW-HA) is important component in extracellular matrix. It can be degraded into low molecular weight hyaluronic acid (LMW-HA) by reactive oxygen molecules (ROS). The later can coordinate with ROS to activate the immune system and induce inflammation reaction through toll-like receptors. Hyaluronic acid, as internal signal of tissue damage, can be recognized by TLRs and TLRs can be activated, thereby producing a series of physiological and biochemical reaction. Different kinds of TLRs can make different reactions on hyaluronic acid in segments of different sizes. Study of relationship between hyaluronic acid and toll-like receptors can provide new concept and means for physiological and pathological mechanism of immune response and inflammatory response.

Keywords: Hyaluronic acid; TLR-2; TLR-4.

1. Introduction

TLRs was firstly reported in drosophila adult antifungal reaction of Lemaitre first et al[1]. In 1996, and then TLRs of mammals was found. Currently, at least 10 TLRs are discovered among human beings, namely TLR1-10. However, TLR11-13 is only found in mice[2]. Wherein, TLR-2 and TLR-4 belong to TLRs with the closest relation with hyaluronic acid fragments, which are studied most thoroughly. They not only play an important role of signal transduction in the immune response and inflammatory response, but also can mediate a wide range of pathogenic molecular model and recognition of various endogenous antigens such as heat shock protein, hyaluronic acid fragment, fibronectin, etc [3-4]. It is the key molecule for connecting natural immunity and acquired immunity. Hyaluronic acid fragments in different sizes play different roles on TLRs[5]. In the paper, function relation among hyaluronic acid fragment, TLR-2 and TLR-4 is described aiming at study of TLR and HA.

2. Function Relation between Hyaluronic Acid Fragment and TLR-2

2.1. *sHA can start inflammatory immune response through TLR-2*

HMW-HA is provided with negative charge in extracellular matrix. It can combine with CD44 and other inflammatory cytokines for producing and inhibiting inflammation reaction. It even has function of inhibiting tumor, which plays an important role in maintaining homeostasis[6]. However, when strong inflammation is available in the body, in the area of reaction, HMW-HA can be degraded into small molecular fragment HA (sHA) by oxygen free radicals, hyaluronidase, β-glucuronidase and hexosaminidase, for example tumor necrosis factor (TNFa) can stimulate lung fibroblasts to produce a large number of HA segments [7]. sHA can activate the expression of inflammatory genes in epithelial cells, endothelial cells, fibroblasts, dendritic cells and macrophages. Meanwhile, it also can improve the response ability of T cells on dendritic cells (DCs). The significance of HA important function in the body lies in that it not only can play a role on inflammation, in addition, it can further enhance pathological process of inflammation induced reaction [8] because it is not removed. When protective barrier in the body is damaged, HMW-HA can be degraded into small molecules capable of the ability of inducing positive regulation of inflammatory genes. However, sHA has the ability of inducing rearrangement of inflammatory chemokines, cytokines and various enzymes in macrophages. In addition, sHA also can stimulate other types of cells, including dendritic cells, epithelial cells and endothelial cell [5]. After sHA is activated by TLRs, inflammatory response reaction process can be started. However, sHA also can be used as a signal to activate TLR-2 [8]. In addition, sHA can induce NF-kB to produce activity in cells expressing TLR-2. Similarly, when the cells are stimulated by TLR-2 ligand HKAL, NF-kB also can be activated [9]. Therefore, TLR-2 is the receptor for both HA induced inflammatory gene and aHA.

2.2. *sHA and HMW-HA produce different effects on TLR-2*

TLR-2 is the receptor of activated HA segments. However, HMW - HA can prevent TLR-2 from producing signals. However, sHA can assist in activating Ag-specific T cells. Namely, sHA, as a danger signal extracellular, can activate TLR-2 and make it produce signals. However, HMW-HA can exacerbate inflammation by preventing TLR-2 from sending out signals. When sHA is expressed through TLR-2 induced inflammatory gene, complete HMW-HA can be used as sHA competitor to prevent TLR-2 from producing signals, thereby weakening the ability of response to inflammation on risk [5].

2.3. *sHA can promote TLR-2 to combine with its composite receptor thereof*

TLR plays an important connection role between congenital immune response activation and acquired immune induction. TLR-2 plays an important role in host resistance to virus, gram-positive organisms, helix, mycobacteria, protozoon and mold. However, lipoprotein and peptidoglycan are TLR-2 characteristic ligands [9]. It is interesting that when TLR-2 produces signal through its ligands, a dimer can be formed through TLR-1 or TLR-6. Expression level of endogenous TLR-1 and TLR-6 is very low in human embryonic kidney cells. However, when sHA produces signals through inducing TLR-2, TLR-1 or TLR-6 can be moved to the surface, thereby being used as TLR-2 composite receptors [10]; It is also possible that polymer repeating disaccharide which composed of HA can promote crosslinking of TLR-2 receptor with dimers, and it still should be further studied.

3. Function Relation between Hyaluronic Acid Segments and TLR-4

3.1. *sHA sends out signals through TLR-4, thereby inducing DCs maturation*

TLR4 is related with intracellular signal production and DCs maturation under the induction of sHA. Exogenous application sHA can induce activation of DCs in vivo. Meanwhile, the activation is mediated by TLR-4-dependent mechanism. Namely, sHA is an independent inducer of DCs activation, which can send out signals through TLR-4. DCs without sufficient TLR-4 can not produce TNF-α on sHA response. One antibody resisting TLR-4 can inhibit TNF-a release of wild-type DCs after sHA induction. However, after wild-type DCs were treated by sHA for seven hours, antibody resisting TLR-4 can not play any role on production of TNF-α. Meanwhile, TLR-4 expression also can be lowered after being treated with sHA for 24 hours. Though there is still TLR-4 on the DCs surface [11]. The experiments show that TNF-α produced by DCs under sHA induction can produce signals and produce more TNF-α after being combined with TNFI receptors on the same cell. In addition, there is a transmembrane domain on TLR-4. The transmembrane domain is linked with intracellular receptor protein MyD88. MyD88 is reacted with IRAK for mediating signal transduction induced by TLR [12]. When human beings and rat DCs are activated by sHA, TLR-4 plays a critical role in vivo and in vitro. In addition, sHA stimulation can induce translocation change of p38/p42–44, MAPKs and NF-kB in the process of TLR-4 signal transduction.

3.2. *sHA can induce TLR-4 to produce signals in the inflammatory response*

Glycosaminoglycan hyaluronic acid is a kind of inducer activating TLR-4. It can lead to release of inflammatory cytokines [13]. Damaged tissue can lead to extracellular matrix to release small molecular weight HA fragments. It can be recognized by TLR-4, CD44 and MD-2 compounds so that sHA can be regarded as internal signal of inflammation and tissue damage [14]. Many experimental results show that aseptic intrinsic inflammation reaction process is dependent on the activation of TLR-4 and signals activated by HA can be sent out [15]. TLR-4 is the carrier of dendritic cells to identify HA fragments, which can make DC produce inflammatory cytokines and make them mature. However, concentration of sHA demanded for inducing TLR-4 to produce signals is higher than required LPS concentration by several magnitudes since only sHA with high concentration appears in the parts with inflammation, thereby inducing signals of inflammation promotion response [16].

3.3. *sHA can activate melanoma cells through TLR-4*

sHA can induce expression of inflammatory factors and cytokines in macrophages. It also can stimulate blood vessel primary response, including proliferation and migration of endothelial cells. It is discovered that expression of matrix metalloproteinases (MMPs) can be improved after NF-kb activation in tumor cells [17]. Protein in extracellular matrix can be degraded by including similar protease, thereby promoting tumor growth and metastasis. TLR-4 is an important regulator of inherent immune response. It can reply products of many microorganisms such as bacteria cell wall component LPS and peptidoglycan, thereby leading to transcription factor NF-kB activation and production of antibacterial cytokines and chemokines. sHA can transfer signals through TLR-4 and make dendritic cells mature through release of interleukins IL-1b, IL-12 and tumor necrosis factor (TNF) as well as NF - kB activation. Furthermore, Release of sHA after tissue damage can stimulate production of endothelial cells IL-8 through TLR-4 dependent approach.

Hyaluronic acid fragment induces positive regulation of human melanoma cell cytokines and metalloproteinases, and signals are sent out through TLR-4 [18]. NF-kB is main component of TLR-4 signaling pathway, IL-8 and MMp-2 transcription are controlled by NF-kB control [10]. Participation of TLR-4 is required in activating melanoma cells by sHA since IL-8 transcription and translation are suppressed after TLR4-specific siRNA is used for treatment. In addition, expression of melanoma cells treated by sHA is increased, activity of MMP-2 precursor is increased, TLR-4 produces signal through transcription of sHA induced by IL-8. Therefore, possible signal transduction cascade response (including TLR-4 activated by sHA) in melanoma cells can be reasoned out after NF-kB activation and subsequent activation of gene expression.

4. Causes of TLR-2 and TLR-4 on different function of HA

Structure of TLR-2 is slightly different from TLR-4 structure. Their downstream pathways and affinity for a variety of ligands are slightly different [19]. Some studies suggest that oligosaccharides digested by polymer HA produces signal through TLR-4. Other studies showed that cells of rats without TLR-4 and cells of mice with complete TLR-4 have the same response ability on small molecule HA. However, HA produces its function through TLR-2. Some studies also believe that HA acts through both TLR-2 and TLR-4. For example, interaction between hyaluronic acid TLR-4 and hyaluronic acid TLR-2 can stimulate corresponding signal transduction pathways to start repair inflammation response. These disputes are produced by HA in different sizes which produce different signals in TLR-2 and TLR-4.

Scheibner et al [8] believe that TLR-2 can be used as an HA segment receptor triggering inflammation gene expression. Jiang et al. [19] also demonstrated that TLR-2 and TLR-4 were related with signal production in lung injury. However, HA segments in moderate size (200 and 135 kDa) were used in the studies. By comparison, the study which proved TLR-4 as sHA receptor used oligonucleotides to chitosan sized HA. Therefore, different TLR receptors had different responses on HA in different sizes possibly because that TLR-2 and TLR-4 had different affinities, other researches also showed that the dimension of HA fragments also can be used for restricting subsequent physiological reaction.

5. Conclusion

In summary, function relation between hyaluronic acid and toll-like receptors has very important role in tissue injury, inflammation reaction, signal transduction, etc. The function mechanism is also more and more emphasized. It is believed that further study on hyaluronic acid and toll-like receptors can provide new thought and means for immune response and inflammatory reaction physiological and pathological mechanism as well as clinical application.

References

1. Lemaitre B, Nicolas E, Michaut L, et al. The dorsoventral regulatory gene cassette spatzle/Toll/cactus controls the potent antifungal response in Drosophila adults. Cell. 1996; 86(06): 973-83.
2. Marshak-Rothstein A, Rifkin I R. Immunologically active autoantigens: the role of toll-like receptors in the development of chronic inflammatory disease. Annu Rev Immunol. 2007; 25: 419-441.
3. Chen C, Zibiao H, Ming Z, et al. Expression pattern of Toll-like receptors (TLRs) in different organs and effects of lipopolysaccharide on the expression of TLR2 and 4 in reproductive organs of female rabbit. Developmental and comparative immunology. 2014; 46(2): 341-348.
4. Chen KQ, Huang J, et al. Toll-like receptors in inflammation, infection and cancer. International Immunopharmacology. 2007; 7(10) 1271-1285.
5. Ruppert SM, Hawn TR, Arrigoni A, et al. Tissue integrity signals communicated by high-molecular weight hyaluronan and the resolution of inflammation. Immunologic research. 2014; 58(2-3): 186-192.
6. Eberleinl M, Scheibner KA, Black KE, et al. Anti-oxidant inhibition of hyaluronan fragment-induced inflammatory gene expression. Journal of Inflammation. 2008; 5: 20, 1-10.
7. Scheibner KA, Lutz MA, Boodoo S, et al. Fragments Act as an Endogenous Danger Signal by Engaging TLR2. The Journal of Immunology. 2006; 177(02): 1272-1281.
8. Abe T, Fukuhara T, Wen X, et al. CD44 participates in IP-10 induction in cells in which hepatitis C virus RNA is replicating, through an interaction with Toll-like receptor 2 and hyaluronan. Journal of virology. 2012; 86(11): 6159-6170.
9. Dusio GF, Cardani D, Zanobbio L, et al. Stimulation of TLRs by LMW-HA induces self-defense mechanisms in vaginal epithelium. Immunology and cell biology. 2011; 89(5): 630-639.

10. Termeer C, Benedix F, Sleeman J, et al. Oligosaccharides of Hyaluronan Activate Dendritic Cells via Toll-like Receptor 4. J. Exp. Med. 2002; 195(01) 99-111.
11. Zhai Y, Shen XD, O'Connell R, et al. Cutting edge: TLR4 activation mediates liver ischemia/reperfusion inflammatory response via IFN regulatory factor 3-dependent MyD88-independent pathway. J Immunol. 2004;173(12): 7115-7119.
12. Pagliara T, Csontos K, Das S, et al. Role of hyaluronic acid and toll-like receptor 4 in regulation of inflammatory liver injury. Journal of the American College of Surgeons. 2007; 205(3): s29.
13. Taylor KR, Yamasaki K, Radek KA, et al. Recognition of Hyaluronan Released in Sterile Injury Involves a Unique Receptor Complex Dependent on Toll-like Receptor 4, CD44, and MD-2. The Journal of Biological Chemistry. 2007; 282(25): 18265–18275.
14. Zhang Y, Bliska J B. Role of macrophage apoptosis in the pathogenesis of Yersinia. Curr Top Microbiol Immunol. 2005; 289:151-173.
15. Prince JM, Levy RM, Yang R, et al. Toll-Like Receptor-4 Signaling Mediates Hepatic Injury and Systemic Inflammation in Hemorrhagic Shock. J Am Coll Surg. 2006; 202(03): 407–417.
16. Barton GM, Medzhitov R. Toll-like receptor signaling pathways. Science, 2003; 300(5625): 1524-1525.
17. Voelckerl V, Gebhardt C, Averbeck M, et al. Hyaluronan fragments induce cytokine and metalloprotease upregulation in human melanoma cells in part by signalling via TLR4. Experimental Dermatology.2007; 17(02): 100–107.
18. Liu Y, Yin H, Zhao M, et al. TLR2 and TLR4 in autoimmune diseases: a comprehensive review. Clinical reviews in allergy & immunology. 2014; 47(2): 136-147.
19. Jiang J, Arp J, Kubelik D, et al. Induction of indefinite cardiac allograft survival correlates with Toll-like receptor 2 and 4 downregulation after serine inhibitor-1 (Serp-1) treatment. Transplatation. 2007; 84(9): 1158-1167.

Study on Algae Inhibition Experiments by Multi-Parameter Tunable High Voltage Pulser

Jiang Weiqiang
CNOOC Guangdong LNG LTD, Guangdong, China

Zhang Deqing, Ma Long, Xiong Lan[a] and Yang Zikang
State Key Laboratory of Power Transmission Equipments & System Security and New Technology, Chongqing University, Chongqing, China
[a]E-mail: lxiong@cqu.edu.cn

In this paper, we cultivated microcystis aeruginosa to do PEF experiments. The layout of experiments was orthogonal design including four parameters, namely peak value, duration and frequency of rectangular pulse and also treatment period. After treatment, we measured the algae cell density every 24 hours till the end of 6 days' solution cultivation. Experimental data proved the feasibility of PEF's effect on the micro-algae. In addition, peak value of pulse was the major impact parameter of PEF algae sterilization, pulse duration ranked No. 2. However, treatment period and frequency played tiny influences. Finally, we did confirmatory experiments with the parameter deduced from orthogonal layout. It was also proved that the optimum electric parameter combination could be deduced for algae inactivation from experimental data as few as possible.

Keywords: Pulsed electric field (PEF); algae inactivation; orthogonal experimental design; algae cell density (ACD).

1. Introduction

Due to eutrophia of the water and exposion to sunlight or living in warm environment, water blooms occurred on the surface of water bodies like lakes and agricultural ponds frequently and extensively, which has posed more and more serious environmental problems worldwide.

Recently, a number of studies focus on the mechanism, electromagnetic parameters of micro-organism inactivation under pulsed electric field (PEF) and also its industrial applications in effluent, foodstuffs and beverages [1]-[2]. However, research reports [3]-[4] on PEF's inactivation effect on the algae in water body are not abundant enough. Although it is a common confess that PEF has irreversible breakdown effect on cellular membrane which leads to the death or inactivation of micro-organism, there are many contrary conclusions about the effectiveness difference between monopolar and bipolar pulses [3], [4], between rectangular and exponential decaying waveforms, it is also unclear about the dominant inactivating process and the most superior treatment parameter among electric field intensity, frequency, duration and treatment time etc.

This paper aims at looking for a proper method to find optimum combination of electric parameters for the best microalgae inactivation effectiveness within the parameter scope of the pulse generator, make clear the superior position among four parameters such as peak value, duration, frequency of pulse and treatment time.

2. Material and Method

2.1. *Microalgae culture and preparation*

We cultivated microcystis aeruginosa to do PEF experiments, it was bought from fresh water algae species base of Institute of Hydrobiology, Chinese Academy of Sciences. Microcystis aeruginosa was cultivated in BG11 medium where there were Trace elements, Macronutrient and vitamins. After high pressure sterilization processing several brown Reagent bottles, it was poured into the concentrated mother liquor with Trace elements, Macronutrients. Then, these bottles and vitamins were refrigerated at 40℃. When the broths were mixed in sterile distilled water with proper proportion of concentrated mother liquor and vitamins, the algae experiments were well prepared.

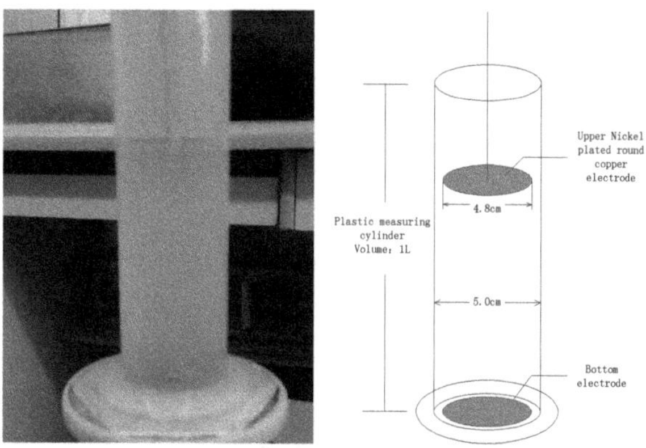

Fig. 1 The experimental treatment chamber.

2.2. *Treatment chamber*

Figure 1 shows the picture and also draft of the chamber for PEF treatment experiments which is a cylinder with 1 L as volume and 5 cm as inside diameter. There were two circular plate electrodes in parallel, the distance between two electrodes is up to 10cm. In this paper, the distance is fixed to 5cm. The bottom electrode is fixed, the upper electrode is hung by an insulation bracket to put on the surface of the solution. The diameter of latter one is 4.8cm in order to move up and down easily accordance with the liquor height. The electrodes are made of nickel-plated copper in case electrolysis and corrosion happen during the PEF treatment experiments.

2.3. *Experimental procedure*

The pulse generator we used is a self-made 7-stage generator has an output voltage of up to 6 kV provide with repeated bipolar/monopolar rectangular pulses whose duration and frequency are up to 5 μs and 1000 pps respectively under the condition of liquid loads.

The layout of experiments is orthogonal design including three levels and four factors, namely four parameters such as peak value, duration and frequency of rectangular pulse and also treatment period. Orthogonal experimental design is helpful to obtain credible and satisfactory results through less experiment than ordinary experimental design [9]. Table 1 shows the orthogonal experimental table, where there are 9 test groups and a control group or blank group, the number 1-3 of test groups represents the level of different factors.

Table 1 The orthogonal experiment table.

Number	Voltage	Pulse width	Frequency	Processing time
1	1	1	1	1
2	1	2	2	2
3	1	3	3	3
4	2	1	2	3
5	2	2	3	1
6	2	3	1	2
7	3	1	3	2
8	3	2	1	3
9	3	3	2	1
10			Blank control	

It is very important to choose a proper parameter correspondence with different level in Table 2. Otherwise, the difference of algae inactivation effectiveness among different groups is not significant enough. Therefore, we did several pre-experiments to settle down the proper values of 3 electric parameters and one processing time shown in Table 2.

Table 2 The electrical parameters as different levels.

Parameters	Level 1	Level 2	Level 3
Voltage (kV)	1	3	5
Pulse width (μs)	1	3	5
Frequency (Hz)	200	400	800
Processing time (min)	5	10	15

Note, the distance between two electrodes was fixed as 5cm, only monopolar pulses were imposed on the electrodes.

According to Table 1, nine PEF experiments were done with different parameters on the microalgae solution, one untreated "zero-pulse sample" was taken from each of the nine microbial medium to be the control group before the start of every test. During PEF treatment, temperature of the solution was online monitored.

The microalgae solution of 9 test groups was displaced into the labeled 150 mL erlenmeyer flask after PEF processing. Then, they were cultivated in the same condition and detected with instruments constantly. According to the pre-experiments, we found that the death and sterilization of microalgae appeared significantly only if the solution was cultivated for a certain period after PEF treatment. Therefore, we settled down the 12th hour after treatment as the first detection time, then detection was done every 24 hours after that, which was lasted for 6 days. Algae cell density (ACD) was the important indicator for microalgae inactivation effectiveness.

We measured the absorbance curves of the microalgae solution with UV-Vis Spectrophotometer of Purkinje General company. We found that corresponding wavelengths of the maximum absorption peak of the absorbance curves were 688nm of microcystis aeruginosa. Meanwhile, we observed that ACD of the microalgae versus absorbance is of linear correlation by plotting a standard absorbance curves. Then, the standard equation was listed in Table 3 by regression analysis.

Table 3 Standard equation of algal cell density versus absorption value.

Microalgae	Equation of Standard curve	Correlation coefficient R2
microcystis aeruginosa	Y=19.76X-0.09	0.992

Therefore, the data of ACD which we recorded was calculated by the standard equation with absorbance values measured with spectrophotometer. If some data was too small, we adopted microscopic counting method individually for verification and correction.

The diameters of the microalgae is less than 10μm, we applied microscopic counting method for counting the amount of microalgae cell in the counting board with XSZ-G optical microscope of Changchun Chongguang company. In fact, the recorded data was the average value of counting number three times. In addition, we defined the microalgae inactivation ratio θ for clear comparison among different test groups. Equation 1 shows the calculation formula of θ with ACD data.

$$\theta = 1 - C_e / C_o \quad (1)$$

Where, C_e is the ACD after PEF treatment, C_o is the ACD of the control group. Then, θ indicates the degree of inactivation effectiveness of PEF treatment.

During the experiments, the chamber had been cooled with fan, the temperature of algae solution was online monitored with Optris infrared thermometer. The ambient temperature was 12℃, the maximum temperature rise of all test groups was 11℃. Therefore, the solution temperature was less than 23℃ within short treatment time, which meant that thermal effect of continuous pulses on the microalgae inactivation was negligible.

3. Results and Discussion

Figure 2a shows the growth curves of 10 groups namely 9 test groups and 1 control group. The curves were plotted by the discrete values of ACD measured in different time. Excluding the curve of the 5th group because of the obvious measurement error, all values of the other eight groups were smaller than that of the blank group at corresponding detection time. Obviously, the growth inhibition of microalgae under PEF treatment was proved by only No. 6 to No. 9 test groups because microalgae of the other groups reproduced gradually. Moreover, the appearance of algae medium in the 6th days after PEF treatment was shown in Figure 2b, from left to right order, that is, the blank group as green color, the 2nd group (1 kV, 3 μs, 400 Hz, 10 min) as green color, the 6th group (3 kV, 5 μs, 200 Hz, 10 min) as light green color and the 8th group (5 kV, 3 μs, 200 Hz, 15 min) as almost transparent. The color showed the difference from each other.

Then, variance analysis was made to get the data in Table 4. Significant level was chosen as $p<0.05$. When confidence probability was 0.95, the sig values of voltage and duration were both less than 0.05, on the contrary, that of frequency and treatment time were bigger than 0.05. Statistically, pulse voltage and duration have major impacts on the microalgae inactivation, and the latter two have not any impacts. Moreover, F value of voltage factor was much bigger than that of duration factor, which meant that peak value of pulse voltage or electric field intensity was the main factor.

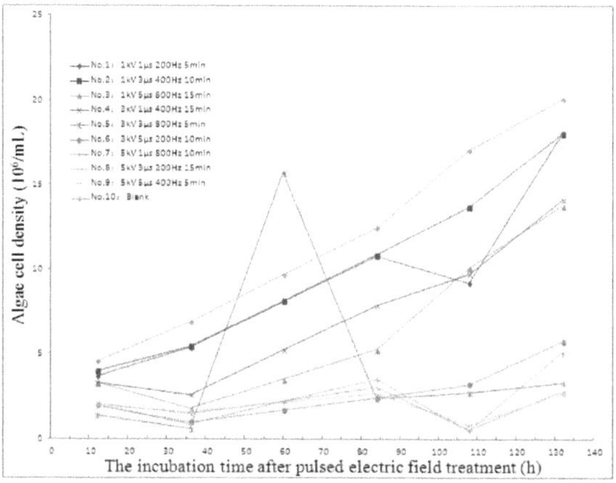

(a) The growth curve

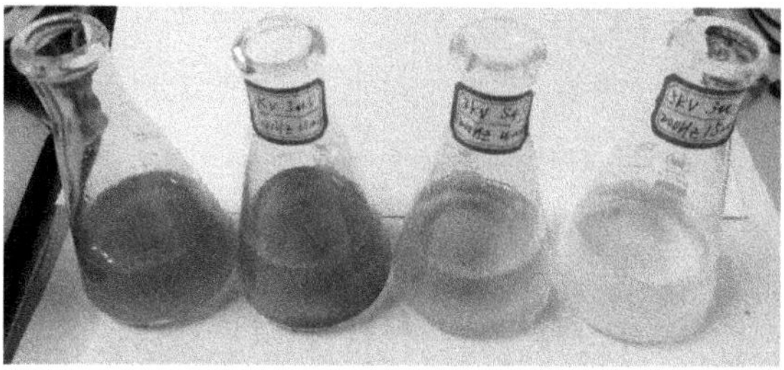

(b) Appearance of solution

Fig. 2 Experimental results after PEF treatment of Microcystis aeruginosa.

Table 4 Variance analysis for ACD inactivation ratio.

	Factor	Quadratic sum	freedom Degree	Mean square error	F	Sig.
A	Voltage	21 232.32	2	10 616.16	19.541	0
B	Pulse width	4 526.70	2	2 263.35	4.166	0.022
C	Frequency	2 403.52	2	1 201.76	2.212	0.121
D	Treatment time	243.72	2	121.862	0.224	0.8
	Aggregate	28 406.026	8			

Furthermore, we applied the Duncan SSR method to test each factor levels of above four parameters which was helpful to obtain the optimum combination of four parameters for the best algae inactivation effectiveness. Figure 6 shows the analysis results of each parameter.

Obviously, the factor level for the best treatment effectiveness is voltage as 5kV, duration as 5 μs, frequency as 800 Hz and treatment time as 10 min. It means that the optimum combination of four parameters is A3B3C3D2 (5 kV, 5 μs, 800 Hz and 10 min).

Supplementary experiments were done to test if this deduced test group had the best algae inactivation effect or not. A blank group was set for microalgae experiments too. The results showed that the microalgae inactivation ratio of the optimum groups was as high as 94.1%, the above data were bigger than the best results of the original experiments as 82.37%.

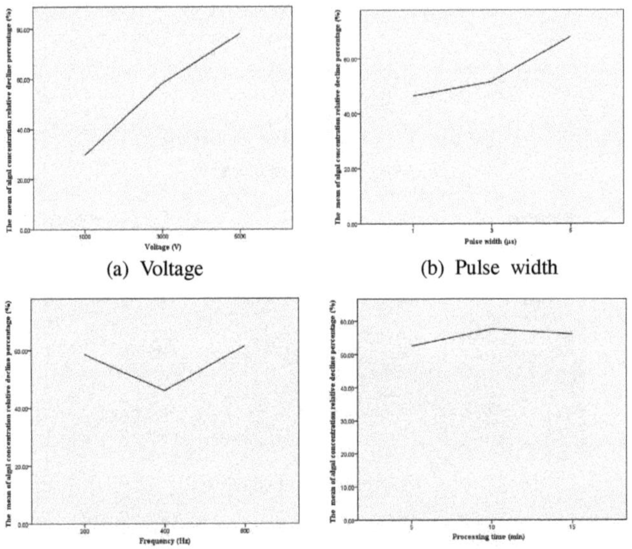

(a) Voltage (b) Pulse width

(c) Frequency (d) Processing time

Fig. 3 Duncan test for each factor levels of different parameters.

4. Conclusion

We made the orthogonal experimental design of three levels and four factors, namely pulse voltage, duration, frequency and treatment time. The algae inactivation experiments of PEF were done for the microcystis aeruginosa with the self-made high voltage pulse generator. The growth inhibition of microalgae under PEF treatment was proved. Meanwhile, the data proved that the pulse voltage or electric field intensity was the major impact parameter of PEF algae sterilization, and pulse duration ranks No. 2. However, treatment period and frequency played tiny influences. Finally, we did confirmatory experiments with the optimum parameter deduced from orthogonal layout and Duncan SSR method. It was proved that the optimum electric parameter combination could be deduced for PEF algae inactivation from experimental data as few as possible.

Acknowledgment

Project supported by the National Natural Science Foundation of China (No. 51077139); China Scholarship Council; cstc2011pt-gc70009.

References

1. Bing, S., A. Nyein Nyein, et al. Eradication of Invasive Organisms From Ballast Water With Electrodeless Pulsed-Discharge Hybrid Reactor. IEEE Transactions on Industry Applications, 2011, 47(3): 1079-1085.
2. Sato M, Ohgiyama T, Clements J.S. Formation of chemical species and their effects on microorganisms using a pulsed high-voltage discharge in water [J]. IEEE Transactions on Industry Applications, 1996, 32(1):106-112.
3. I. V. Timoshkin, S. J. MacGregor, R. A. Fouracre, B. H. Crichton, et al. Transient Electrical Field across Cellular Membranes: Pulse Electric Field Treatment of Microbial Cells, Journal of Physics D: Applied Physics. 2006, 39(3): 569-603.
4. P. S. Brito, H. Canacsinh, J. P. Mendes, et al. Comparison Between Monopolar and Bipolar Microsecond Range Pulsed Electric Fields in Enhancement of Apple Juice Extraction, IEEE Transactions on Plasma Science, 2012, 40(10): 2348-2354
5. Lin Yu, Yang Xiaoguang, Ma Yingying. An Analysis of Factors Causing Congestion with the Application of Orthogonal Experimental Design Method [J]. Systems Engineering, 2005, 23(10): 39-43.

Joint Meta-Sample Extraction and Classifier Learning for Tumor Classification*

Jianhua Wu[a], Mindan Wei and Li Zhu
Department of Electronic Information Engineering, Nanchang University, Nanchang 330031, Jiangxi Province, China
[a]*E-mail: jhwu@ncu.edu.cn*
www.ncu.edu.cn

Fei Guo[b] and Yang Liu
Burns Institute, First Affiliated Hospital of Nanchang University Nanchang 330006, Jiangxi Province, China
[b]*E-mail: guofei2005@126.com*

Sparse representation based classification (SRC) has been extensively and successfully applied to tumor classification due to its effectiveness in classification. Different from many existing SRC methods which emphasize on strong representational ability, our proposed method takes the discriminative ability into account, i.e. joint meta-sample extraction and classifier learning, which may be favor to better performance. In addition, a novel decision rule, in relation to both the minimal reconstruction residual and the minimum classification error, is presented and used during the classification stage. Experiments using several publicly available microarray gene expression data demonstrate that the proposed algorithm is efficient and achieves comparable accuracies with the state-of-the-art sparse coding techniques for tumor classification.

Keywords: Tumor classification; meta-sample extraction; sparse representation; classifier learning.

1. Introduction

Many methods have been applied to tumor classification, such as discriminant analysis, support vector machine, etc. Sparse representation (SR) has been widely used and shown to be an effective technique for classification recently. For instance, J. Wright et al. [1] applied SR to face recognition successfully. Its

* This work is supported by the National Natural Science Foundation of China (61162014, 61210306074), the Natural Science Foundation of Jiangxi Province (20122BAB201029), the Science & Technology Project of Jiangxi Provincial Department of Education (GJJ13008) and the Graduate Student Innovation Special Funds of Jiangxi Province (YC2012-S016).

application to classifying gene expression data was proposed in [2]. Taking the original training samples as the basis vectors might not be effective enough to represent the test samples owing to the noise in the original data. Another drawback of SRC is its high computational cost once the size of training set becomes large. To address these issues, Zheng et al. [3] presented an SRC based on meta-samples. Their experimental results on some publicly available MGED indicated that meta-sample based sparse representation classification (M-SRC) is feasible and valid. By replacing l_1- norm regularization with non-negative least squares (NNLS), Li presented a method that performed sparse coding via solving an NNLS optimization problem [4].

M-SRC algorithm pays close attention to the representational capability only. In this case, the extracted meta-samples may not be optimal for specific classifying tasks. In reality, the discriminative ability of the classifier is of the same importance as the representational capability. Inspired by this fact, we propose an algorithm for tumor classification on MGED in this paper. Our approach takes both strong representational ability and classifier's discriminative ability into account by unifying the meta-sample extraction and classifier learning as one optimization problem. Performing two tasks jointly would result in a discriminative sparse representation suitable for classification. We name the algorithm as sparse representation classification based on meta-sample extraction for classifier learning (MC-SRC). In addition, to further improve the performance of MC-SRC method, a novel decision rule has been proposed. Different from the established SRC methods whose classification are achieved directly through the sparse representation coefficients of each sample, our decision rule keeps a watchful eye on the classification error as well as the reconstruction residual. In this way, more accurate decisions would be made.

2. Preliminary

Mathematically, MGED can be denoted as a matrix $\mathbf{X} \in \mathbf{R}^{m \times l}$ ($m \gg l$). The vector $\mathbf{x}_i \in \mathbf{R}^m$ represents the i- th ($i = 1, 2, \cdots, l$) sample and the value of x_{ji} means the expression level of the j- th ($j = 1, 2, \cdots, m$) gene in the i- th sample. Given a set of basis vectors $\mathbf{a}_i$ ($i = 1, 2, \cdots, k$), approximately represent a test sample $\mathbf{x} \in \mathbf{R}^m$ as $\hat{\mathbf{x}} = s_1\mathbf{a}_1 + s_2\mathbf{a}_2 + \cdots + s_k\mathbf{a}_k = \mathbf{As}$, where $\mathbf{s}$ is the coefficient vector representing $\mathbf{x}$ and ideally, it is a vector whose entries are zeros except for those associated with the class which $\mathbf{x}$ belongs to. $\mathbf{s}$ can be achieved by introducing a sparsity term which leads to fewest non-zero coefficients in $\mathbf{s}$. l_0- norm $\|\mathbf{s}\|_0$, which equals to the number of non-zero entries in $\mathbf{s}$, is the first choice. On account of the nature of combinational optimization, to find the solution to sparse representation problem: $\hat{\mathbf{s}} = \arg\min_{\mathbf{s}} \left\{ \|\mathbf{x} - \mathbf{A}\mathbf{s}\|_2^2 + \lambda \|\mathbf{s}\|_0 \right\}$ is NP-hard. In most cases, l_1- norm is applied to take place of l_0- norm to obtain the approximation solution. l_1- norm is defined as $\|\mathbf{s}\|_1 = \sum_{i=1}^{k} |s_i|$ and the sparse representation of $\mathbf{x}$ is reduced to solve an l_1- regularized least square problem:

$$\tilde{G}(\mathbf{s}, \lambda) = \arg\min_{\mathbf{s}} \left\{ \|\mathbf{x} - \mathbf{A}\mathbf{s}\|_2^2 + \lambda \|\mathbf{s}\|_1 \right\} \tag{1}$$

where λ is a regularization parameter that balances reconstruction error and sparsity.

To classify a test sample $\mathbf{x}$, the reconstruction residual when $\mathbf{x}$ is assigned to class j should be computed by:

$$\mathbf{r}^j(\mathbf{x}) = \|\mathbf{x} - \mathbf{A}\delta(\hat{\mathbf{s}}, j)\|_2 \tag{2}$$

where $\hat{\mathbf{s}}$ represents the sparse representation obtained by solving (1) and $\delta(\hat{\mathbf{s}}, j)$ is constructed by keeping the entries related to class j ($j = 1, 2, \cdots, c$) in $\hat{\mathbf{s}}$ and assigning other entries as zeros, and c denotes the number of classes. Then the class label of $\mathbf{x}$ is determined by minimizing the residual:

$$\text{class}(\mathbf{x}) = \arg\min_{j} \mathbf{r}^j(\mathbf{x}) \tag{3}$$

Meta-samples, which may capture the inherent structures of training samples and provide biological insight, are extracted to be the basis vectors instead of the original samples in training data. Mathematically, the matrix $\mathbf{X} \in \mathbf{R}^{m \times n}$ can be approximately factorized into two matrixes:

$$\mathbf{X} \approx \mathbf{A}\mathbf{P} \tag{4}$$

where each of the k columns of $\mathbf{A} \in \mathbf{R}^{m \times k}$ defines a meta-sample. Each column in $\mathbf{P} \in \mathbf{R}^{k \times n}$ shows the meta-sample expression pattern of the corresponding sample. In this paper, NMF method is used to obtain the meta-samples $\mathbf{A}$.

3. Proposed Method MC-SRC

We present a sparse representation classification based on meta-sample extraction for classifier learning, considering the fact that the discriminative ability of a classifier is as important as the representational capability. Unifying the meta-sample extraction and classifier learning as one optimization problem would result in a discriminative sparse representation suitable for classification.

Given $\mathbf{X} \in \mathbf{R}^{m \times l}$, we suppose that the l samples belong to c categories.

Firstly, $\mathbf{X}$ is divided into two subsets, a training set and a test set: $\mathbf{X} \rightarrow \left(\mathbf{X}^{train} \in \mathbf{R}^{m \times n}\right) \cup \left(\mathbf{X}^{test} \in \mathbf{R}^{m \times p}\right)$. Secondly, meta-sample extraction and classifier learning are unified as one optimization problem, which can be formulized as:

$$\tilde{J}(\mathbf{A},\mathbf{B},\mathbf{S}) = \arg\min_{\mathbf{A},\mathbf{B},\mathbf{S}} \left\{ \left\| \mathbf{X}^{train} - \mathbf{AS} \right\|_F^2 + \beta \left\| \mathbf{Y} - \mathbf{BS} \right\|_F^2 \right\} \quad s.t. \quad \mathbf{S} \geq 0 \tag{5}$$

where the first term and the second term represents the reconstruction residual and the classification error, respectively. β is a tradeoff parameter controlling the two terms. $\mathbf{A} = [\mathbf{A}_1, \mathbf{A}_2, \cdots, \mathbf{A}_c] \in \mathbf{R}^{m \times k}$ is a set of meta-samples and matrix $\mathbf{A}_j \in \mathbf{R}^{m \times k_j}$ denotes the meta-samples extracted from the samples in class j ($j = 1, 2, \cdots, c$). Matrix $\mathbf{B} \in \mathbf{R}^{c \times k}$ represents the classifier parameters which would be learned together with $\mathbf{A}$. $\mathbf{Y} = [\mathbf{y}_1, \mathbf{y}_2, \cdots, \mathbf{y}_n] \in \mathbf{R}^{c \times n}$ is the class label matrix and each column $\mathbf{y}_i = [0, 0, \cdots, 1, 0, \cdots, 0]^T \in \mathbf{R}^c$ denotes the label vector of $\mathbf{x}_i$. The non-zero position indicates the class to which $\mathbf{x}_i$ belongs.

To achieve the optimal meta-samples $\mathbf{A}$ and classifier parameters $\mathbf{B}$, the first step is to initialize them. Here, non-negative matrix factorization (NMF) is introduced to get the initial $\mathbf{A}$ [4]. Given $\mathbf{A}$, the initial coefficient matrix $\mathbf{S}$ can be computed via solving the NNLS optimization:

$$\arg\min_{\mathbf{S}} \left\| \mathbf{X}^{train} - \mathbf{AS} \right\|_F^2 \quad s.t. \quad \mathbf{S} \geq 0 \tag{6}$$

In this study, fast combinatorial non-negative least squares algorithm (FCNNLS) [5] has been applied to solve this optimization problem: $\mathbf{S} \leftarrow \text{FCNNLS}(\mathbf{A}, \mathbf{X}^{train})$. And the initial classifier parameters $\mathbf{B}$ can be obtained through $\mathbf{B} \leftarrow \mathbf{YS}^{\dagger}$, where $\mathbf{S}^{\dagger}$ denotes the pseudo-inverse of $\mathbf{S}$.

Updating the initial $\mathbf{A}$, $\mathbf{B}$ and $\mathbf{S}$ in equation (5) is a crucial step to find the joint optimal solution. If the data are non-negative, the following multiplicative update rules, which are exactly the same as those rules in [6] when all elements in the weight matrixes equal to one, are used in our approach:

$$\mathbf{A} \leftarrow \mathbf{A} \odot \frac{\mathbf{XS}^T}{(\mathbf{AS})\mathbf{S}^T}, \mathbf{B} \leftarrow \mathbf{B} \odot \frac{\mathbf{YS}^T}{(\mathbf{BS})\mathbf{S}^T}, \mathbf{S} \leftarrow \mathbf{S} \odot \frac{\mathbf{A}^T\mathbf{X} + \beta\mathbf{B}^T\mathbf{Y}}{\mathbf{A}^T(\mathbf{AS}) + \beta\mathbf{B}^T(\mathbf{BS})} \tag{7}$$

where $\odot$ means product element by element. When the data are of mixed signs, we apply the following multiplicative update rules to alternatively renovate $\mathbf{A}$, $\mathbf{B}$ and $\mathbf{S}$:

$$\mathbf{A} \leftarrow \mathbf{XS}^{\dagger}, \mathbf{B} \leftarrow \mathbf{YS}^{\dagger}, \mathbf{S} \leftarrow \mathbf{S} \odot \sqrt{\frac{(\mathbf{A}^T\mathbf{X})^+ + (\mathbf{A}^T\mathbf{A})^- \mathbf{S} + \beta(\mathbf{B}^T\mathbf{Y})^+ + \beta(\mathbf{B}^T\mathbf{B})^- \mathbf{S}}{(\mathbf{A}^T\mathbf{X})^- + (\mathbf{A}^T\mathbf{A})^+ \mathbf{S} + \beta(\mathbf{B}^T\mathbf{Y})^- + \beta(\mathbf{B}^T\mathbf{B})^+ \mathbf{S}}} \tag{8}$$

where $(\bullet)^+ = \frac{|(\bullet)|+(\bullet)}{2}$ and $(\bullet)^- = \frac{|(\bullet)|-(\bullet)}{2}$. Multiplicative updates for A, B and S are easily derived from those in [7] and the convergence property of the rules was proved in the work. Iterate these update processes until convergence is guaranteed: $\frac{\left\|\tilde{\mathbf{J}}-\tilde{\mathbf{J}}_{pre}\right\|_F}{\left\|\tilde{\mathbf{J}}_{pre}\right\|_F} < \rho$, where $\tilde{\mathbf{J}}_{pre}$ denotes the previous value of $\tilde{\mathbf{J}}$. ρ is the termination criterion for iteration and we assign it an empirical value of 0.01.

After learning the meta-samples and the classifier parameters jointly, the next work is sparse coding, i.e., representation of each test sample as a linear combination of the learned meta-samples:

$$\mathbf{x}_i^{test} = s_1\mathbf{a}_1 + s_2\mathbf{a}_2 + \cdots + s_k\mathbf{a}_k = \mathbf{As} \tag{9}$$

where $\mathbf{x}_i^{test} \in \mathbf{R}^m$ is the i-th sample in test set $\mathbf{X}^{test} \in \mathbf{R}^{m\times p}$ ($p = l - n$). Sparse representation coefficients of a test sample can be computed via solving the following l_1-regularized least square problem:

$$\mathrm{G}\left(\mathbf{s}_i^{test},\lambda\right) = \arg\min_{\mathbf{s}_i^{test}}\left\{\left\|\mathbf{x}_i^{test} - \mathbf{A}\mathbf{s}_i^{test}\right\|_2^2 + \lambda\left\|\mathbf{s}_i^{test}\right\|_1\right\} \tag{10}$$

The rule to decide the label of the test sample $\mathbf{x}_i^{test}$ is critical to the performance of classification. To match the proposed method better, we present a novel decision rule and compare it with nearest subspace (NS) rule and a rule that directly uses the learned classifier parameters (hereafter we denote it BS rule) [8]. The NS rule, which takes advantage of the discriminative property of sparse coefficients, computes the reconstruction residual when $\mathbf{x}_i^{test}$ is assigned to class j by applying (2). And then the class label of $\mathbf{x}_i^{test}$ is determined by minimizing the residual: $\mathrm{class}(\mathbf{x}_i^{test}) = \arg\min_j \mathbf{r}^j(\mathbf{x}_i^{test})$. The BS rule, which simply uses the learned classifier $\mathbf{B}$ to assign the label j to $\mathbf{x}_i^{test}$, can be formulated as following: $\mathrm{class}(\mathbf{x}_i^{test}) = \arg\max_j (\mathbf{B}\mathbf{s}_i^{test})_j$.

Different from the existing decision rules, our proposed new decision rule makes decision depending on both the learned classifier $\mathbf{B}$ and the reconstruction residual $\mathbf{r}^j(\mathbf{x}_i^{test})$ ($j = 1, 2, \cdots, c$). As a matter of convenience, we denote the proposed rule as BS-NS rule:

$$\mathrm{class}(\mathbf{x}_i^{test}) = \arg\max_j \left\{\frac{\left(\mathbf{B}\mathbf{s}_i^{test}\right)}{\mathbf{r}(\mathbf{x}_i^{test})}\right\}_j \tag{11}$$

4. Experimental Results

In order to investigate the classification performance of MC-SRC, we use six datasets available in [3,9]. 10-fold cross validation is employed to divide each dataset into ten parts, and ten trials are performed. In the ten trials, each part would be used as a test set in turns and the remaining parts are incorporated into one training set. We compare our method with SRC [2], and M-SRC (applying SVD to extract meta-samples) [3]. Accuracy is the performance metric used in our study. In the experiments, we set parameters as λ=0.1, ρ=0.01 and β=0.1. As the partition files achieved by cross validation deeply affect the accuracies, we repeat 10-fold cross validation 10 times and for fair comparison, the obtained ten partition files are unified in all approaches. The experimental results are listed in Table 1.

Table 1 Classification accuracies on multi-category and binary-category datasets (%).

	Multi-category datasets			Binary-category datasets		
Dataset	Lung	11_Tumors	Brain_Tumor1	Colon	Prostate	DLBCL
SRC	94.57	95.41	90.94	82.40	92.35	95.21
M-SRC	95.39	95.88	90.38	85.88	88.80	96.86
MC-SRC(NS)	94.10	96.19	88.46	85.69	87.52	95.48
MC-SRC(BS)	94.54	96.36	90.92	87.81	88.88	96.73
MC-SRC(BS-NS)	94.93	96.42	91.10	87.95	88.98	97.25

From the results, it can be seen that the classification accuracies of MC-SRC are comparable or even higher than that of SRC and M-SRC. Sometimes, the extracted meta-samples cannot represent the substantial information well, so methods based on meta-samples may be not so good as SRC method. Prostate dataset is an example. From the comparative experiments of different decision rules on MC-SRC, we notice that the BS-NS rule indeed matches MC-SRC better than individual BS rule or NS rule.

5. Conclusions

In this paper, we have presented an approach called MC-SRC and the contribution of it lies in jointing meta-sample extraction and classifier learning, which results in sparse representation of the test samples and an optimal classifier for classification. Experimental results of tumor classification over several sets of microarray gene expression data show that MC-SRC approach has better performance than SRC and M-SRC.

References

1. J. Wright, A.Y. Yang, A. Ganesh, et al., Robust face recognition via sparse representation, Pattern Analysis and Machine Intelligence, IEEE Transactions on 31 (2009), 210-227.
2. X. Hang and F.X. Wu, Sparse representation for classification of tumors using gene expression data, Journal of biomedicine and biotechnology, 2009.
3. C.H. Zheng, L. Zhang, T.Y. Ng and C.K. Shiu, Metasample-based sparse representation for tumor classification, Computational Biology and Bioinformatics, IEEE/ACM Transactions on 8 (2011), 1273-1282.
4. Y. Li and A. Ngom, Supervised dictionary learning via non-negative matrix factorization for classification, Machine Learning and Applications (ICMLA), 2012 11th International Conference on. IEEE (2012), 439-433.
5. M.H. Van Benthem and M.R. Keenan, Fast algorithm for the solution of large-scale non-negativity-constrained least squares problems, Journal of chemometrics 18 (2004), 441-450.
6. T. Goldstein and S. Osher, The split Bregman method for L1-regularized problems, SIAM Journal on Imaging Sciences 2 (2009), 323-343.
7. H. Lee, J. Yoo and S. Choi, Semi-supervised nonnegative matrix factorization, Signal Processing Letters, IEEE 17 (2010), 4-7.
8. Z. Jiang, Z. Lin and L.S. Davis, Learning a discriminative dictionary for sparse coding via label consistent k-svd, Computer Vision and Pattern Recognition (CVPR), 2011 IEEE Conference on. IEEE (2011), 1697-1704.
9. A. Statnikov, C.F. Aliferis, et al., A comprehensive evaluation of multi-category classification methods for microarray gene expression cancer diagnosis, Bioinformatics 21 (2005), 631-643.

Application of Inherent Safety and TRIZ in the Innovation Design of Intelligent Pacifier

Shu-Chen Yang
Doctoral student, Institute of Allied Health Sciences, College of Medicine, National Cheng Kung University, Central Taiwan University of Science and Technology, No.666, Buzih Road, Beitun District, Taichung City 40601, Taiwan (R.O.C.).
sjyang@ctust.edu.tw

Kuo-Yi Li
National Chin-Yi University of Technology, No. 57, Sec. 2, Zhongshan Rd., Taiping Dist., Taichung 41170, Taiwan (R.O.C.).
kyli@ncut.edu.tw

Ying-Ju Chang
National Cheng Kung University, No. 1 University Road, Tainan701, Taiwan (R.O.C.)
yxc2@mail.ncku.edu.tw

This study proposed a novel design of intelligent pacifier, in order to help the caretakers knowing when to feed the newborn infants or premature infants who do not have sufficient sucking ability. By adopting the inherent safety and TRIZ methods, the inherent safety analysis and design could effective prevent the injuries caused by improper feeding. Furthermore, Su-Fields Analysis was performed to identify the problems, and 76 Standard Solutions were used to find the possible design structure for systematic innovative design. The intelligent pacifier was designed with a distortion sensor to detect the changes of sucking ability and frequency of the infants. The data were transmitted via the wireless transmitter to a remote receiver, and the computing module of the intelligent pacifier would display the actual sucking force and frequency on the screen. Then, the caretakers could refer to the data and provide proper care for the infants.

Keywords: Intelligent pacifier; sensor; wireless transmission; inherent safety; TRIZ.

1. Introduction

Due to immature body function and lack of coordination between sucking and swallowing, premature infants rely on nasogastric tube feeding. They are not fed orally until their sucking ability is developed, in order to prevent possible complications, such as over-fatigue and dyspnoea due to their poor sucking ability

[Boiron et al., 2007; Capilouto et al., 2014]. At present, the American Academy of Pediatrics has included oral feeding as an indicator of discharge [Lau and Smith, 2011]. Hence, accurate evaluation of the premature infants' sucking ability has become an important issue in clinical care. A conventional method of testing the infants' sucking ability is to place the finger into the infant's mouth, and subjectively evaluate whether the infant has sufficient sucking ability based on the infant's suction on the finger [Holloway, 2014; Rocha et al., 2011]. This method is based on subjective judgment, and the results may vary due to the sensitivity of different testers. Hence, there is no given standard for the test result. Other studies have adopted behavioral observation method and descriptive scales (e.g. Neonatal Oral-Motor Assessment Scale, Early Feeding Skill assessment) [Howe et al., 2007; Wrotniak et al., 2009] to evaluate the premature infants' sucking ability. Those methods lack objective data, thus, the accuracy is doubted. Therefore, the evaluation of premature infants' sucking ability requires a more objective and quantitative measuring tool. This study designed a set of suction sensing device, which uses a strain gauge to detect the distortion of the pacifier. The computing module of the intelligent pacifier can convert the distortion data into sucking force and frequency. The measured data are transmitted via a wireless transmitter to a remote receiver, and are displayed on the screen. This objective evaluation tool is expected to help the medical staffs learning about the developmental stages of the premature infants' sucking ability, find the best feeding time, and prevent the complications due to improper feeding.

2. Literature Review

Sucking ability is the key factor determining whether premature infants can be orally fed [Wrotniak et al., 2009]. The action of sucking can be divided into two parts: 1) suction: oral cavity forms negative pressure to suck milk into the mouth; 2) expression: when the oral cavity presses milk, it forms positive pressure [Capilouto et al., 2014; Holloway, 2014]. A mature sucking action starts with suction, and proceeds with a good coordination between suction and expression [Lau et al., 2000]. Sucking force increases with the growing maturity of premature infants [White-Traut et al., 2013a]. Generally, the development of sucking ability can be divided into five stages: 1) occasional sucking, with sucking pressure between -2.5 and -12.5mmHg; 2) irregular sucking, with sucking pressure between -7.5 and -15.0mmHg; 3) some regular sucking, with sucking pressure between -15 and -75mmHg; 4) regular sucking, with sucking pressure between -50 and -75mmHg; 5) highly regular sucking, with sucking pressure between -110 and -160mmHg [Holloway, 2014; Lau, 2006; Lau et al., 2000]. In the fourth and fifth stages, the oral feeding success rate for premature infants are higher, and the complications due to improper feeding are less likely to occur [Lau et al., 2000; Mizuno and Ueda, 2003]. However, the premature infants would have different sucking frequencies due to varied levels of maturity, generally from occasional sucking to regular sucking. When the premature infants are able to maintain continuous and regular sucking, their sucking ability is considered good, and would not encounter problems of bradycardia and polypnea [Fucile et al., 2009; White-Traut et al., 2013].

Based on the above, the evaluation of sucking ability includes two key indicators, namely sucking pressure and sucking frequency. Thus, a pacifier that could collect information on sucking ability could help medical staffs evaluate and understand the sucking ability of the premature infants. Our previous study designed an air flow sensor to detect the air pressure, in order to detect the sucking ability of the infants objectively. The current study designed a distortion sensor to detect the sucking ability and frequency, thus solving the problem of sucking and pressure for premature infants.

3. Methods

In order objectively measure the sucking force and frequency of infants, and allow infants to be fed safely, this study adopted inherent safety and TRIZ methods to design an intelligent pacifier. The concept of inherent safety is improper operation does not lead to damages, thus, is an effective approach to prevent accidents. It is a protection technology that ensures the electronic devices to be safely operated even in a flammable environment or under abnormal operating conditions. The design method is to prevent the release of energy that will lead to explosion. The aim of inherent safety is safe operation in a dangerous environment, such as the gas platform in Pakhoi [Elvik, 2010; Hansson, 2010; Leong and Shariff, 2008]. The common techniques of inherent safety include Intensification, Substitution, Attenuation, Limitation of Effects, Simplification, Avoiding Knock - on Effect, Making Incorrect Assembly Impossible, Making Status Clear, Tolerance, Ease of Control, Software, Isolation and Inter-lock. Those methods can allow the production process to achieve the objective of inherent safety [Elvik, 2010; Hansson, 2010; Lu, 2012].

Under the premise of inherent safety, the design procedures for the chemical industry, which is subject to hazards of explosion or corrosion, the mechanical industry, which is prone to the risks of rolling-in or cutting, or other highly dangerous industries are as follows: (1) identify the hazards: to discover the sources of hazard in the system; (2) prevent or eliminate the hazards: strengthen, replace, adjust, and simplify; (3) control the hazards: such as limit the impacts of the errors, prevent the collision effect, avoid assembly errors, and ease-to-control;

(4) alleviate, isolate, and ring-fence; (5) deal with the hazards: diminish the dangers and toxins of the hazardous substances. Although the above procedures are proposed for the inherent safety design of the chemical industry, they are also adopted by the mechanical industry. The inherent safety design in the mechanical industry refers to the ergonomic considerations during the design, and the preventive measures taken during the design stage to eliminate the potential hazards. Thus, even with improper operation or mechanical failure, accidents could be avoided. For example, when working on the stamping press, if the sliding block drops and the operator's hand is still in the stamping mold, injury will occur. Thus, if the activation of the stamping press requires two buttons to activate, and the operator needs to use both hands to press the button, the injury could thus be avoided. This is an example of inherent safety design [Shariff et al., 2012; Srinivasan and Kraslawski, 2006].

TRIZ is an abbreviation of Theory of Inventive Problem Solving. When Altshuller served as a patent reviewer, he discovered that most patents are not the outcome of ingenious work due to random inspiration, but systematic use of prior art or cross-field knowledge to solve the problems. Hence, he chose 40,000 representative patents from over 200,000 patents to analyze the approaches of problem-solving [Sung, 2009]. The main solving approach of TRIZ is Paradigm Shift, which shift specific problems into general problems, then find general solutions from the models of general problems, and finally shift the general solutions to specific solutions. There are various tools to solve problems, including contradiction matrix, 40 Inventive Principles, Su-Fields Analysis, 76 Standard Solutions, Trend of Evolution, and universal design [Sheu and Hou, 2013].

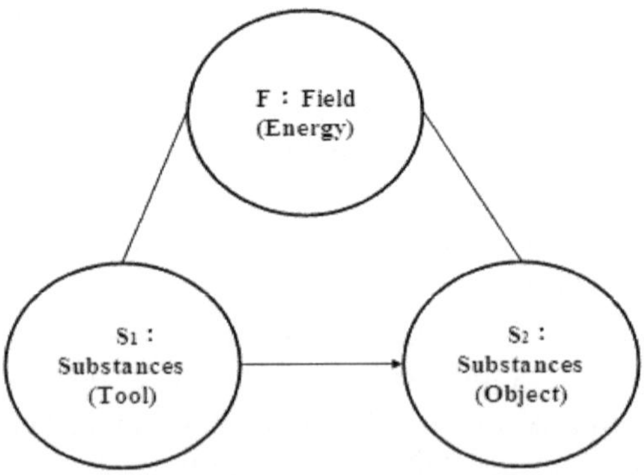

Fig. 1 Basic Su-Fields Triangular Model Source: [Lin, 2011].

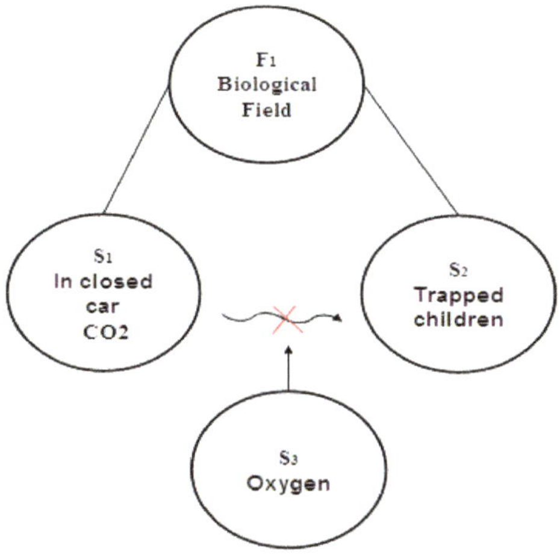

Fig. 2 Advanced Su-Fields Model Source: [Lin, 2011].

Table 1 Five types of 76 Standard Solutions.

Type	Explanation	Standard solutions
Type 1	No change or minor change to improve the system	13
Type 2	Change the system for improvement	23
Type 3	System conversion	6
Type 4	Examination and measuring	17
Type 5	Simplification and modification strategies	17

Source: [Sung, 2009].

When applying TRIZ in design, several problems must be clarified first. Su-Fields Analysis Modeling, which uses simple symbols and conversions for problem solving, should be used to identify the problems, and determine the type of Su-Fields Analysis that it belongs to. A complete Su-Fields structure is comprised of three elements, namely S1 as the object substance, S2 as the tool substance, and Field (F). If the problem is complex, the Su-Fields Triangular Model can be modified into an advanced Su-Fields Model, as shown in Fig.1 and Fig. 2. The substance can be any material, environment, tool, component, or even person. It may refer to a single element or a complex system. Field is a type of energy generated among the substances, including mechanical force, gravity, audible force, thermal force, chemical force, electric force, and magnetic force. Then, 5 types of solutions, totaling 76 Standard Solutions, can be substituted into the system, and find the most appropriate solution [Yan et al., 2013]. After constructing the Su-Fields Analysis Model, Altshuller proposed 76 Standard Solutions, which can be used when the system has flaws, hazards, excess or insufficient effect. After the model is converted into an effective and complete system model path, the solving direction can thus be obtained. The details of the

76 Standard Solutions are shown in Table 1. The six steps of innovative design using the Su-Fields analysis and 76 Standard Solution are: (1) describe the main problem; (2) list all relevant interactive elements; (3) construct the systematic Su-Fields Model; (4) list corresponding standard solutions; (5) construct the new Su-Fields Model; and (6) find the solutions [Lin, 2011; Song et al., 2012].

This study applied the inherent safety concept to analyze the design of pressure sensing pacifier, and found that infants may suffer injuries due to poor sucking ability. This problem can be solved by fool-proof design and simplification. In terms of the TRIZ method, Su-Fields Analysis and 76 Standard Solutions were adopted to analyze the feeding risks, specifically the problems of difficulty and lack of objectivity in determining the infants' sucking ability. A strain gauge sensor and computing module were used to obtain the sucking pressure and frequency, as detailed below.

As premature infants have poor sucking ability, they tend to feel over-fatigue or dyspnoea when sucking milk. Thus, determining whether the infants' sucking ability has sufficiently developed to be fed with breast milk or formula is an important task for the caretakers. First, the inherent safety method was applied to design the intelligent pacifier, and fool-proof design (Making Incorrect Assembly Impossible) simplification was adopted to solve the problem of feeding risks. A strain gauge sensor was used to detect the distortion of the pacifier to avoid the human errors when judging the sucking ability of the infants. The measured data were displayed on the screen for the caretakers to determine the sucking ability.

In the Su-Fields analysis, S1 is the "finger used for feeding", S2 is "feeding", and F is the pressure in the mechanical force. The Su-Fields Model is shown in Fig. 3. As there exists a hazardous system in the Su-Fields Model, subjective judgment and human errors may occur, thus leading to infants' complications due to improper feeding. Moreover, the caretakers' fingers may be injured. Type 3 system in the 76 Standard Solutions was used for conversion, in order to generate two or more system according to the different characteristics of the elements, and enhance the performance. In Type 3, there are 6 standard solutions available, which are 3.1) converting into two or multiple systems, with 5 standard solutions; 3.2) convert to microscopic level, with 1 standard solution. The usable standard solution is 3.1.3 system conversion, which adds different characteristics among the elements to enhance the performance. In the design structure of intelligent pacifier, a strain gauge sensor is added to detect the distortion of the pacifier when the baby is sucking. The data are analyzed by the computing module of the mainframe, and converted into the sucking force. The signals are transmitted via a wireless transmitter to a remote receiver, and the information is displayed on the screen. For the convenient use of the caretakers, the transmission of the signals is achieved wirelessly. The framework is shown in Fig. 4.

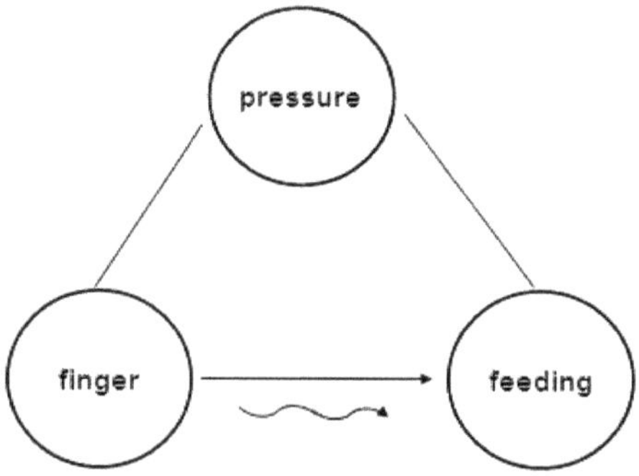

Fig. 3 Su-Fields Analysis of the traditional finger test.

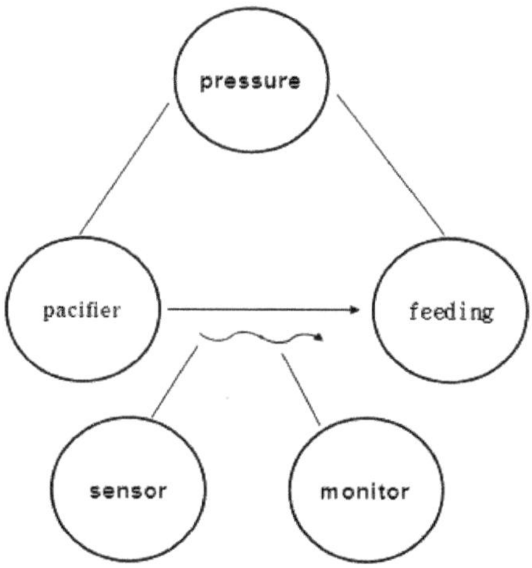

Fig. 4 Su-Fields Analysis of the intelligent pacifier.

4. Product Design

According to the above inherent safety and Su-Fields Analysis, the intelligent pacifier can accurately measure the sucking force of the infants. The strain gauge sensor inside the pacifier can detect the distortion of the pacifier when the infant is sucking. The distortion value is converted by the computing module of the intelligent pacifier into pressure values, so that the caretakers can learn about the correct sucking pressure and frequency. The data shown in the display screen can allow the caretakers to determine the best time of feeding. The intelligent pacifier is comprised of a pacifier, a base plate, a strain gauge sensor, a computing module, a display unit, a wireless transmitter, and a remote receiver. The structure and the operating status of the strain gauge sensor are shown in Fig. 5 and Fig. 6. The distortion of the strain gauge sensor is shown in Fig. 7. The structure and assembly diagram of the intelligent pacifier are drawn by Solidworks. Perspective diagrams and operational schematics are used to illustrate the component structure and functions. After turning on the power of the intelligent pacifier, the caretaker can enter the information of gender, age, weight, illness, division, language, and curves on the lower left corner of the screen. The caretaker then places the pacifier in the mouth of the infant, and the sucking force of the infant is shown on the screen. The pacifier with a strain gauge sensor is shown in Fig. 8. The pressure values measured by the strain gauge sensor are transmitted via a wireless transmitter, such as wi-fi, Bluetooth, and Internet, to a remote receiver. Thus, the caretaker can learn about the sucking status of the infant, and determine the best feeding time, as shown in Fig. 9. Compared with the conventional finger test, the proposed design can accurately determine the sucking force, and allow for objective determination of the pressure standard, thus providing best care to the premature infants.

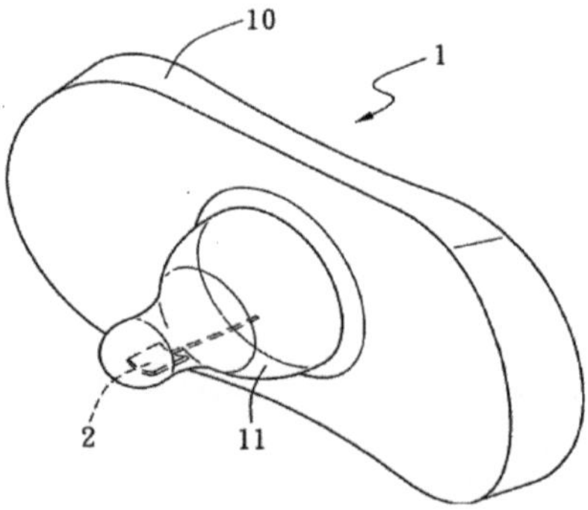

Fig. 5 A perspective view of the intelligent pacifier.

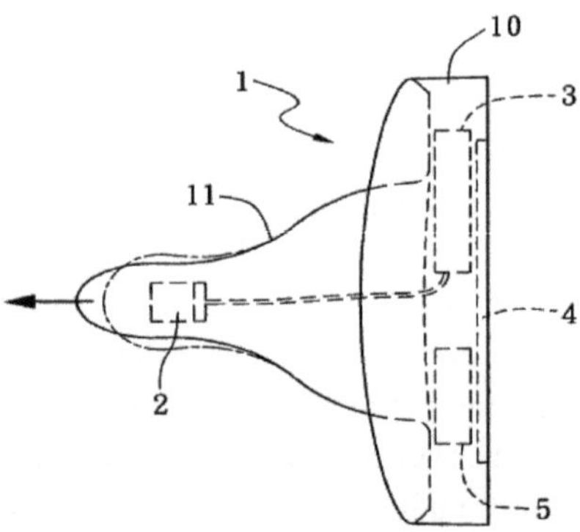

Fig. 6 The strain gauge sensor under pressure and in use.

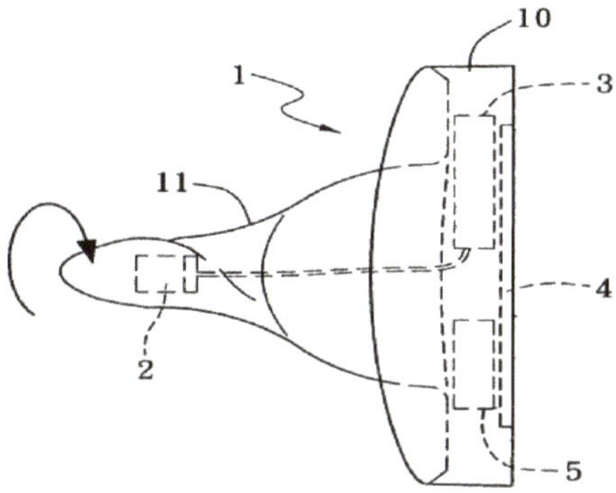

Fig. 7 The strain gauge sensor under distortion.

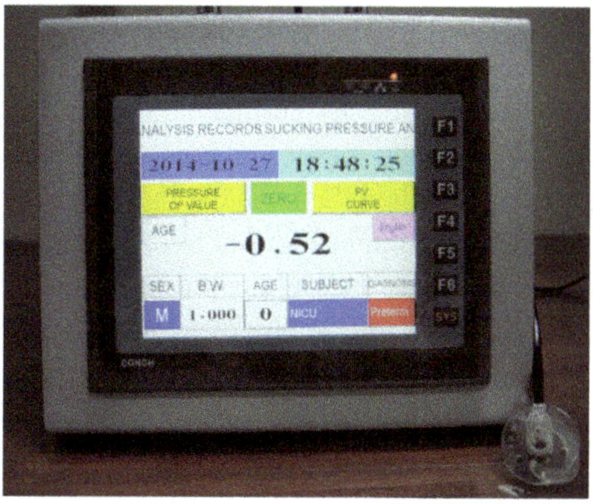

Fig. 8 Embodiment of the intelligent pacifier.

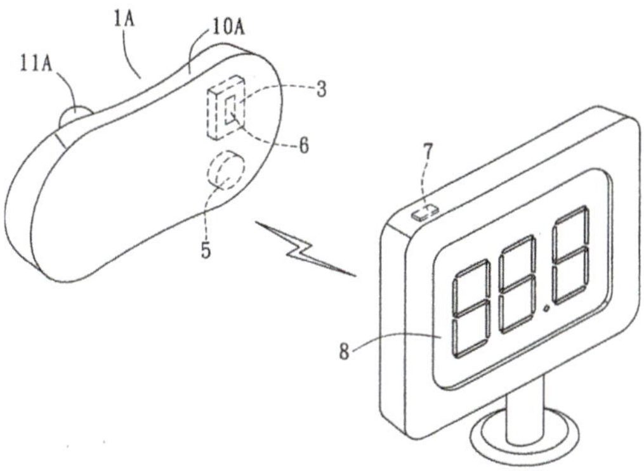

Fig. 9 Wireless transmission of the intelligent pacifier.

5. Conclusion

This study proposed an intelligent pacifier that can accurately detect the sucking pressure and objectively judging the pressure standard, in order to solve the problem of determining the best feeding time for newborn infants or premature infants who have sufficient sucking ability. The inherent safety method and Su-Fields Analysis of the TRIZ method were applied to design a pacifier sensing device. Fool-proof and (Making Incorrect Assembly Impossible) and simplification were adopted to prevent the feeding hazards. Su-Fields Analysis and 76 Standard Solutions were applied to provide a reference basis for the components of the intelligent pacifier. Solidworks was used to design the prototype. The strain gauge sensor could detect the distortion of the pacifier during sucking, and the computing module was used to find out the accurate sucking pressure of the infants. The measured data were displayed on the screen, allowing the caretakers to determine the best feeding time. This is a useful tool for infant care. The features of the proposed design include: (1) accurately determine the sucking pressure: the strain gauge sensor and computing module can accurately record the sucking pressure of the infants, allow the caretakers to determine the best feeding time, and prevent complications of over-fatigue and dyspnoea during feeding; (2) objectively determine the sucking pressure standard: the strain gauge sensor is a precise sensing device that can implement a consistent standard for all infants, thus making the measured sucking pressure highly objective, and prevent the human errors in finger test.

References

1. Boiron M., Da Nobrega L., Roux S., Henrot A., and Saliba E. (2007) "Effects of oral stimulation and oral support on non- nutritive sucking and feeding performance in preterm infants." *Developmental Medicine & Child Neurology,* 49(6), pp. 439-444.
2. Capilouto G. J., Cunningham T., Frederick E., Dupont-Versteegden E., Desai N., and Butterfield T.A. (2014) "Comparison of tongue muscle characteristics of preterm and full term infants during nutritive and nonnutritive sucking." *Infant Behavior and Development,* 37(3), pp. 435-445.
3. Elvik R. (2010) "Sources of uncertainty in estimated benefits of road safety programmes." *Accident Analysis and Prevention*, 42(6), pp. 2171-2178.
4. Fucile S., Gisel E., Schanler R. J., and Lau C. (2009) "A controlled-flow vacuum-free bottle system enhances preterm infants' nutritive sucking skills." *Dysphagia*, 24(2), pp. 145-151.

5. Hansson S.O. (2010) "Promoting inherent safety." *Process Safety and Environmental Protection,* 88 (3), May, pp. 168-172.
6. Holloway E. M. (2014) "The dynamic process of assessing infant feeding readiness." *Newborn and Infant Nursing Reviews,* 14(3), pp.119-123.
7. Howe T. H., Sheu C. F., Hsieh Y.W., and Hsieh C. L. (2007) "Psychometric characteristics of the Neonatal Oral- Motor Assessment Scale in healthy preterm infants." *Developmental Medicine & Child Neurology*, 49(12), pp. 915-919.
8. Lau C. (2006) "Oral feeding in the preterm infant." *NeoReviews*, 7(1), pp. e19-e27.
9. Lau C., Alagugurusamy R., Schanler R., Smith E., and Shulman R. (2000) "Characterization of the developmental stages of sucking in preterm infants during bottle feeding." *Acta Paediatrica*, 89(7), pp. 846-852.
10. Lau C. and Smith E. (2011) "A novel approach to assess oral feeding skills of preterm infants." *Neonatology*, 100(1), pp. 64-70.
11. Leong C.T. and Shariff A.M. (2008) "Inherent safety index module (ISIM) to assess inherent safety level during preliminary design stage." *Process Safety and Environmental Protection*. 86 (2), pp. 113-119.
12. Lin Y.C. (2011) "Applying Su-Fields Analysis and Morphological Analysis on Rescue Ventilation Device for Vehicles." *Minghsin Journa,* 37(2),
pp. 39-49.
13. Lu H.C. (2012) "Try to Improve Equipment and Facility Inherent Safety." *Industrial Safety and Health*, 277, pp. 57-62.
14. Mizuno K., Nishida Y., Taki M., Hibino S., Murase M., Sakurai M., and Itabashi K. (2007) "Infants with bronchopulmonary dysplasia suckle with weak pressures to maintain breathing during feeding." *Pediatrics*, 120(4), pp. e1035-e1042.
15. Mizuno K. and Ueda A. (2003) "The maturation and coordination of sucking, swallowing, and respiration in preterm infants." *The Journal of Pediatrics*, 142(1), pp. 36-40.
16. Rocha A. D., Lopes J. M. D. A., Ramos J. R. M., Gomes S. C., Lucena S. L., Medeiros A., and Moreira, M. E. L. (2011) "Development of a technique for evaluating temporal parameters of sucking in breastfeeding preterm newborns." *Early Human Development*, 87(8), pp. 545-548.
17. Shariff, A.M. Leong C.T. and Zaini D. (2012) "Using process stream index (PSI) to assess inherent safety level during preliminary design stage." *Safety Science*, 50(4), pp. 1098-1103.

18. Sheu D.D. and Hou C. T. (2013) "TRIZ-based trimming for process-machine improvements: Slit-valve innovative redesign." *Computers & Industrial Engineering*, 66(3), pp. 555-566.
19. Song, M. J. Lee J. G., Park J. M. and Lee S. (2012) "Triggering navigators for innovative system design: The case of lab-on-a-chip technology." *Expert Systems with Applications,* 39, pp. 12451–12459.
20. Srinivasan R. and Kraslawski A. (2006) "Application of the TRIZ creativity enhancement approach to design of inherently safer chemical processes." *Chemical Engineering & Processing*, 45(6), pp. 507-514.
21. Sung M. H. (2009) TRIZ Systematic Innovation Theory and Application. Ting Mao Publishing, Taipei.
22. White-Traut R., Rankin K., Lucas R., Shapiro N., Liu L., and Medoff-Cooper B. (2013) "Evaluating sucking maturation using two pressure thresholds." *Early Human Development*, 89(10), pp. 833-837.
23. Wrotniak B. H., Stettler N., and Medoff-Cooper B. (2009) "The relationship between birth weight and feeding maturation in preterm infants." *Acta Paediatric*, 98(2), pp. 2
24. 86-290.
25. Yan W., Zanni-Merk, C. Rousselot F., Cavallucci D. and Collet P. (2013) "A New Method of Using Physical Effects in Su-field Analysis based on Ontology Reasoning." *Procedia Computer Science*, 22, pp. 30-39.

Medical Fluorescence Imaging Processing System Based on 2CCD Camera

Yanxiang Wang*, Mingquan Wang , Yu Wang
Key Laboratory of Instrumentation Science & Dynamic Measurement, Ministry of Education, Key Laboratory of Electronic Test Technology, North University of China, Taiyuan, 030051, China
*757116245@qq.com

Xiaofeng Yang,
Shanxi Medical University Taiyuan, 030051, China

In this paper, the 2CCD camera AD-080CL of the JAI company was studied, design of visible light and near infrared image fusion algorithm for the fluorescence imaging system. And use MFC application architecture built the supporting software system in VS2010 environment. The system consists of the same optical path for visible light and near infrared image, ensure the two lines of the same vision, it's convenient to set up and adjust and more practical and low cost. Image processing better fusion results achieved the purpose of the display area of fluorescent tags in visible light image, and possesses the advantages of simple rapid and suitable for engineering development. Software has achieved the basic functions such as real-time display and save the video image.

Keywords: 2CCD; fluorescence imaging; picture processing; software system.

1. Introduction

This subject use living creatures injected with fluorescent markers as the research object, the system software is based on 2CCD camera, it's function is fluorescence image fusion. We achieve real-time detection of an injection of fluorescent markers of organisms, display fluorescent area and related process.

At present, there are various optical molecular imaging detection system, general with computed tomography (CT) technology as a major means of detection, often using single channel CCD camera for optical signal receiver [1], most of these systems is an external light source excitation in fluorescent markers for image signal [2], using filter combined with CCD camera used for single fluorescence images [3]. In order to realize visible light and near infrared shows at the same time, the traditional solution, is still expensive [4,5], difficult to deploy. AD-080CL uses the prism spectroscopic technology, collects near infrared and visible light at the same time, enables users to ensure the road visual unity, thus the software will be developed more easily.

2. Systematic Hardware Components and Their Operation Principles

The camera is equipped with the base, bracket, bearing beam, when used, the experiment bench under the camera. The hardware system include mobile armrest which drives the camera under the support of loading arm horizontal or vertical movement. Around the camera installed circular LED lights, including fluorescent excitation light source and lighting light source.

When system is working, excitation light exposure on the tested organism, fluorescent markers launch near infrared light, light of emission and lighting light is reflected to the camera at the same time, filter in front of the lens filter out the excitation light. Optical signal through the prism is divided into visible light and near infrared light, two optical signals respectively through the corresponding light-sensitive chips and be converted to electrical signals transmitted to the computer, processed by the software.

3. Image Processing Algorithm Design

3.1. *Visible light and near infrared image fusion directly*

The visible light image is three-channel, but the near infrared image is stored in a matrix. Different data types cannot be operated for the same type of operation. So we define a three-channel image, then replace the value of each channel with the value of gray image.

The fusion algorithm can use weighted average method, Fourier transform method and wavelet transform fusion method, the wavelet transform fusion method gets the image whose brightness is good, better retain the information in the visible light image. However, such fusion cannot highlight the fluorescent part of near infrared image.

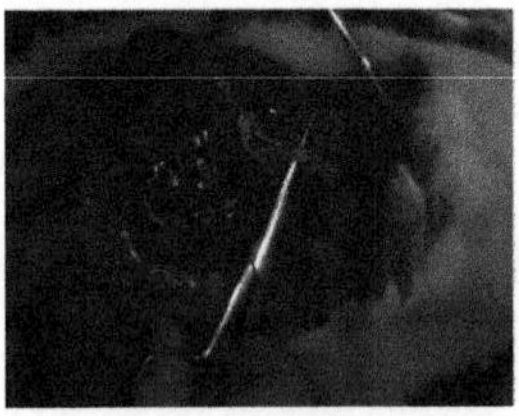

Fig. 1 Visible light image.

Fig. 2 Near infrared image.

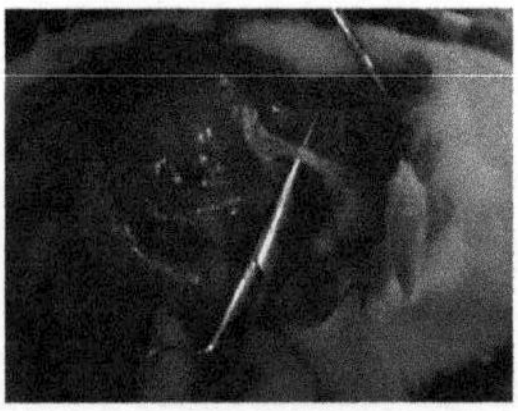

Fig. 3Wavelet transform fusion image.

3.2. *False color fusion*

At first, use frequency domain pseudo color fusion to process the near infrared image. then deal with the output filter with appropriate processing, make it as the three primary input, the finally completed image is formed according to frequency distribution characteristics of the original gray image.

Gray image after dealing with the pseudo color image and fusion with visible light image can achieve better fusion result, but the detail information in the near infrared image is weakened, and more complex fusion algorithm will be waste more time, that is not conducive to real-time display.

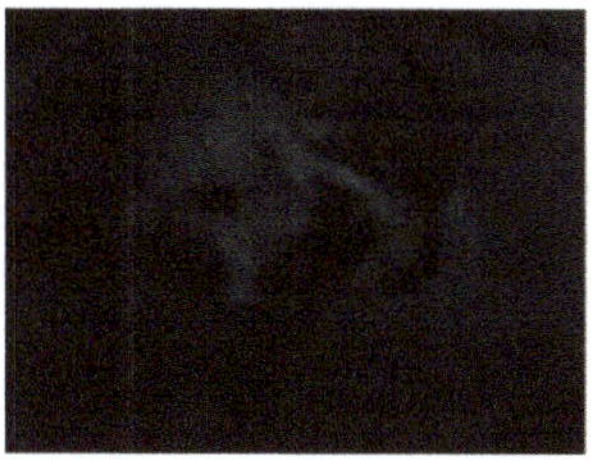

Fig. 4 This is the pseudo-color image.

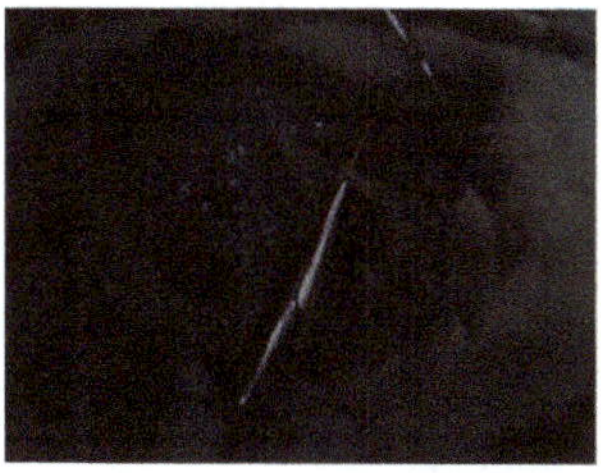

Fig. 5 This is the fusion image.

3.3. *Color component replacement*

To reflect information of gray image the color image, we can change color image using the gray scale information of a single color in the color values. Use near infrared image grey value directly replace the green component of the visible light image color values. The follow-up handling is to fuse with visible light image in order to correct fluorescent influence in other areas.

After changing color image using the gray scale information, the area of visible light image without fluorescent tags has also been replaced the green component, so result in chromatic aberration. Fuse the image with visible light image using original fusion methods in order to correct this problem. We choose weighted average fusion method.

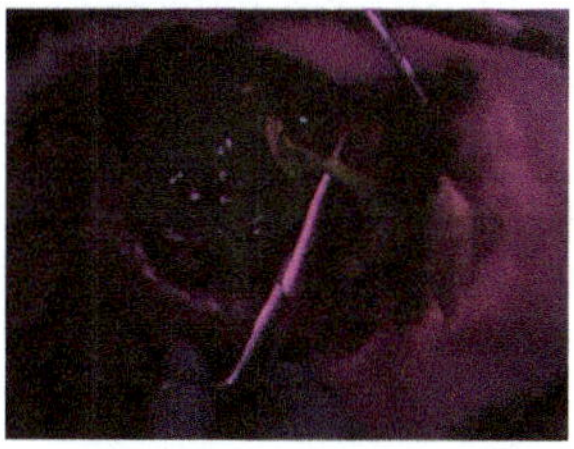

Fig. 6 This is the color replaced image.

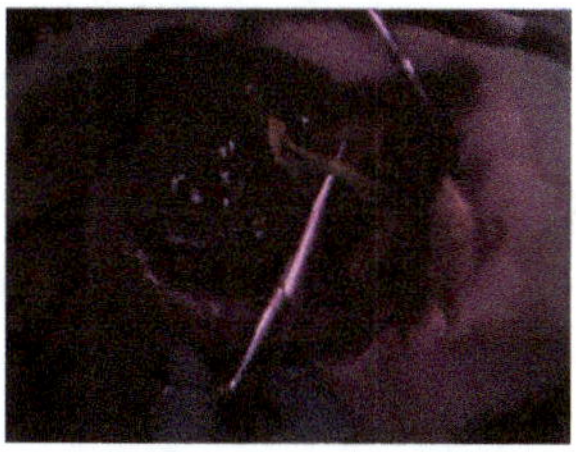

Fig. 7 This is the weighted average fusion image.

4. Software System Development

JAI SDK provides interface function, each interface function through its specific protocol can achieve its specific function such as camera connection, close and imaging, correction, image transmission, etc.

The software requests to carry on the real-time display and operations such as data acquisition, save pictures, record video and so on. Besides, there are three different windows respectively show visible light image, near infrared image and fusion image. In order to solve the real-time and multitasking, multithreaded programming is an ideal choice [6].

Establish a MFC project, add header files and link library files and control sources to the project, explicit reference the interface functions provided by JAI SDK. After open the camera, we need to call interface function for the following information of image. The callback function will realize the variable transformation from the data stream to image, we need to define image variables use Iplimage format, used to hold and handle collected images. The subsequent image processing, storage, video, and other functions are realized by using OpenCV.

Acknowledgments

This work was supported by Projects from National Natural Science Foundation of China (No. 61171177) and Natural Science Foundation for Young Scientists of Shanxi Province (No. 2012021011-1, 2015021086).

References

1. Jing Liu, Optical molecular imaging technology and its application in the field of drug development, *Acta Biophysica Sinica*, **8**, 27 (2011).
2. Y. Nakayama, P. J. Pauzauskie, A. Radenovie et al, Tunable nanowire nonlinear optical, *Nature*, **7148**, 447 (2007).
3. Dawei Deng, et al, Two kinds of near-infrared fluorescent probe synthesis and tumor targeted research, *Chinese Journal of Lasers*, **11**, 37 (2010).
4. Susan L. Troyan, Vida Kianzad, et al, The FLARETM Intraoperative Near-Infrared Fluorescence Imaging System: A First-in-Human Clinical Trial in Breast Cancer Sentinel Lymph Node Mapping, *Ann Surg Onco*,16 (2009).
5. Alec M. De Grand, John V. Frangioni, An Operational Near-Infrared Fluorescence Imaging System Prototype for Large Animal Surgery, *Technology in Cancer Research & Treatment*, **6**, 2 (2003).
6. Faliang Chang, Multithreading under multimedia timer in the application of fast data acquisition, Computer Technology, 2003, 23: 176-178.

Identification and Characterization of E. Coli Producing ESBLs Isolates from Pediatric Settings

Li Qu[a] and Mingcheng Li[b]
College of Public Health, Beihua University, Jilin, Jilin, China
E-mail: [a]chenning_qu@163.com, [b]Limingcheng1964@163.com
www.Beihua University.edu

To study the genotype and antimicrobial mechanism of ESBLs among E. coli. The strains that produced the ESBLs were tested by the disk diffusion; plasmid spectrum were used to detect the genotype of E. coli. There were 53 isolates producing ESBLs. The number of natural plasmid was 4 to 5, the size is about 2.0-40kp.

Keywords: Escherichia coli; extended-spectrumβ-lactamases; resistance plasmid.

1. Introduction

Escherichia coli is the most common clinical pathogens, it infected widely. ESBLs can hydrolyze β-lactam broad-spectrum antibiotics such as the first, second and third-generation cephalosporins and aztreonam, it can spread by plasmid mediated between bacteria [1]. The author collected the resistant strains from pediatric respiratory infections samples and preliminary discussed on distribution characteristics of resistance genes producing by E. coli with ESBLs.*

2. Materials and Methods

2.1. *Bacteria*

Escherichia coli was isolated from children with respiratory tract specimens and collected in Jilin three level hospitals from January 2010 to December 2012 during antibiotic therapy for more than three days. 149 strains of E. coli by cultivated and identified were advantage bacterium or pathogenic bacteria. Operating in accordance with the requirements of the third edition of the

* Work partially supported by the Health Department Funding Research Project in Jilin Province, China (20112108).
† Corresponding Author.

national clinical test procedures [2].

2.2. *Phenotypic identification*

Initial screening experiments according to the standard disk diffusion method [3]. Phenotypic confirmatory test uses both ceftazidime (30μg), ceftazidime/clavulanic acid (30/10μg) and cephalosporin cefotaxime (30μg) and cephalosporins, cefotaxime/clavulanic acid (30/10μg), any one put in clavulanic acid, inhibition zone diameter increased ≥5mm, can confirm the strains producing ESBLs.

2.3. *Drug resistant plasmid extraction*

Plasmid were extracted with a QIA quick plasmid extraction kit according to the instruction book (5ml system, room temperature). Agarose gel electrophoresis using 0.6% agarose gel electrophoresis for 12 h, using pBR322 as Marker, photographic gel imaging system is analyzed.

3. Results

3.1. *Detection Rate of Strains Producing ESBLs*

149 strains of E. coli isolated from clinical according to NCCLS recommended standard , 53 strains were confirmed producing ESBLs strains by phenotype confirmation experiment, ESBLs detection rate is 35.6%.

3.2. *Analysis of plasmid spectrum*

Plasmid spectrum of E. coli strains isolated from clinical is diversiform, plasmid spectrum of E. coli producing ESBLs is similar. General the number of natural plasmid was 4 to 5, the size is about 2.0-40kp, plasmid spectrum of no producing ESBLs strains is a single, only two types of plasmid (Figure 1).

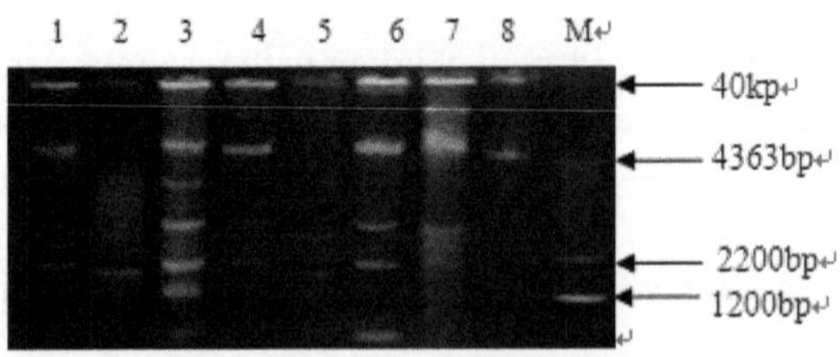

Figure 1 Agarose gel electrophoresis detect plasmid spectrum of E. coli

Lane 1,3,4,6,7: ESBLs; lane2,5,8:non- ESBLs; M: pBR322

4. Discussion

E. coli is one of the most common clinical gram-negative pathogenic bacteria, which is the most common producing ESBLs strains. ESBLs can hydrolyze penicillin, cephalosporin and aztreonam, make its loss of bactericidal activity. It can make the sensitive bacteria become resistant bacteria and cause severe nosocomial cross infection, make the spread of drug-resistant bacteria. In this study, the positive strains in phenotypic confirmatory test wereamplified by PCRusingspecific β-lactamase geneprimers, Which of blaTEM, blaSHV and blaCTX-M were amplified the expected size fragment.

There were different mechanisms in the nosocomial infection pathogens to β-lactam antibiotics resistance. Beijing, Shanghai and Taiwan with producing extended-spectrum epidemic strains mainly, the type of CTX-M ismore commongenotypebecause of cefotaxime and ceftriaxonebeingthe most important third-generation phalosporinsinclinical[4]. The type of CTX-M enzyme has powerful hydrolytic activity to cefotaxime and ceftriaxone, but poorhydrolytic to ceftazidime. ESBLs genotype were mostly of type CTX-M as the most common extended-spectrum β-lactamase in Beijing, Shanghai, Zhejiang and Guangzhou, the detection rate has exceeded the type of TEM and SHV ESBLs[5].

It is an important content of epidemiological investigation to analysis plasmid mass spectrometry of infection strains. The investigation helps to determine popular root and to find infection way. So it can prevent and control the occurrence of hospital infection effectively[6]. This study collected 149 strains of E. coli, producing ESBLs isolates have the same plasmid spectrum, they were from the same period or the same hospital, department, may be the same clone strains. The clone strains may cause small nosocomial infection of epidemic in local hospital. Clinical should pay attention to the producing ESBLs strains the homology of monitoring and to prevent the spread of the same clone strains.

Because of selectivepressurein antibiotics,rationaluse of antibioticsisan important meanstofight against multi-resistant. Therefore, the first is rational use of β-lactam antibiotics especiallybroad-spectrumcephalosporins.Strictly limited andreasonableuseof the third and the fourthgeneration cephalosporinsin order to reduce the emergenceand prevalence of strainsproducing ESBLs. We shouldavoidtheapplicationofinadequate dosage. The second, the patientinfection strains producing ESBLs should be immediatelyisolatedtopreventcross-infectioncaused bythe outbreak, andthe doctor selects of effective drugsas soon as possible, pay attention todose, and enough treatment. We should proper applicate themedical devices suchasintubation and ventilator, detect antimicrobial resistance in hospital of high-riskareas. It needs the joint efforts of clinical laboratories and clinicians to prevent and control prevalent of ESBLs[7].

The study revealed the source and mechanism of E. coli drug resistance in jilin area from molecular level for the pediatric respiratory tract infection, to reveal the spread of antibiotic resistance, to put forward the control strategy of drug resistance generation and transmission, to prevent or reduce hospital infection effectively, to guide the clinical reasonable application of antibiotics. So this study has important and far-reaching significance.

References

1. Gootz TD. The forgotten Gram-negative bacilli: What genetic determinantsare tellingus about the spread of antibiotic resistnace. Biochem Pharmaco, 2006, Vol. 71, pp. 1073-1084.
2. China's ministry of health department. 2006. National clinical test procedures. The third edition.
3. National Committee for Clinical Laboratory Standard, 2002 Performance Standards for Antimicrobial Susceptibility Testing. NCCLS, Wayne, Pa
4. Wu J L, Gu H G, Yu Y S.The drug resistance strains producing ESBLs and the genotype distribution of β-lactamases. Zhejiang medicine, 2005, Vol. 27, pp. 401-403.
5. Cao J G, He X F, Wu D. The Distribution and Drug Resistance of the Common Clinical Gram-Negative Bacillus. Microbiology journal, 2006, Vol.33, pp.188-191.
6. Zhang J, Bao Q Y, Zhang H Q. Antibiotic plasmid profile and genotypes of extended-spectrum β-lactamase producers in multi-drug resistant Escherichia coli. Chinese journal of antibiotics, 2006, Vol. 31, pp. 198.
7. Molecular clone [M]. Cold Spring, 2006.

Experimental Study on Human Knee Joint Instantaneous Center*

Run Ji and Lifeng Li
National Research Center for Rehabilitation Technical Aids
Beijing, 100176, China
E-mail: zhegeshuiyong@163.com

Sa Wang and Jianfeng Li
College of Mechanical Engineering and Applied Electronics Technology,
Beijing University of Technology, Beijing, 100124,China
†*E-mail: everywhere0823@163.com*
www.bjut.edu.cn

The research on instantaneous center of human knee joint is one of more important research areas of knee joint biomechanics research. In this paper, NDI OPTOTRAK optical motion capturing system was adopted to measure the movement information of knee joint of one adult male. A simple and efficient method about calculating instantaneous center of human knee joint was provided. To avoid experiment error caused by improper operation, Planar fitting and cubic polynomial fitting was applied in processing data. The result provide reference for assembling and designing clinical prosthetic knee.

Keywords: Human knee joint; instantaneous center; planar fitting; motion capture.

1. Introduction

The theoretical foundation of human motion biomechanics, includes mechanics, anatomy, physiology and other subjects, is a subject to study mechanics problems in the human body. In recent years, the research on biomechanics of knee joint has aroused great biomechanics and rehabilitation engineering experts' attention. Establishment and application of human knee joint motion simulation model is an important method for knee joint biomechanics research. The development and application of computer technology and its software and hardware makes building, analyzing and calculating of model more fast and

* This work is supported by National Research Center for Rehabilitation Technical Aids basic scientific research expenses (1181400900101); National Natural Science Foundation of China (61273342); Beijing Natural Science Foundation (3132005).

† Email to the Corresponding author.

accurate. With the development of related technologies, the research on the biomechanics of the model of knee joint enable promote development of the biomechanics of the knee joint, pathology of knee joint and rehabilitation guidance, and prosthetic knee.

The research on biomechanics of knee joint mainly includes the impacts of joint motion and stress on movement, joint contact, deformation and stress of muscles and ligaments. Interface movement of femoral and tibial is Rolling of the femoral condyle relative to the tibial and relative shift of the contact surface. Zuppinger attributed and confirmed the mechanism of knee movement to cross four-link mechanism formed by ligament [1]. Kettlekamp studied the tibiofemoral joint contact on the dead body in 1972 [2]. Muller et al. found that the length of the profile curves of articular surface of the femoral condyle articular surface is much larger than the length of the tibial plateau, and femoral movement in the tibial plateau is the rolling movement and sliding movement. O'Connor et al. drew a conclusion: flexion of bilateral contact surfaces are backward shift, just the lateral shift is greater than medial shift, and it is different from femoral condyle movement. However, there is a doubt that PCL are not in the state of tension [3]. His conclusion is no clear that the impacts and relationships between flexion and changes of instantaneous center of knee. Blacharski et al. applied of photographic technology to calculate the instantaneous center axis of knee joint angle of the continuous stretch. But, they only studied a particular way of bearing, so their results have not been widely used. In 1979. Van Dijk et al used data in Blacharski's paper and provided a method that marks the ACL and PCL and calculated the motion of the femoral-tibial [4]. However, this method also applied in the dead body.

Due to the practical experiments on the dead body lacks physiological environment of the human body and the structures and motion characteristics of knee joint, contact between the parameters of knee motion is highly dependent on the load conditions: constraints of muscles and ligaments. Several studies have investigated the instantaneous center of human knee joint. Marta Kordasz et al. [5] provided a method that based on X-ray scan image and calculated he instantaneous center of human knee joint. Stefan Moser [6] developed a variable knee, using the instantaneous center of cross four-bar mechanism simulated the instantaneous center of human knee. Radcliffe [7] built mathematical model of centorde of four-link knee and stability, and conducted common four-bar linkage knee joint gait analysis. Jin et al have further investigated in the field of human gait and intelligent knee joint [8, 9, 10]. However, algorithms for the human knee joint are often complex. X-ray methods have large limit and X-ray have undesirable effects. Designing prosthetic knee requires reference of instantaneous center of human knee joint. There is less literature giving valves of centrodes.

This paper through NDI OPTOTRAK optical motion capturing system measure movement information of knee joint of one adult male and obtain the spatial position coordinates of thigh and shank. And this paper will provide a simple and efficient method about calculating instantaneous center of knee joint.

2. Materials and Methods

2.1. *Subjects*

One adult male (aged: 24 weight: 85kg, height: 1.80 m, leg length: 970mm,) with no neurological disorders and heart and lung disease, and no lower limb muscles, bone disorders performed gait sit the chair. The volunteer was told steps and purpose of this experiment.

2.2. *Methods*

The measurements were realized in Human Biomechanics laboratory of National Research Center for Rehabilitation Technical Aids using NDI OPTOTRAK optical motion capturing system. NDI optical motion capturing system determine the trajectory of an object during motion using optical positioning method, Optical positioning method is widely used, mainstream and high precision positioning method [2]. Its advantages are high accuracy, flexible and convenient for handling, the disadvantage is susceptible to be blocked, the influence of ambient light and specular reflection from metal objects. Optical positioning method observes the target area through CCD-array camera, and then reconstructs the spatial location of the target based on the stereoscopic principle. CCD-array measuring system consist two CCD-array cameras at least using a standard lens. each light point in the image defines the projection line of space, the intersection of the space and the projection line can be calculated using camera, and three-dimensional coordinates of the point that regarded as experimental data are obtained. To ensure the accuracy of the experimental results, the experiment carried out with the subject who chose his own feel-good condition. Marks were attached to the thigh and the shank respectively. Four small marks exists on each big mark, which attached to the rigid body, In order to eliminate the errors from the undesired movements, the upper leg is firmly wrapped on a chair using plastic tape. During the experiment, each data acquisition time is 5 seconds, the acquisition frequency of 100Hz, subjects continuously curved leg and continuous acquired 5-6 groups of data. The location of the markers is illustrated in Fig. 1 and Fig. 2.

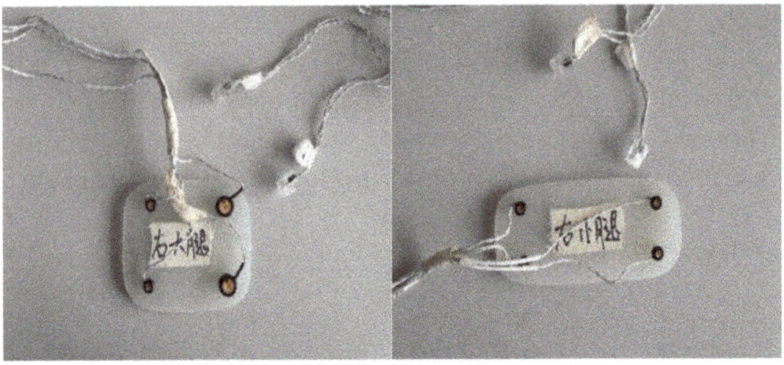

Fig. 1 Markers of thigh and shank.

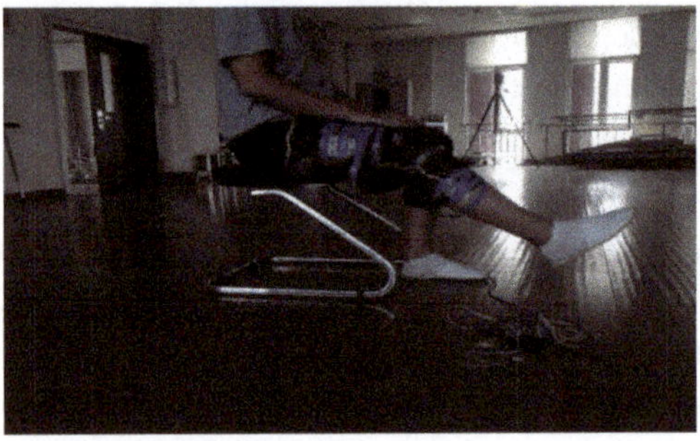

Fig. 2 Location of markers.

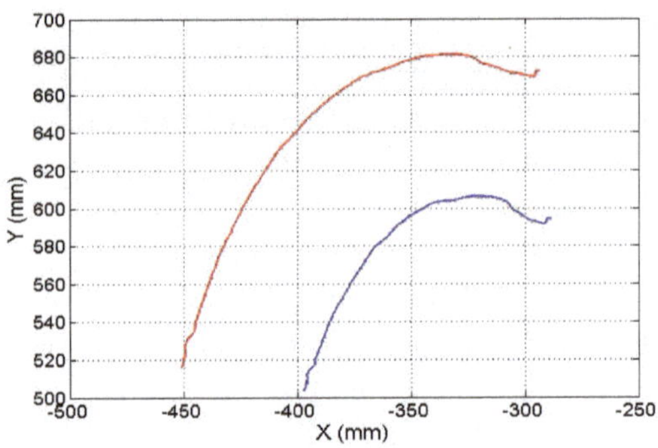

Fig. 3 Trajectory of markers.

3. Experiment Results and Processing

The first stage of keypoint detection is to identify locations and scales that can be repeatably assigned under differing views of the same object. Detecting locations that are invariant to scale change of the image can be accomplished by searching for stable features across all possible scales, using a continuous function of scale known as scale space. It has been shown by Koenderink [14] and Lindeberg [15] that under a variety of reasonable assumptions the only possible scale-space kernel is the Gaussian function. Therefore, the scale space of an image is defined as a function, $L(x, y,\sigma)$, that is produced from the convolution of a variable-scale Gaussian, $G(x, y, \sigma)$, with an inpuExperimental data include spatial position coordinates X, Y, and Z directions of the mark point, According to the experimental program settings, the thigh remain intact throughout the experiment and markers on the shank form a trajectory in space. X, Y direction of location coordinates of two landmarks were selected from four markers. Trajectory is illustrated in Fig. 3.

Due to deviations caused by attaching position of landmarks on the thigh and the shank. In order to reduce this error, MATLAB was used to programming, regress function was adopted to fit 'sagittal plane' using eight landmarks from the thigh and the shank. Plane equation can be expressed as follow.

$$Z_{fit} = a * Y_{fit} + b * X_{fit} + c \tag{1}$$

Where, a , b , c are constant. Plane fitting are illustrated in Fig. 4.

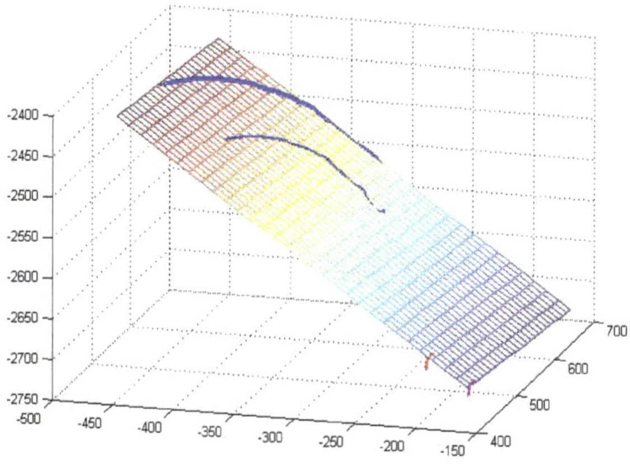

Fig. 4 Plane fitting-'sagittal plane'.

The two small landmarks from the shank were projected onto 'sagittal plane'. Specific steps as follows: spatial coordinates of random landmark is set to $U_{shank} = (U_x, U_y, U_z)$.

$$n = \sqrt{a^2 + b^2 + c^2} \tag{2}$$

$$m = -(a * U_x + b * U_y + c * U_z) \tag{3}$$

$$k = m / n \tag{4}$$

According to equation (1), (2) and (3), we get new coordinates of random landmark in the 'sagittal plane': $I_{shank} = (I_x, I_y, I_z)$.

Where,

$$I_x = U_x + k * a \tag{5}$$

$$I_y = U_y + k * b \tag{6}$$

$$I_z = U_z + k * c \tag{7}$$

In order to get intersection of normal of two curves on the shank, we need use curve fitting techniques. Although there are many types of curve fitting methods, only the polynomial function type are chosen for this study. Cftool Fitting Toolbox in MATLAB was adopted to fit curves. Index of assessment include: R-square is close to 1, indicating that the model fits the data are better. Adjusted R-square is close to 1, indicating that the better fit. RMSE is closer to 0, indicating that the data fit better. The loci of the marked points can be described as continuous functions as equation (8) and (9), curves are illustrated in Fig. (5), Indexes of assessment are presented in Table 1.

$$f_1(x) = 1.56 * 10^{-4} * x_1^3 + 9.07 * 10^{-2} * x_1^2 + 25.49 * x_1 + 2929 \tag{8}$$

$$f_2(x) = 6.11 * 10^{-5} * x_2^3 + 5.6 * 10^{-2} * x_2^2 + 16.93 * x_2 + 2355 \tag{9}$$

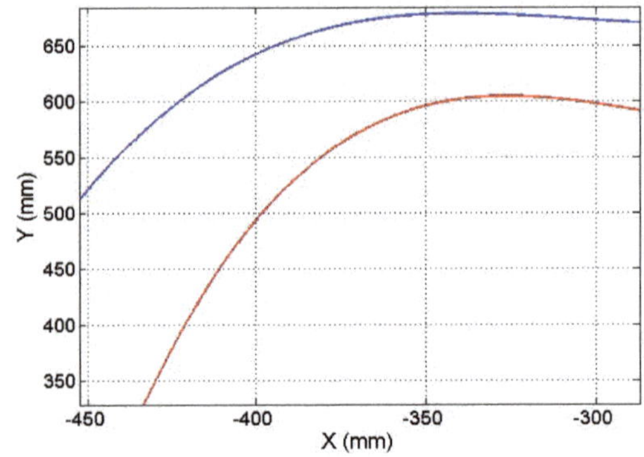

Fig. 5 Curve fitting by polynomial function.

Table 1 Results of goodness of fit.

	R-square	Adjusted R-square	RMSE
$f_1(x)$	0.9983	0.9983	1.567
$f_2(x)$	0.9991	0.9991	1.942

According to Table 1, three Indexes of assessment are close to the ideal value, which indicates the curve fitted better.

For the equation ($y = f(x)$) fitting by polynomial, the slope of the tangent at any point (such as, point $(a, f(a))$), the slope of the normal is $k = -1/f'(a)$. So, the normal equation of the curvecan be described as follows:

$$y = f_1(x) + k*(x-a) \tag{10}$$

Use of Equation (8)-(10), we can get intersection of normal of two curves and plot data what we have obtained in MATLAB. The centrode of knee joint is illustrated in Fig. 6, coordinate values of centrode of knee joint are presented in Table 2.

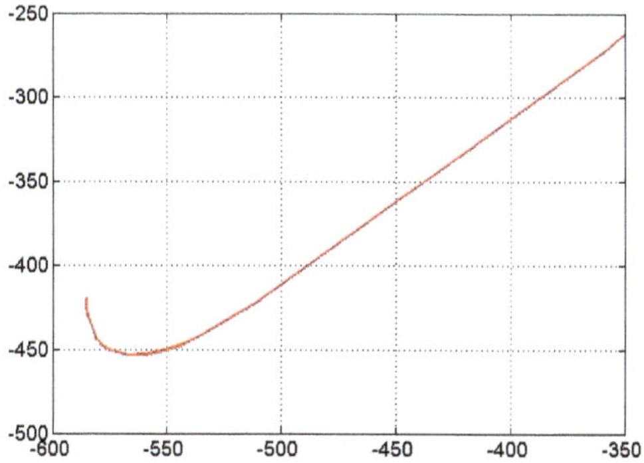

Fig. 6 The centrode of knee joint.

Table 2 Coordinate values of centrode of knee joint.

	1	2	3	4	5	6
X(mm)	-358.9	-511.0	-535.9	-542.2	-550.5	-599.1
Y(mm)	-272.2	-422.7	-442.8	-446.7	-450.6	-453.2
	7	8	9	10	11	12
X(mm)	-567.0	-575.1	-577.7	-579.9	-580.8	-584.2
Y(mm)	-453.6	-450.3	-447.7	-444.6	-443.0	-430.2
	13	14	15	16	17	18
X(mm)	-584.6	-584.8	-584.9	-584.7	-584.6	-584.7
Y(mm)	-427.1	-426.7	-426.4	-420.8	-420.1	-420.8

4. Conclusion

NDI OPTOTRAK optical motion capturing system was adopted to measure the movement information of knee joint of one adult male. Multiple linear regression function was adopted to fit plane, which reduced experiment error caused by improper operation. Equation of the loci of the marked points was obtained from fitting curves by polynomial function type. Through intersection of normal of two curves, we get centrode of knee joint. This method is simple and efficient. The result provide reference for assembling and designing clinical prosthetic knee.

References

1. J. Goodfellow, J. O'Connor, The mechanics of the knee and prosthesis design. Journal of Bone and Joint Surgery, 3, 358 (1978).
2. D.B. Kettelkamp, A.W. Jacobs. Tibiofemoral contact area-determination and implications. Journal of Bone and Joint Surgery, 54, 349(1972).
3. S. Nakagawa, The posterior cruciate ligament during flexion of the normal knee. Journal of Bone and Joint Surgery. Vol. 86, pp. 450-456, Apr. 2004.
4. X.S. Wang, R.P. Bai, REVIEW ON BIOMECHANICAL MODELLING FOR HUMAN KNEE JOINT. ADVANCES IN MECHANICS, 29, 244 (1999).
5. M. Kordasz, P. Sauer, Automatic determination of knee kinematics for lower limb rehabilitation manipulator design, 2013 9th Workshop on Robot Motion and Control (RoMoco), 86 (2013).
6. S. Moser, Development of a variable knee joint, bachelor thesis, Swiss Federal Institute of Technology Zurich, (2013).
7. C.W. Radcliffe, M.S. Deg, Biomechanics of Knee Stability Control with Four-Bar Prosthetic Knees, ISPO Australia Annual Meeting Melboume, Australia, (2003).
8. R.C. Wang, Q. Shen, D.W. Jin, Advances in intelligent prosthetic knee joint. Chinese Journal of Rehabilitation Medicine, 22, 1093 (2007).
9. Y.Y. Yang, R.C. Wang, Y.L. Wang, D.W. Jin, S.Y. Tian, Humanoid Design and Movement Simulation of a New Knee Prosthesis, 19, 72 (2008).
10. F. Cheng, R.C. Wang, X.H, Jia, J.C. Zhang, Advances in partial weight support treadmill training. Chinese Journal of Rehabilitation Medicine, 23, 366 (2008).

CHAPTER 4

Technology for Education

Flipping Language Study in Classroom Instruction

Guimei Xie
Beijing Wuzi University, School of Foreign Languages and Cultures,
Beijing, China, 101149
E-mail: xieguimei@bwu.edu.cn
www.bwu.edu.cn

The way we teach and learn is at a once-a-millennium turning point. Language study is improved mostly through mastery learning both in classroom and routine life. The traditional classroom instruction is no longer as effective as before with the advancement of modern information technology. This is where the flipped classroom model could function well. Flipped classroom instruction model can both improve students' achievement and classroom performance and bring a very fundamental and significant effect: the good cultivation of critical thinking in high education classroom which is critical in bring forth both the teacher's and students' potential and creativity.

Keywords: Flipped classroom instruction model; language learning; mastery learning.

1. Introduction

While everyone has a say in education, we agree that we should not limit our students to our own learning, for they were born in a totally different world from ours and they are more equipped in this modern world with loads of information and the internationally connected internet world. And there are a lot of free education programs all around us through internet media. While the traditional classroom model is too often a passive and simple way of learning for students where there are less active processing of information with the teacher disseminating almost all the knowledge and information unilaterally to students in the classroom. Students behaved passively and were pushed in groups with a one-pace-fits-all style. Meanwhile, new technologies offer options for more effective ways of teaching and learning. That is the reason why flipped classroom instruction model come to us. This paper is about the advantages and benefits of flipped classroom instruction in college English classroom teaching.

2. Flipped Classroom Instruction in English Instruction

Flipped classroom is a new instructional strategy and a type of blended learning that reverses the traditional educational arrangement by delivering instructional content outside of the classroom and moves activities, including those that may have traditionally been considered homework, into the classroom. Simply speaking, flipped classroom study is the one whose main contents are done independently at a student's free time at home/dorm at his own pace, and the thing that teachers and students do in classroom is problem-solving. The flipped classroom intentionally shifts instruction to a learner-centered model in which class time is dedicated to exploring topics in greater depth and creating meaningful learning opportunities. In a flipped classroom content delivery may take a variety of forms. Often teaching materials recommended by the teacher are used as a content delivery mechanism (cited from Wikipedia).

In my instruction for my *College English Reading and Writing Course*, I borrowed the flipped classroom model particularly and accustomed it to my own instruction by assigning the task of passage reading before the classroom instruction, including students' own understanding of every word, every sentence, every phrase and then try to converse with their group members what they have learned from the text after class with the help of modern information technology including modern multimedia through internet. My students are not used to language self-study since after graduating from their middle school where the first and main purpose of language study is to pass the college entrance exam and be enrolled by a key university. About 50% of the students are not used to self-study and always rely on teachers to lead them and force them to study and explain every points of English grammar, sentence structures and ways of conducting a passage or a writing. They are relieved in some degree after being accepted by a local municipal university and what most of them want is a diploma. They are expecting teachers to tell them all the things with the same expectation as before. The thing that is urgent to be changed for them is to alter the old thinking.

During the after-class activities, university students may consult any materials available and helpful to understand the text. In the classroom time, me as a teacher would ask questions about one particular sentence, one particular word, or some long sentences and their structures. Sometimes, a long sentence would be asked to be shortened into a few words by deleting supplemental clauses or attributive phrases. I trained students to read fast in this way and grasp the main meaning of sentences, paragraphs and finally the main idea of the whole text. Sometimes, a dictation is given to students to check the preview work they have done.

As a college English teacher in university, I have been feeling better about using flipped classroom instruction in teaching and my role as a teacher. Because when students prepared themselves before class, they are well prepared and are challenging in receiving my information. They could take in the concept in a very positive way when I explained the long sentences, the complicated meaning of a phrase, and even a long passage. Too often, English words have different connotations in different contexts and it is hard for an individual student to decide the real meaning of a word, phrase, or even associate the synonyms in a text. For the grammatical rules, different students have different understanding and mastery, the reflection beforehand is provoking. The gap between the teacher's lips and the students' ears is fixed and bridged effectively than the traditional way. Students always argue a lot in understanding the contents of the text and thus very helpful in constantly improving their classroom achievements and critical thinking.

3. Consolidation of Mastery Learning in Flipped Classroom Model

According to constructivist approach, knowledge should be given and acquired step by step with the new and different one on the basis of the old and easy one. At the core of the constructivist theory is the idea of mastery learning which is closely related to contents of each unit or section and thus content-based. Mastery learning means that students should comprehend the comparatively easy given knowledge firstly before they are expected to understand a more advanced concept or knowledge point. This fundamental applied to both adult and young learners. There are two radicals in mastery learning: one is the belief that all students could learn if provided with conditions appropriate to their needs; the other is that mastery learning structured its curriculum in terms of certain target levels of comprehension and achievement, not in terms of time. We often divide different subjects into different parts and smaller sections which go like a ladder from the lower one to the upper one.

In a traditional classroom model, a certain amount of time is devoted to a particular topic, concept or unit. When one unit is finished, another unit will be progressed on, the entire class moves on. Considering the fact that individual student has various degrees of mastery over the learning of a certain concept or unit, Students proceed at different rates toward the same level of mastery. Those who learn more quickly can move ahead while those who learn slowly should be helped along by either individual tutoring or peer assistance, or additional homework. Otherwise, the next step would not be based on the solid previous basis and thus influence greatly the afterwards performance and classroom achievement. The shortcoming of the traditional classroom model is that the time allotted to learning stuff is fixed while the comprehension and mastery of a unit is practically and individually variable. So, what should be fixed is a high level of comprehension and what should be variable is the amount of time students have to understand a concept. Whatsmore, some students may like some topics much more than the others, so they can enjoy the specific unit by themselves after class and thus get a more profound understanding of the content which may be closely related to his own personal experience which means more to him considering his own personalities. Flexibility is greatly required in the process of learning according the theory of mastery learning and structuralism.

Based on the basic principles mentioned above, both adult and young students learned at their own pace, that's why we should advocate flipped classroom instruction model, because this model takes individuality and variety into consideration and it is learner-oriented model in a very human way. Learners learned at their own pace, proceeding to the next knowledge point and combining the old points into the new ones only after reaching a prescribed degree of mastery over the previous concept. The role that teachers plays is that they served primarily as guides and mentors rather than lecturers.

In Chinese classrooms, teachers are too often dull lecturers which more or less discouraged students' interests and enthusiasms in learning. Peer communications and instructions in small groups are advocated in this process and are beneficial not merely academically but also positively in establishing and forming a friendly atmosphere among members in contributing cooperatively to a common task.

The results of mastery learning is impressive in that students in all levels "increased gains in achievement over those in traditional instruction programs… and students retained what they had learned longer under mastery learning both in short-term and long-term studies"[1]. And it was proved that it can reduce academic gap between the slower and faster students without bringing a negative influence to the faster students[2].

Strengths of flipped classroom model were enhanced with the advance of modern information technology. Technology has radially lowered the cost of formerly expensive learning approach. For there are no more paper workbooks. This is especially good for college students and university students who have a good mastery of modern information technology and could take full advantage of the them. Once the task is given , they know how to get there and finish their task efficiently. There is no pricey printings of different exercises with most of the stuff related to the task is in the computer through internet. People have a lot of access to the content needed through the internet and could also gather more information and have an insight reflection on them. For learning without thought is labour, and thought without learning is perilous. Lots of opinions and arguments on internet lead people to be discernable and critical in agreeing or disagreeing. True learning occurs only when one get information in a logical way, accept and internalize the content in his own critical way. In some degree, personal responsibility is also well developed and autonomy and self-education is formed gradually. Learners could reap the benefits of learning in a more broader and effective way.

References

1. B. Bloom, Learning for Mastery, *Evaluation Comment* 1(2), 1968.
2. D. Levine, Improving in Elementary and Secondary Classrooms, *Education Leadership* 43(8), 1986.

Mobile Phone Brands Preference Analysis of Post-90s with Multidimensional Scaling*

Shi-qiong Meng†, Zhi Yin and Jia-qing Xu
College of Science, Ningbo University of Technology,
Ningbo, 315211, China
†E-mail: tougao56777@163.com

Ying Du
College of Humanities, Ningbo University of Technology,
Ningbo, 315211, China

The brands preference analysis research draws lots of attention recently. It is useful for marketing, personal recommendation, etc. We utilize an effective statistical analysis method called multidimensional scaling to study the brands preference of mobile phones. The results show that there are four distinct groups of brands and one outliers brand based on our post-90s preference data. Finally, we represent the results visually.

Keywords: Brands preference analysis; post-90s; multidimensional scaling.

1. Introduction

The analysis of preference of users about products is a hot topic in psychology, marketing science and statistical analysis. The expression of people about some brands can be used for target marketing, personal recommendation, etc.

Statistical analysis skills are useful performing brands preference analysis. Out of many multivariate statistical analysis methods, multidimensional scaling (MDS) is a effective way to cluster and detect the distinct groups of products or people based on the features (in the most common case, voting scores or rating data) they have.

MDS can map the data into a low-dimensional space, especially two or three dimensions. We can see the structure of the data more clearly. This is some kind like principle component analysis while the primary objective of MDS is to

* This research was financially supported by the Scientific Research Project of Ningbo University of Technology, National Undergraduate Training Programs for Innovation and Entrepreneurship 2013, Natural Science Foundation of the City of Ningbo, China, under Contract 2012A610029 and Department of Education of Zhejiang Province (Y201120179).

fit the original data into a low-dimensional coordinate system such that any distortion caused by a reduction in dimensionality is minimized [1].

The remainder of our paper is organized as follows. In Section 2, we review the related work about brands preference analysis and MDS. In Section 3, we describe the data set we want to analysis. In Section 4, we present the basic algorithms of MDS. In Section 5, we use MDS to study the brands preference and conclude the paper in Section 6.

2. Related Work

In this section, we review several major researches about brands preference analysis and the applied MDS methods which including metric MDS and nonmetirc MDS.

Traditionally, brands preference analysis is from the perspective of marketing and advertising. [2, 3, 4] study the methods and practices of brands preference in marketing and advertising research. There is also research about the brand preference from an experimental view [5]. In the work [6], D. I. Padberg et al. discuss the consumer brand preference measurements. In recent work [7] researchers review the perceptual mapping by MDS in which use classical MDS and weighted MDS to discuss the brands.

On the hands, MDS as a useful tools for analysis is studied a lot itself in recent years. Andreas BUJA et al. [8] discuss the interactive techniques for MDS. Tynia Yang et al. [9] present an approximation algorithm for MDS for use with large datasets and interactive applications. Arvind Agarwal et al. [10] propose a unified algorithmic framework for solving many known variants of MDS.

3. Dataset Description

Our data is from an Internet survey. We perform a survey to ask 178 young post-90s (the age distribute between 17 to 25) 73 of whom are female. The survey record their rating for the 14 brands of mobile phones which reflect their preference about the brands. The mobile phone in our survey cover all the consumption levels including iPhone, MI, Samsung, etc. The subjects fill in the survey with score between 0 and 1 point. Generally speaking, if subject own the brands of mobile phone, they should rate 1 point. If subject like the phones and do not own them, they can rate like 0.5, 0.6, etc. 0 point means subject do not like the brands of phone. So the rating data can reflect the post-90s preference about the brands and definitely influence the future purchase of the customers when they are about to buy a brands they rated high and not own it yet.

4. Methodology

The methodology we used in this paper to analysis the mobile phone brands preference is called multidimensional scaling. It was developed by Shepard [11], Kruskal [12] and others. With such methods, we can reduce the dimensions of the data, map it into a low-dimensional space and visually plot it in a figure. This helps researchers to understand the brands better.

First, we define a $n \times n$ matrix Z.

$$Z = XX^T \tag{1}$$

Next, we want to get the matrix of Euclidean distances. With the elements of matrix Z, we get the distance matrix which is the squared Euclidean distance as

$$d_{ij}^2 = z_{ii} + z_{jj} - 2z_{ij} \tag{2}$$

Utilize the methods of singular value decomposition (SVD), we reduce the dimension of the data. Here we can set the dimension k according to the restriction of the MDS algorithms.

Usually, our results is given by the k eigenvectors of Z corresponding to the k largest eigenvalues. We can choose the dimension to be represented by the criterion of Mardia et al. [13] Generally, we can sum up the MDS method process as in Table 1.

Table 1 The running steps of multidimensional scaling method.

1. Formulating the research problem.
2. Getting the original data usually rating matrix and preprocessing.
3. Choose the dimension k and use the suitable type of MDS methods
4. Showing result usually with data visualization

5. Data Analysis and Visualization

To study the preference of our brands, we first see the basic statistics of the data. we sum up the points of every brands of mobile phone. The points of each brands is illustrated as Figure 1.

As we can see from Figure 1. The highest points is OPPO and lowest points brand is TCL. As we known from the design of our survey, the points just reflect the preference of people to the brands. One person can just like the brands while not own that kind of mobile phone. This may be caused by some reason like it is too expensive to buy or it is a new style of products and people cannot make decision to buy it right now. We will see later that the order of the score do not reflect the exact preference of the brands.

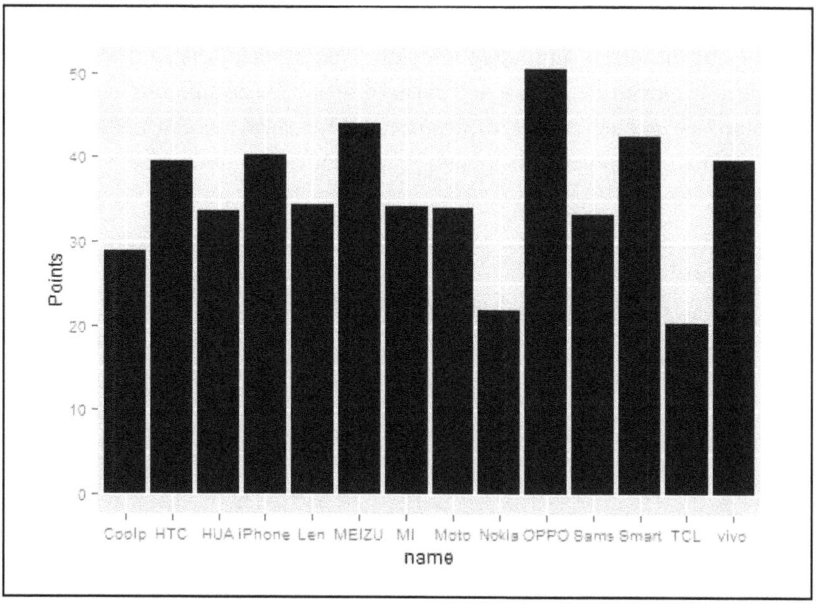

Fig. 1 Points of each brands (some names are shorten considering plot clarity).

Next, we discuss the brands preference with MDS. To use MDS, we should transform the original data. Since we want to discover the structure of the mobile brands while our original data describe the user's rating of the brands. So we transpose the original rating matrix to get the preference of brands rating by users. And based on the flow in Table. 1, we can get the MDS results. Since we want to show this visually, we pick the dimension k = 2. This also can satisfied the demands of the algorithm. We illustrated the result in Figure 2.

As we can see from the Figure 2, there are approximately four distinct groups of brands in the picture. OPPO, MEIZU are denoted as group 1. MI, iPhone and HTC are denoted as group 2. Motorola, TCL and Nokia are denoted as group 3 and Lenovo et al. are denoted as group 4. We can see from the view of post-90s, the brands in the same groups are similar and from the analysis of the product data, these grouping make some sense. Take group 1 as example, OPPO and MEIZU both have the characteristics of pretty and elegant appearance and these kinds of traits attract young people a lot and many people use them.

Interestingly, there are two outliner in Figure 2. They are vivo and Smartisan respectively. Although vivo is near the group 1, Smartisan seems separated from every group in the picture. As a result, we dig out that Smartisan is a new brand of mobile phone and the company behind the product is fairly young. On the other hand, the appearance and user experience seems nice according to the demo and advertisement. This attracts lots of young people. However, the price of this brand is relative high, few people buy it right now. This cause the unique position of this brand. Moreover, we can figure out from Figure 1. that the points Smartisan get is very high, this also verifies our analysis.

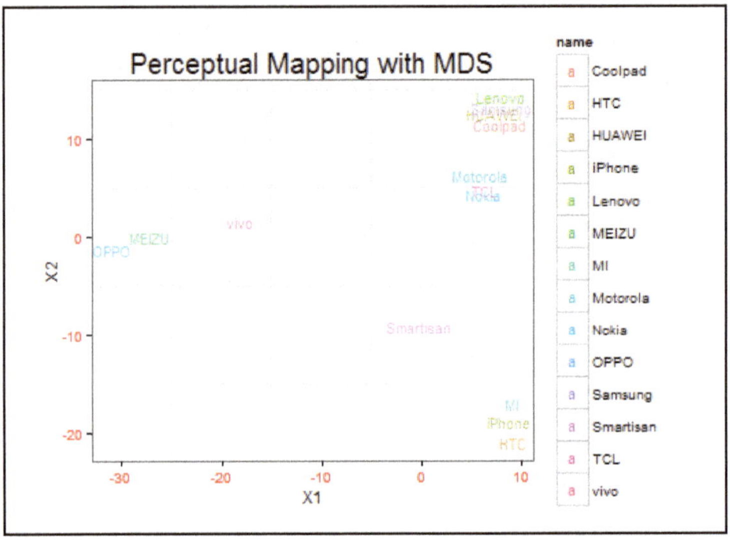

Fig. 2 The perceptual mapping with multidimensional scaling of mobile phone brands.

6. Conclusion

In our paper, we analysis the mobile phone brands preference of post-90s whose ages distribute between 17-24. We got the mobile phone brands preference of them under the methods of MDS. We can see the distinct groups of the mobile phones visually under the method of MDS. The interpretation of the result consistent with the real-world consumption situation. The results help us to understand the post-90s preference about mobile phone brands better.

Acknowledgments

This research was financially supported by the Scientific Research Project of Ningbo University of Technology, National Undergraduate Training Programs for Innovation and Entrepreneurship 2013, Higher education research project of Ningbo University of Technology, Natural Science Foundation of the City of Ningbo, China, under Contract 2012A610029 and Department of Education of

Zhejiang Province (Y201120179).

References

1. Richard A. Johnson and Dean W. Wichern, *Applied Multivariate Statistical Analysis*, 6th edn. (Pearson, Prentice Hall, 2007).
2. Blair, Margaret H., and Allan R. Kuse, *Better Practices in Advertising Can Change a Cost of Doing Business to Wise Investments in the Business, Journal of Advertising Research* **44**, 01 (2004), pp 71-89
3. Shepard, Barry., *Developing and Managing Advertising for StarKist Tuna in a Pouch., Quirk's Marketing Research Review* (2003).
4. Stewart, David W, *Advertising Wearout: What and How You Measure Matters, Journal of Advertising Research* **39**, (1999), pp. 39-42.
5. Reham Ebrahim, A Study of Brand Preference: An Experiential View, Doctoral Symposium, Brunel Business School (2011).
6. D. I. Padberg, F. E. Walker and K. W. Kepner, *Measuring Consumer Brand Preference, Journal of Farm Economics* **49**, 3 (1967), pp. 723-733.
7. Brian F. Blake et al., Perceptual Mapping by Multidimensional Scaling: A Step by Step Primer, Methodology Series, Cleveland State University (2003).
8. Andreas Buja, et al., *XGvis: Interactive Data Visualization with Multidimensional Scaling* (2001).
9. Tynia Yang, Jinze Liu, Leonard McMillan, et al, *A Fast Approximation to Multidimensional Scaling* (2006).
10. Arvind Agarwal Jeff M. Phillips Suresh et al., *Universal Multi-Dimensional Scaling, KDD'10* (2010), Washington, DC, USA.
11. Shepard, R.N., *Multidimensional Scaling, Tree-Fitting, and Clustering, Science,* **210**, 4468 (1980), pp. 390-398.
12. Kruskal, J.B., *Multidimensional Scaling by Optimizing Goodness of Fit to a Nonmetric Hypothesis, Psychometrika* **29**, 1(1964), pp. 1-27.
13. Mardia, KV, Kent, JT, and Bibby, JM, *Multivariate Analysis*, (London: Academic Press, 1979).

Current Issues on the Education of Professional Degree Postgraduate Students in China

Jing Zhang
School of Electrical Engineering, Guizhou University,
Guiyang, 550025, China
E-mail: ee.jzhang@gzu.edu.cn
www.gzu.edu.cn

Peijia Yu
College of Computer Science and Information, Guizhou University,
Guiyang, 550025, China

The Chinese education status of the postgraduate degree is described in this paper. The characteristics of the professional degree postgraduate students are compared with those of the academic degree postgraduate students in detail. Finally, in order to provide reference for education of professional degree postgraduate students, the current difficulties during the education is discussed.

Keywords: Professional degree; academic degree; education of postgraduate students.

1. Current Situation of the Development of the Postgraduate Degree in China

Since 1981, when People's Republic of China Degree Regulations was implemented, China's degree and postgraduate education has made great progress. However, academic degrees are the only type of graduate degree-granting over the years. With the rapid economic and social development and industrial structure adjustment and transformation of economic development, the demand for application-oriented students is greatly increased. In order to meet the needs of China's economic and social development and to accomplish the degree system, the education program of master of engineering is proposed in 1984. And then in 1997, the Fifteenth Degrees Committee of the State Council meeting approved the Master of Engineering Planning. Since 2009, most professional degrees are opened for graduates, in addition to Master of Business Administration (MBA), Master of Public Administration (MPA), Master of Engineering, and Public Master of Health, Master of Sports, and Master of Arts.

Experience from pilot projects to lay the stage of the master training mode, in 2010 the program of the professional degree postgraduate students mentioned as important as that of the academic degree. The universities are required to expand full-time professional degree graduate enrollment, in order to improve the professional degree graduate enrollment proportion. The planning is that the ultimately ratio of professional degree to academic degree is 7 to 3. In the notice about the recruitment of master in 2011, the Chinese Ministry of Education said that China should vigorously promote the development of the professional degree in education, promote structural adjustment and optimization of postgraduate education.

According to reference [1], the number of the postgraduate education institutes reached 811 in 2012. The number of enrollment students was 589,673, including 390,790 academic degree students and 198,883 professional degree students. The ratio of professional degree students to academic degree postgraduate was 5.09 to 4.91. From the data above, the number of professional degree enrollment has exceeded that of the academic degree enrollment. Training applied postgraduate students characterized with stronger ability of application has become an important part of postgraduate education in China.

2. Comparison of the Characteristics of the Professional Degree and That of the Academic Degree Postgraduate Students

At present, there are two types of degree of postgraduate education. One is the traditional academic degree postgraduate students, the characteristic of which is the emphasis on theory and research. The education target of the academic degree postgraduate students is primarily to develop high-level expertise with good theoretical foundation and adaptive ability to specific industries or occupations. The other type is professional degree postgraduate students, the characteristic of which is the emphasis on practice and application. It features both academic and occupational closely. The training target of this kind of students is to develop a professional practice-oriented complex high-level engineering and project management expertise mainly for corporate training applications [2]. Professional degree postgraduate students include full-time students and part-time students. During the training, the students with different kind of degree have obvious difference [3].

2.1. *The difference between the training targets*

The academic degree education is primarily to foster teaching and research personnel. And the education target of professional degree students is defined very clearly in Professional Degrees approval of the Interim Measures, which is approved by the fourteenth meeting of the Academic Degrees Committee of the State Council. It is defined that professional degree postgraduate students are to foster to be specific high-level expertise and professional with training of occupational backgrounds.

2.2. *The difference between the recruit criteria*

Recruit of the academic degree and full-time professional degree postgraduate students does not require applicants to have work experience. However, full-time professional degree requires applicants to be graduating students. Part-time professional degree requires applicants to have work experience generally.

2.3. *The difference between entrance examinations*

Academic degree entrance examination is only once a year. Professional degree entrance examination is twice a year. One examination is carried on in October, and the other examination is carried on at the same time of the academic degree entrance examination. Part-time professional degree candidates may participate in the examination in October, and full-time professional degree candidates participate in the examination at the same time with academic degree candidates. The professional examinations are all different and arranged by education institutes.

2.4. *The difference between training methods*

Academic degree students and full-time professional degree students study full-time. A academic degree student is supervised by a supervisor in the university, but a full-time professional degree student is supervised by both a supervisor in the university and a supervisor in industry. A part-time professional degree student studies in part time and is supervised by both a supervisor in the university and a supervisor in industry.

2.5. *The difference between study fees*

At present, study fees are charged for all academic degree students and full-time professional degree students. The academic degree students and full-time professional degree students can apply for both scholarship and state loans or business loans in order to ease financial burden. Study fees vary greatly due to the various training institutes and there are no scholarships or state loans for part-time professional degree students.

2.6. *The difference between diploma issued*

Academic degree and certificate will be issued to academic degree and full-time professional degree students. However only academic degree will be issued to part-time professional degree students without any diploma.

2.7. *The difference between recognition*

Because the training of academic degree is very accomplished and Academic degree and certificate will be issued, social acceptance of such students is very high. However these kinds of students get high theoretical knowledge but they are lack of experience generally. The program of full-time postgraduate degree has implemented since 2009. Although there are a small number of graduates entering although society, social recognition needs to be improved, however. Only academic degree is issued, so the acceptance of part-time professional degree is low.

3. The Main Problem of Professional Degree Postgraduate Students Training

Like that of many countries, the professional degree in China is developed after the academic degree. Postgraduate education originally granted different degree levels, but there are only single academic degrees. As the fast development of division of labor in society, the demand for talent is getting variable and complex. Currently, with the rapid development of postgraduate education in China, it becomes consensus that academic degree postgraduate students and professional degree postgraduate students adapt to different demand of the society. However, due to the program of the professional degree started lately, there are still some problems in its development.

3.1. *Misunderstanding about the professional degree*

First, it has been fully recognized by university that the professional degree education is the same importance as the academic degree education. But time is needed to peoples to understand the professional degree education.

Secondly, although the full-time professional degree postgraduate students can get Academic degree and certificate, but because the full-time professional degree postgraduate students was approved in 2009 and its formal enrollment began in 2010, the employers do not understand the professional degree very well.

3.2. *Training methods and evaluation criteria are similar to each othor*

Firstly, the training targets are similar to each other. The key quality of academic degree students is aimed to academy. The students can carry out basic research independent. The key quality of professional degree students is aimed to application. The students can carry out the application of research. However, due to the impact of long-term academic degree postgraduate students training mode, academy is considered as the criteria to evaluate the quality of the postgraduate students. This leads to similar training targets to each other.

Secondly, the curriculum is similar to each other. Generally, the curriculum reflects the knowledge structure of the students. Professional degree education is to train the ability of high-level technical and management, so the corresponding curriculum should aim to improve the students' professional competence, rather than to master a discipline of knowledge as the goal. And therefore a distinguished course features should be developed for professional degree students. However, in facts, many aspects, such as the curriculum and teaching conditions, are all similar to each other.

Thirdly, the evaluation criteria is similar to each other. The professional degree education aims to train high-level application-oriented talents, and writing paper is to enhance the ability to study and solve practical problems. The features of the dissertations focus on social value, economic value and practical value. Therefore, the evaluation criteria for the dissertation of professional degree students should emphasize the integration of the application value and the academic value. At present, this has been a broad consensus. But in practice, there is still more or less to evaluate the dissertation of professional degree students by the criteria of the dissertation of the academic degree.

3.3. *Inadequate education resources*

Firstly, the supervisor team of professional degree students is not inadequate. The quality of the education depends largely on the quality of the supervisor team. The characteristics of the professional degree education require that the supervisor must have rich practical experience and industry background. The supervisors should strengthen the training of the academic research. At the same time they must address the characteristics of professional degree postgraduate education in order to update training content and improve education methods. Finally the students' practical ability can be enhanced. The implementation of dual tutorial makes the supervisors to do their best. But in the actual process of postgraduate training, the dual tutorial is of mere formality. An efficient and professional supervisor team should be built up.

Secondly, the practice fields for professional degree students are not accomplished. The most important difference between the professional degree and the academic degree is that postgraduate degree education focuses on the training of the practical application ability. In order to obtain this kind of ability, practice is one of the most important training methods. However, establishing the practice fields and the mechanism of students practice still requires the joint efforts of the government, universities and industries.

4. Conclusion

From the number of current enrollment, the training of the professional degree students has become a very important part of postgraduate education in China. Therefore, accomplishing the professional degree education has important significance. There are many difficulties and problems during the education process because the professional degree education started lately and we must handle seriously, although the professional degree education has achieved good results. Fully understanding the difficulties and problems and solve them, the quality of the professional degree education can be ensured and the healthy development of graduate education can be promoted.

Acknowledgments

We would like to thank the project supported by the Graduate Education Reform Foundation of Guizhou Province (2012003).

References

1. National Bureau of Statistics of China. China Statistical Yearbook. (China Statistics Press, 2014).
2. Shuang Ying, Jun Kang, Liang Zhen, Xuemei Ding. Exploration and Practice: Innovation of the Postgraduate Training Model in China, Journal of Graduate Education, 1, (2014).
3. Linglin Hu. Comparison of Academic Degree and Professional Degree Graduate Education mode. Academic Degrees & Graduate Education, 4, (2006).

The Exploration of Practical Education in Universities

Wanmi Chen
School of Mechatronic Engineering and Automation, Shanghai University,
Shanghai, 200072, China
E-mail: Wanmic@163.com
www.shu.edu.cn

What is the best means for students to acquire knowledge, Practice! How to practice education of executive in the university, is the main problem to be solved in this paper, through the curriculum, students' independent experiment and classroom discussion, college students to participate in competition in science and technology and other aspects of the comprehensive. Proposed to explore practical education in colleges and universities.

Keywords: Practical education; self experiment; classroom discussion.

1. The Generation of Problems

I often encounter students for learning confusion, they do not know How can use so many courses they studied during the university, also do not understand their own professional direction. This is not only a freshman, even in the year two, year three or year four students have the situation.

Indeed in the university curriculum, curriculum between mostly scattered, little contact, most of the teaching theory mainly, the combination of practical application less, so if you can have one or several courses, can take some courses on up to the unity of theory and practice?

2. Implementation Plan

With this problem of the students confusion, after nearly ten years of practice, I finally in mechatronic specialty opened courses of combination of theory and practice, the tentative course called "The Technology of Robot Controled", the curriculum introduces the robot's mechanical design, manufacturing, and is taught in robot motion control part, the combination of machine and electricity, simultaneously also is the theory and practice of combining.

The course in the lecture form using a variety of ways, Flashback taken parlance, such as from the robot's function, to realize the function of theoretical knowledge and mathematical derivation. Let the students feel obtained prior to the study of some courses, such as advanced mathematics, ordinary physics, circuit and electronic technology, computer theory, automatic control theory, motor and so here to find the actual application, the students suddenly enlightened that the originally learn the course is to be used.

3. Self Experiment

All obtained by experimental verification of the knowledge, will get more profound memory. The experiment in the course "The Technology of Robot Controled", does not provide uniform experimental guide books, and presented by the students themselves as experimental, each student in the course of study, what is not entirely clear, or what need is verified by the experiment, students can carry out, write their own experimental procedures, after get the teacher's approval can themselves alone, but is completely open (managed by the students), so in a curriculum, each student's experiment will appear the phenomenon is not the same.

Secondly, according to the college students' innovative and practical project, and college students' science and technology competitions such as development, lets the student can keep up with the world in the forefront of the latest, more broad display platform.

Figure 1 and Figure 2 are shown the basketball robot and home service robot designed and manufactured by students.

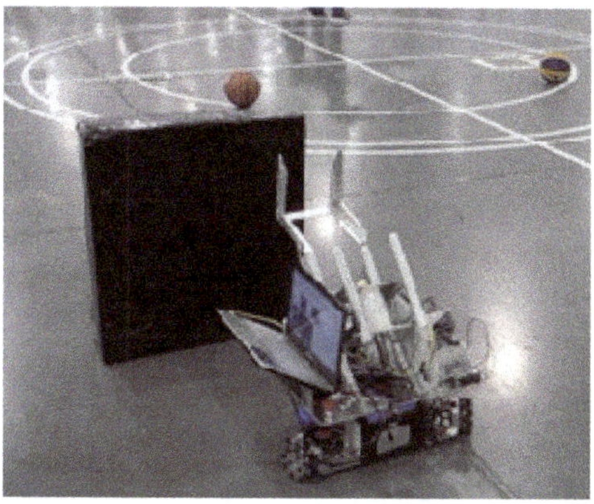

Fig. 1 The basketball robot.

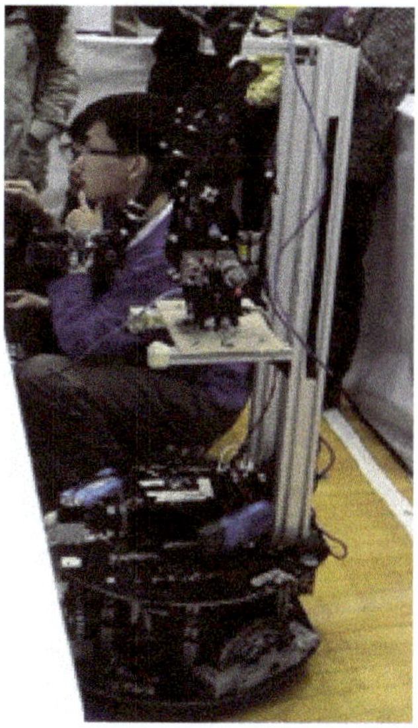

Fig. 2 Home service robot.

4. Classroom Discussion

Teaching process is consist the process of teaching and learning, the classroom discussion, can deepen the knowledge intensive, give an example here, such as "Agent" and " Robot", to the class discussion, let students to the differences or similarities of the freely.

The discussion was carried out very smoothly, the class to speak, the following is a comprehensive result on the blackboard by the students, as shown in Figure 3.

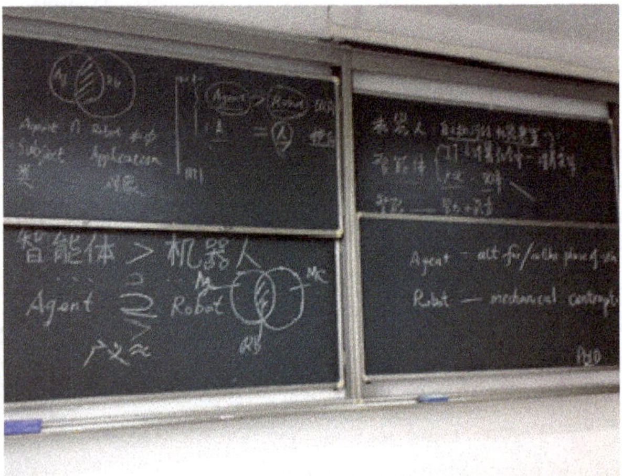

Fig. 3 The discussion result on the blackboard in classroom.

In Figure 3, the students in the course of the discussion on the blackboard record.

The point of view 1, "Agent" category is greater than the (>) " Robot ".

The point of view 2, "Agent" category including (⊐) "Robot".

The point of view 3, "Agent" is equivalent to the "Class", "Robot" is the equivalent of "Object".

The point of view 4, "Agent" is "Subject", "Robot" is "Application".

Agent and Robot have the intersection, are not included in part.

The point of view 5, Agent $\cap$ Robot $\neq \emptyset$, as shown in Figure 4.

The point of view 6, Agent $\cap$ Machinery = Robot, as shown in Figure 5.

The point of view 7, the concept of each keywords,

The concept of "Agent": Agent is an intelligent entity, including intelligence and ability. The agent is a very important concept in the field of artificial intelligence. Any independent thought and with environment interaction entities can be abstracted as an agent.

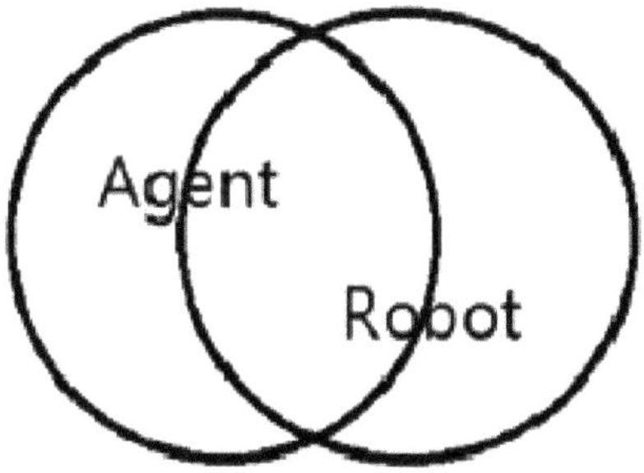

Fig. 4 Relationship between Agent / Robot 1.

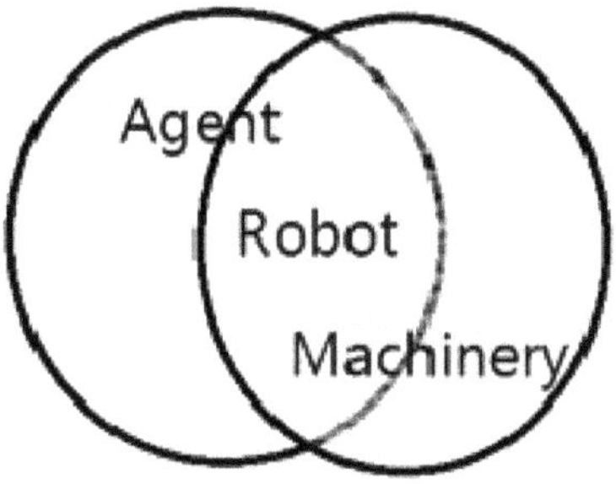

Fig. 5 Relationship between Agent / Robot 2.

"Robot" concept: The robot is a machine device automatically performing work. It can accept human command, and can run pre programmed procedures, also can according to the principle of developing artificial intelligence technology platform for action. Its mission is to assist or replace human work.

Agent: Autonomous entity which observes and acts upon an environment and good its activity towards achieving goals, agent refers to the independent activities of software or hardware entity.

Robot: A robot is a mechanical contraption which can perform tasks on its own, or with guidance that can be executed automatically machines.

Although the students have different opinions, debate, but through this discussion, that students have a deeper and more comprehensive understanding for intelligent "Agent" and "Robot", this discussion has very practical significance, students can fully express and modify their views, let the facts more clearly.

5. Conclusion

After more than 10 years of exploration, from the curriculum, teaching methods change, from the open experiment to the students' self-design experiment, students actively participate in the competition of science and technology and the implementation of certain effect.

References

1. W.M. Chen, *Innovation and practice of competition robots*, the press of Shanghai University, 2014.

Internet of Things Experimental Equipment Innovation: A New Internet of Things Teaching Instrument Based on Android Mobile Phones*

Fan Liang†, Fenghui Dai, Shigang Cui, Li Zhao and Jiabao Liu

Tianjin Key Laboratory of Information Sensing and Intelligent Control, Tianjin University of Technology and Education, Tianjin, 300222, China

†E-mail: bachelormd10@163.com

With the rise of the Internet of Things (IoT) and increasing application, the IoT teaching instrument demand of colleges and universities is increasing. Traditional IoT teaching instrument integratesa lot of hardware components, not only with the high cost but also with poor portability. Besides, the update of IoT technology leads thata lot of IoT teaching instrument have been eliminated without full use. Facing these problems, we propose a new design pattern to realize the diversity, modernization and informatization of the IoT teaching instrument. The experimental instrument is small and convenient to operate, which saves cost with extendable interface. According to the analysis of the traditional teaching instrument and the experimental equipment design principle, the IoT teaching instrument based on the Android mobile phone has been designed to optimize the structure and improve performance.

Keywords: Android phone; IoT; Teaching instrument; Structure optimization.

1. Introduction

In China, with the widely application of the modern information technology in the education industry, a large number of information technology application software and the high technology of modern equipment have broken the original pattern in the field of education[1]. Due to the deepening of curriculum reform, the diversity of teaching methods and the enrichment of classroom information sources, the increasing role of IoT teaching instruments for modernization and informatization in the vocational education should not be underestimated. With the continuous development of internet technology, the Android smart-phone gradually turns into the IoT terminal equipment. Current versatility of IoT

*The research was sponsored by Undergraduate Teaching Quality and Teaching Reform Planning Program of Tianjin Colleges (No. C03-0803), "Twelfth Five" Investment Planning for Major Construction Program of Tianjin Colleges, Tianjin Science and Technology Foundation (No. 14JCQNJC04300) and College Fund (No. KYQD13022).

instrument and equipment has been keeping pace with the times. Although the auxiliary means of teaching have diversity forms, IoT teaching instruments designed for Android smartphone have not yet appeared. The renewal speed of traditional IoT teaching instrument causes that a lot of teaching instruments and equipment have not yet make full use. In this paper, how to make good use of the IoT teaching instrument of modernization and informatization to assist teaching and improve the teaching quality is considered, at the same time, how to make use of modern means of science and technology to design and optimize the traditional teaching instruments is also considered. In order to solve the lack of IoT teaching instrument for Android mobile and collective elimination of a large number of teaching instrument, a new kind of IoT teaching instrument is designed.

2. Problems of Current IoT Teaching Instrument Design

(1) IoT teaching instruments is a kind of Internet of things product that fuse sensor technology, embedded technology, distributed information processing technology, wireless communication technology, network security technology, intelligent control technology and a series of advanced technology. This instrument involves many peripheral devices, such as WiFi module, ZigBee module, RFID radio frequency module, camera module, blue-tooth serial port module and various sensors[2-3]. In order to achieve the goal of profit maximization and shorten the development cycle, the different peripheral equipment and the different hardware of IoT teaching experiment board is designed by manufacturers in the same circuit boards. As a consequence, the circuit board is big, inconvenient to carry and operation is not flexible, and the cost is high, the hardware is not configured.

(2) The IoT teaching instrument has many peripheral devices. Developers have left a unique interface for them in the design. The interface is fixed on the experimental board and wiring has been determined in factory. If any interface is failure, the whole board function will be fixed, that will influence the experiment teaching. In addition, the device replacement is also very troublesome, and even some can not change, that contribute to the difficulty in maintenance. The problems increase the cost and affect the service life of the instrument.

(3) Currently, the IoT teaching instrument design is still within traditional idea that is not innovative. The function of each part of teaching instrument is designed by manufacturer first. Due to the manufacturer's propaganda and

equipment factory packaging, students will think that a pin is fixed peripherals in the subconscious. It's so hard for them to be digested and the teaching effectiveness become worse.

3. Development Trend of the Future IoT Teaching Instrument

(1) IoT emphasizes the commonality in the form of teaching instruments. A complete set of IoT teaching instrument has many components. The main control chip is designed to independent core board. The core board combines with different components, assembling into various laboratory equipment, to complete the different experiment task[4]. If a component fails, they can replace each other.

(2) The content of IoT teaching instrument is not only confined to the scope of the textbook. Teaching instruments will be the appliance of autonomous learning and development in extracurricular based on students' personal hobby. IoT teaching instrument provides hardware support for IoT teaching. The students can buy some special peripherals according to their own conditions or interest in learning, and combine system according to their own ideas.

(3) IoT teaching equipment should be enhanced visual, and as much as possible in the experimental exploration and the basic operation process. The equipment can provide different experimental scheme, and should make full use of information technology. IoT teaching instrument should increase teaching instrument "transparency", avoiding black-box operation of equipment.

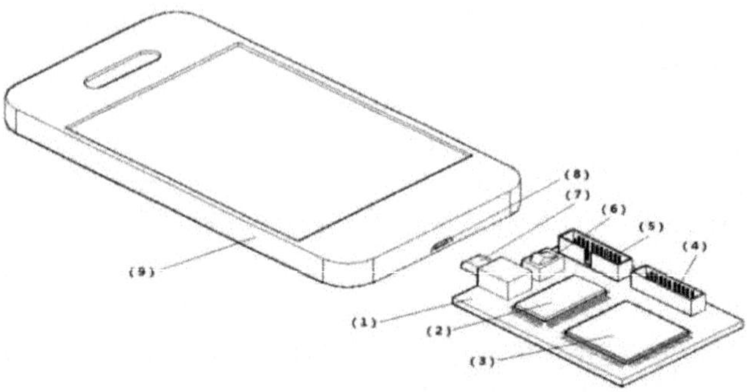

Figure. 1 IoT teaching instrument module.

4. IoT Teaching Instrument and Modular Design

IoT teaching instrument existed on the market at present is designed by the traditional idea. All peripheral equipment and the core chips are on one circuit board, such that the experimental board is big and inconvenience to operate. The interface isn't extendable. Due to a lot of unnecessary hardware, the instruments increase costs and waste resources[5-6]. Therefore, a modular design idea of IoT teaching instrument is put forward to design and optimize structure. And a IoT teaching instrument module for Android smartphone is designed according to the idea. The connection diagram of IoT teaching instrument module and mobile phone is shown in Figure 1.

Figure 1 is the diagram of Android smartphone and the IoT teaching instrument module, including IoT teaching instrument module circuit board (1), PL2303HXD chip (2), STM32f103zet6 chip (3), I/O port pin (4), simulator download mouth (5), the power switch (6), Micro USB connector (7), the Android mobile phone Micro USB interface (8), the Android mobile phone (9), etc. The IoT teaching instrument module function is realized control of different peripheral devices by programming based on the core chip STM32f103zet6 and instruction will be delivered to the mobile phone in real-time by means of the usb serial port and OTG technology. The IoT teaching instrument module with special structure and circuit design realizes two-way communication between mobile and embedded devices. The interface is designed as a standard Micro USB connector, which is consistent with mobile phone cable interface and compatible with physical interface of Android smartphone. The module has the simulator interface to download the software to the core chip. To meet the experimental operating flexibility, cost savings and improving the utilization ratio of IoT teaching instrument, the module provides the peripheral interface and all peripherals are optional. Through the combination of different peripheral devices on the interface pins, IoT experiment hardware structures can be constructed.

The design has the following features. Firstly, in the structure design, the core chip circuit independent of instrument board reduces the complexity and cost of circuit board. Instrument parts function is clear and internal structure is prominent and intuitive. The IoT instrument can attract the students attention and inspire students' thinking. Secondly, in the design process, the principle of standardization, generalization and serialization is carried out, not only can improve the quality of the components, but easy to maintain and change[7]. Thirdly, on the teaching effect, hardware sensor and transmission module can be effectively tested, the IoT experiment about dynamic network and mobile monitoring more easily are realized. Finally, the design thought is conform to the development trend of the reform of teaching instrument and the teaching instrument design is the inevitable requirement of era development. Mainly embodied in the following two aspects: (1) The students construct the system hardware with the teaching experiment module combination according to their need. It can greatly improve the efficiency of classroom teaching, the students' interest in learning and promote the students' ability. (2) With the update of science technology and knowledge, a module out of teaching instrument instead of the elimination of the entire experiment box and the same module between different experiment box can replace each other in use process. That saves the investment in teaching instrument and reduces the waste of resources. And to really achieve the aim "burden lighten and Efficiency increased", we also need to continue to improve in terms of reform and promotion of teaching equipment, which is the orientation that we continue to work toward.

References

1. Feng Zhuqin. Conform to the requirements of times, reduce burdens and increase efficiency -- The discussion of modernization and informationization of teaching instruments and equipment to improve the experiment teaching quality of primary school [J]. The winner papers of the fifth China education technology equipment forum (top), 2014. 11.
2. Li Hong. Internet of things: The transformation of the productivity [M]. Binjing: Postsand Telecom Press, 2010, 7-11.
3. LIU Jia, LIU Bai-quan, et al. The Design and Realization of an Internet of Things Teaching Experiment System [J]. Journal of Electrical & Electronic Education, 2010, 32(6): 89-92.
4. Jiang Jinlong, Ren Weide. Develop conventional teaching instrument with the goal of educational reform [J]. China Educational Technology & Equipment, 2002.
5. Zeng Chuixing, Liang Yilong, et al. Effect and significance of independent development of the experimental teaching equipment [J]. Experiment Science and Technology, 2010, 8(4).
6. Li Ruqi, He Qiuli, et al. Homemade experimental teaching instruments and equipment to promote experimental teaching reform [J]. Higher Education of Sciences, 2009 (1): 71-74.
7. He Shengjing, Li Pu. The first theory of basic principles of teaching instrument design [J]. Teaching instruments and experiments, 1989, 5(5).

On the Generation Mechanism of Occupational Emotion of University Counselors Based on Emotion Generation Theories

Li Jiang[†], Ke Xiaohua and Zhu Qianyu
Faculty of Chinese Language and Culture, Cisco School of Informatics, Guangdong University of Foreign Studies, Guangzhou, Guangdong 510420, China
[†]E-mail: ck0900@hotmail.com
www.gdufs.edu.cn

The cultivation of university counselors' occupational emotion is an important part of constructing professionalism among counselors. This study will explore the generation mechanism of university counselors' occupational emotion from the perspectives of individual, university, and society on the basis of such emotion generation theories as cognitive theory of emotion and behaviorism so as to further expand the horizon of studies on occupational emotion and counselor.

Keywords: Emotion generation theory; counselors; occupational emotion; generation mechanism.

1. Introduction

Counselors, an important part of university's faculty and administration team, are the driving force of university students' ideological and political education. As organizers, educators and supervisors of university students' daily ideological education and management, they play a significant role in fostering students' moral character and supervising their study, maintaining the stability of universities, and promoting the all-round development of students. The counselors' work is comprehensive and direct. Since they have to involve themselves in college students' study, life and work, their ideas, behaviors and habits will definitely exert a subtle influence on these students. Moreover, their sense of identity and sense of responsibility toward their occupation as well as their working attitude and enthusiasm will directly influence students' sound development. Occupational emotion is the emotion toward one's occupation. The occupational emotion of counselors refers to an attitudinal experience formed in their judgment of whether their occupation could satisfy their personal needs, and also to a special feeling based on their knowledge, evaluation and reflection of their occupation [1]. Positive occupational emotion makes counselors view their work as their career and arouses a mental dependence on and a deep understanding of their occupation. As a result, they will love their occupation and position, and carry out their work with passion. Negative occupational emotion makes counselors view their work only as a living, and care a lot about their personal gains and material benefits. Consequently, they will have little sense of identity and sense of responsibility toward their occupation, and frequently show slackness or even resistance to their work. In other words, counselors' understanding and acknowledgment of their occupation have a great impact on their enthusiasm and performance in work, and their occupational planning and development.

It is essential and necessary to carry out a study on counselors' occupational emotion which has both theoretical importance and practical value. In recent years, more and more scholars pay close attention to the issue, making it a hotspot in the research area of student affairs. The study on counselors' occupational emotion involves a lot of theoretical knowledge in disciplines such as management, organizational behavior, psychology and pedagogy. But seen from relevant literature up to now, researchers only focused on empirical study without conducting a deep exploration of the theoretical foundation and generation mechanism of counselors' occupational emotion. Without solid theoretical support, these studies fail to present the issue with clear concepts, processes, and mechanisms, which is a defect in the field of counselor occupational emotion research. This paper tries to take emotion generation theories in psychology—the cognitive theory of emotion and behaviorism—as its theoretical foundation, and deduct and interpret the generation mechanism of counselors' occupational emotion so as to further expand the horizon of studies on occupational emotion and on counselors from theoretical perspectives.

2. Theoretical Basis

2.1. *The cognitive theory of emotion*

According to the cognitive theory of emotion in psychology which is represented by Arnold, Schacht, Lazarus, Siminoff, etc., emotion results from the evaluations of stimulus situations or events. In the 1950s, Magda Arnold, an American psychologist put forward the appraisal-emotion theory. The theory goes that stimulus situations do not define the property of emotion, and from the exposure to stimulus to the emergence of emotions, estimations and evaluations are required. The sequence of emotion embraces three steps: stimulus situations, evaluations and emotions. Usually, different evaluations of the identical stimulus situations lead to different emotional responses. In the 1960s, the American psychologists Stanley Schachter and Jerome Singer proposed the two-factor theory of emotion, stating that two factors are necessary for particular emotions. The first one is that the individual should have experienced the high level of physiological arousal such as tachycardia, sweating hands, gastric contraction, and tachypnea. The other is to have cognitive arousal to the physiological changes. In the 1970s, Richard Stanley Lazarus came up with the cognition-appraisal theory which deemed emotion as the outcome of interactions between human and the environment. In emotional activities. When information exceeds the demands of the organism, positive emotions arise; otherwise, negative emotions emerge. But both positive and negative emotions can promote behaviors [2].

2.2. *Behaviorism*

Born at the turn of the 20th century and represented by Watson, Skinner, James, Langer and Bandura, behaviorism embraces two main features: the first one is the denying of consciousness and advocating of psychological researches, the other is about methodology, opposing introspection, it embraces experiment. In the eyes of behaviorists, it is impossible to carry out objective researches on consciousness which is invisible and untouchable. The objects of psychological studies should be observable events, namely, behaviors, instead of consciousness.

3. Generation Mechanism of Counselors' Occupational Emotion

3.1. *Generation mechanism of counselors' occupational emotion based on cognitive theory of emotion*

Occupational emotion is not formed naturally, but generated by certain environment and events. According to the cognitive theory of emotion, emotion generation is caused by people's cognitive appraisal of outside stimulus events, since positive or negative emotions can only be triggered after people are aware of the good and the bad sides of the stimulus events. It also applies to the generation of counselors' occupational emotion.

Counselors' occupational emotion refers to counselors' attitudinal experience formed on the basis of whether the counselors' occupation meets their personal needs. This attitudinal experience is actually a process of cognitive appraisal. In accordance with the cognitive theory of emotion, a cognitive process is a process involving people's accepting, storing, processing and understanding various kinds of information, and namely a reflective process of human brains on the form and nature of objects and events. When performing their duties, counselors will certainly experience a growth in understanding of their occupation. This process involves the counselors' evaluation and estimation of their occupation, and their judgment on its value. Generation mechanism of counselors' occupational emotion mainly lies in individual factors, including the following four cognitive appraisals:

3.1.1. *Cognitive appraisal of occupation*

According to cognitive theory of emotion, the word "cognition" refers to the individual's knowledge and opinions on a particular event, including appraisals of past events, interpretations of present ones and expectations of future ones. As a rational mental activity, cognition exerts a strong regulatory effect on people's emotion, sentiment, motive and behavior. Counselors' understanding of their work is closely related to whether occupational emotion arises and what kind of emotion it is. Counselors' judgment on their work is primarily based on whether relevant conditions, including the nature, environment, objects, duties and payment of their work, conform to their demands and expectations.

(1) Cognitive appraisal of occupational values

Cognition involves an appraisal of the significance of information. Therefore, counselors' appraisal of their occupational significance counts a great deal. They need to know about and reflect on essential issues like the value and significance of life and the mission of education. And they cannot develop a passion for student affairs and realize their self-worth unless they become fully aware of the fact that their job is of major significance for bringing up socialist builders and successors featuring an all-round development in morality, intelligence, physique and art.

(2) Cognitive appraisal of occupational knowledge and competence

Cognitive theory of emotion regards emotion as the interactive result of human and environment. In emotional activities, humans not only reflect the influence of stimulus events in the environment, but also adjust their own response to the stimulus. While getting to know their occupation, counselors need to select and evaluate various kinds of information. Undoubtedly, their emotion will be intensified when there is information calling for high-level knowledge and competence concerning their work. Such emotion will induce counselors to select appropriate behavior responses, that is, improving their occupational knowledge and competence so as to meet the demands of the job. At this point, desire becomes an important constituent of emotion triggering motives, and motivated counselors begin to organize certain behaviors to adapt to their desire.

3.1.2. *Cognitive appraisal of the outside world*

Emotion and sentiment play a driving role in cognitive activities. People's positive or negative cognitive appraisal of outside stimulus events may generate positive or negative emotion respectively.

(1) Cognitive appraisal of social identity

Generation of counselors' occupational emotion is based on the cognitive appraisal of the job of counselors. Commendatory cognitive appraisal produces positive occupational emotions, while the opposite produces negative ones. According to the cognitive theory of emotion, outside influence evokes emotion through people's appraisal. Although the source of emotion and the experience of it comes from the influence of environment, stimulus events in the environment alone cannot cause or determine the emotion directly. Whether the appraisal of their job from the society can provoke their emotions and what emotions it will provoke are only determined through counselors' cognitive appraisal. Such cognitive appraisal of outside evaluation is a process of defining the meaning of outside evaluation for counselors, which primarily involves value judgments (good or bad, satisfactory or dissatisfactory). Only when counselors have developed their own view of the outside evaluation of their work can they make corresponding response and produce positive or negative occupational emotion.

(2) Cognitive appraisal of family factors

According to the cognitive theory of emotion, emotion is the individual's response to a perception of an outside event appraised as harmful or beneficial. In emotional activities, people need to continuously appraise the relationship between stimulus events and themselves. There are appraisals of three levels: first-appraisal, second-appraisal and third-appraisal. Family factors also influence the counselors' cognitive appraisal of their job, for counselors spend most of their spare time with their families whose understanding and supports will affect their emotion. Once conflicts arise between family and work, counselors will have a first-appraisal of whether their families' attitude plays a simulative or an impeditive role in their work, regulate their own emotion and strike a balance between family and work, and at last make an appraisal of the effectiveness and appropriateness of their own behavior response. Actually, that is a feedback behavior.

4. Conclusion

The cultivation of occupational emotion has become an indispensable part in the process of promoting the professionalism construction of counselor teams. Besides, counselor occupational emotion is a prerequisite for the achievement of counselors' sustainable development. Researches indicate that we can use the cognitive theory of emotion in psychology, or the principle of changing individuals' emotional experience by shifting their view of outside stimuli, to interpret the generation mechanism of counselors' cognition appraisal of their professional value, professional knowledge and capability, social recognition, family, pressure and their personality differences. We can accurately grasp the essence of the generation mechanism and patterns of counselors' occupational emotion and actively adopt intervention measures to control and eliminate negative factors, so as to guide counselors to generate a positive occupational emotion.

Acknowledgments

The authors would like to express their sincere appreciation to the University Innovation Projects of Guangdong province (2014), and the financial sponsorship of Ideological and Political Education of Guangdong Province under the Research project (2014ZK023).

References

1. Yang Changrui, Sun Li, Shen Bo, On the value and expression of counselors' occupational emotion [J]. School Party Development and Ideological Education, 2012(5): 123.
2. Meng Zhaolan, The Development of Contemporary Emotion Theories[J]. Acta Psychologica Sinica, 1985(2): 209-212.
3. Guo Nianfeng, The Coursebook of National Professional Qualification Training: Psychological Counselor [M], Beijing: National Publishing House, 2012: 434-435.
4. Fei Meiping, Behaviorism and its Research Paradigm. [J], Journal of East China University of Science and Technology (Social Sciences), 2000(4): 61-63.

Instructional Design of Cultural Arts and Crafts Program for Atayal High School in Taiwan

Chao, Jen-Yi* and Yao, Lo-Yi
Graduate School of Curriculum and Instructional Communications Technology, National Taipei University of Education, Taiwan(ROC), Taipei
**E-mail: jenyichao@gmail.com*
www.ntue.edu.tw

Xu, Rui-Yan
Nan Oau Senior High School Taiwan (ROC), Yilan
E-mail: 1434@tmail.ilc.edu.tw

Chang, Lin
Nan Oau Community Development Association, Taiwan (ROC), Yilan
E-mail: nanao0921@gmail.com

Through a three-way collaboration between an Atayal community high school, a community society and the research team, this study adopted the five-stage model of ADDIE instructional design for conducting the analysis, design, development, implement and evaluation of an Atayal cultural arts and crafts program. The 21 high school seniors who participated in the program completed works of Atayal cultural arts and crafts, such as strings of millet beads, Atayal woven fabric, flip-flops, leather carving and ramie key rings. We hope this study may become a reference for the instructional designs of humanities and social sciences for other tribes.

Keywords: ADDIE; Atayal; Tribe Culture; Indigenous Senior High School Students.

1. Introduction

The researchers worked with a local community society and high school, and designed an Atayal cultural arts and crafts program for high school seniors using the ADDIE instructional design model.

The collaborating high school is a community high school, of which most students belong to the Atayal Tribe, located in Yilan County, Taiwan. Though most of the students come from neighboring villages, they did not understand much about Atayal cultural arts and crafts. Thus, the research team, along with resources from the local community society and the high school, integrated the elements of Atayal cultural arts and crafts into program design and used the integrate program for guiding students in completing works of cultural arts and crafts. Finally, through contents of students' feedback records and interviews with teachers, this study understood the merits and flaws of the instructional design of the cultural program to provide a reference model for instructional designs of humanities and social sciences.

The purposes of this study include: (1) understanding the ADDIE instructional design processes of cultural arts and crafts programs; (2) understanding the opinions of teachers and students of the Atayal community high school toward the implementation of such instructional design model.

2. Atayal Culture of Arts and Crafts

Among the aboriginal tribes in Taiwan, the Atayal is a tribe with the second highest population and the most expansive distribution. A third of uplands in Taiwan have Atayal habitants [1,2].

Atayal traditional arts and crafts are mainly about weaving, of which materials used include ramie, makino bamboo and rattan. Works created using these materials are necessities (clothes, hats, mambo baskets, back baskets, etc.) in the daily lives of Atayal people[2,3].

The Atayal community tribe collaborating with this study is located in Yilan County, Taiwan. This tribe has recently been developing actively multiple arts and crafts products with Atayal cultural elements, such as flip-flops, Atayal woven bags, stone paintings, hanging ornaments made of bead strings, neckties, wallets, quilts, woven bamboo baskets, table cloths and leather carvings (http://sixstar.moc.gov.tw/blog/nanao0921). The research team will participate in the program design and teaching by means of qualified teachers from the community tribe, and teach accordingly high school seniors to complete productions of multiple Atayal arts and crafts to understand the suitability of the design of Atayal cultural program.

3. ADDIE Instructional Design Model

ADDIE is a model that designs or develops systematically instructional or curricular activities. Such instructional design is divided into five stages: analysis, design, development, implement and evaluation [4]. The five stages are summarized below [5,6].

(1)Analysis: analyze the learners' required learning performance and demands toward goal of course teaching, structure of learners' cognition and cultural properties to define the type and difficulty of program contents.

(2)Design: design the learning tasks to be completed by learners in teaching units based on the teaching objectives, learner traits, teaching procedure, teaching materials and resources, and evaluation methods determined by the analysis stage.

(3)Development: develop evaluating tools and aid materials for use during teaching to evaluate whether learners can achieve the set learning objective.

(4)Implement: apply the teaching objectives, teaching procedure, materials and contents established in the previous stages in actual teaching activities.

(5)Evaluation: through conclusive and formative evaluation, discover and review whether any improvement is required for programs, teaching materials and contents.

Based on the abovementioned literatures, this study adopted the ADDID instructional design model for the design and development of an Atayal cultural arts and crafts program, as summarized below:

3.1. *Analysis*

The research subjects are 21 students who are high school seniors at an Atayal community high school, including 15 Atayals and 6 Hans. These students do not understand much about the production process of Atayal cultural arts and crafts, and they are tending to employment after graduation. Thus, the teaching objective of this cultural arts and crafts program is to provide an opportunity for passing on Atayal cultural arts and crafts as well as promote the students' identification and learning interests toward Atayal cultural arts and crafts.

3.2. *Design*

The program is designed to include six teaching events, three hours per course, and the Atayal cultural arts and crafts courses are carried out at the site of the community society for students to experience more profoundly local cultures. Display of works and sharing of after-program thoughts are conducted at the high school at the end of the semester so that other students who did not participate in the program can have the opportunity of coming in contact with local culture. The planning and contents of the program are as shown in Table 1:

Table 1 Planning of Atayal cultural arts and crafts program.

Planning	Contents	Location
Atayal Cultural Arts and Crafts Course	Strings of millet beads; Atayal woven fabric; creative shoes; leather carving; ramie key ring	Community society
Accomplishments sharing at end of semester	Exhibition of works and sharing of after-program thoughts	Community high school

3.3. *Development*

Through discussions with the society's arts and crafts experts as well as with the high school teachers, the contents of the teaching unit designed based on students' capabilities include courses on the making of strings of millet beads, Atayal woven fabric, flip-flops, leather carving and ramie key rings.
The suitability of the instructional design is evaluated using students' feedback records and contents from teachers' interviews as assessment tools.
The coding and classification of assessment tools are as follows: "L (learn)" represents students' feedback records; "T (teach)" represents teachers' interview records; and S1-S21 indicates student codes.

3.4. *Implement*

The following explains the teaching processes and end items of part of cultural arts and crafts works.

3.4.1. *Strings of millet beads*

Production process: 1. Select colors of beads; 2. Cut string for making the connection of the hanging ornament; 3. Complete all bead treading and cut the string; 5. Use a lighter to burn and melt the string to prevent beads from falling out ; 6. The product is complete (Figure 1).

3.4.2. *Atayal fabric*

The processing of traditional Atayal weave and ramie fiber is quite complex and the weaving tool is huge. Therefore, the string materials, weaving tools and procedures of modern Atayal weave have been simplified and improved. The production process of weaves: 1. Sort the required strings, "tie string", "load string", and entwine the strings back and forth on the wooden weaving tool; 2. Use a string organizer to fix the required strings back and forth on the weaving tool; 3. Commence weaving ; 4. Complete weaving and cut the string (Figure 2).

3.4.3. *Flip-flops*

Production process: 1. Make webbing for vamp; 2. Cut out length of vamp webbing and apply adhesive; 3. Apply adhesive on "insole" of vamp; 4.Complete making of vamp webbing; 5. Adhere rush vamp stereotype and insole, inset and fix the vamp webbing to present a "semi-finished vamp"; 6. Adhere "semi-finished vamp" and rubber sole; 7. Use machine to compact the shoe to ensure it is adhered tightly, and the shoe is complete (Figure 3).

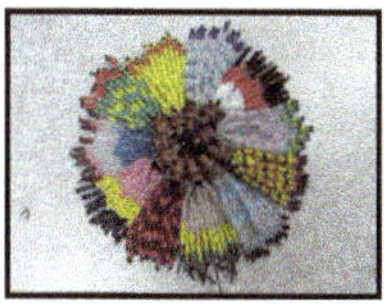
Figure 1.

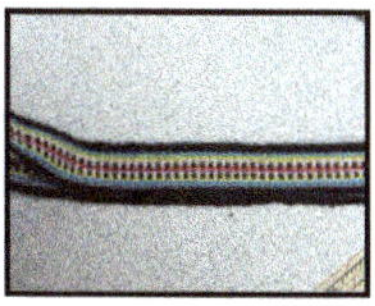
Figure 2.

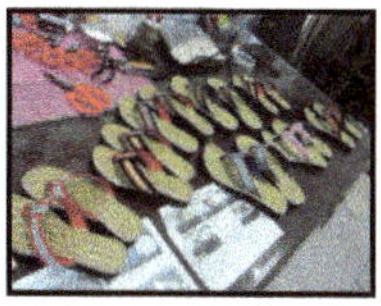
Figure 3.

The patterns of these five works of cultural arts and crafts are design by the students. The products of each student are creative and colorful, indicating individual differences and characteristics.

3.5. *Evaluation*

In order to understand the suitability of the instructional design of this cultural arts and crafts program, the students' feedback and teachers' interviews are analyzed as follows:

(1)The high school teachers approve of such instructional design model through three-way collaboration. They hold that the arrangement of a cultural arts and crafts program can arouse students' identification and interests toward the culture, and that the program allows both students and teachers to attain new thoughts and learning contents, benefiting from the process.

I think the teaching method carried out by working with the community society and the research team of National Taipei University of Education is very good. The students like it and are interested. They often ask me before class, "What are we making in the next class?" It makes them expectant of the next class. (T)

Some of our students have learned Atayal woven fabric in elementary school but, though many students are Atayals, they have no experience in learning Atayal arts and crafts. I feel that the students indeed did gain much experience and identification toward Atayal cultural arts and crafts, and this helps promote their identification toward Atayal culture. (T)

Because woven fabrics require more time to produce, some students take time after class to make them. I discovered that other classmates were willing to assist when they saw those students making the woven fabrics. It was during the time when mock exams were about to start, but a lot of people were making woven fabrics, no matter whether or not they were students who selected to take the course. (T)

(2)Most students say they like the arrangement of the program, and they think the arts and crafts program is fun. Not only do they gain a sense of achievement from making the products, but their interest in learning Atayal cultural arts and crafts is also enhances.

I like the program pretty much. It can be considered as a kind of passing on, otherwise I would not know how so many products are made. Though it is a little time consuming, but the sense of achievement is overwhelming. (LS15)

I feel that this program is very interesting and I can understand more about the skills and diversity of Atayal cultural arts and crafts. (LS18)

4. Conclusion

Through three-way collaboration with a community society and a community high school, this study developed an instructional design for an experiencing course on Atayal culture. The instructional design received positive feedbacks from interviews and after-program thoughts of teachers and students, indicating that it can not only promote students' identification toward and learning interest in Atayal cultural arts and crafts, but also provide teachers with new thinking toward instructional designs for teaching courses related to cultures and societies. Thus, it indeed is worthy.

Acknowledgments

This article is one of the phased results of "A Study on the Teaching of Digital Project-Based Learning at Atayal High Schools" (No.: NSC 102-2514-S-152003-MY3) and "A Study on the Teaching of Digital Storytelling of Handmade Creative Arts at Atayal High Schools" (No.: NSC 101-2515-S-152-003) of the Ministry of Science and Technology.

References

1. Wang, M.H., *Atayal* (San Mim Book, 2007).
2. Rimuy • Aki., *The Rainbow's Judgment: Stories of the Atayal Tribe* (Third Nature Publishing, 2013).
3. Y.Y. Zheng & Y.F. Pan, *Atayal Weave Knowledge and Talent Development, Ethnic Consciousness and Cultural Identification,* Taiwan Aborigine Research Review, vol. 7 (Taiwan, Hualien, 2010), pp. 209-242.
4. Hodell, Chuck, *ISD from the Ground Up: A No-nonsense Approach to Instructional Design* (Natl Book Network, 2011).
5. Shih, M.J. A Study of Designing and Developing Chinese Digital Teaching Materials with Fortune Poems in Chinese Culture, Thesis, National Taipei University of Education, (Taiwan, Taipei, 2010).
6. Lin, C. M, Theoretical Basis and Key Model of Instructional Design, *TAECT: Theory and Practice of Educational Technology* (Pro-Ed Publishing, 2009).

Research and Practice on Specialty Construction of Medical and Rehabilitation Engineering*

Liqing Geng†, Li Zhao, Chunxiao Han and Ying Cui
Tianjin Key Laboratory of Information Sensing and Intelligent Control,
Tianjin University of Technology and Education, Tianjin, 300222, China
†E-mail: genglq2004@126.com

Medical devices belong to one of national strategic emerging industries, in need of numerous professionals. Practice is explored on medical and rehabilitation engineering construction aspects. The distinctive talent training program is developed. The relevant curriculum system is established. The practical teaching system and the subject characteristic specialty laboratory are designed. The academic structure, age structure, professional structure, discipline more rational structure of the teaching staff are constructed. The new path of medical an rehabilitation engineering specialty construction is explored.

Keywords: Medical devices; rehabilitation engineering; training program.

1. Introduction

With rapid develop of our country medical industry [1], the professionals of medical and rehabilitation instrument design development, sales and technical support etc. are shortage. Therefore, medical and rehabilitation engineering specialty is established. There are practical significance in culturing medical and rehabilitation professionals.

As the guiding ideology of facing medical instruments industry, uniting medical institutions and medical equipment enterprises, forging excellent specialty, social needs and occupational demand-oriented, higher vocation college to rely, the high-skilled talents and integration vocational education teachers are cultivated. With fundamental of improving teaching quality, focusing on teaching reform, the personnel training mode and the framework of content adapting social need are established. A high-level characteristic teacher team is activated. Below, talent training program, curriculum system, laboratoryroom construction and teacher team are expounded.

* The research was sponsored by Undergraduate Teaching Quality and Teaching Reform Planning Program of Tianjin Colleges (No. C03-0803) and "Twelfth Five" Investment Planning for Major Construction Program of Tianjin Colleges.

2. Talent Training Program

Combining development tendency of our country medical apparatus and instruments and school-running characteristics of "cultivating applied advanced special talents and all-in-one vocational education teachers" [2]. The talent training program of medical and rehabilitation engineering is developed. The training objective is cultivating applied advanced special talents of medical professionals union and electromechanical union having comprehensive ability to design, to develop, to apply, to maintain, to detect and manage medical and rehabilitation instrument.

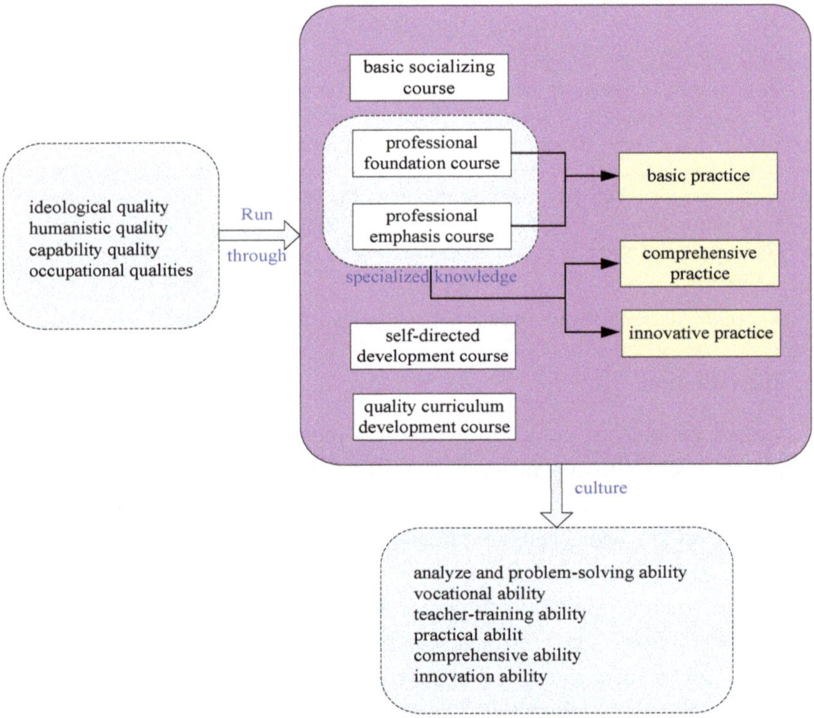

Fig. 1 This is talent training programfigure.

The personnel training objective system includes six modules, such as basic socializing course, professional foundation course, professional emphasis course, self-directed development course, quality curriculum development course and practical training. In the talent training program (Fig. 1) professional foundation course and professional emphasis course are to extend basic practice training, such as course experiment and curriculum project. The specialized knowledge is permeated in comprehensive practice such as integrated curriculum project, skill training, graduation field work and graduation project etc. and innovative practice such as engineering practice, competition, scientific research project etc. students comprehensive ability and innovation ability are cultured. Students' ideological quality,humanistic quality, capability quality and occupational qualities are running through each teaching program.

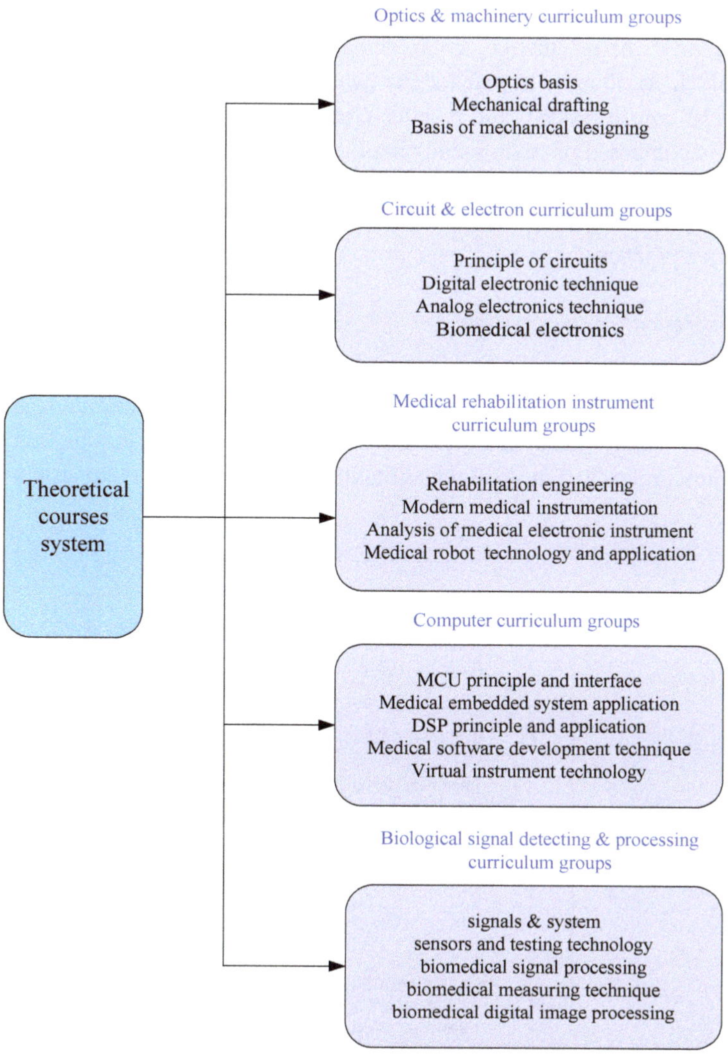

Fig. 2 This is theoretical courses system figure.

3. Curriculum System

According to "double-certificate integration" talent cultivation demand [2]. The layering, modularization and serialization curriculum structure is formed. The course content combines various aspects. The relation of basis and specialty, theory and practice, main subject and related subject is solved. To combine liberal education and specialist education, stand out teaching characteristics of application engineering undergraduate education. The modularization specialty training system of mutual complementation and organic integration is established, standing out practice module. The curriculum system includes theoretical courses system and practice courses system. The theoretical courses system is composed of basic socializing course, professional foundation course, professional emphasis course, self-directed development course. The practice courses system is composed of basic practice, comprehensive practice and innovative practice.

3.1. *Theoretical courses system*

The theoretical courses system includes five curriculum groups which include optics & machinery curriculum groups, circuit & electron curriculum groups, biological signal detecting & processing curriculum groups, computer curriculum groups and medical rehabilitation instrument curriculum groups (Fig. 2).

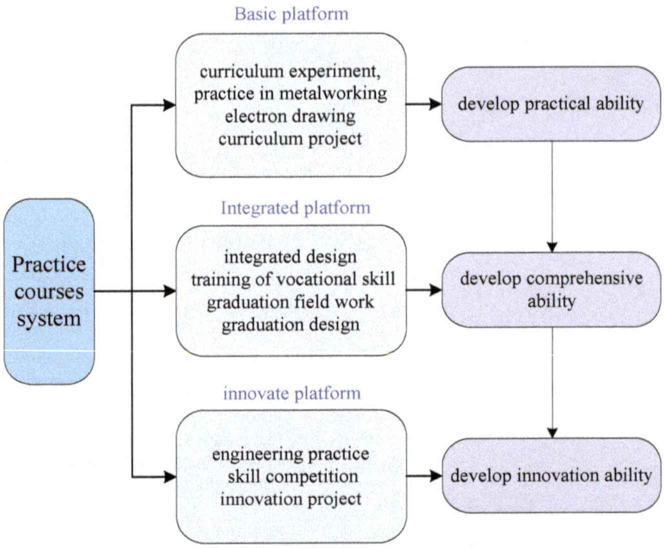

Fig. 3 This is practice courses system platform figure.

3.2. *Practice courses system*

Practice courses system includes basic platform, integrated platform and innovate platform (Fig. 3).

4. Teaching Staff Construction

Teaching staff construction is fundament of improving teaching quality and promoting talents quality. The project team do a lot of work on teaching staff construction. The high-level talents are introduced. Sending out and bringing in methods should be adopted together to build up a reasonable talent team of discipline staff. An academic structure, age structure, professional title structure, discipline more rational structure of the teaching staff is constructed.

To implement "pass three barriers" engineering for young teachers [3], that is teaching, skill and scientific research. The feature double teachers teaching staff. Specific measures are as follows.

(1) The teaching aspect: the implementation of one-on-one old with the new model, Old teachers with rich experience mentor young teachers. To cultivate young teachers on aspect of teaching method, teaching process and teaching method etc. whose teaching ability and culture of teaching are increased.

(2) The skill aspect: new young teachers are trained on skill and learn skills training courses. Improving young teachers' practical teaching abilities.

(3) The scientific research aspect: leading young teachers into the scientific research team to study on scientific research and teaching; training young teachers to carry out the scientific research work independently.

5. Conclusions

Aim at national strategic emerging industries related specialty [4], the connotation construction of medical and rehabilitation engineering specialty is researched. To the talented person and medical equipment industry market demand as the guidance, the distinctive talent training program is developed. The relevant curriculum system is established. The practical teaching system and the subject characteristic specialty laboratory are designed. The teachers echelon of reasonable teachers structure, high teaching level, strong scientific research ability and having development potential is completed. Achieved research achievement has the very good practice guidance significance and promotion value.

References

1. Peiran Chen, Ministry of Science and Technology puts forward to develop new TCM diagnosis and treatment equipment in the 12th five-year plan, Journal of Traditional Chinese Medicine Management (China, 2012) pp. 16.
2. Cuiqin Liu, The exploration and thinking of double certificate integration cultivation model, Vocational and Technical Education, (China, 2000) pp. 12-13.
3. Dexin Zhang, Xiwu Yang, Xihai He, Preliminary study of the training mode: teachers in vocational institutes should pass three barriers, Journal of Shiyan Technical Institute, (China, 2005) pp. 11-14.
4. Jianhua Yu, About thinking of universities developing strategic emerging industries related specialty, China University Teaching, (China, 2011) pp. 43-45.

A New Type of Machine Learning Based Gamified Examination System*

Zhi Yin† and Shi-qiong Meng
College of Science, Ningbo University of Technology,
Ningbo, 315211, China
†E-mail: tougao56777@163.com

Ying Du
College of Humanities, Ningbo University of Technology,
Ningbo, 315211, China

Examination is significant for education. Effective style of examination makes students learn better. We propose a new type of machine learning based gamified examination system which benefits from the intelligence of machine learning algorithm and attractiveness of gamification. The new type of examination system helps students learning happily and effectively.

Keywords: Examination system; machine learning; gamification.

1. Introduction

Examination takes an important role in education. It is used to not only verify the performances of the study, but also push students study effectively. The better type of examination which attracts students more often makes students learn better.

Gamification is a new kind of methodology. It means using games or technology in the games to attract users so as to make the users use constantly and accumulate both experience and skills meanwhile obtain better user experience. It utilizes the concept of games, put the work and joy together. There are many instances of gamification applied in various domains, such as E-commerce, social network, collaborative working system, etc.

* This research was financially supported by the Scientific Research Project of Ningbo University of Technology, National Undergraduate Training Programs for Innovation and Entrepreneurship 2013, Higher education research project of Ningbo University of Technology, Natural Science Foundation of the City of Ningbo, China, under Contract 2012A610029 and Department of Education of Zhejiang Province (Y201120179).

Machine learning is a kind of technique can teaches machine to learn. With data and algorithms, it can make system intelligent. Especially, it can predict and interpret the system behaviors based on the massive history records.

In this paper, we apply the gamification concept and machine learning skills into the examination system. The examination is considered as a two-dimensional role play game. We utilize the machine learning algorithms to make the examination more intelligent. We make the examination more suitable to specific students and improve their study effects.

The remainder of this paper is organized as follows. In Section 2, we sum up the related work. Section 3 presents our work on machine learning based gamified examination system. The further discussion of the system are presented in Section 4, followed by the conclusion of our work in Section 5.

2. Related Work

In this section, we review some new kinds of examination and several works on gamification and machine learning, especially for some real-world systems cases.

There are lots of work discussing new kinds of examinations in the world. [1, 2, 3] study new kinds of examination and analysis the pros and cons of these methods from the perspective of cognitive psychology. Some application based on gamification and machine learning emerges. Codecademy [4] is an online interactive platform that offers free coding classes for people around the world. They have reward system when you finish some lectures, you can level up and have badges. Duolingo [5] is also a free language-learning platform. The gamification of the system makes people enjoy the app and learning a lot unwittingly.

As the cases mentioned above, the concepts of gamification is gradually developed. Researchers study gamification from various perspective. [1] defines the gamification from the view of marketing. Research [2] talks about gamification from the point of human behavior. And many people from game areas also give analysis about gamification [3]. We can see gamification everywhere. There is a report says that we should get ready for the decade of gamification [6].

On the other hand, machine learning is also a topic nowadays [7]. There are lots of systems running machine learning algorithms. Technical giants like Google and Amazon utilize machine learning to solve their extremely difficult problems [8, 9].

3. Machine Learning Based Gamified Examination System

3.1. *Gamified functionality of the examination system*

Our system is designed to be a 2-dimensional adventure role playing game. Students can login the system using student's number or names of them. Then they can choose an avatar as his/her role. Every student has health bar (health points) at the beginning of the examination. And the attendance rate will be considered as the reference of health points. The examination of different kinds of disciplines can be different adventure scenarios.

Students can pick a scenario and go into the adventure (examination) process. In the main examination situation, the character walks around and picks a problem to answer. Problem here is asked by a monster or enemy. The harder the problem is the big the monster is. As in the common examination, there are required questions and alternative questions. You can buy some hints in the stores in the game. The money in the game can be you attendance rate. If you can neither answer the questions nor have enough money. You health points will be reduced. Once health bar is empty, you are dead in the game which means you failed the examination. This kind of real time feedback system benefits the process. We can choose difficulties of the system and we can adjust difficulties of the system. This is similar to the GRE computer-based test system. The difficulty of the problem can be adjusted dynamically during the test process. As a plus, in some examinations you can also build a team to solve some difficult problems.

3.2. *Architecture of the examination system*

Our system is based on rich Internet application (RIA) architecture [10]. This kind of technology can work better in the game scenario which means smoothness, interactiveness, feedback in the real time, etc. All the waiting and refreshing processes are time consuming. Especially in our case, machine learning algorithms of the system using data to fit the difficulties of the examination, data always push back and forth between the front-end and back-end of the system. This makes the process more complicated. RIA is based on the browser and take advantages of both web based application and desktop based application. As desktop software, the RIA can response rapidly. As the web base application, we can deploy the system easily and update the system easily. Technically, it is asynchronous communication system and the problems caused by synchronous communication system such as the long time waiting and so on can be solve by this.

We choose FLASH technology [11] to be our choice for RIA implementation. As a game engine technology, FLASH has lots experiences and best practice. We can find many massive users online games with FLASH and they are running fast let alone having lots of mature frameworks to implement such online system. The characteristics of cross-platform also benefits us a lot.

The back-end of our system is based on PHP [12]. The data transferring standard we chosen is NOSQL [13] schema – MongoDB [14] which is a widely used standard NOSQL database. Consider the machine learning part of our system, these choice make our system more scalable. From the software perspective, we use objective oriented design and development process to guarantee the whole system maintainable and components reusable. The simple system architecture illustrated as Figure 1.

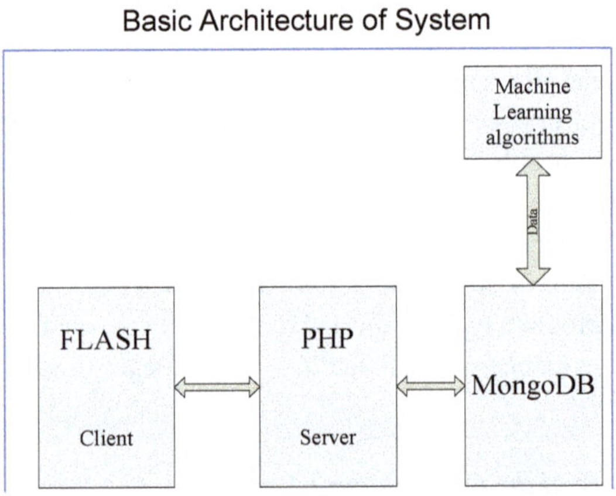

Fig. 1 The simple architecture of the examination system.

3.3. *Machine learning techniques used in the examination system*

As time goes on, based on the massive students data of their clicks and results answers, the system can accumulate lots of data and we can consider them as modes of the students' learning situation. We use machine learning skills of clustering to cluster the students based on their answer data. With the cluster analysis on the test data, we can put the students who have the similar answers together. Moreover, we take the different clusters out and profile each cluster. We got the statistics of each clusters and then store all the result above in a table. When the system is running, initially we can distribute the same problems set to the students. This is based on his/her previous history data. We gather the data during this time of game and use the data to fit the suitable profiles for the students, updating the problem difficulties dynamically.

4. Further Discussion of the System

Since we have analysis the advantage of the system in the former section from the perspective of technique. We will discuss the pros and cons of this kind of system from the perspective of the exam effectiveness and study the restriction to let the system working better.

First, gamification of the exam is a kind of auxiliary skill in order to make the exam test students better and study better. These are the fundamental of our system. So our design of the game is to test all the test of the class, and every game task is served for the exam. Second, although our system is a game, it is not a real game for entertainment. Like the gamification in the human computation tasks, this is "games with a purpose" [15]. We should restrict some negative parts of the game, so as to make the students focus on the exam itself. Third, machine learning algorithms underlying should take a great part in. More and more exam data emerge and machine learning algorithms will work better on the massive data. We can fit the learning curve of the students and get the most valuable study effect.

5. Conclusion

In this paper, we propose a new type of machine learning based gamified examination system. This system not only utilize the joy of gamification but also the intelligence of machine learning algorithm. These traits of this examination system can make the examination more attractive and improve learning effect of students.

Acknowledgments

This research was financially supported by the Scientific Research Project of Ningbo University of Technology, National Undergraduate Training Programs for Innovation and Entrepreneurship 2013, Higher education research project of Ningbo University of Technology, Natural Science Foundation of the City of Ningbo, China, under Contract 2012A610029 and Department of Education of Zhejiang Province (Y201120179).

References

1. Huotari, K., Hamari, J., Defining Gamification - A Service Marketing Perspective, in *Proceedings of the 16th International Academic MindTrek Conference* (Tampere, Finland, 2012).
2. Koivisto, J., Hamari, J., Demographic differences in perceived benefits from gamification, *Computers in Human Behavior* **35**, (2014), pp. 179–188.
3. Fuchs, Mathias, Ludic interfaces. Driver and product of gamification, *The Italian Journal of Game Studies* **1**, (2012).
4. Codecademy (2015), http://www.codecademy.com/
5. Duolingo (2015), https://www.duolingo.com/
6. O'Brien, Chris, Get ready for the decade of gamification, *San Jose Mercury News* (October 24, 2010).
7. C. M. Bishop, *Pattern Recognition and Machine Learning*. (Springer, 2006).
8. Markoff, John, How Many Computers to Identify a Cat? 16,000, *New York Times*, (June 25, 2012).
9. Greg Linden, Brent Smith, Jeremy York, Amazon.com Recommendations Item-to-Item Collaborative Filtering, *IEEE INTERNET COMPUTING* **3**, (2003), pp. 76-80.
10. Fraternali. Piero, Politecnico di Milano, Rossi. Gustavo et al., Rich Internet Applications, *IEEE INTERNET COMPUTING* **14**, 3(2010), pp. 9-12.
11. George Lawton, New Ways to Build Rich Internet Applications, *Computer* **41**, 8(2008), pp. 10-12.
12. PHP (2015), http://php.net/
13. Michael Stonebraker, SQL databases v. NoSQL databases, *Communications of the ACM* **53**, 4(2010), pp. 10-11.
14. mongoDB (2015), https://www.mongodb.org/
15. Luis von Ahn, Games with a Purpose, *Computer* **39**, 6(2006), pp. 92-94.

The Application of Materials Studio in the Teaching of Crystal Structure in Solid State Physics

Qian Zhao, Jianmin Wang and Zhihua Xiong
Communication and Electronic College, Jiangxi Science & Technology Normal University,
Key Laboratory for Optoelectronics and Communication of Jiangxi Province, Nanchang, Jiangxi Province, People's Republic of China
†*E-mail: xiong_ zhihua@126.com*

In views of the crystal structure and symmetry, the key points and difficult points of crystal structure section in the curriculum of solid state physics, we use Visualize module of Materials Studio (MS) software to stimulate and analyze the typical diamond structure listed in the textbook, thus the study situation that constructivism theory advocates is established, which not only clearly shows the characteristics of atomic arrangement and lattice periodicity and symmetry, but also vividly describes some abstract conception of the related parameters about crystal structure and symmetrical characteristic. Eventually, the efficiency and quality of teaching can be improved effectively. Moreover, the application of software in teaching can enhance integration of multimedia technology and constructivism theory, and improve the development of modern education.

Keywords: Materials studio software; simulation; crystal structure.

1. Introduction

Solid state physics is the subject of studying the solid structure, interaction between constituent particles as well as their motion law, and clarifying the solid performance and application.[1-3] It is an important branch in physics with rich contents and wide applications, and an elementary and compulsory course with great importance. Therefore, it's particularly important to teach solid state physics well. But this curriculum researches materials from the electronic or atom level, which is not visual and intuitive. Lots of problems, such as crystal structure and symmetry, demand highly for the ability of space imagination. Because these parts involve in 3D space transformation.

Recently, with the popularity of multimedia technologies, some softwares have been used to show the crystal structure, such as 3D Max[4-5], VRML[6] and Materials studio and so on. Their introduction all can visually show the abstract and complex things for students, and help to develop students' ability of space imagination and abstract thinking. Among them, MS, a material simulation software that can be run on the PC, is developed specially for the field of materials science by the Accelrys company, the leader of the molecular simulation software. Although, there are already reports about MS being applied to the teaching of solid state physics.[7-8] Both briefly describe the application of MS in crystal structural teaching and band structural calculation. But the function of MS is especially powerful, so it is necessary, aiming to one of the modules, to illustrate the subsidiary function of MS in the understanding of related concepts, characteristics in full detail. For instance, Materials Visualizer, the core modules of MS, can provide the tools for modeling, visualization and analysis. We can carry on some simple operations on the Visualizer module to construct 3D models of all kinds of crystal, so that its characteristic such as structure and symmetry, etc. can be revealed visually.

In this paper, taking Materials Studio 6.0 for example, we will show the subsidiary function of MS in the teaching of crystal structure by building the typical diamond crystal structure listed in the textbook.

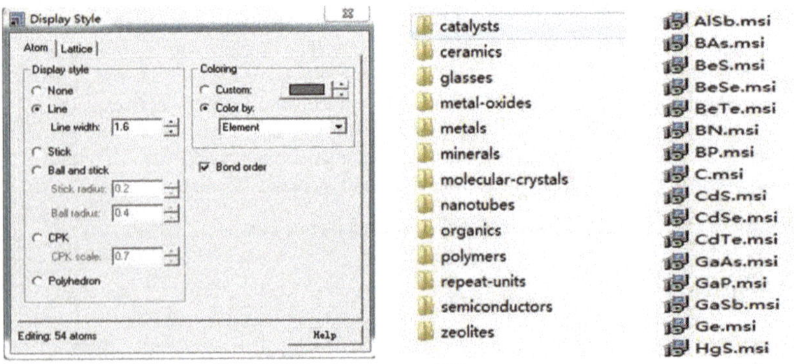

(a) (b) (c)

Fig. 1 Display style (a), data of molecules (b, c).

2. Features of MS software

MS can provide a comprehensive simulation environment, can help researchers to build, display and analysis the structural model of molecular, solids and surface, and predict the relevant properties of materials. Its characteristics are following.

(1) Using the software can construct and display crystal model in various forms, such as linear, ball stick, CPK, etc., and the model can be freely rotated, moved, and zoomed in the three-dimensional space.

(2) It can use different color schemes and instructions to indicate and emphasis some part, according to need, by the setting of molecular displaying style, logo and other functions provided by the software, as shown in Fig. 1(a).
(3) Many data of molecules are included in this software, which can be used directly, as shown in Figs. 1(b) and (c).

3. The Application of MS in the Teaching of Crystal Structure

3.1. *Building crystal configurations by MS to grasp the characteristics of atomic arrangement in crystal*

The form of atomic arrangement in a solid, being defined as lattice, is the basis of studying the macroscopic properties and various micro processes for solid materials. Diamond lattice structure formed by carbon atoms is one of the important basic crystal structures. Its structure is that 8 diagonals are made from the center of the face-centered cubic unit to apex Angle, then add an atom to the midpoint of every 4 diagonals which are not adjacent in the 8 diagonals. Or its structure can be described as a two stagger face-centered cubic structure and the staggered range is a quarter of the length of the diagonal in the cube. But these two descriptions are not intuitive and the structure is relatively difficult to understand among the typical crystal structures listed in the textbook.

While diamond structure can be imported directly by clicking "File| Import| Structure| Semiconductor| C" in the MS Visualize module. And carbon atoms in the midpoint of diagonal are modified white colours specially, as shown in the Fig. 2, which is simple and visualized. So we can understand diamond structure quickly. Moreover, we can clearly find an important feature of diamond that each atom has four nearest neighboring atoms and they are just in the apex angle position of a tetrahedron, that is, each carbon atom forms covalent bond with the other four carbon atoms by SP_3 hybrid orbitals and a regular tetrahedron is constituted.

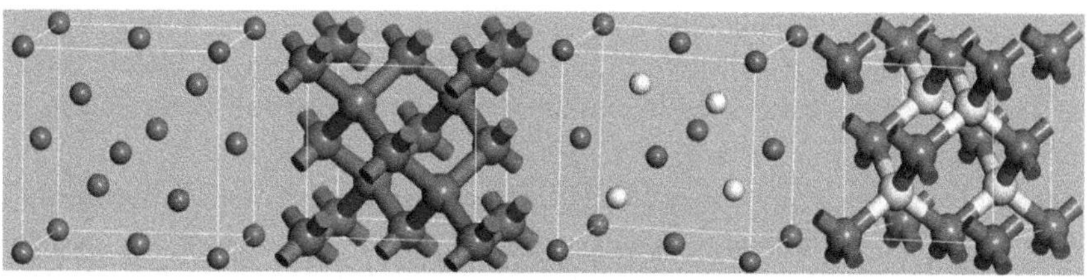

Fig. 2 Lattice structure of diamond in different perspective and style.

3.2. *Using simple operations on MS helps to understand the periodism*

Periodism, a common feature of all lattices, is usually described by primitive cell and basis vector. The primitive cell can be got directly via the steps from build, symmetry to primitive cell. Then the base vector can be got easily. As seen in the picture, for diamond structure (Fig. 3(a)), two atoms are contained in each primitive cell (Fig. 3(b)) and their coordinates are (0, 0, 0) and (1/4, 1/4, 1/4) respectively. While eight atoms are included in each space unit and their coordinates are (0, 0, 0), (0, 1/2, 1/2), (1/2, 0, 1/2), (1/2, 1/2, 0), (1/4, 1/4, 1/4), (1/4, 3/4, 3/4), (3/4, 1/4, 3/4) and (3/4, 3/4, 1/4).

Through graphical comparison and respective coordinates in the above, two concepts, primitive cell and space unit, can be easily understood. What's more, periodism of lattice can also be accessible through the qualitative displaying of the primitive cell and the quantitative presentation of base vector.

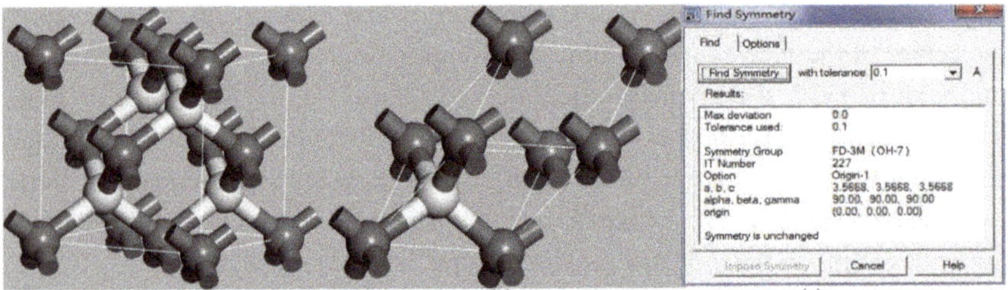

(a) (b) (c)

Fig. 3 Unit cell (a), primitive cell (b), symmetry information (c).

3.3. *Combing with the crystal structure model and simple operations on MS to further understanding the symmetry*

Periodicity of crystals, also being called translational symmetry, and macroscopic symmetry are two sides for describing crystal symmetry. A collection of translational symmetry operations is called the translation group, a collection of rotation or rotation plus inversion symmetry operations form point group, usually expressed in R. While a collection of all the lattice symmetry operations is called the space group and a combination of a translation group and a point group is called points space group, generally represented as $(R|t\ t_{l_1 l_2 l_3})$.

Similarly, the symmetry can be got directly by clicking "Build| Symmetry | show symmetry". Besides, the accuracy of search for symmetry can be improved through "Build| Symmetry| Find symmetry| with tolerance". As shown in Fig. 3 (c), diamond has a cubic point group and Oh symmetry. Combining with the analysis of crystal structural characteristics, the symmetry operations can be written as $(R|T_R+ t_{l_1l_2l_3})$.

Comparing diamond with Sodium chloride, their macroscopic symmetry is the same. But their lattice symmetry is different, that is, all R, T_R in the symmetry operation for Sodium chloride are zero. We say that they have the different space group. Therefore, we can deeply understand the point group and space group.

4. Conclusion

From discussion in the above, the application of MS in the crystal structural teaching can effectively build the study situation that constructivism theory advocates, and realize meaning construction about relevant knowledge, involving not only characteristics of atomic arrangement, lattice periodism and symmetry, but also some abstract conception of the related parameters about them. This teaching method can effectively enhance the integration of multimedia technology and constructivism theory and improve the development of modern education.

Acknowledgments

This work was supported by National Natural Science Foundation of China (Nos. 51062003, 61264005), Natural Science Foundation of Jiangxi Province (No. 20151BAB202005), Science & Technology Support Program of Jiangxi Province (Nos. 20111BBE50001, GJJ14587), Young Scientist Program of Jiangxi Province (No. 20122BCB23030), and Innovation Team in JXSTNU (2013CXTD001).

References

1. K. Huang, *Solid State Physics* (Higher Education Press, 1988).
2. J.F. Wang, Solid State Course (Shandong University Press, 2003)
3. S.S. Yan, *Solid State Basis* (Beijing University Press, 2011).
4. J.Y. Lei, L.P. Guo and P.W. Zhang, The development for the teaching software of 3 d computer animation. *Computers and Applied Chemistry* **4**, 19 (2006).
5. Shi Y.L, The creation and application of 3 ds model about crystal structure in the Solid state physics, *Higher Science Education* **5**, 33 (2000).
6. Li G.W, The application of VRML in crystal structural teaching and analysis. *Computer and Modernization* **7**, 95 (2003).

7. Wu Y.H, Wu. P and Li Y.T, The application of Materials Studio in the teaching practice for solid state physics. *Gakuen.* **33**, 17 (2013).
8. Du Y.S, The application of Materials Studio in the solid state physics teaching. *Technical Physics Teaching* **33**, 54 (2009).

The Combination of Audience Response System and Network-Aided Teaching Platform

Xiaodong Wu[a] and Ronghai Wang[b,*]
Faculty of Mathematics and Computer Science, Quanzhou Normal University,
Fujian Provincial Key Laboratory of Data Intensive Computing,
Key Laboratory of Intelligent Computing and Information Processing,
Fujian Province University, Quanzhou, 362000, China
E-mail: [a]xdwu@foxmail.com, [b]wrhai@163.com
www.qztc.edu.cn

With the development of information technology and the popularity of internet, network aided teaching has been widely applied in colleges and universities. Moreover, audience response system, which allows instructors to ask questions and immediately obtain responses from students through response devices, has also been widely adopted in higher education. In this paper, we suggest that the conventional face to face tutoring should be combined with the audience response systems and the network aided teaching technologies, so that the teaching efficiency can be improved, the teacher-student interaction could be promoted and the performance of the student could be comprehensively evaluated.

Keywords: Audience response system; network aided teaching; teacher-student interaction.

1. Introduction

Along with the speed development of information and communications technology during the past decades, more and more colleges are making use of the network and electronic technologies to improve the effectiveness of their teaching. As a result, computer-aided education and network-based education have played an important role in higher education. The introduction of new technologies has been regarded as the most important innovations in educational systems [1, 2].

Because of the ubiquity of internet, a network-based teaching platform can be established so that the teaching resources can be put onto the server for share. For example, we can build a web site platform onto which the teaching

* Corresponding author.

resources, e.g., audios, videos, documents and other form of teaching media can be uploaded so that students could visit those resources according to their actual learning situation. Moreover, it is also a platform for promoting the communication between the instructors and the students. Via the forum or BBS module of the web site, communications and discussions can be conveniently implemented without the limit of space and time.

On the other hand, the use of Audience Response System (ARS) has grown in recent years. Typical ARS allows instructors to present questions to the audience, and individual audience members respond with a keypad. Then, the responses data can be automatically collected [3]. In this paper, we suggest that these two techniques should be combined together with the conventional teaching so as to make it convenient for the students to access the study materials as well as promote the interactive between instructors and audiences.

2. Audience Response Systems

There are many different labels for Audience Response System (ARS) in the literature, such as Student Response Systems (SRS), Electronic Voting Systems (EVS), Personal Response System (PRS), Audience Paced Feedback (APF), Classroom Communication System (CCS) and voting-machines, clickers [4]. ARS allows teachers to present questions to audiences, then each of the audiences can respond to the questions by a remote control devices. With the development of electronics, ARS is becoming cheaper, more user-friendly and more sophisticated [3].

Using an Audience Response System can improve the students' activity during lectures, enhance their learning and make instructors easily to find out what topics are not well understood by students during the lectures [5]. In order to suit the audiences' actual levels in the course of a class, the instructors can adjust their teaching process and methods according to how well the students can follow, which is indicated by the feedback. For instance, the teacher can stop to discuss misconceptions and difficulties after the feedback is collected.

The feedback is usually anonymous. However, the teacher can assign individual remote devices to specific students in the class [6]. Thus, the statistics data of the students' learning state can be saved to a database for purpose of later evaluation.

Though there are some less positive evaluations of ARS, such as the influence on preparation for class [7], ARS still plays a positive role in the view of many teachers and students.

3. Network-Aided Teaching System

Since there are some disadvantages in the conventional classroom teaching, such as inefficient, monotony in forms of teaching, lack of audios, videos, animations and so forth, the network-aided instruction in higher education emerges, and its popularity has risen in recent years.

Generally, when using a network-aided teaching platform, various forms of teaching materials are uploaded onto a website in the campus network so that they can be accessed by all students. Furthermore, each course is associated with a teaching space and the materials are organized based on courses. Therefore, the limitation of space and time in the conventional teaching classroom is broken, and the workload of the teacher is alleviated because the students could look up the materials after class without the interference of the teacher.

In addition to the resource management, these systems often provide the services of BBS, homework management, online test, and so on. Hence, students can communicate with teacher or other students by BBS, paperless homework can be conducted and even the examination can be taken without paper.

Nevertheless, network instruction also has its disadvantages. A common disadvantage is it provides little higher level thinking and application and lack of higher order thinking [8]. In addition, the platform is often used by students after the class and the feedback from the student is not in time. As a result, the instructor cannot adjust the teaching immediately in accordance with the students' learning situation. Further, the homework usually cannot be checked automatically and the statistic scores cannot be analyzed by our teaching platform.

4. Combining ARS with Network-Aided Teaching Platform

While ARS has been regarded by the students as a positive influence on their attention, interest and involvement during the class [9] with regards to classroom engagement, the integration of ARS with classroom does not necessarily result in improvement of student learning [10]. What eventually influences learning effects is the implementation of pedagogical strategies combining with the teaching technology [11].

In order to improve the learning effects, we suggest that the conventional face to face teaching mode should combined with the above mentioned technologies, e.g., the network-aided teaching system and ARS. Consequently, in the course of class, ARS could be integrated with good pedagogy so as to enhance the classroom teaching effects. Likewise, the network-aided teaching system plays its part mainly after class. For example, by the platform, a student can submit his homework to the system, or post to a certain course forum when he has difficulty in learning this course after class, then discuss with instructor or other students. Similarly, instructor can mark homework with a paperless manner, and be aware of the students' learning situation. Therefore, both instructors and students are able to manage or obtain the learning resources in and after class without limitation. In addition, flipped classroom teaching reform has grown in recent years. The successful probability of flipped classroom will be improved when the ARS and network-aided teaching system apply in it.

Moreover, the students' learning can be evaluated comprehensively in this mode. Figure 1 shows the three aspects that mainly decide the synthesized performance, which come from the ARS statistic, network-aided teaching system, and the everyday face to face instruction. Since some of those data are automatically generated, the workload of the teacher can be relieved.

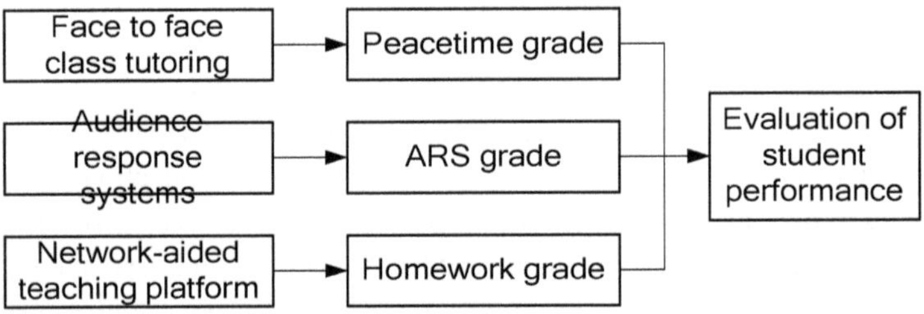

Fig. 1 Evaluation of the students' performance.

5. Conclusion

With the development of the information and electronic technology, the audience response system and network-aided teaching system have been applied in the colleges and universities to assist teaching in higher education. In this paper, we suggest that the conventional teaching should be integrated with these two technologies, so as to improve the students' positivity, enhance the teaching efficiency and relieve the workload of the teacher.

Acknowledgments

This work was supported in part by the Natural Science Foundation of Fujian Province, China (Grant No. 2015J01663), Key Project of Quanzhou City Science and Technology Program (No. 2015Z121), Quanzhou Normal University Scientific Research Initiative Foundation, and the Teaching Reform Project of Quanzhou Normal University (Grant No. JAX14013).

References

1. Ha, Sung Ho and Bae, Sung Min and Park, Sang Chan. 2000. "Web mining for distance education," International Conference on Management of Innovation and Technology, 2000, ICMIT 2000, pp. 715-719.
2. Romero, Cristobal and Ventura, Sebastian. 2007. "Educational data mining: A survey from 1995 to 2005," Expert systems with applications, 33(1): 135-146.
3. Boscardin, Christy and Penuel, William. 2012. "Exploring benefits of audience-response systems on learning: a review of the literature," Academic Psychiatry, Springer, 36(5): 401-407.
4. MacArthur, James R and Jones, Loretta L. 2008. "A review of literature reports of clickers applicable to college chemistry classrooms," Chemistry Education Research and Practice, 9(3): 187-195.
5. Uhari, Matti and Renko, Marjo and Soini, Hannu. 2003. "Experiences of using an interactive audience response system in lectures," BMC Medical Education, 3(1): 12.
6. Kay, Robin and Knaack, Liesel. 2009. "Exploring the use of audience response systems in secondary school science classrooms," Journal of Science Education and Technology, Springer, 18(5): 382-392.
7. MacGeorge, Erina L and Homan, Scott R and Dunning Jr, John B and Elmore, David and Bodie, Graham D and Evans, Ed and Khichadia, Sangeetha and Lichti, Steven M and Feng, Bo and Geddes, Brian. 2008. "Student evaluation of audience response technology in large lecture classes," Educational Technology Research and Development, Springer, 56(2): 125-145.
8. Fish, Wade W and Gill, Peggy B. 2009. "Perceptions of Online Instruction," Online Submission, ERIC, 8(1).
9. Rice, Ronald E and Bunz, Ulla. 2006. "Evaluating a wireless course feedback system: The role of demographics, expertise, fluency, competency, and usage," SIMILE: Studies In Media & Information Literacy Education, UT Press, 6(3): 1-23.
10. Kay, Robin H and LeSage, Ann. 2009. "A strategic assessment of audience response systems used in higher education," Australasian Journal of Educational Technology, 25(2): 235-249.
11. Simpson, V and Oliver, M. 2007. "Electronic voting systems for lectures then and now: A comparison of research and practice," Australasian Journal of Educational Technology, 23(2), 187-208.

Novel Communication System Teaching Method Exploiting Android Based RFID System *

Zhou Ronghua†, Ye Neng and Lu Jihua
School of Information and electronics, Beijing Institute of Technology, Beijing, 100081, China
†E-mail: zhrh@bit.edu.cn

Universities are experiencing significant growth in international students' enrollment, which makes the teaching innovations are urgently needed. Practical and systematic experiments are suitable for some traditional theory teaching courses, like data communication, control theory, communication theory, and digital communication, et. al. However, they are not suitable to the emerging enrollment of international undergraduate students, for the complex theories cannot easily absorbed or grasped by different education-background students. An android based "Radio Frequency identity" (RFID) "Objects' Searching System" (OSS) is designed to demonstrate the transmission and controlling of signals through the user-friendly Android apps, and also explain easily the information exchange and signal processing. The proposed OSS has a flexible mobile keyboard control center, which is suitable to non-native international students to operate. Also, the proposed android RFID system combines Bluetooth, serial, and SPI communications together, which are designed to promote the efficiency of finding small objects and has preliminary higher level network interfaces for the students to extend the system functions and further improve the efficiency.

Keywords: Communication theory course; android based radio frequency identification; bluetooth; information exchange and transmission; electronic product code.

1. Introduction

Innovation is an important ingredient of development under the trend of emerging growth of international students' enrolling into modern colleges. Faster paced changing impact gradually the conventional courses, for example, the digital communication system. Android based algorithms has been proposed and applied in teaching methodologies [1-3]. However, most of these platform are more devoted to the software functions and are lack of hardware control and transmission modules [1]. With the rapid development of information

* The work has been supported by the National Science Fund (61002014, 6097201 and 60972018), Foundation for Distinguished Young Talents in Beijing Institute of Technology (X01011), National Major Scientific and Technological Special Project for Next-generation broadband wireless mobile communication network (2010ZX03002-003-03).

technology and increasing number of undergraduates, curricular teaching reformation of 'digital communication theory' becomes increasingly important, because it is one of the most important specialized course for students of undergraduate degree programs in fields of communication, information and electronics, et. al. [4]. Moreover, the teaching effects of digital communication theory course has large influence on the students' professional qualities [4-5]. However, as the rapid development of wireless communication technology, communications with the RFID tags bundled through the I/O (like Bluetooth) interfaces are emerging with the appropriate user applications, such as finding the missing small objects [6]. Thus, combined teaching schemes with software/hardware experiments are more and more popular in digital communication theory courses. On the one hand, the "Information and Internet" era bears characteristics of well comprehension, quick development, flexible migration, and expansion abilities to other radio fields. On the other hand, conventional 'digital communication experimental platforms are lack of extensibility and flexibility and also hard for an international student to understand, let alone to grasp those experimental instructions and carry out the experiments smoothly.

Small objects are easily missing or lost in our fast-pace modern life. We propose an android based "Radio Frequency identity" (RFID) "Objects' Searching System" (OSS), which bears high extensibility and flexibility, comparing with traditional hardware and software experiment platforms, is useful for experimental teaching, improving students' interests and awareness of digital communication. This system can demonstrate the digital signal transmission process through the user-friendly Android apps, which combines digital signal processing, Bluetooth communication, and SPI applications. The basic experiment skills of C++ language and practical abilities could be enhanced through the proposed system. Moreover, the extensibility of the new platform allows students to design extra components, which is helpful for improving their practice and innovation ability.

The main features of proposed platform are that it generously bears a time-driven architecture, built from the bottom to up, and includes a variety of subsystems. Accordingly, the coexisting of model-driven and features driven approach enable the system to add new nodes quickly [7]. Also, the system functions can be simulated and verified by software, then verification can be realized based on software and hardware simultaneously. This features could enable students acquire knowledge profoundly and intuitionally. In this way, the students can master the basic principle of digital communication theory and basic operation firmly, which would be helpful for developing the interests of students, especially international students.

Teaching practice shows that the proposed android based RFID experimental platform can enhance students' mastery of the digital information transmission process and can obtain the actual hardware signal measurements and software design process. Moreover, the students' interests in learning and motivation can be improved by independent design, debugger the program, and in contrast with measures of the hardware platform.

2. System Design Model

Current experiment teaching of digital communication theory was mainly based on modular hardware platform, whose experiments could only contain little parts of an integrated digital communication system, such as sampling theory, modulation/demodulation and channel coding. The proposed designation combines communication, control and information transmission of a full-featured, flexible and extensible digital communication platform which can validate and complement the expansion the existing course's contents and improve the teaching effects.

2.1. *Overview of designation*

A novel design of OSS is proposed as follows:

1) Replace the central controller by android Operating System (OS) to make the system connect with the Internet; 2) Design the mobile applications that allow users to name the serial number for each tag, which means the user only need to name new tag on Smartphone, instead of buying a new set of controller and tags, which can greatly enhance the reusability of the proposed OSS; 3) Frequency band of 2.4GHz to assure the compatibility with the other generally used personal wireless devices. 4) RAM of RF tags and functions are defined with the standard EPC GEN2, which strengthen the compatibility [8].

2.2. *Diagram of objects' searching system*

There are three main modules "User Interface", "Gate Module", and "RF Tag" marked with A, B, C in the proposed objects' searching system, shown in Fig. 1.

The aforementioned functions are described as follows:

(1) User interface: Bluetooth and NFC are used in Android operating system (OS), written in Java. Two kinds of technologies can be applied here; one is to use Bluetooth as the signal L_{ab}, the other is to use NFC as L_{ab}. The former is well established, and the second is common in the up-to-date

cellphones and is more popular today. Using NFC can reduce a lot of trouble in the section B.

(2) Gate Module: This module receives control and data packets from Android OS, and then decodes them and transmitted to the RF tags.

(3) RF Tag: initialize and number the tags and set searching mode. When receiving the relevant signals, the tag enables local power and drives the buzzer.

Using the aforementioned modules, the user can find small objects through the buzzer, and then the user turn off the buzzer's power manually.

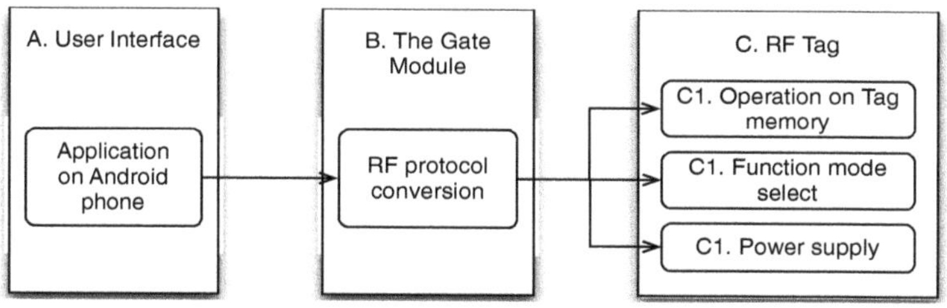

Fig. 1 Block diagram of proposed android based RFID system.

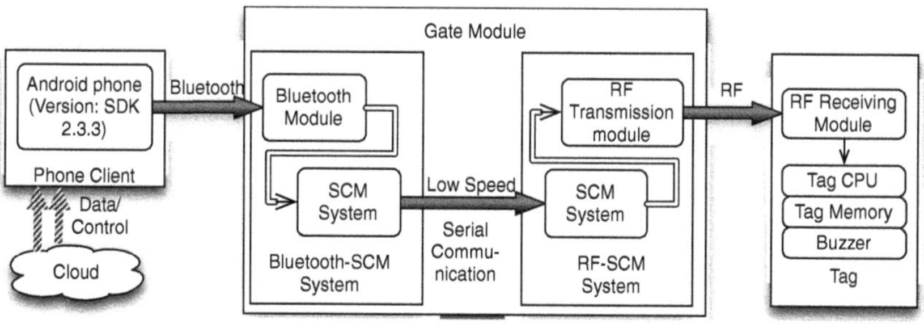

Fig. 2 Hardware diagram of objects searching system.

3. Hardware Design of Objects' Searching System

The system block diagram with the specific hardware is shown in Fig. 2.

Figure 2 shows that several things should followed to fulfill the OSS functions. First, we develop the application on Android Software Development Kit 2.33 (SDK 2.33). Then, Bluetooth module along with the MCU is used to form the Bluetooth-MCU system. Third, choose NRF24L01 module to transmit radio signals and another NRF24L01 module as the tag, which can be further developed to achieve wireless charging and storing electricity.

3.1. *Hardware design of gate module*

Gate module contains Bluetooth-SCM and RF-embedded SCM modules.

nRF24L01 is a highly integrated, ultralow power (ULP) 2Mbps RF transceiver IC in the ISM (Industrial, Scientific and Medical) 2.4GHz band, which integrates a RF transceiver, RF synthesizer, and a baseband logic module with enhanced ShockBurst™ hardware protocol accelerator, which support a applicable high-speed SPI interface controller. The connections between nRF24L01 and MCU modules are defined in Fig. 3.

nRF24L01 module first uses ShockBurst mode to connect with MCU module. Then, the MCU send data by using nRF24L01 RF protocol based on the "address" and "data" of nRF24L01, i. e. add header at the beginning and CRC check code at the end. During the data's receiving, RF module will do calibration and verification first, and then prompt MCU to accept high-speed data streams, which greatly reduces the burden of MCU and enables the low speed MCU to adapt to high data transmission requirements.

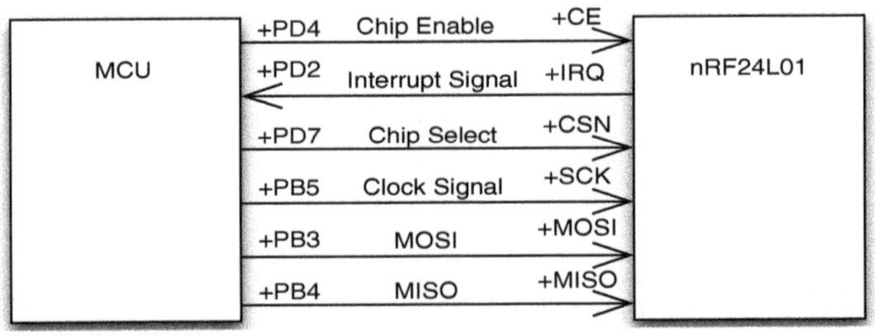

Fig. 3 Connections between nRF24L01 and MCU.

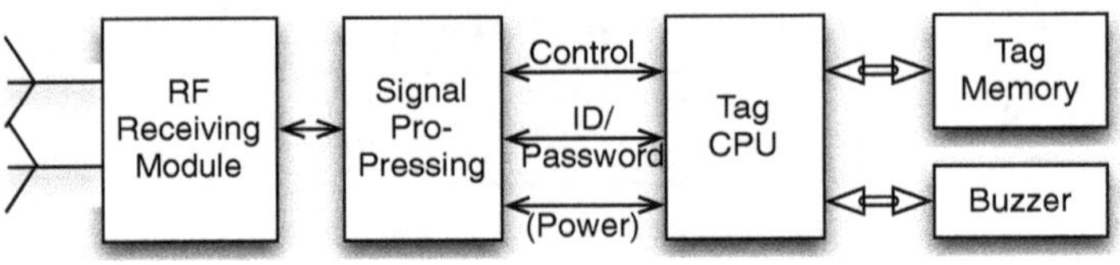

Fig. 4 Hardware structure of RF Tag.

3.2. *Structure of RF Tag*

Combining ISO/IEC 18000, EPC global, and UID standards, the RF Tag bears the following logical structure.

The storage unit in Fig. 4 having four chunks, here are their names and functions: 1) Reserved memory: contain system commend and system password; 2) EPC memory: store the Tag ID information and password; 3) TID Memory: store the Tag vendor information; 4) User storage: for users to customize the information stored. The processing unit operates with built-in power supply, and controls the behavior of the Tag depending on the control signal and system commend, for example, change the content of the storage or start the buzzer.

4. Software Design of Proposed Android Based RFID System

4.1. *Software design of the Android User Interface*

Except for interacting with user, the software will be designed to enable communication and data transmission between Android smartphone and other Bluetooth modules [12-13]. The Android platform includes support for the Bluetooth network stack, which allows a device to wirelessly exchange data with other Bluetooth devices. All the Bluetooth APIs are available in android Bluetooth, through which the main Bluetooth communication can be realized.

4.1.1. *Setting up Bluetooth*

1) Get the Bluetooth Adapter which represent the device's own Bluetooth adapter (the Bluetooth radio); 2) Enable Bluetooth by setting the Bluetooth Adapter. Then, a dialog appears to request the user permission of enable Bluetooth.

4.1.2. *Searching the object device*

Using method packaged in Bluetooth Adapter, such as start Discovery() function which will scan for about 12 seconds, and then return a page scan of each founded device to retrieve its Bluetooth name, we can find remote Bluetooth devices either through device discovery or by querying the list of paired (bonded) devices.

4.1.3. *Connecting devices*

When we see the feedback device list of the start Discovery() function, we cannot actually communicate with any of the device on the list without Bluetooth socket. In order to create a connection, one device must open a server socket through Bluetooth Socket packaged in android Bluetooth, and the other one must initiate the connection (using the server device's MAC address to initiate a connection). A request will be on the screen in following Fig. 5.

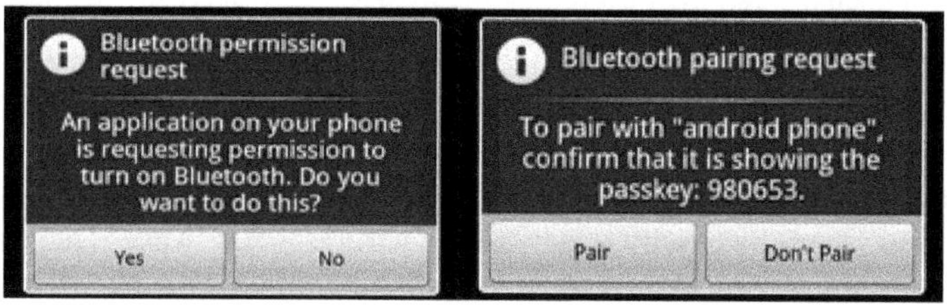
Bluetooth permission request
An application on your phone is requesting permission to turn on Bluetooth. Do you want to do this?
Yes
No
Bluetooth pairing request
To pair with "android phone", confirm that it is showing the passkey: 980653.
Pair
Don't Pair

Fig. 5 The prompt interface.

4.1.4. *Managing a connection*

After the connection is established, we open the serial port. The smart phone can communicate with outer Bluetooth module in the framework of Bluetooth Socket.

4.2. *Workflow design of gate module*

4.2.1. *Bluetooth-MCU system*

We have made the hardware design of the Bluetooth-MCU system, and now we employ serial port communication to enable data transmission between the Bluetooth module and the MCU. The MCU in Bluetooth-MCU system connects the Bluetooth module and the lower machine.

4.2.2. *RF embedded MCU system*

We use SPI to realize the inner connection between nRF2401 and MCU, which act as a process unit in RF embedded MCU system [9-10].

4.3. *The workflow design of the Tag*

The workflow diagram of the Tag is shown in Fig. 6. The Tag will be test the ID series and the password for further operations. This method follows the trend of the RFID development.

4.4. *Protocol design and strategy improvement*

Communication Protocol between the Bluetooth-MCU and RF-MCU system uses low-speed serial I/O ports to enable communication between the Bluetooth-MCU and RF-MCU system [11].

The communication occurs between the two MCUs between Bluetooth-MCU and RF-MCU system. We choose 2 I/O ports (Pa and Pb) as control ports, 3 I/O ports (Pc1,Pc2 and Pc3) as data ports and another I/O port Pd as check digit in each MCU, and then we define the interfaces between the two MCUs.

We can design different sizes' tags to support different applications. For example, the Tag on the key should be smaller and less powerful than the Tag on a casket. Then if we take advantages of some novel technology such as wireless charging technology and advanced electrical storage media, we may extract and store electricity from the electromagnetic wave and use this electricity to support the Gate module.

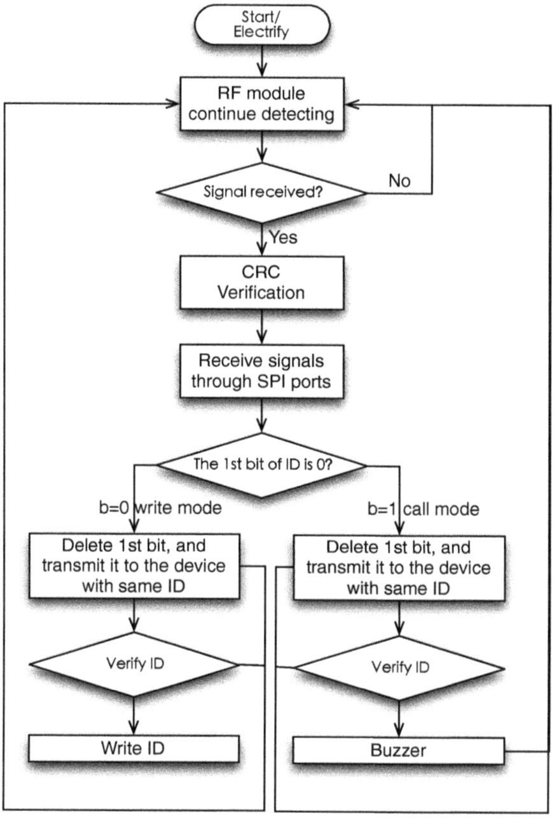

Fig. 6 Control flow of RF Tag.

5. Conclusion

A novel Android objects' searching system with Bluetooth and RFID interfaces embedded are designed to enhance the teaching effects, and promote the study of communication series' courses, including data communication, communication principal, and digital communication, etc. The system workflow starts from the user command on a smart phone, which makes it suitable to use. The phone send Bluetooth signals to communication with the Gate, while the Gate can control the Tag to buzzer by RFID. Focusing on the user experience and industrial production, which is synchronized with major international standards and allows further upgrade. The user-friendly system interface achieves sufficient Internet accesses and cloud controls. Moreover, the SPI based communication is universal and easy to be exploited. The realizations of this objects' searching system enhances the quality of life. Also can stimulate the study and research interests of both home and abroad students.

References

1. Srivastava, D.K., Mathur, R., "Innovation and technology in engineering education system based on Android," 2013 IEEE International Conference in Innovation and Technology in Education (MITE), 2013, pp. 285 - 288.
2. Karakus, M., Uludag, S., Guler, E., Turner, S.W., Ugur, A., "Teaching computing and programming fundamentals via App Inventor for Android," 2012 International Conference on Information Technology Based Higher Education and Training (ITHET), 2012, pp.1-8.
3. Setiabudi, D.H., Tjahyana, L.J., Winsen, "Mobile learning application based on hybrid mobile application technology running on Android smartphone and Blackberry," 2013 International Conference on ICT for Smart Society (ICISS), 2013, pp. 1-5.
4. Zhou youbin. The design of the teaching and research model of communication principal [D]. Jiang su, Suzhou University, 2006.
5. Jiang hong, Mo xiulin, Kang jian, et al. Research of the teaching model of "Digital mobile communication principal" [J]. Journal of electrical and electronic education, 2011, 33(4): 23-24.
6. Yubo Song, Xiaoyun Zhu, Yelin Hong, Haoyue Zhang, Hangbo Tan, "A mobile communication honeypot observing system," 2012 Fourth International Conference on Multimedia Information Networking and Security (MINES), 2012, pp. 861-865.
7. Mary Catherine O'Connor (7 January 2008). "RFID Is Key to Car Clubs' Success". RFID Journal. Retrieved 9 May 2011.
8. Luigi Atzori, IOT: A survey. Computer Networks. (2010).
9. Nordic. nRF2401 Product Specification. Nordic Corporation, 2004.
10. Haiyong Luo, Jintao Li, Junbo Guo, et. al. "New generation high-frequency wireless access standard, Study of EPC CLASS-1/Gen-2," [J]. Journal of Electronic technologies application. Vol. 32, No. 5, pp. 131-135, 2006.
11. Chia Patent, No. CN201120380615.3[P]. 2012-5-30.
12. Li Shaosong, Yin Dong, Mu Dejun, Dai Guanzhong. The design and implementation of extensible Mapreduce based on FPGA [J]. Computer technology and development. 2012, 2,103-106.
13. Fan Changxin, Cao Lina, Communication Principal [M]. Beijing, National Defence of Industry Press, 2011.

Research on the Computer Specialty Construction: From the Perspective of Oriented Computing

Xu Cui[a], Jing Yin[b] and Ran Chen[c]
Shandong Urban Construction Vocational College,
250103, Jinan, China,
[a]cuixu20021981@163.com, [b]yinjing_163@163.com, [c]chr_hl@163.com

The construction of a specialty determines the life of the specialty. And the quality of the computer specialty construction scheme plays an important role in the cultivation of computer specialty students. But in the course of implementation of the existing computer specialty construction scheme, we find three significant questions: the teachers are lack of practical experience; the students have no chock-a-block professional knowledge; the students are lack of practical ability and innovative consciousness. Aiming at these questions, we do some investigation and research first, and then draw up a new computer specialty construction scheme based on the perspective of oriented computing and reform the curriculum construction scheme based on working process. After the implementation of the new schemes, the problems above can be weakened. And the evaluation of students, experts, teachers, and enterprise and industry is more satisfactory.

Keywords: Computer specialty construction; the perspective of oriented computing; working process.

1. Introduction

Along with the information level unceasing enhancement, the demand of the society to high-quality skilled talents is growing. Accompanied with the high-quality skilled talents is Vocational Education which cultivates high-quality skilled talents. In this article, we pay attention to the Higher Vocational Education only.

In recent years, Higher Vocational Education as a form of higher education is paid more and more attentions. A large number of national and provincial Demonstrative Higher Vocational Colleges and Special Higher Vocational Colleges emerged. And a great number of system policies and economic policies come on to support the construction of the projects above. After finishing the projects, the specialty construction and curriculum system showed obvious advantages than common Higher Vocational Colleges which did not been constructed. Our college - Shandong Urban Construction Vocational College is one of the provincial Special Higher Vocational Colleges, and it is under the construction period. In the process of construction, we also have some experience to share with all experts and teachers.

2. Related Works

In the process of specialty construction, three aspects which are training objectives, training specification and curriculum system are the most important contents. In order to obtain first-hand materials, investigation and research have become the most important tasks. We prepare and conduct research data mainly from four aspects as follows:

The first, we use a variety of ways of investigation and research including the questionnaire, E-mail, Micro-blog, Micro-letter, Bulletin Board System (BBS), Telephone and QQ etc to collect data and information. And according to the different objects of investigation and research, we use proper investigation and research methods.

The second, according to each kind of investigation and research way, we design suitable questionnaires which must include all questions we need and convenient forms to fill in. And taking into account the special situation, we add some flexible design to questionnaire investigation in order to get a more appropriate one hand data.

The third, before the investigation and research are going on, we carefully chose researched targets. National and provincial Demonstrative Higher Vocational Colleges and Special Higher Vocational Colleges are the first choices. And the enterprises and institutions that have accepted graduates are the first choices also.

The fourth, we collated and classified all investigation and research data referring to the three aspects of the specialty construction: training objectives, training specification and curriculum system.

The results are regarded as the first hand references of the specialty construction.

3. The Specialty Construction Scheme at Present and the Exiting Problems

3.1. *The specialty construction scheme at present*

At present, most specialty construction scheme is based on the progressive four learning fields. Then design the corresponding courses to support every learning field. For example, the specialty construction is going on according to the basis learning field, individual occupation ability learning field, comprehensive occupation ability learning field, and development occupation ability learning field. And in every learning field, we set up some courses to support the cultivation of the students' ability to reach the ultimate objective-cultivating high-quality skilled talents. Figure 1 shows the process of training professional talents.

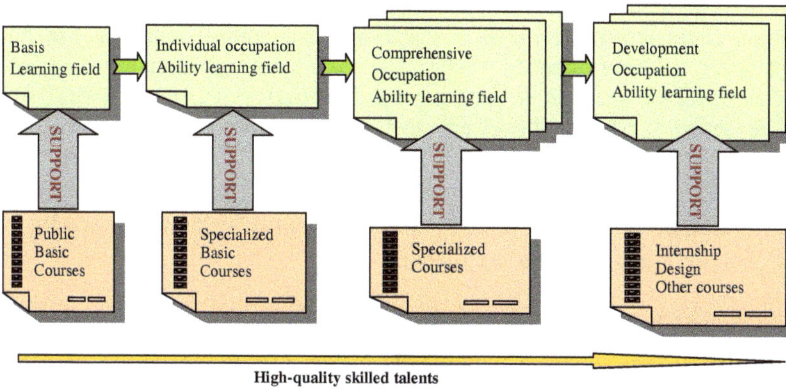

Fig. 1 The process of training professional talents.

Based on the process of training professional talents, we accord to the sequence of courses – public basic courses, specialized basic courses, specialized courses, Internship, and design to cultivate students. But in most cases, we teach more theoretical knowledge and less practical knowledge to students according to the cultivation mode.

3.2. *The existing problems*

If we see from all specialties, the process of training professional talents is tolerable. But for a certain specialty which has unique characteristics of itself is not appropriate. Such as Computer Specialty, the main character is compute. But in the exiting specialty construction scheme, the thought of compute is not exit. Of course, there are other urgent questions from the results of investigation and research aiming at the specialty construction. Let us list and analyze them:

(1) The teachers are lack of practical experience (coming from colleges and universities)

Most teachers in Higher Vocational College have no much practical experience because they are university graduates who do not participate in the training practice. So to practice going to the enterprise is one of the most important tasks.

(2) The students have no chock-a-block professional knowledge (coming from

enterprises)

The main question is the length of schooling of the Higher Vocational Educational system. There are only four semesters to finish all teaching tasks and the rest two semesters are used to Internship and graduation design. It is very possible that some professional knowledge is lost.

(3) The students are lack of practical ability and innovative consciousness (coming from enterprises)

Lower grades, poorer foundation, and less learning enthusiasm are the common characters of the Higher Vocational Educational students. We must adopt better teaching methods to stimulate their learning enthusiasm, and then they will meet the needs of the enterprise and industry.

The three questions above put forward some requirements of specialty reform.

4. The Perspective of Oriented Computing of Computer Specialty Construction and Problems Solved

4.1. *Computer specialty construction*

The Perspective of Oriented Computing has been proposed as a teaching method since 2003. And Shandong University launched a MOOC [1-3] (Massive Open Online Courses) "University Computer Foundations - A Computational Thinking Perspective" which is enlightenment to our computer specialty construction.

Borrowing from the thoughts of the MOOC, the computer specialty construction facing to the working process comes from the following main line of thoughts:

Information society needs information skills,

Information skills come from software and hardware computational thinking,

Computational thinking comes from software and hardware computer knowledge.

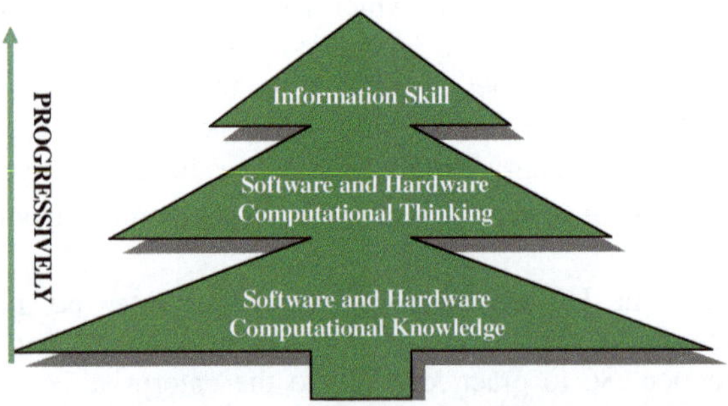

Fig. 2 The specialty requirement model of the computer specialty construction.

Figure 2 shows the specialty requirement model of the computer specialty construction.

In order to meet the specialty three layer requirement models, we set two professional learning lines which are software learning line and hardware learning line.

(1) The software learning line (after analyzing the questions exiting)

In this line, the main courses include Algorithm Design, Data Structure, Data Base, and Computer Program and so on. Figure 3 shows the organization of all the courses related to software.

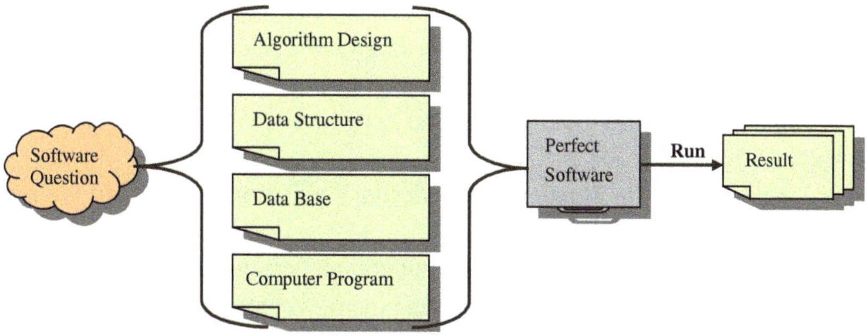

Fig. 3 The software learning line.

(2) The hardware learning line (after analyzing the questions exiting)

In this line, the main courses include System Design, Project Cost, Project Supervision, and Wiring Engineering and so on. Figure 4 shows the organization of all the courses related to hardware.

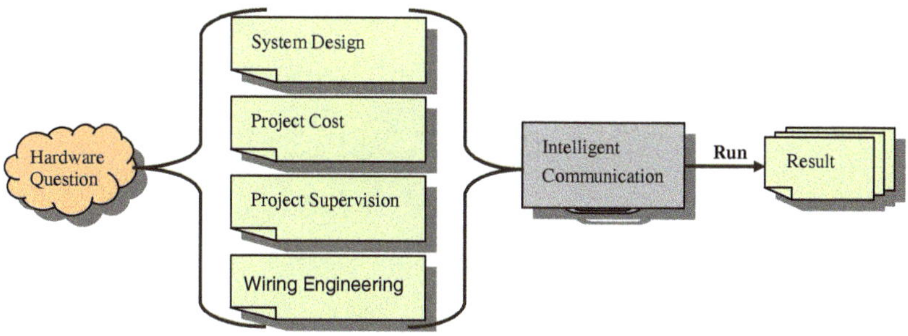

Fig. 4 The hardware learning line.

In the process of software and hardware learning line, a number of relevant courses are designed to support the computer specialty. And in the process of explanation and implementation of these courses, a number of knowledge points [4, 5] and knowledge unites [4, 5] are extracted to support the courses. At the same time, we refer to the relevant MOOCs which are one of the most important information technologies in future [6] in website [7-10]. And we also join some edge courses in our learning process to broaden the vision of all students. For example, we give lectures to our students by inviting famous scholars coming from relevant specialties.

4.2. *Computer course construction*

Following the process of training professional talents, we adopt teaching method based on working process, and indeed it is well worked. For example, the course of *the Comprehensive Wiring Engineering* is designed including four progressive engineering projects:

(1) Single layer, single room design and construction of comprehensive wiring system (SLSR),

(2) Single layer, multiple rooms design and construction of comprehensive wiring system (SLMR),

(3) A building design and construction of comprehensive wiring system (AB),

(4) Building group design and construction of comprehensive wiring system (BG).

In every project, we design optional six subsystems which are different according to different engineering project. And the six subsystems are:

The work area subsystem (WS)
Horizontal subsystem (HS)
Vertical subsystem (VS)
Management subsystem (MS)
Equipment room subsystem (ES)
Building subsystem (BS)

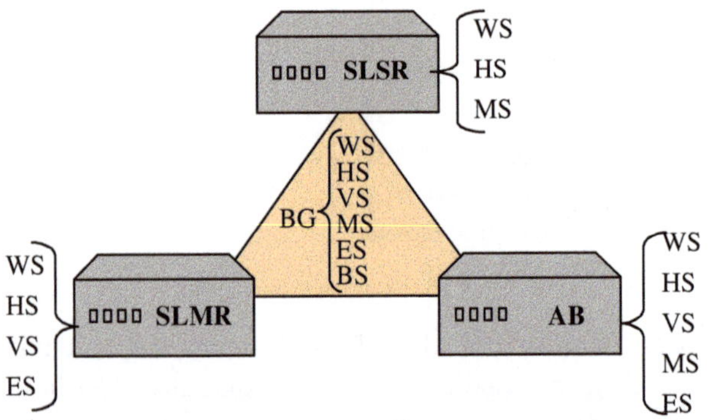

Fig. 5 The teaching process of the comprehensive wiring engineering.

Figure 5 shows the teaching process of *the Comprehensive Wiring*

Engineering. In the Figure 5, SLSR includes three subsystems which are WS, HS and MS; SLMR includes four subsystems which are WS, HS, VS and MS; AB includes five subsystems which are WS, HS, VS, MS and ES; BG includes six subsystems which are WS, HS, VS, MS, ES and BS. All four engineering projects are progressive and every engineering project can cultivate the students' design and construction abilities step by step.

4.3. *Problems solved*

According to *the Perspective of Oriented Computing of Computer Specialty Construction,* which includes specialty construction and course construction, we can weaken the three questions proposed in section 3:

(1) The teachers are lack of practical experience (practicing in enterprises)

If teachers want to finish the course design based on working process, they must gain practical experiences. The reform forces them to increase the practical experience by some feasible measures such as listening to the lectures, learning or doing part-time jobs in enterprises.

(2) The students have no chock-a-block professional knowledge (enriching the course contents)

In order to enrich students' professional knowledge, we also join some edge courses in our learning process to broaden the vision of all students. For example, we give lectures to our students by inviting famous scholars coming from relevant specialties.

(3) The students are lack of practical ability and innovative consciousness (adopting diversified teaching methods)

We adopt diversified teaching methods such as method based on working process and talking about and so on. The ultimate objective is to improve the students' practical ability and stimulate the students' innovation ability.

5. The Evaluation of Students

Every expert and teacher knows that there is a specialty introduction to fresh students and a specialty feedback to former students every year. After doing some adjustment to the specialty construction, we still do these works. From the feedback of the two kinds of students we gain the results as follows:

(1) The feedback of the fresh students (including the fresh students' asking questions)

To the specialty, we know that the learning objectives after listening to the specialty introduction. And according to the characteristics of ourselves, we find the direction that we should try hard.

To the courses, we understand the learning scheme of every course and we look forward to learning all courses.

(2) The feedback of the former students (including the second and third grade students)

Before the adjustment, we only know the four fields in section 3 and the courses in every field, but we do not know the relationships between curriculum. We are confused about the whole curriculum system.

After the adjustment, we not only know the four fields and the courses in every field but also know the relationships between curriculum. We are aware of the whole curriculum system. And we know the direction that we should try hard. And to every course, it is more practical.

And some former students said: if we listen to the new specialty introduction earlier, maybe we will study harder. Although there is a *maybe*, when we hearing the words above, we regret that we do not do the adjustment earlier, then we will cultivate more excellent students.

We do some statistics to the former students about the recognition to the specialty and courses. The average rate rose from 63.4 percent before reform to 70.1 percent after reform.

6. The Evaluation of Experts and Teachers

We have invited some professors and experts of university and college to evaluate our specialty construction and curriculum implementation.

Professor Xingwei Hao of Shandong University evaluates our reform: the computer specialty construction that facing to the perspective of oriented computing is very appropriate.

Researcher Dayuan Jiang of the ministry of Education Occupation Technology Education Center Research Institute directed the curriculum reform of our college in November 4, 2014, and he said that the reform and exploration based on working process is well done.

Our teachers said: we have a thread in the process of teaching and have the key contents. And the same time, the curriculum reform compels us to learn more knowledge and to increase practice experiences. By doing so, we can improve our own self-cultivation and improve the teaching level.

7. The Evaluation of Enterprise and Industry

We have no graduates after the reform, but we have some students who are working in some enterprise and industry. The executive director of the internship enterprise and industry evaluate that this group of students have more practice and construction ability than students in the past. And the following is the feedback of the practice unit.

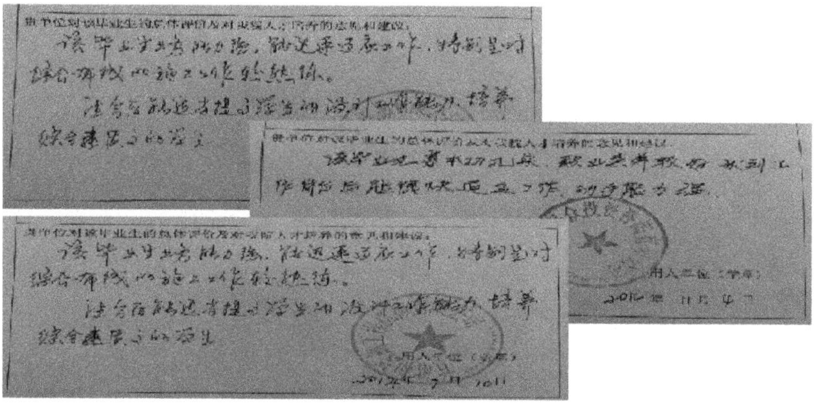

References

1. MOOCs Directory. http://www.moocs.co/
2. John Daniel, Making Sense of MOOCs: *Musings in a Maze of Myth, Paradox and Possibility*, (25 September 2012).
3. McAuley A, Stewart B, Siemens G, Cormier D (2010) *Massive open online courses. Digital ways of knowing and learning. The MOOC model for digital practice* (2010) *Massive open online courses. Digital ways of knowing and learning. The MOOC model for digital practice* (2010).
4. Xingwei Hao, Xiangxu Meng, and Xu Cui, *Knowledge Point Based Curriculum Developing and Learning Object Reusing*, ICWL 2007, LNCS 4823, pp. 126-137, (2008).
5. Xingwei Hao, Xiangxu Meng, and Xu Cui, *A New Layering Architecture of E-learning System*, ICWL 2007, LNCS 4823, pp. 218-229, (2008).
6. http://redarchive.nmc.org/publications/2013-horizon-report-higher-ed
7. http://www.icourses.cn/imooc/
8. Coursera. http://www.coursera.org
9. Edx. http://www.edx.org
10. Udacity. http://www.udacity.com

CHAPTER 5

Building Material and Civil Engineering

Effect Mechanism of Metakaolin on the Hydration Process of Cement

Hou Yunfen†, Peng Xiaodong and Xu Bochao

Beijing High Institution Research Center for Engineering Structures and New Materials, Beijing University of Civil Engineering and Architecture, Beijing, China,
†E-mail: houyunfen@163.com
www.bucea.edu.cn

The thermal analysis and DTA are used to study the effect of metakaolin on the hydration process and mechanism of cement. The result shows that the second exothermal peaks are in advance which means metakaolin can accelerate the hydration speed. DTA and strength result show that metakaolin can increase the strength observably, especial for 28 days strength.

Keywords: Metakaolin; activity; thermal analysis; hydration.

1. Introduction

Metakaolin is produced by heated kaolin to dehydrate at proper temperature [1-3]. A lot of studies about production and usages in concrete of metakaolin have been done [4-5], which show that the structure of activity for metakaolin is different from fly ash and slag which are glass structures formed by rapid cooling melt [6-7], but structure of metakaolin is amorphous. Metakaolin can increase strength more than fly ash and slag can. In order to make clear the reason, pure cement as a comparison, the hydration process and mechanism of cement with metakaolin are studied by thermal analysis and DTA, and the strengths of different ages are measured too.

2. Raw Materials and Test Method

2.1. *Raw materials*

P.O 42.5 manufactured in Jinyu is used. Metakaolin is made by calcined kaolin for 2 hours at 750°C.

2.2. *Test method*

ToniCAL-Technik thermal analyser is used to analyse hydration heat and WCT-

2C differential thermal analyser is used.

3. Results and Analysis

3.1. *Thermal analysis for metakaolin-cement system*

The first exothermal peaks of five pastes during hydration process are showed in Fig. 1. It shows in Fig. 1 that the first exothermal peaks appear in five to six minutes after mixed with water because of reaction of C_3A, and the first exothermal peak of pure cement is highest which is 106J, but it declines inordinately when adding four metakaolins, and it declines least for metakaolin JY and it declines more for other three metakaolins which is 60J. And then the heat release speed reduces quickly because of delayed coagulation of gypsum and hydration reaction is into induction period.

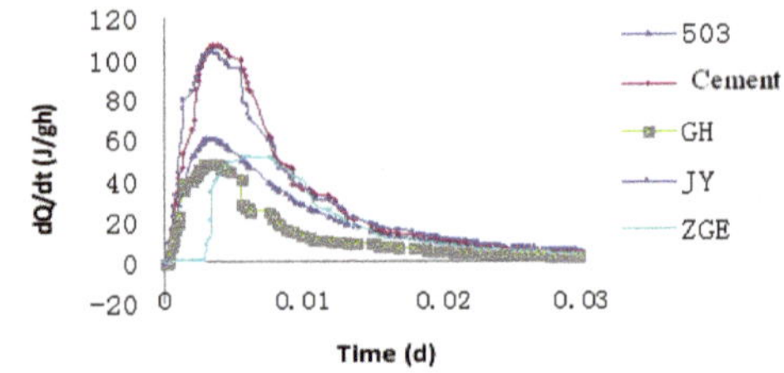

Fig. 1 The first exothermal peaks curve f pastes during hydration process.

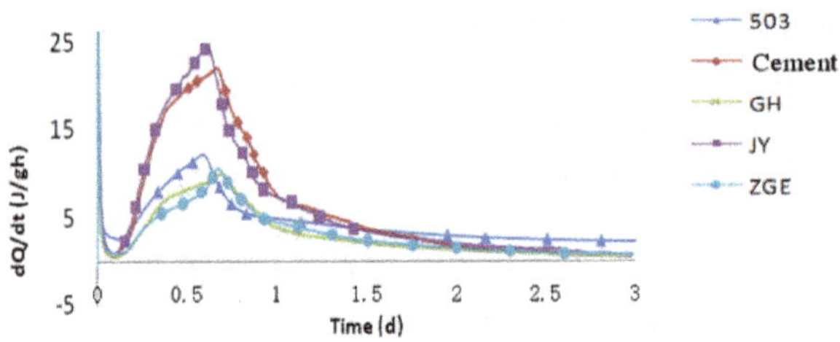

Fig. 2 The 3 days exothermal peaks curve f pastes during hydration process.

Fig. 2 shows the second exothermal peaks. Making a comparison for the five peaks, the peak is highest for metakaolin JY that is about 24J and exceed that of pure cement which is 21J, the second peaks for other metakaolins are lower which are 21J and is half of that of pure cement. Comparing the time of the second exothermal peaks appeared, it can find that it is in advance when adding metakaolin which indicates that metakaolin can accelerate the hydration speed, in especial for metakaolin of JY and 503.

In conclusion, metakaolin adding in cement can reduce the hydration heat amount and shorten induction period and bring forward the second exothermal peak.

3.2. *DTA analysis for metakaolin-cement system*

Fig. 3 is DTA curve of five pastes hydrating for 2 days. The endothermic peaks at temperature 460℃ due to $Ca(OH)_2$ decomposing shows the hydration process. From Fig. 3, it can be seen that the endothermic peaks of metakaolins-cement are sharper than that of pure cement which shows that metakaolin can accelerate hydrate of cement to form more $Ca(OH)_2$, and shows that the extent of the second reaction of metakaolin is low during that time.

When hydration for 3 to 7 days (seen Fig. 4 and Fig. 5), the endothermic peaks due to $Ca(OH)_2$ decomposing of metakaolin-cement are lower than that of pure cement which means that the second reaction of metakaolin with $Ca(OH)_2$ proceeds to a certain extend.

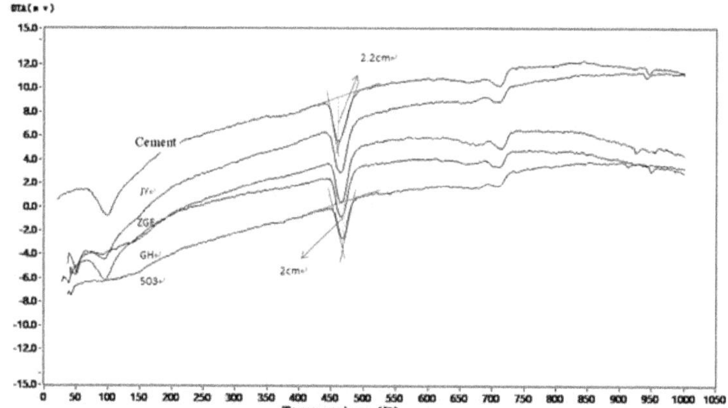

Fig. 3 The DTA curve of metakaolin-cement for 2 days.

3.3. *Influence of metakaolin to mortar strength*

In order to study the influence of metakaolin to strength of long time, the strengths of cement mortars with 10% metakaolin are measured listed in Fig. 6.

Fig. 6 shows that metakaolin can increases compressive strength of cement mortar at a certain degrees. Comparing 3 days strength, it can be seen that the strength of sample with metakaolin ZGE is up to 48MPa which is 2.6 times to that (is 18MPa) of pure cement, and then strength of sample with metakaolin JY is up 133% than that of pure cement, and strength of sample with metakaolin 503 is 28MPa, which is the smallest of all sample with metakaolin, but it still is bigger than that of pure cement.

By comparing 28 days strength, it shows that the compressive strengths are increased more than that of 3 days by metakaolin, especial for metakaolin ZGE whose strength is up to 110MPa, but the strength of pure cement is only 48MPa. For other metakaolin, the results are the same.

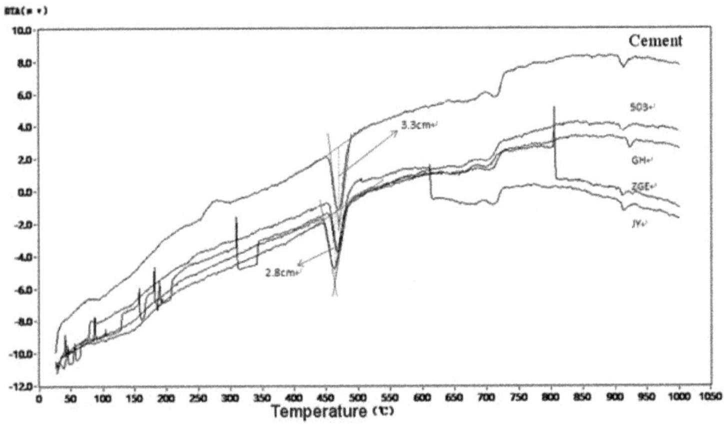

Fig. 4 The DTA curve of metakaolin-cement for 3 days.

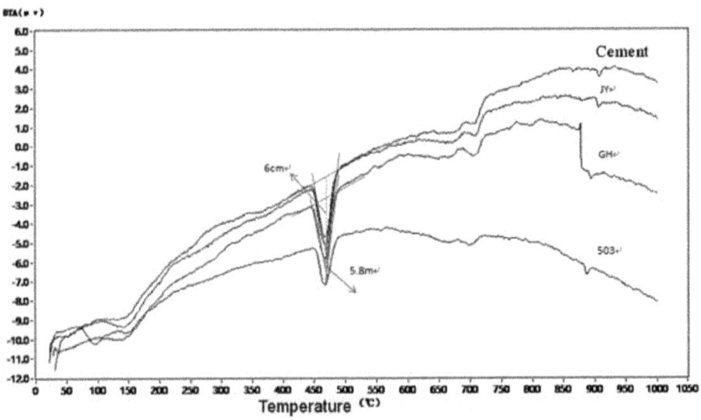

Fig. 5 The DTA curve of metakaolin-cement for 7 days.

3.4. *Discussion*

After dehydration treatment by heating, the $[AlO_6]$ octahedral structure of kaolin is distortion, which is coordination number of Al changes to hexa-coordination from penta-coordination, or remains hexa-coordination octahedral structure which is joined by surface instead of by arris. All changes happening in octahedral structure will result in decrease of distance between Al^{3+}, increase of repelling force between Al^{3+}, which will increase the degrees of instability of metakaolin structure. At the same time, although the coordination number of silica tetrahedron is invariability, silica tetrahedron must take place relative rotation and warpage to match the distorted aluminum-oxygen polyhedron which is very difficult to match, which results in irregularity of structure and breakage of partial Si-O bond and Al-O bond. In sum, although metakaolin maintains stratified structure like kaolin after dehydration treatment, the degree of crystallinity of metakaolin is poor which means that the structure of metakaolin is amorphous state which makes metakaolin with pozzolanic activity.

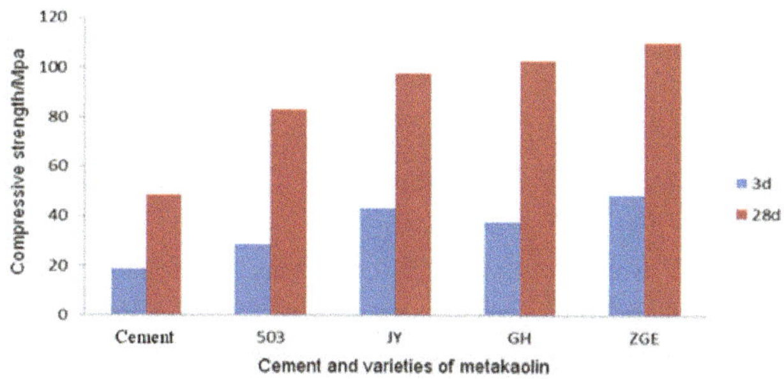

Fig. 6 The compressive strength of different mortar.

When metakaolin is added in cement, it can be as a crystal nucleus to accelerate the hydration of cement and can react with $Ca(OH)_2$ which is produced by cement hydration to form C-S-H and hydrated calcium aluminate to increase the strength for long ages.

4. Conclusion

Basing on the result of thermal analysis and DTA, it concludes that metakaolin can accelerate the hydration speed to bring the second exothermal peak forward before 3 days, and reduces the content of $Ca(OH)_2$ after 3 days. The result of compressive strength of mortar shows that metakaolin can increase the strength observably, especial for 28 days.

References

1. H. Changling, B. Osbaeck, E. Makovicky, Pozzolanic reaction of six principal clay minerals: Activation reactivity assessments and technological effects, *Cem. Concr. Res.* 25(8) (1995) pp. 1691–1702.
2. M.H. Zhang, V.M. Malhotra, Characteristics of a thermally activated alumino-silicate pozzolanic material and its use in concrete, *Cem. Concr. Res.* 25(8) (1995) pp. 1713–1725.
3. Desilva P S, Glasser F P. Hydration of cements based on metalaolin: thermo chemistry. *Adv. Cement Chem,* (1990), 3(12) pp. 167–177.
4. S. Wild, J.M. Khatib, A. Jones, Relative strength, pozzolanic activity and cement hydration in superplasticised metakaolin concrete, *Cem. Concr. Res.* 26(10) (1996) pp. 1537–1544.
5. Xiaoqian Qian, Zongjin Li, The relationships between stress and strain for high-performance concrete with metakaolin, *Cem. Concr. Res.* 31 (2001) pp. 1607–1611.
6. Uchigawa H. Effect of blending components on hydration and structure formation. *Proc. Of the 8th International Cement Chemistry Conference. Rio de Janeiro.* (1986). pp. 249-280.
7. Smolczyk H.G. Slag structure and identification of slags. *Proc. of the 7th International Cement Chemistry Conference.* Paris, France. (1980.1, pp. 3-17).

Structure Calculation and Analysis of the Intake Tower Being Impacted By Landslide*

Zhang Xuhui†, Yuan Mingdao and Pan Zhanzhao
Guangdong Research Institute of Water Resources and Hydropower, Guangdong Technical Research Centre of Flood Disaster Emergency, 116#, Tianshou Road, Tianhe District, Guangzhou, 510635, China
†E-mail: 30408932@qq.com

Zhong Zhihui
College of Civil and Architecture Engineering, Wuhan University Wuhan, 430072, China
E-mail: lufeezhong@yahoo.com.cn

The intake tower of a dam is impacted by landslide during the process of reinforcement. The inlet of culvert pipe is pulled open from the connection with the intake tower for about 30cm. Through measurement of the site of intake tower, non-destructive detection of pile foundation, and the engineering monitoring, it preliminarily analyzes the influence of the landslide on the structure of the intake tower.

Keywords: Structure calculation; landslide impact; engineering monitoring; passive pile.

1. Introduction

In China, the drought and flood disasters happen quite frequently. In order the eliminate the damage and initiate affairs good for the people, plenty key water-control projects have been established, and the task of reinforcement is very arduous and urgent. A reservoir in Guangdong was built in 1966, which is a comprehensively key water-control project focusing on prevention of flood integrating the functions of irrigation, electricity generation and water supply. The reservoir has homogeneous earth dam, with the crest elevation of 260.0m, maximum height of 46m, length of dam crest of 400m, and width of 5.0m. In October 2009, the reinforcement officially started. And in March of the next year, during the filling construction of the clay sloping core wall, landslide occurs at the clay sloping core wall being newly filled at the left side of the

* This work is supported by open funds from Guangdong Technical Research Centre of Flood Disaster Emergency (201405002).

upstream batter of dam, causing the obvious displacement of the inlet of the culvert pipe.

After being impacted by landslide, the inlet of the culvert pipe is pulled open from the connection with the intake tower for about 30cm. Limited by the lack of the monitoring materials of the construction and the precision of the monitoring instrument, especially the complexity and variability at the construction site, the horizontal displacement and sedimentation of the intake tower caused by the landslide, and the safety status of the tower structure can not be precisely confirmed. The safety of the intake tower during the flood season should be guaranteed by adopting effective and scientific methods to discuss the completeness and reliability of the pile foundation based on the geological conditions, and developing the safety assessment of the tower structure.

2. Intake Tower Being Impacted by Landslide

On March 20th 2010, landslide occurs at the clay sloping core wall being newly filled at the left side of the upstream batter of dam, and the number of the pile of landslide is about 20+095.000~0+255.000. The length of the landslide is about 160m and width is about 10m. The entire height of slide is about 2m. A strip of wide longitudinal crack occurs at the surface of filling. The finished concrete revetment has entirely slipped down, and there exists partial crack. Obvious upheaval has been found at the bottom of the concrete revetment and the filling in the groove of foundation trench, and the inlet of the culvert pipe has obvious displacement, the relative displacement of about 30cm at most as shown in Fig. 1.

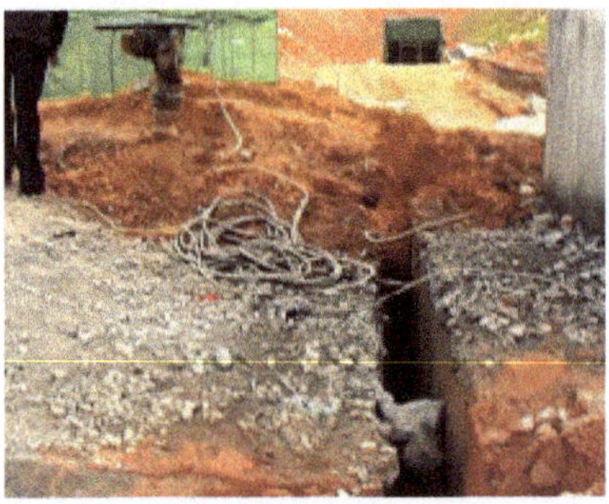

Fig. 1 Displacement and crack of the inlet of culvert pipe.

3. Drill of Crack Structure of Intake Tower

As shown in Fig. 2, the pile foundation of the intake tower comprises four concrete piles with diameter of 1m, allocated in the four corners of the intake tower. To avoid the damage to the integrality of the pile foundation of the intake tower, and also to reflect the actual safety performance of the pile foundation, we decide to conduct spot check of the pile foundation (Drill ZC) by selecting the first pile close to the upstream at the right side of the most unfavorable position affected by the landslide. The designed length of pile is 18.8m.

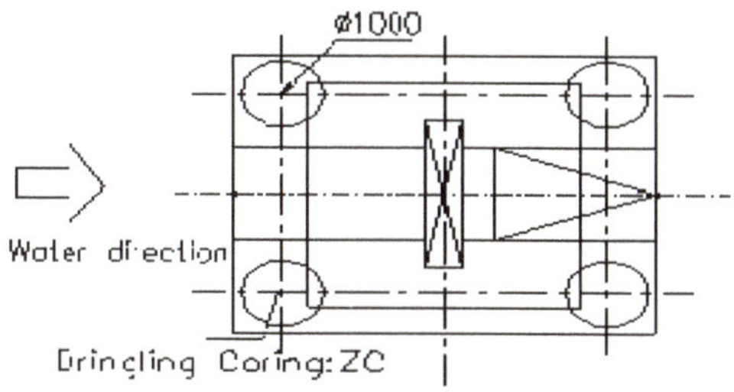

Fig. 2 Schematic diagram of drilling position of the spot check of pile foundation.

The drill locates close to the center of pile, about 30cm to the outer wall of the tower. The single-action and double-barrelled drilling machine of 101mm for geology is adopted. Keep vertical during drilling. The depth of drilling is 16.6m.

3.1. *Drilling Coring of the Pile Foundation*

The results of the drilling of pile foundation shows that the sample concrete cores are continuous and complete with good cement. The samples are columnar, with smooth side surface. The distribution of the aggregate is mostly even and there exist honeycomb and pores at the side of partial sample cores. The drilling sample cores are presented in Fig. 3 and Fig. 4.

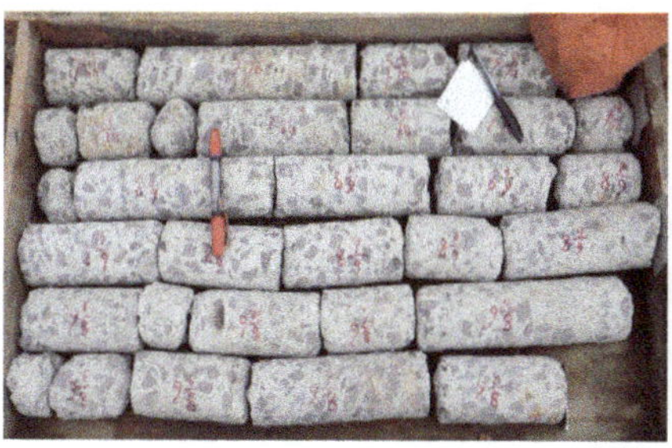

Fig. 3 Sample cores of site drilling(1.0~8.0m)

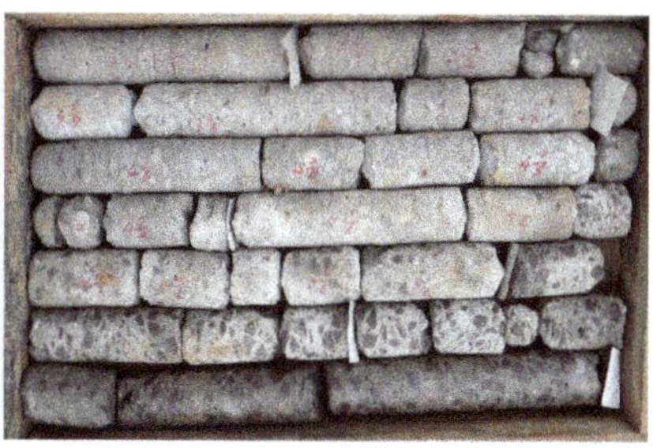

Fig. 4 Sample cores of site drilling(8.0~16.6m)

3.2. *Pressure Water Test*

After the drilling ZC, according to the rules of Regulations for Pressure Water Test of Water Resources and Hydropower Engineering (SL 31- 2003), the pressure water test shall be conducted for every 5m drilling.

As shown in Fig. 5, three sections of pressure water test shall be conducted to detect the drilling, of which the features of the curve are that "the boosting curve is the straight line passing the origin, and the drawdown curve and boosting curve basically coincide". Corresponding to the A (laminar flow) type P-Q curve of the Regulations for Pressure Water Test of Water Resources and Hydropower Engineering, the obtained permeable rate of the three sections of pressure water test are respectively 0.16Lu, 0.14Lu, and 0.14Lu as shown in Table 1.

Table 1 Data of Pressure Water Test.

Footage [m]	Length[m]	Piezometer [MPa]	Water manometer [MPa]	Total pressure [MPa]	Quantity of flow [L/min]	Permeable rate [Lu]	Curve types
-4.0~-9.0	5	0.8	0.068	0.868	0.68	0.16	A
-9.0~-14.0	5	0.8	0.118	0.918	0.65	0.14	A
-12.6~-16.6	4	0.8	0.149	0.949	0.55	0.14	A

We can conclude that within the range of the drilling of the pile close to the upstream at the right side of intake tower, the permeable rate is not bigger than 0.16Lu. It's preliminarily estimated that there is no crack of the pile within the range of drilling and the pile keeps complete.

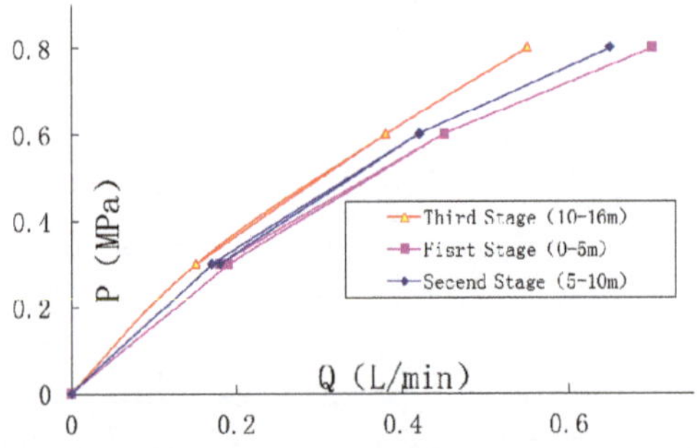

Fig. 5 Pressure water test P~Q curve.

3.3. *Monitoring of Deep Displacement of Pile*

After finishing the spot check of the pile foundation of the intake tower, imbed inclinometer in the selected drilling holes to monitor the displacement of the pile foundation. The monitoring has obtained stable data of 6 times of pile foundation (including 2 times of original value). The result of the monitoring of pile foundation's inclinometry shows that there is no abnormal displacement of the pile foundation. Shows as Fig. 6.

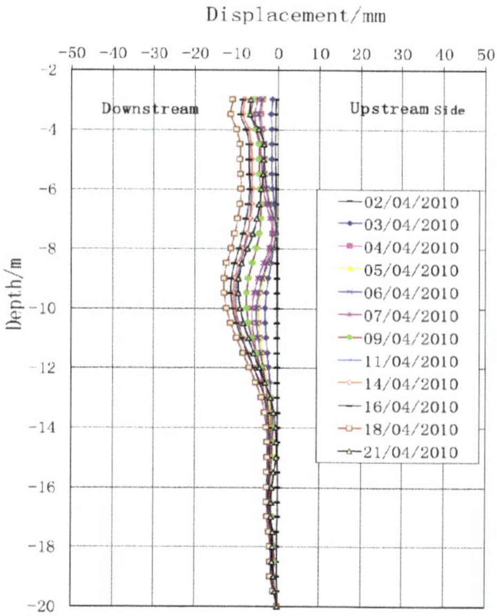

Fig. 6 The monitoring of pile foundation's inclinometry result.

3.4. *Computational Analysis for Passive Pile Structure*

The pile foundation of the intake tower comprises four concrete piles with diameter of 1m, allocated in the four corners of the intake tower. After the landslide happens to the upstream slope, at the beginning of April 2010, the units concerned have conducted site retest on the position of the pile foundation. And the result indicates the position of the first pile at the upstream of the right side deviates about 3cm from the designed value. Now, we assume that the passive pile moves for 3cm, then we conduct analysis of re-check according to the pile foundation, to verify whether the pile foundations meet the designed requirements.

As for the analytical calculation of the passive pile, the difference method proposed in 1973 by Poulos is mostly adopted, which uses the Mindlin solution of the elastic mechanics. The designed diameter of the pile in this method is D, length is L, and rigidity is EpIp. It divides the pile into n+1 different sections, each with the length of δ, and sections at top and bottom with the length of δ/2. The side pressure bore by the pile caused by the lateral displacement of soil mass is {P}, and the horizontal distortion of the pile is {ρ}. The difference equation of the displacement of the pile is:

$$[D]\{\rho\} = -\frac{dL^4}{E_p I_p n^4}\{P\} \cdot \tag{1}$$

In Eq. (1), {ρ}: vector of horizontal displacement of the pile; {P}: vector of horizontal pressure force on the pile; [D]: differential coefficient matrix; n: all the units of pile (the top and bottom of pile belong to one unit).

Due to the external conditions, the displacement of soil along the length of pile is $\{\rho_e\}$, and the counter-force of soil given by the pile during lateral displacement is {P}. The displacement {ρ} equation of soil on the contact surface with pile is:

$$\{\rho\} = \frac{d}{E_{sr}}\{\frac{E_{sr}}{E_s}\}[I]\{P\} + \{\rho_e\} \cdot \tag{2}$$

In Eq. (2), Esr: relative modulus value of soil; Es: modulus of soil at nodes; [I]: displacement coefficient matrix of soil, it equals to add a unit force at i point. The displacement coefficient at j point can be calculated by Mindlin solution. $\{\rho_e\}$: refers to the lateral displacement of soil by external reasons, namely, the lateral displacement not considering pile.

The compatibility of deformation by displacement will happen at the contact surface of pile and soil, that is, the displacements of pile and soil at the contact surface are equal, then:

$$[D + \frac{[II]}{K_R n^4}]\{\rho\} = \frac{[II]}{K_R n^4}\{\rho_e\} \cdot \tag{3}$$

In Eq. (3), $[II] = [I]^-$ refers to the inverse matrix of the soil's displacement coefficient matrix; $K_R = E_p I_p / (E_s L^4)$ is the flexibility coefficient of pile.

The $\{\rho_e\}$ is known, and the displacement of pile, {ρ}, can be obtained by solving the Eq. (3). With {ρ}, the load, {P} (stress on the pile), on the pile can be obtained from Eq. (1). When {P} exceeds the yield stress of soil, the iteration modification is needed. After obtaining {P}, the values like internal force can be obtained by the method of mechanics of materials.

By calculation, under the impact, the maximum bending moment of the passive pile is 561kN•m. But according to the design drawing of pile, the flexural capacity of it is M=886kN•m, and the corresponding displacement of the top of pile is 3cm. From the result, we can see that the flexural capacity of pile can almost meet the requirements.

4. Conclusions

Through the drilling detection, pressure water test, deep displacement monitoring and preliminary structural analysis about the pile foundation of the intake tower of the culvert pipe, we can conclude that there is no crack of the pile within the range of drilling and the piles remain intact; No abnormal displacement of the pile foundation is found; Flexural capacity of pile meets the requirements.

References

1. Zhu Bofang, On expansive concrete dam construction technique, *Journal of Hydroelectric Engineering*, 3 (2000).
2. Cheng Yonghui, Rao Xibao and Li Qingyun, Analysis of main dam landslide and treatment of certain dangerous reservoir, *Journal of Yangtze River Scientific Research Institute*. **129**, 26 (2009).
3. Yang Guanghua, *Practical calculation method and application of deep foundation pit supporting structure* (Geological Publishing House, Beijing, 2004).

Impact of Soil Frost Heave on Supporting Structures*

Chao Sun[a] and Yansheng Zhou[b*]
College of Surveying & Prospecting Engineering, Jilin Jianzhu University, Changchun, Jilin, China
[a]sunchaobox@163.com, [b]zhouyanshengbox@163.com

Effect of frost heave on overwintering foundation pit supporting structure cause a large number of engineering accidents, the research topic is paid more and more attention by researchers. Based on the finite difference analysis software FLAC3D, earth pressure back continuous wall and the impact of Frost Heave on the forced deformation of Supporting Structures are studied by numerical simulation method; theoretical calculation value and simulation value of earth pressure back continuous wall, displacement of retaining structure before and after the frost heave and the change value of soil temperature under different time of frost heave; the influence law of frost heave deformation of foundation pit supporting structure by frost heave is revealed.

Keywords: Frost heaving; supporting structure; forced deformation; earth pressure; numerical simulation.

1. Introduction

Foundation pit engineerings in our country in recent years, especially the past 10 years get rapid development, a large number of engineering practice greatly enrich and improve the technical level in the field of foundation pit engineering in our country. But in the cold regions such as in north and the west China, with the reducing of land resources, construction engineerings demand space form the underground constantly. More and more deep and large foundation pit, as well as the complexity of geological conditions, the particularity of the obvious difference of four seasons climate temperature, building foundation pit damage by frost and circulation, cause large hidden danger for the security of foundation pit supporting engineering in the cold area [1]. The article uses the finite difference analysis software FLAC3D for numerical simulation analysis, research of frost heaving on the foundation pit supporting structure is simplified as a plane strain problem for elastic-plastic numerical simulation analysis. Step 1: by gravity stress balance of soil mass and the supporting structure, the initial

* This work is supported by Housing and Urban research and development projects.

stress state and initial deformation caused by gravity stress are obtained in computing simulation study area; step 2: the stress and displacement of the retaining structure are obtained by excavating foundation pit; step 3: by frost heave simulation, it is concluded that the displacement of supporting structure and the change of soil temperature under the action of frost heave. Through the numerical simulation of foundation pit supporting structure cold expansion, the effect on the deformation of supporting structure is analyzed and studyed.

2. Calculation Model And Model Parameters [2, 3, 4]

The model X direction is 45 m, points of 75 units, Y direction is 1 m, divided into 2 units, Z direction is 28 m, divided into 56 units, carries on the excavation, excavation depth is 10 m, continuous wall is adopted for foundation pit supporting structure, the wall thickness is 0.6 m, the wall under the pit bottom is 8 m, the geometric model after the completion of excavation is shown in Fig. 1. Soil is Mohr model, continuous wall is the Elastic model, physical and mechanical parameters of the soil and continuous wall are shown in Table 1. Thermodynamic parameters of soil and the continuous wall, are shown in Table 2. Boundary conditions: the surrounding of model is normal fixed free boundary, the bottom is three direction constraints by degrees, and the top surface is free surface and the overall limit Y direction displacement; Coupling effect, the surface, side wall, bottom of the foundation pit, are applied fixed temperature boundary-10°C, its mechanical boundary is constant.

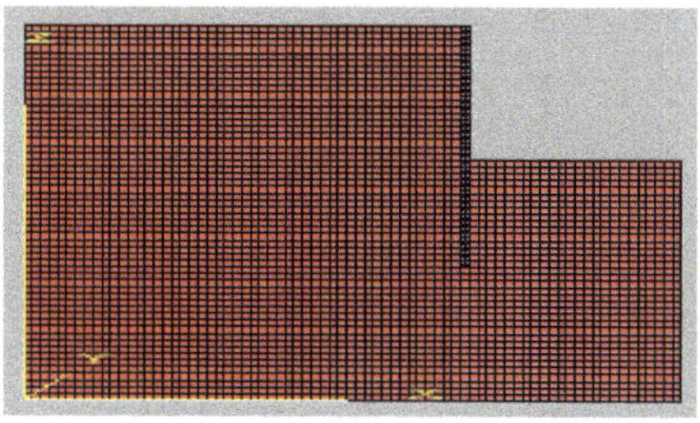

Fig. 1 Geometric model.

Table 1 Physical and mechanical parameters of the soil and continuous wall.

	Thickness of the soil [m]	Severe [KN/m³]	Bulk modulus [Gpa]	Shear modulus [Gpa]	Cohesion [Kpa]	Internal friction angle [°]
Soil1	0.0~3.5	15	10.3×10^{-3}	3.9×10^{-3}	16	20
Soil2	3.5~13.5	16	10.5×10^{-3}	3.9×10^{-3}	20	25
Soil3	13.5~28.0	17.5	11×10^{-3}	3.9×10^{-3}	20	30
Continuous wall		25	15.9	10		

Table 2 Thermodynamic parameters of soil and continuous wall.

	Specific heat [J/(kg℃)]	Thermal conductivity [W/(m℃)]	Thermal expansion coefficient[1/℃]
Soil and the continuous wall	500	1.5	-8×10^{-5}

3. Calculation Results Analysis

3.1 *Simulation Value Compared with the Theoretical Calculation Value*

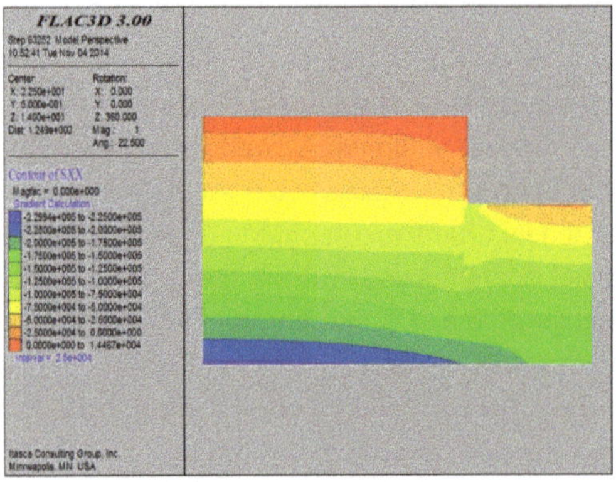

Fig. 2 Horizontal stress nephogram.

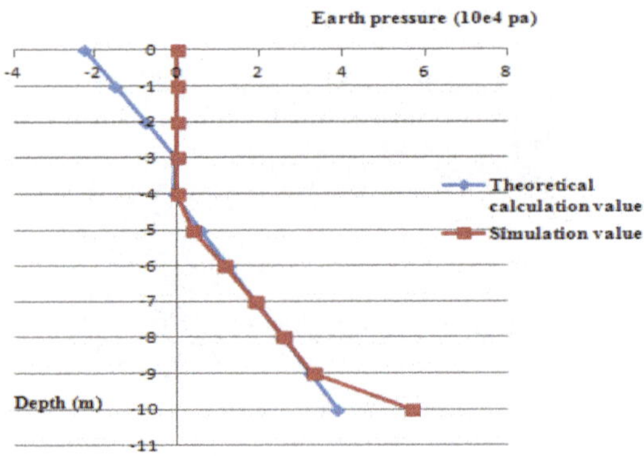

Fig. 3 Earth pressure back continuous wall of x direction.

At present, due to the complex stress state and influencing factors, earth pressure theory is not perfect, we still adopt traditional Coulomb soil pressure theories or Rankine soil pressure theories. In this paper, obtaining earth pressure by the finite difference numerical simulation software FLAC3D; theoretical calculation values are compared with the simulation values, as shown in Fig. 3.

3.2 *Displacement Comparison Under No Frost Heave and Frost Heave*

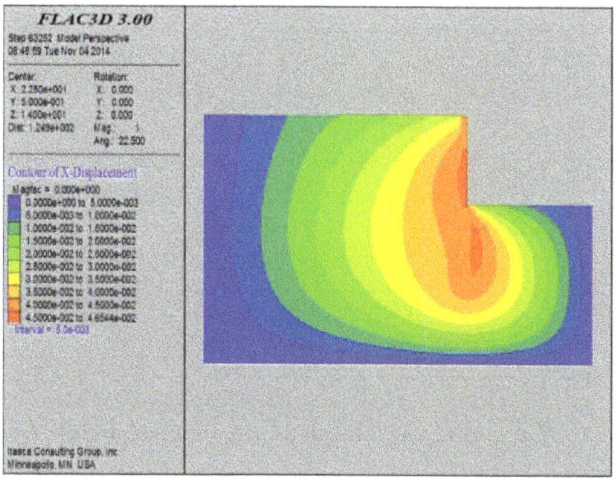

Fig. 4 Horizontal displacement nephogram of x direction under no frost heave.

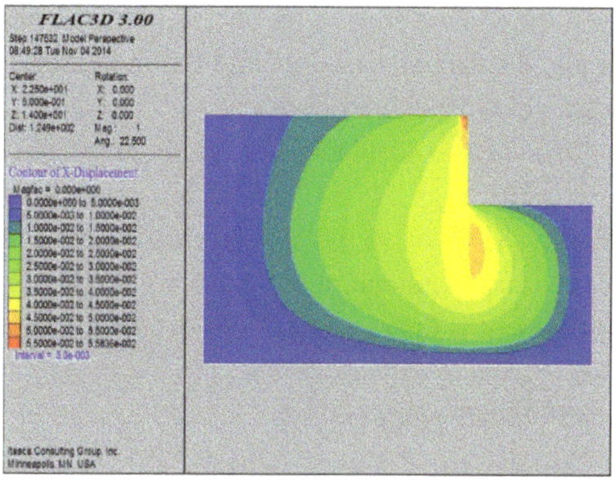

Fig. 5 Horizontal displacement nephogram of x direction under frost heaving 30 days.

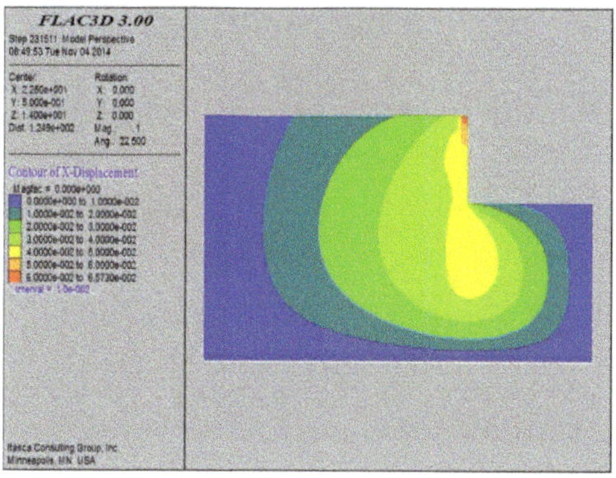

Fig. 6 Horizontal displacement nephogram of x direction under frost heaving 60 days.

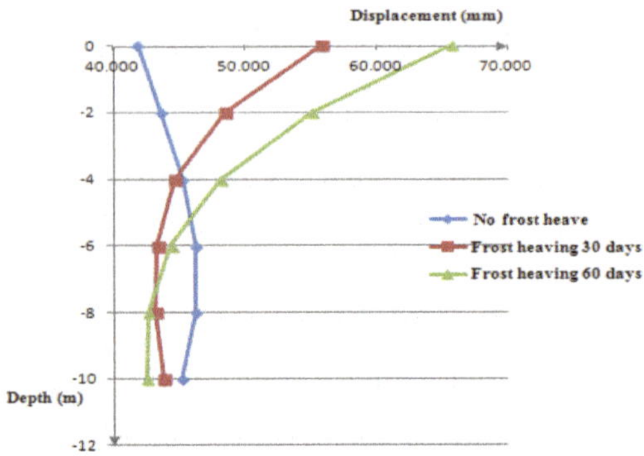

Fig. 7 Horizontal displacement of x direction.

No frost heave and frost heave 30 days, 60 days of displacement nephogram and displacement value comparison showed that:

(1) The Fig. 7 shows that each point of retaining structure (0 ~ 4 m depth of foundation pit) displacement value with the increase of the frost heaving days, the displacement value increases.

(2) By no frost heave displacement nephogram (Fig. 4) shows the maximal displacement is 4.654 cm; The frost heave displacement nephogram 30 days (Fig. 5) shows the maximal displacement is 5.584 cm; The frost heave displacement nephogram 60 days (Fig. 6) shows the maximal displacement is 6.573 cm.

3.3 *Temperature nephogram comparison*

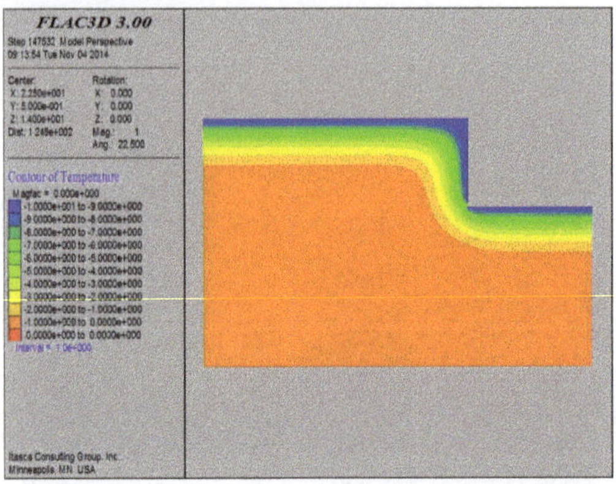

Fig. 8 Temperature nephogram under frost heaving 30 days.

The temperature nephogram of the frost heave 30 days, 60 days shows: Under the effect of thermal coupling, the frozen depth reach 5 m along the surface after 30 days frost heaving; the frozen depth reach 8 m along the surface after 60 days frost heaving. That states along the increase of freezing days, frozen depth increasing, the soil temperature is falling.

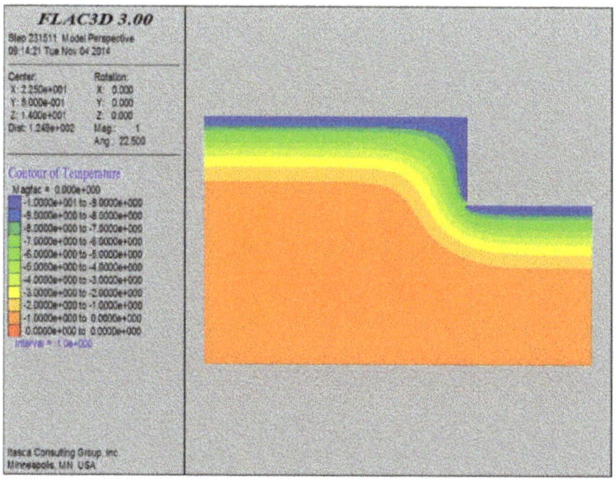

Fig. 9 Temperature nephogram under frost heaving 60 days.

4. Conclusions

Earth pressure value of the theoretical calculation and simulation value is different. Theoretical calculation earth pressure can't reflect that the dynamic variation of the earth pressure along with displacement, time; numerical simulation need to establish appropriate actual numerical simulation model, strive to various assumptions truly. Due to the frost heave force, the displacement value increases along the increase of the frost heaving days. In order to further explore the researches of frost heave on frost heaving force, mechanism of retaining structure, should strengthen research of the frozen soil physical properties, mechanical behavior and mechanism. Scientific and effective anti-freezing expansion measures are put forward, and strengthen the strength and stability of the supporting structure, in case of damage.

References

1. Luzhong Li. Foundation Pit Support Project Affected by Freezing Earth Expanding in Winter and Deal with Measure. (Engineering Quality. 2012 (10): 75-78).
2. Zhibiao Xiong. Building Foundation Pit Supporting (the Second Edition). (Beijing: China Architecture & Building Press, 2013).
3. Shuwei Sun, Hang Lin, Lianwei Ren. The Application of FLAC3D in

Geotechnical Engineering. (Beijing: China Water Power Press, 2011).
4. Yumin Chen, Dingping Xu. FLAC/FLAC3D Foundation and Engineering Examples (the Second Edition). (China Water Power Press, 2013).

Evaluation on Creep and Stress Relaxation Properties of Epoxy/Rubber Modified Bitumen Using Experiment and Simulation†

Wen-Long Li
Traffic Engineering Bureau of Tongliao City, Tongliao, 028000, China
Email: liwenlong201411@163.com

To evaluate the creep properties and viscosity of bitumen, dynamic shear rheometer (DSR), Burgers model and viscometer were used to measure these properties. Finite element analysis (FE) were used to measure the stress distribution on the stress relaxation process. Results indicated that curing time decreases with the increasing epoxy content and viscosity decreases with the increasing temperature. The viscosity parameters of low and high temperature is not consistent because of the different test methods. Burgers model showed that the viscoelastic characteristic parameters of modified asphalt are available and elastic parameters E_1 and E_2 increase when the contents of epoxy resins increased and the viscosity parameters η_1 and η_2 decrease when the contents of epoxy resins increased.

Keywords: Modified bitumen; epoxy and rubber; burgers model; creep properties.

1. Introduction

Epoxy modified bitumen (EMB), which has high-temperature stability, high strength and waterproof, has proved to be a special material because it appears viscoelastic and thermosetting properties before and after curing[1,2]. In civil engineering, epoxy modified bituminous are widely used in orthotropic steel bridge deck pavement because of its performances[3]. The first application of EMB in the deck pavement was on the San Mateo-Hayward bridge, US. in 1967[4]. As a high performance application material, harsh environments, especially environments temperature, it meet low-temperature cracking resistance and high-temperature rutting resistance's need[5]. EMB is brittle and flexibility is poor at low temperature[6]. Rubber plays an important role in flexibility of modified bitumen. The addition of rubber is contributed to improve the high-temperature stability of bitumen and low-temperature brittleness of EMB[7]. However, owing to the special requirements of deck pavements for the material performance, epoxy and rubber modified bitumen may be a good choose.

The major objective of this research is to prepare and develop a kind of bitumen that can be used in steel deck pavement. First, the viscosity changes of epoxy and rubber modified bitumen (ERB) was measured by viscometer and dynamic shear rheometer (DSR), and then creep and relaxation performance was investigated by DSR. The stress and strain distribution of ERB was simulated by Finite element analysis (FE) at the creep process.

2. Materials and Experiments

2.1 *Compositions and preparation of modified bitumen*

Bitumen with $70^{\#}$ penetration grade (dmm), Ring and Ball temperature of 47.2°C, which was measured according to ASTM D36-76, was used. Epoxy resin bought from Wuhan XingZhengYuan Co. Ltd. Rubber particles with a size less than 80 mesh sieve was used to increase the flexibility of the EMB binder, offered by Hunan Deli Alwayseal Technology Ltd. Anti-UV light additive Mg-Al layered double hydroxides (LDHs) with a density of 2.7g/cm^3 was supplied by Ruifa Chemical Co. Ltd., China, with a median diameter (D50) of ca.200um. Fundamental properties of epoxy resin were summarized in Table 1.

500g base bitumen was firstly heated to 135 °C in a container located on a thermoelectric heater. At this temperature, 25 wt. % of rubber particles and 3% and 5% epoxy resin were then added into the bitumen, and a high-shear mixer was used to mix the composite at a speed of 4000rpm for 1 hour. Then, curing agent was added and mixed with the composite for 15 minutes with manually stirring. These binders' experimentally rheological properties were given in Table 2.

Table 1 Fundamental properties of epoxy resin.

Sample	Appearance	Peel strength	Tensile bond strength	Volume ratio for mixing	Curing time
epoxy resin	viscous liquid	22MPa	>20MPa	1:1	3-4h

Table 2 Experimentally rheological properties of ERB binder.

Sample	Bitumen composition (wt)	Softening point, [°C]	Penetration at 25°C, [dmm]	Ductility at 5°C,%
1	Base bitumen(B)	47.2	61.8	15
2	ERB3%	81.5	58.0	79
3	ERB5%	>100	53.2	88

2.2 *Tests methodology*

FE on stress distribution was conducted cylinder that diameter is 25mm at 60°C with a height of 2mm. The mass density of bitumen is 1.021, elastic modulus is 1.4e9 and Poisson ratio is 0.35. A Coulomb-Mohr plasticity like criterion in combination with shear and normal stresses is proposed to deal with the extreme thin bitumen layer. 5% strain and 0.7MPa pressure was applied in bitumen.

3. Results and Discussions

3.1. *Viscosity-temperature characteristic curves*

The viscosity-temperature characteristic curves were used to measure the best mixing temperature (Bitumen's viscosity is 0.2 Pa.s during mixing with aggregate), construction temperature and resistance of fluids at different epoxy resin contents, due to its importance in mixing and construction for bitumen mixtures. As is evident from Figure 1, viscosity increased significantly with the increased contents of epoxy and viscosity decreased when heating temperature increased. The viscosity-temperature characteristic curve of 5wt% epoxy resin is very special, which may be due to ERB is to form the cross-linked structure and leads to the fast increasing of bitumen viscosity. At the same time, the viscosity-temperature characteristic curves tended to smooth when the temperature rose up to 150 or 160°C. Viscosity test results also showed that bitumen rheology was remarkably changed when epoxy doped.

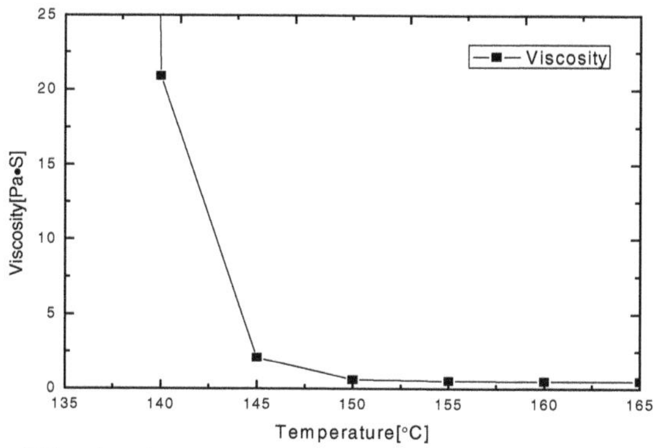

Fig. 1 The viscosity-temperature characteristic curves of ERB5%.

3.2. *Creep performance*

The high temperature creep performance represent the slowly changes of stress at a content value. These tests were conducted at 60°C by using DSR with 8mm diameter and 2mm height specimen. Firstly, a constant shear stress of 10kPa was applied for 1200s. Secondly, after the loading cycle, the shear stress was removed and the creep deformation was allowed to recover for another 400s. The relaxation rate ($R\%$) is defined as Eq. (1):

$$R\% = \frac{S_{1400} - S_{1800}}{S_{\max}} \times 100\% \tag{1}$$

Where, S_{max} is the maximum strain, [%], S_{1400} and S_{1800} is the strain at the 1400s of test and the 1800s of the test, respectively [%].

As shown in Figure 2, epoxy bitumen appeared greatly linear elasticity, but elastic recover is too slow and recover rate is too low. The elastic recover rate of Sample 1, 2, 3 is 6.5%, 10.4% and 41.3%, respectively. The elastic strain of Sample 1, 2, 3 is 113.2%, 30.4% and 22.8%, separately. The elastic strain decreased with the increase of the epoxy resin contents.

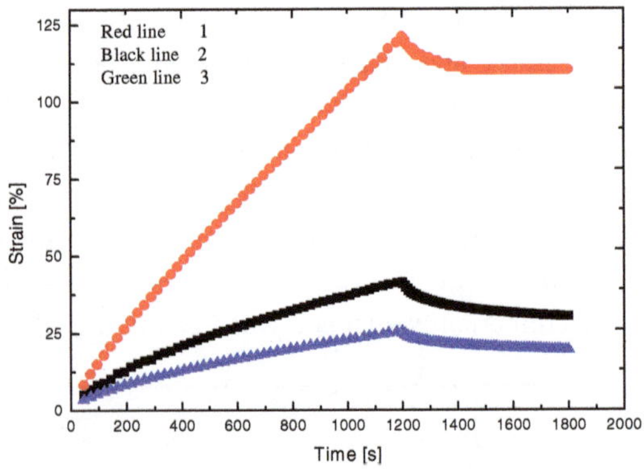

Fig. 2 Creep curves of ERB at -5°C.

3.3. *Rheological response modelling*

Using Burgers model parameters obtaining from the master curves, relaxation tests for whole binders were simulated. The mathematical representation of the model for the stress is given by Figure 3:[3]

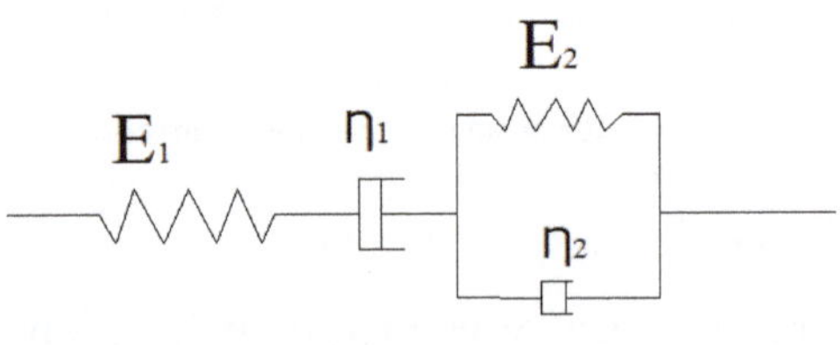

Fig. 3 Burgers model of ERB.

The Burgers model generalized constitutive equation show in equation (2) and the solution of all parameters show in equation (3)-(6).

$$\sigma + p_1\sigma_1 + p_2\sigma_2 = q_1\varepsilon_1 + q_2\varepsilon_2 \tag{2}$$

$$p_1 = \frac{\eta_1}{E_1} + \frac{\eta_2}{E_2} + \frac{\eta_1}{E_2} \tag{3}$$

$$P_2 = \frac{\eta_1\eta_2}{E_1E_2} \tag{4}$$

$$q_1 = \eta_1 \tag{5}$$

$$q_2 = \frac{\eta_1\eta_2}{E_2} \tag{6}$$

Burgers model parameters were solved by following equation (7)-(10).

$$E_1 = \frac{\sigma_0}{\varepsilon_0} \tag{7}$$

$$\eta_1 = \frac{s_0}{k_1} \tag{8}$$

$$E_2 = \frac{s_0}{d_{(0)t}} \tag{9}$$

$$\eta_2 = -\frac{E_2}{k_2} \tag{10}$$

Table 3. The ERB of Burgers model viscoelastic properties parameters at 60°C.

Sample	E_1(MPa)	η_1(MPa·S)	E_2(MPa)	η_2(MPa·S)
1	5.78	2090.59	0.154791	0.96054
2	6.82	2360.35	0.25729	8.60214
3	10.14	3857.14	0.782473	8.21667

The E_1 and E_2 increased with the increase of the epoxy resin contents, which approved that epoxy resin can improve the elastic components. The η_1 and η_2 also increased with the increase of the epoxy resin contents, which indicated that viscosity components increased.

3.4. *Stress relaxation performance simulation*

To understand the stress distribution of bitumen at the stress relaxation process, stress relaxation was simulated by ABAQUS. As shown in Figure 4, the stress distribution of the front and side of bitumen cylinder were studied and nodes stress distribution of two path were selected. It indicated that one side of the bitumen cylinder appears stress concentration and the stress is very little in the middle of the front of bitumen cylinder. The stress distribution curves showed that the stress of central displacement is very little and the stress of side displacement appears stress concentration to some certain extent.

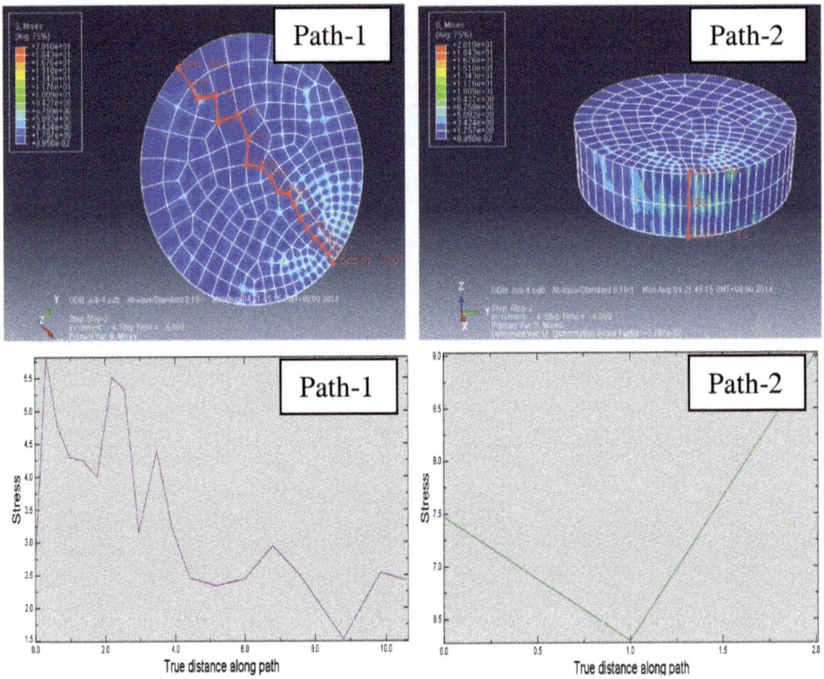

Fig. 4 Stress relaxation path and relaxation curves.

4. Conclusions

In conclusion, viscosity test results also showed that bitumen rheology was remarkably changed when epoxy doped. The dynamic viscosity increased slowly with the increased epoxy resin contents and the relationships between dynamic viscosity and temperature are also consistent with the viscosity-temperature characteristic curves. The elastic strain decreased with the increase of the epoxy resin contents. Burgers model indicated that the viscosity and elastic performance increased with the increased the epoxy resin contents. The rubber particles were more uniform than that in other image and the increase of epoxy resin can improve the compatibility of rubber in the ERB. Moreover, the rubber particle will expand in the bitumen when it absorbs some oil component. Under a certain epoxy resins content level the effect of curing mechanisms for epoxy resins is improved with the increased content of epoxy resin.

Acknowledgments

The authors acknowledge the financial supported by the National Key Scientific Apparatus Development Program from the Ministry of Science and Technology of China (No. 2013YQ160501).

References

1. X. X. Zhou, S. P. Wu, G. Liu, P. Pan, Molecular simulations and experimental evaluation on the curing of epoxy bitumen, *Materials and Structures*. (2014).
2. L. Chen, Z. Qian, H. Hu, Epoxy asphalt concrete protective course used on steel railway bridge, *Construction and Building Materials*. **411,** 25 (2013).
3. Z. Qian, C. Chen, C. L. Jiang, A. D. F. Smit, Development of a lightweight epoxy asphalt mixture for bridge decks, *Construction and Building Materials*. **48,** 516 (2013).
4. D. Q. Yuan, *Study on epoxy modified bitumen and mixtures*, Southeast University Nanjing. (Nanjing, Reading, MA, 2006).
5. B. Yao, G. Cheng, X. Wang, C. Cheng, S. Y. Liu, Linear viscoelastic behaviour of thermosetting epoxy asphalt concrete-experiments and modeling, *Construction and Building Materials*. **48,** 540 (2013).
6. Z. Qian, L. L. Chen, C. L. Jiang, S. Luo, Performance evaluation of a lightweight epoxy asphalt mixture for bascule bridge pavements, *Construction and Building Materials*. **25,** 3117 (2011).
7. M. Cubuk, M. Gürü, M. K. Çubuk, Improvement of bitumen performance with epoxy resin, *Fuel*. **88,** 1324 (2009).

Study on Physical Performance of Steel Slag and Rice Husk Ash Composite Cementations Materials

Ying Han

Huanyu Highway Supervision and Consulting Co., Ltd of Tongliao City, Inner-Mongolia, 028000, China

E-mail: lipingli2014@foxmail.com

With the resource recycling concept putting forward, all kinds of industrial waste have been applied in cement industry. The relatively common steel slag and rice husk ash were selected as raw materials to study the physical properties of steel slag and rice husk ash composite cementations materials. Cubic compressive strength, water absorption and drying shrinkage performance were studied and the results showed that the high contents of composite cementations materials met the building mortar strength requirements. Meanwhile, the drying shrinkage of steel slag and rice husk ash composite cementations materials is improved. While the water absorption is higher than pure cement.

Keywords: Steel Slag; rice husk ash; composite cementations material

1. Introduction

Steel slag, a by-product from the processing of iron to steel, is a waste residue. Steel slag accounted for 15-20% of crude steel production. Steel slag is mainly composed of calcium, silicon, magnesium, iron, and small amounts of other elements, and the content of CaO is about 35-60%, the content of SiO_2 is about 10-15%, the content of MgO is about 3-13%, the content of Fe_2O_3 is about 3-9%, and the content of FeO is about 7-20%. The mineral composition of steel slag is similar with cement. The main composition of steel slag and cement are C_3S and C_2S, C_4AF. Owing to the existence of C_3S, C_2S, and C_4AF, the activity of steel slag and cement is relatively high. There are no appropriate methods to deal with steel slag except that a part of ashes is used as fertilizer and hollow brick; the vast majority of ashes are discarded, resulting in wasted resources. Rice husk ash includes a significant amount of SiO_2 with a high activity, and the SiO_2 belongs to nanoparticles under the lower combustion temperature, so rice husk ash has a high volcanic activity in low temperature. It can be used as modifier or reinforced phase using in cement.

Wang et al. [1] studied the influence of steel slag on the hydration of cement and found that steel slag decreased the early hydration rate of cement and promoted the hydration of cement in late ages. Li et al. [2] investigated the workability and mechanical properties of steel slag concrete with different types of steel slag and different dosages of admixtures, and the results showed that steel slag can greatly enhance the properties of concrete and durability of concrete. Zhang et al. considered that the rice husk ash is highly pozzolanic and can be used as a supplementary cementing material to produce high-performance concrete and showed excellent performance under freezing and thawing conditions, and its resistance to deicing salt scaling was similar to that of the control concrete and marginally better than that of the silica fume concrete [3]. Gemma et al. [4] investigated the effects of partial replacements of Portland cement by rice husk ash on the autogenous shrinkage. The result showed that the volume shrinkage of concrete decreased with the increase of the content of rice husk ash, and the rice husk ash can effectively improve the volume stability of concrete under the lower combustion temperature [4]. Al-Khalaf et al. [5] considered that the addition of 40% rice husk ash can be made with no significant change in compressive strength compared with the control mix. Mehta [6] investigated the blended properties of rice husk ash cements. The results demonstrated that a unique property of the cements containing rice husk ash is their excellent resistance to dilute organic and mineral acids.

2. Experimental

2.1. *Materials*

Table 1 Chemical compositions of steel slag.

Composition	SiO_2	MgO	Fe_2O_3	CaO	Al_2O_3	P_2O_5
content(%)	13.85	5.82	28.8	43.58	3.34	1.51
Composition	TiO_2	MnO	Cl	SO_3	Loss	
content(%)	0.62	0.01	0.04	0.37	2.06	

Table 2 Chemical compositions of rice husk ash.

Composition	SiO_2	Fe_2O_3	Al_2O_3	MgO	K_2O
content(%)	89.45	1.26	0.71	0.64	1.39
Composition	P_2O_5	CaO	MnO	Cl	SO_3
content(%)	0.46	4.35	0.45	0.87	0.42

Steel slag and rice husk ash have been reprocessed, which meet requirements on its fineness and pozzolanic activity. The compositions of steel slag and rice husk ash are shown in Table 1 and Table 2. The Portland cement was used with 42.5MPa.

2.2. *Compositions of concrete*

This paper mainly studied the performance of concrete with a high addition of steel slag-rice husk ash. Table 3 shows the fundamental compositions of steel slag, rice husk ash, and cement.

Cubic concrete specimens with dimensions of 70.5mm×70.5mm×70.5mm were prepared to determine the compressive strength of steel slag-rice husk ash concrete. After casting, the specimens were left in the casting room at a temperature of 20±2°C for a period of 24 h. Then the physical properties of concrete were measured.

Table 3 Compositions of different binders.

Sample	steel slag (%)	rice husk ash (%)	Cement (%)	water reducer (%)
0	0	0	100	0.5
1	20	40	40	0.5
2	30	30	40	0.5
3	30	40	30	0.5
4	40	20	40	0.5
5	40	30	30	0.5

3. Results and Discussions

3.1. *Cubic compressive strength of cementations materials*

Figure 1

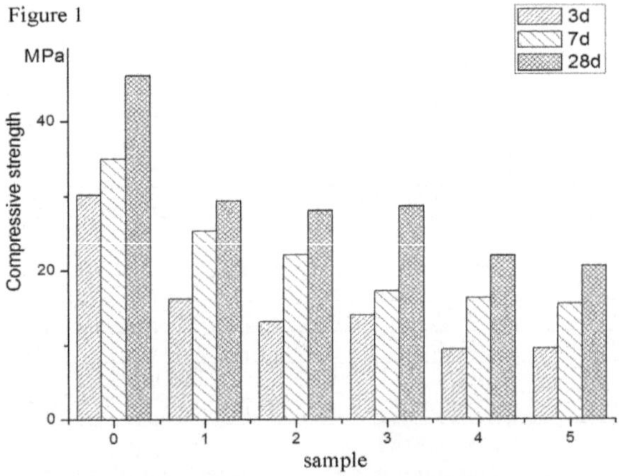

Fig. 1 The compressive strength of concrete.

In Fig. 1, the strength of the blank sample (0) is obviously higher than composite cementations material, and the 28d strength reaches to 46.15MPa. The strength of composite cementations material also have reached to 20MPa. The high content of composite cementations material can be satisfied with the requirement of the building mortar strength. Comparing different mixing ratio of specimen, it can be found that the activity of rice husk ash is higher than the activity of steel slag. So the activity of cement is highest, followed by rice husk ash, steel slag is minimum.

3.2. *Water absorption rate of cementations materials*

The water absorption rate of high composite cementations materials reflected the internal pore size and appeared a good waterproof performance. Meanwhile, it can indirectly reflect the erosion resistance, anti-permeability performance in the early stages. The water absorption rate of concrete was measured in Table 4.

Table 4 Water absorption rate of concrete.

Sample	Dry weight			Wet weight			Water absorption (%)			Average
	a	b	c	a	b	c	A	b	c	
0	772.11	779.25	780.02	775.72	782.83	783.62	4.68	4.59	4.62	4.63
1	760.54	758.43	763.68	764.43	762.32	767.61	5.11	5.13	5.14	5.13
2	775.2	780.61	779.32	779.01	784.48	783.15	4.92	4.96	4.91	4.93
3	753.21	759.81	754.65	757.05	763.73	758.53	5.1	5.16	5.14	5.13
4	782.65	784.11	787.13	786.52	787.94	791.01	4.95	4.89	4.93	4.92
5	770.02	768.36	764.27	773.91	772.27	768.18	5.05	5.09	5.11	5.08

In Table 4, the water absorption rate of the blank sample (0) is lower than composite cementations material. Comparing the water absorption rate results of sample 1, 2, and 4, we can conclude that the rice husk ash could reduce the void content of concrete. It indicates that the void content of steel slag concrete is less than the rice husk ash concrete in cementations materials.

3.3. *Drying shrinkage of cementations materials*

It can be seen from Fig. 2, the drying shrinkage of composite cementations materials and pure cement increase obviously with the extension of time. The drying shrinkage of pure cement is larger than composite cementations material in the drying shrinkage of each time period. The drying shrinkage is the largest than other period before 7th day, the drying shrinkage rate is relatively slow after 7th day. Compared to sample 1 and 3, 2 and 4, we can find that equivalent replacement of cement with steel slag reach to 10% and the drying shrinkage of concrete decreases; Compared to sample 1, 2, and 4, we can find that equivalent replacement of rice husk ash with steel slag reach to 10% and the drying shrinkage of concrete decreases; Compared to sample 2 and 3, 4 and 5, we can find that equivalent replacement of cement with rice husk ash reach to 10% and the drying shrinkage of concrete is smaller than the pure cement. Therefore, the result indicates that not only rice husk ash and steel slag can effectively inhibit the drying shrinkage of concrete but also the inhibitory effect of steel slag is better than rice husk ash.

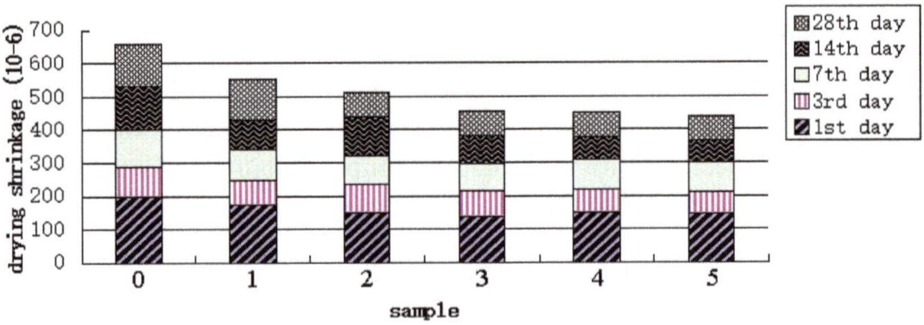

Fig. 2 The drying shrinkage of high composite cementations materials.

4. Conclusions

(1) The strength of the blank sample is higher than composite cementations material and the 28 d strength reach to 46.15MPa. The strength of composite cementations material also have reached more than 20MPa. The results show that high content of composite cementations material can be satisfied with the requirement of the building mortar strength.

(2) The water absorption rate of the blank sample is lower than composite cementations material, and void content of steel slag concrete is less than the rice husk ash concrete in cementations material.

(3) Not only rice husk ash and steel slag can effectively inhibit the drying shrinkage of concrete, but also the inhibitory effect of steel slag is better than rice husk ash.

References

1. Q. Wang, P.Y. Yan, The influence of steel slag on the hydration of cement during the hydration process of complex binder, Science China Technological Sciences. 54 (2011) 388–394.
2. Y.F. Li, Y.O. Yao, L. Wang, Recycling of industrial waste and performance of steel slag green concrete, Journal of Central South University of

Technology. 16 (2009) 768–773.
3. M.H. Zhang, M.M. Wen, High-performance concrete incorporating rice husk ash as a supplementary cementing material, Materials Journal. 93 (1996) 629-636.
4. G.R. de Sensalea, A.B. Ribeirob, A. Gonçalvesb, Effects of RHA on autogenous shrinkage of Portland cement pastes, Cement and Concrete Composites. 30(2008) 892-897.
5. M.N. Al-Khalaf, H.A. Yousif, Use of rice husk ash in concrete. International Journal of Cement Composites and Lightweight Concrete. 6(1984) 241–248.
6. P.K. Mehta, Properties of blended cements made from rice husk ash, Journal Proceedings. 74(1977) 440-442.

Effect of Desulfurization Residues on Moisture Resistance of Asphalt Concrete

Jin Wang[1,a]

[1]*Management Department of Southern Tongliao Section of Tong-Chi Highway Transportation Engineering Department of Tongliao City, Tongliao, 028000, China*

[a]*Email: mashankui@live.com*

Water damage is one of the most common damages for asphalt pavement. Desulfurization residues, cement, and limestone as filler were added into asphalt mixture. In order to study the moisture resistance of asphalt pavement, the asphalt mixture Marshall Immersion test and freeze-thaw splitting test were conducted. AC-16C and AC-20C based on basalt aggregate were designed and used to materials performance test and analysis. It shows that the Marshall stability (MS) and residual stability of adding desulfurization residues are 10.65KN and 96.9%, and compared with limestone added sample, the desulfurization residues sample's value of intensity ratio of frozen and melted (TSR) has increased about 20%, respectively. Meanwhile, desulfurization residues can also improve the moisture resistance of asphalt mixture.

Keywords: Moisture resistance; residual stability; asphalt concrete; desulfurization residues.

1. Introduction

There is a very large coal reserves and coal consumption in china, which increased year by year [1]. With the popularity of the technology and equipment, the number of desulfurization product is more and more [2]. So how to good use the desulfurization has become a key problem of environmental protection and resource recycling. Owing to the complex characteristics of desulfurization residues, only a few desulfurization residues are used and most of it is abandoned or stored [3]. The desulfurization residues applications are on the rise in building materials [4-6].

Since the eighty's century, the highway is developing rapidly, eighty percent of it is asphalt pavement [7]. Water damage has become one of the most serious diseases in our country, because of the complex structure of asphalt pavement [8-10]. Considering the present situation above and based on mature technology, the most effective way for improving moisture resistance of asphalt concrete is to apply desulfurization residues into asphalt concrete. Not only can it improve the moisture resistance but also can effective use of desulfurization residues to realize the recycling of resources.

To better understand the desulfurization residues on moisture resistance of asphalt concrete, AC-16C and AC-20C asphalt concrete grading design and the Marshall stability of two type asphalt mixture were investigated and analyzed.

2. Materials and Experiments

2.1. *Materials*

Asphalt with 70# penetration grade, Ring and Ball temperature of 48°C, which was measured by ASTM D36-76, was used. Limestone powder, which was conforming to the requirements of JTG F40-2004, was used. Cement was bought from Chongqing Kehua Building Materials Co. Ltd. Aggregate was basalt.

2.2. *Experiments*

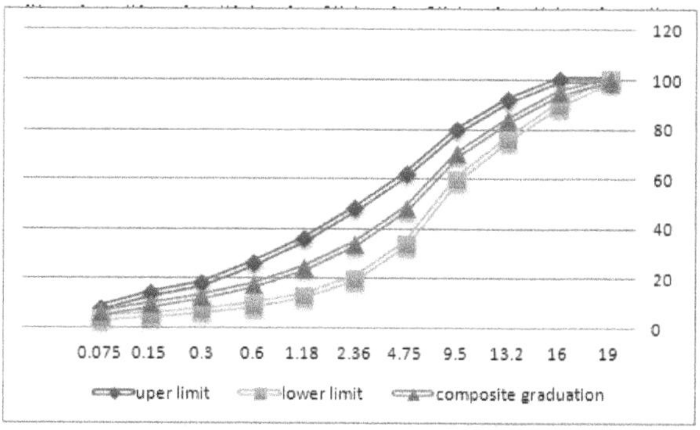

Fig. 1 Basalt AC-16C grading curve.

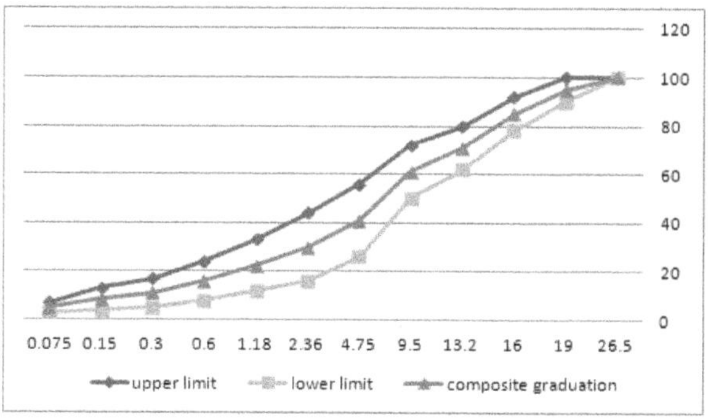

Fig. 2 Basalt AC-20C grading curve.

Cement, desulfurization residues, and ordinary limestone powder were chosen as the filler of asphalt concrete. The 40% limestone powder were replaced by Portland cement in asphalt concrete. Mixed type used basalt AC-16C gradation and AC-20C gradation shown in the Fig. 1 and Fig. 2. It demonstrated that synthesis of gradation is better consistent with asphalt concrete design because the curve of synthesis of gradation lies between upper limit and lower limit.

According to JTG E30-2011, Marshall samples were preparation and the size and porosity of Marshall sample was measured and calculated. Meanwhile, there are two kind of asphalt concrete, which were called groups A and B. Group A is the experimental group, group B is the control group. Put the group B sample into 60ºC water bath holding for 30min, then MS experiments were done. Put the group A sample into 60ºC standard constant temperature water bath holding for 48h, then do the same experiments to contrast the residual stability. The residual stability can be expressed by equation (1):

$$MS_0 = \frac{MS_1}{MS} \times 100\% \quad (1)$$

MS1 is the Marshall stability of experimental group, KN

MS is the Marshall stability of control group, KN

The size of Marshall sample is 63.5±1.3mm×101mm (diameter×height), and the only difference is the compaction times that is 50 (two sides) fewer than Marshall sample. Owing to the larger void fraction, the samples were divided into two groups A (experimental group) and B (control group). The group B sample was put into water which vacuum degree is 97.3kPa for 15min. After that, put the sample into pure water for 0.5h, and then put them into plastic, adding 10ml water and freezing them for 16h at -18℃. At last, put the sample into constant temperature water bath for 24h. Put group A and group B into water with 25℃ for 2h, then do the splitting test. Splitting tensile strength RT can be expressed by equation (2)

$$R_T = 0.006287 P_T / \mathrm{h} \quad (2)$$

RT is the splitting tensile strength, MPa

PT is the experimental load value, N

h is the height of sample, mm

The splitting tensile strength ratio can be expressed by equation (3)

$$\mathrm{TSR} = \frac{\mathrm{R}_{\mathrm{T1}}}{\mathrm{R}_{\mathrm{T2}}} \times 100\% \quad (3)$$

TSR is the splitting tensile strength ratio, %

RT1 is the splitting tensile strength of experimental group, MPa
RT2 is the splitting tensile strength of control group, MPa

3. Results and Discussion

Marshall immersion test results show in Fig. 3 and Fig. 4. In the basalt AC-16C gradation, the Marshall stability reached to 13.55kN when limestone powder was acted as filler, and it is satisfied with the pavement requirement. At the same time, residual stability reached to 89.4% and was also satisfied with the requirement. The residual stability reached to 93.8%, when 40% limestone powder was replaced by cement acted as filler, and the residual stability has even up to 96.9%, when the desulfurization residues acted as filler. In the basalt AC-20C gradation as coarse aggregate gradation, when use limestone powder as filler, the residual stability only is 58.1%, obviously unsatisfied the requirement. When 40% limestone powder was replaced by cement, the residual stability of Marshall sample has improve to 78.9%. Meanwhile, desulfurization residues acted as filler can improve the residual stability to 90.9%.

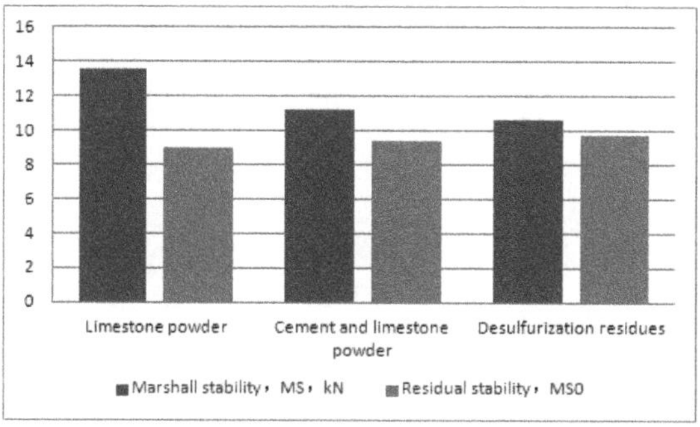

Fig. 3 Basalt AC-16C grading Immersion test results column graph.

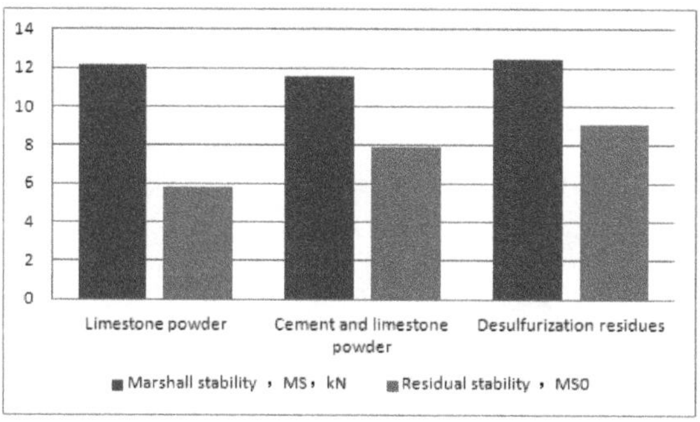

Fig. 4 Basalt AC-20C grading Immersion test results column graph.

Asphalt is also known to be a colloid in which asphaltenes are covered by a stable phase of polar resins and saturate forming complex micelles that are dispersed in the oil phase and is also a kind of weak polar material [11]. When asphalt contacted with acidic stone, the acidic component of asphalt can't form chemical reaction with stone. Therefore, it belongs to physical adsorption and adhesion force is not strong. When asphalt contacted with alkaline stone, they can react to form chemical bonds and the adhesion force is very strong. In this experiments, adding desulfurization residues into mixture can make the aggregate alkalify and increase the surface roughness to improve moisture resistance.

The basalt AC-16C splitting test results show in Fig. 5, the splitting tensile strength ratio has no obvious improvement but all samples are satisfied with the requirements (≥75%). In Fig. 6, the TSR value of the basalt AC-20C asphalt mixture, when limestone powder acted as filler, is 51.4%. When 40% limestone powder was replaced by cement, the value of TSR has up to 65.1%. Meanwhile, desulfurization residues filler can improve the value of TSR to 77.2%.

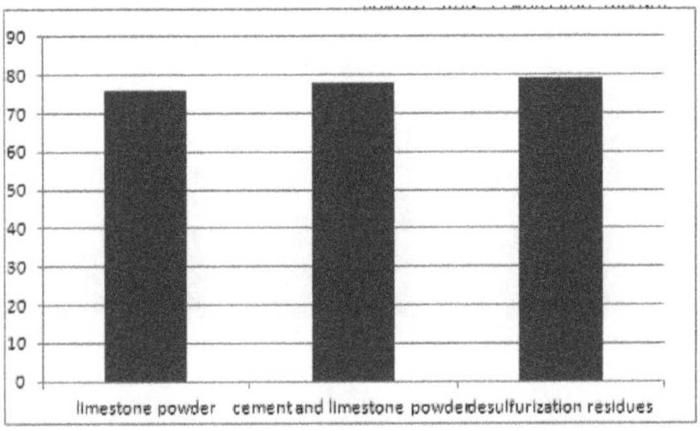

Fig. 5 Basalt AC-16C grading splitting test results column graph.

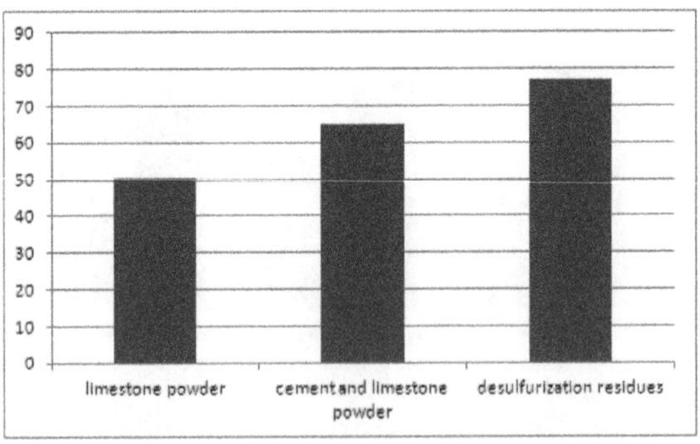

Fig. 6 Basalt AC-20C grading splitting test results column graph.

4. Conclusion

Based on the part of the desulfurization residues to replace ordinary limestone powder added into the asphalt mixture, the Marshall standard sample and the residual stability were studied.

The addition of desulfurization residues could lead to Marshall Stability slightly become lower; however, the desulfurization residues can obviously improve the moisture resistance of asphalt concrete. Its effect is better than cement. When basalt AC-16C grading as aggregate, The residual stability has improved by 7.5%. When basalt AC-20C grading as aggregate, the residual stability has improved by 32.8%.

The addition of desulfurization residues could improve the splitting strength ratio. When basalt AC-16C grading as aggregate, the value of TSR has improved a little. When basalt AC-20C grading as aggregate, the value of TSR has obviously improved by 25.8% and the addition of desulfurization residues can obviously improve the water stability of asphalt mixture.

References

1. Y. Wang, J.W. Li, China's present situation of coal consumption and future coal demand forecast, China Population Resources and Environment. 18 (2008) 152-155.
2. M.Y. Sun, J.A. Hou, T.M. Tang, R.J. Lu, L.H. Cheng, and X.H. Xu, Stabilization of mercury in flue gas desulfurization gypsum from coal-fired electric power plants with additives, Fuel Processing Technology, 104 (2012) 160-166.
3. T. Punshon, A. S. Knox, D. C. Adriano, J. C. Seaman, and J. T. Weber, Flue gas desulfurization residues potential applications and environmental issues, Kluwer Academic/Plenum Publishers, New York, (1999) 7-28.
4. Z.W. Chen, Y. Xiao, L. Pang, W.B. Zeng, and S.P. Wu, Experimental assessment of flue gas desulfurization residues and basic oxygen furnace slag on fatigue and moisture resistance of HMA, Fatigue & Fracture of Engineering Materials & Structures. 37(2014) 1242-1253.
5. Z.W. Chen, S.P. Wu, F.Z. Li, J.Y. Chen, Z.H. Qin, and L. Pang, Recycling of flue gas desulfurization residues in gneiss based hot mix asphalt: materials characterization and performances evaluation, Construction and Building Materials, 73(2014) 137-144.
6. Z.H. Qin, Desulfurization ash content on the influence of steel slag to the moisture resistance of asphalt concrete, Wuhan University of Technology Press, Wuhan, 2014.

7. J.S. Zhang, Y.Y. Zhang, Asphalt materials, Beijing Chemical Industry Press, Beijing, 2009.
8. X.S. Zhang, J.P. Chen, Water damage of asphalt concrete pavement study, Qingdao University of Petroleum Press, Qingdao, 2011.
9. Y.X. Zhang, R.J. Qin, Treatment measures of early water damage on asphalt pavement of freeway, Management and Service Science. (2009)1-4.
10. P.S. Kandhal, C.W. Lubold, F.L. Roberts, Water damage to asphalt overlays: case histories, Annual Meeting of the Association of Asphalt Paving Technologists. Nashville, Tennessee, 1989.
11. G. Polacco, J. Stastna, D. Biondi, F. Antonelli, Z. Vlachovicova, and L. Zanzotto, Rheology of asphalts modified with glycidylmethacrylate functionalized polymers, Journal of Colloid and Interface Science. 280 (2004) 366-373.

Study on Scheme Optimization of Concrete Temperature Control and Crack Prevention During Construction Period*

Wang Zhenhong†, Li Yue, Zhang Guoxin and Liu Yi
Department of Structures and Materials, China Institute of Water resources and Hydropower Research, Beijing, 100038, China
†E-mail: faithzhen@126.com
www.iwhr.com

Cracks of concrete structure during construction are mainly caused by temperature load, but good effect of cracks prevention methods can be achieved if the timely and reasonable scheme of temperature control is selected. Research shows that the method of external heat preservation and internal cooling pipes can prevent cracks, while the type and thickness of the thermal insulating materials, cooling water temperature, cooling lasting days and cooling pipe arrangement influence the effect of temperature control by certain degree. In view of this problem, a case study is presented where the 3-D FEM including water-pipe cooling is adopted to simulate the thermal field and stress field of concrete under different combinations of measures. The result shows that good effect of temperature control and crack prevention is achieved. This research should have great reference signification to similar concrete projects in the future.

Keywords: Scheme optimization; temperature control and crack prevention; stress field; temperature field; numerical simulation.

1. Introduction

With the rapid development of the national economy and infrastructure, there are many sluice, inverted siphon, aqueduct, pump station and other hydraulic concrete structures, subsequent crack problems are more and more worthy of attention. Engineering experience indicates that, the main causes of cracks in concrete structure during construction period are the temperature load, including early basic temperature difference, temperature difference between inside and outside and so on [1-4]. Therefore, the temperature control during construction of concrete structure has become the key of quality assurance.

Surface insulation and pipe cooling combination is a new method to prevent

* This work is supported by National Key Basic Research Program of China (973 Program) (2013CB036406, 2013CB035904), Special Scientific Research Project of State Key Laboratory of Simulation and Regulation of Water Cycle in River Basin.

cracks. Surface insulation can reduce the temperature difference between inside and outside of the structure to prevent early cracks, but will cause concrete temperature rise and increase the shrinkage stress of concrete; pipe cooling can reduce the temperature difference between inside and outside and the early temperature rise, but the cooling time, water temperature and the flow should be appropriate and reasonable. In this paper, based on the large sluice at home, according to concrete thermal parameters obtained by inversion analysis [5-7], the effect of temperature control is analyzed about the combination of different surface heat preservation and cooling mode through 3-D FEM. Then the contrast analysis is carried and the timely and reasonable scheme is selected to guide construction.

2. Scheme Optimization of Concrete Temperature Control and Crack Prevention

2.1. *Survey of project*

Project locates in Shaoxing, Zhejiang province and lies at potamic entrance of one main tributary of Qiantang River, so it belongs to estuarine sluice. This sluice is a diversion junction project in east Zhejiang. According to the engineering standard, the sluice is a grade one project and the main structure also belongs to first-grade structure. The length, height and thickness of sluice pier are 25m, 10.5m, 4m, respectively. Because the concrete of sluice is high-performance slag concrete, the task of temperature control and crack prevention is formidable and complicated. Table 1 is the mix proportion of sluice concrete.

Table 1 Mix proportion of sluice concrete $\frac{1}{m}$ unit: kg/m3.

C30	P0.42.5 Cement	Ground slag	Dihydrate Gypsum	Sand	Gravel stone	Middle stone	larger stone	additive	water
Three-gradation	104.1	181.5	11.9	529.0	451.0	451.0	602.0	2.0	119.0
Two-gradation	138.3	241.0	15.8	588.0	654.0	654.0	-	3.0	158.0

Three-gradation concrete is used for sluice floor; two-gradation concrete is used for sluice pier.

2.2. *Calculation Model*

According to the character of structure and its symmetry, half model is used for the calculation. Because the surface of sluice pier is easily affected by environment temperature and the temperature and stress gradient is also bigger, the temperature and stress of concrete surface is the keystone of research. In order to simulate the pouring process of concrete, reasonable mesh is used in the direction of height and thickness of structure. For the higher precision of results, the element of surface is very thin and the thickness of element is 0.4m which is one lift. After establishment of the model, the number of elements and nodes is 21719, 26177, respect.

2.3. *Scheme of concrete temperature control*

The gate pier concrete belongs to high performance concrete and concrete construction is in all year. Because of limited space, an example of pier concrete construction in a season is introduced. This project takes the temperature control method of surface insulation and internal cooling pipes. In order to achieve the best effect of temperature control, numerical simulation of multiple parameters and schemes is done. Table 2 is different combinations of temperature control scheme.

Table 2 Temperature control scheme.

scheme	Pouring temperature /°C	heat preservation	Water cooling time /d	water temperature /°C	flow /m^3.h-1	form removal /d
1	26	Geotextiles	5	18	3.62	7
2	26	—	5	18	3.62	7
3	26	Geotextiles	2.5	18	3.62	7
4	26	—	2.5	22	8	7
5	26	Geotextiles	2.5	22	8	7

2.4. *Calculation results*

The simulation results are shown in Figure 1-Figure 2. Concrete temperature and stress change process of typical points are analyzed comparatively, as follows:

(1) The water cooling time has great influence on the temperature and stress of concrete, concrete water cooling longer, cooling rate faster and larger, then the tensile stress is larger, as shown in Figure 1 and Figure 2. water cooling for 5 days, pier concrete basic temperature is below 30℃ and concrete temperature decrease obviously which makes concrete tensile stress is significantly greater than cooling water for 2.5 days.

(2) In this situation of water cooling for 2.5 days, to the pier ,concrete temperature has passed its peak when cooling water stops ,so concrete temperature will rebound slightly and then decrease slowly. Whether or not to take the surface heat preservation measures, reducing speed is more than 1°C /d. Therefore, from the perspective of the cooling rate, it is to not continue cooling in the later, because the calculation stress is not large.

To the upper concrete of pier, the temperature continues to rise when cooling water stops because concrete temperature is at or before the peak. Then the highest temperature will exceed now temperature and cooling water cannot cut peak of concrete temperature. So the internal temperature will continue to rise and the temperature difference between inside and outside will increase, resulting in a larger the surface tensile stress. The crux of the problem is the gate pier with one pipe; therefore, it suggested arranging two water pipes, one in 1.50m height, one in above, independent water cooling.

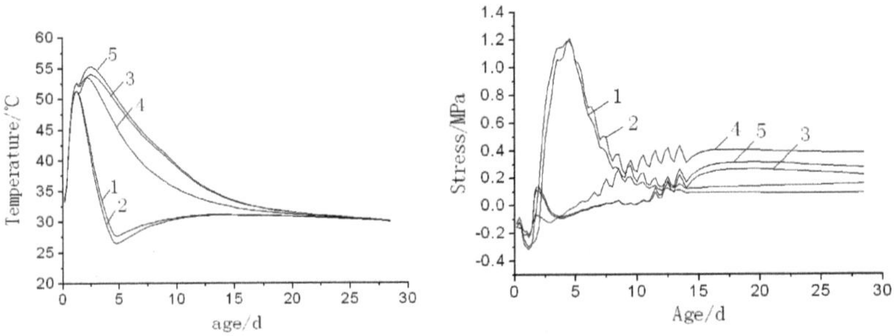

(a) Temperature (b) Stress

Fig. 1 Temperature and stress duration curve of 1 point in each scheme.

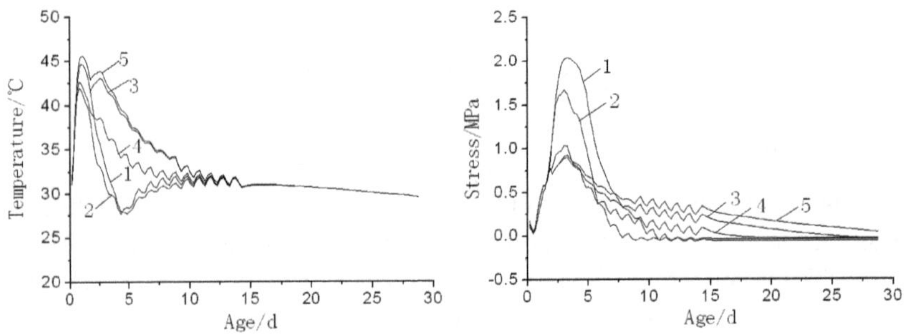

(a) Temperature (b) Stress

Fig. 2 Temperature and stress duration curve of 5 point in each scheme.

(3) Whether or not surface heat preservation measure is used, it is has greater influence on temperature and stress of concrete. Do not using the surface heat preservation, there will be greater temperature difference between inside and outside, if the surface heat preservation is too much, it can reduce temperature difference between inside and outside and early surface crack, but later temperature shrinkage stress amplitude increases. To resolve this contradiction, it recommends the use of insulation strength smaller geotextiles surface coverage. The computing result of stress shows that the surface tensile stress is reduced significantly (scheme 1, 3, 5).

(4) Increasing the cooling water temperature can reduce the temperature difference of water pipe wall; decrease the possibility of cracking in pipe wall. But at the same time the effect of reducing peak is decreased, therefore, increasing water flow is a good choice. The results from the operating case 3 and 5 show that the water temperature is increased from 18°C to 22°C, and flow rate increases from 3.62 m^3/h to 8.00m^3/h, the pier highest temperature rise less than 1°C, but the stress situation has be improved.

3. Conclusions

(1) The temperature difference between inside and outside and based temperature difference is the main cause of cracks, while the surface moderate thermal insulation and internal water cooling are the effective measures to prevent cracks, worthy of promotion and application

(2) To temperature control and crack prevention, the effect of different temperature control measures is different. They have some shortcomings, even contradictory, restrict each other. so more parameters condition should be calculated to select the timely and reasonable scheme for crack prevention

(3) The gate pier is thinner than dam structure, more constraint, so crack easily appear, especially the gate slot. In addition, this paper does not consider the influence of water salinity to stress and temperature, which need further study.

Acknowledgments

The author acknowledges the support provided by National Key Basic Research Program of China (973 Program) (2013CB036406，2013CB035904), Special Scientific Research Project of State Key Laboratory of Simulation and Regulation of Water Cycle in River Basin.

References

1. G. De Schutter. Finite element simulation of thermal cracking in massive hardening concrete elements using degree of hydration based material laws. Computers and Structures, (2002) pp. 2035-2042.
2. Ding Baoying, Wang Guobing, Huang Shuping, et al. A review on causes of cracking in domestic concrete dams and preventive measures., Water Resources and Hydropower Engineering, (1994) pp.12-18.
3. Zhang Zhiming, Guo Xingwen, Du Rongqiang. Analysis of hydration heat-induced stresses and cracks in massive concrete walls. Journal of Hohai University, (2002) pp.12-16.

4. Cao Weimin, Wu Jian, Shan Li. Numerical simulation of temperature field and stress field of sluice piers. Journal of Hohai University, (2002), pp. 48-52.
5. Zhu Bofang. Thermal Stresses and Temperature Control of Mass Concrete. Beijing, (1998).
6. Zhu Yueming, Xu Zhiqing, He jin-ren, et al. A calculation method for solving temperature field of mass concrete with cooling pipes. Journal of Yangtze River Scientific Research Institute, (2003), pp. 19-22.
7. Bofang Zhu. Effect of cooling by water flowing in nonmetal pipes embedded in mass concrete, Journal of Construction Eng. *ASCE.* (1999).

[1]Study on the Impact of Infinite Foundation Radiation Damping Upon Arch Dam Earthquake Response

Heng Cheng[a] and Guoxin Zhang[b]
State Key Laboratory of Simulation and Regulation of Water Cycle in River Basin of China Institute of Water Resources and Hydropower Research
Beijing, 100038, China
E-mail: [a]chengheng1020@163.com and [b]gx-zhang@iwhr.com

Xiaopeng Li
Management Office of Nanhai Spring Region of Anyang
Anyang, 455006, China
E-mail: 13503724509@126.com

The infinite foundation radiation damping effect shall be fully taken into account for the purpose of simulating the earthquake response of arch dam more genuinely. This article studies the border element with consistent equivalent viscoelasticity as well as the method and technology for wave input on this border, realizes the seismic motion input of arch dam-foundation system with the stress time history in correspondence with the incident field at bottom border and free field at side border as border load. With some high arch dam in China as example, it analyzes dynamic response of arch dam-foundation system in three-direction earthquake action, compares it with calculation results of traditional massless foundation model and studies the impact of infinite foundation radiation damping upon arch-dam earthquake response.

Keywords: Radiation damping; arch dam; consistent equivalent viscoelasticity; border element; seismic motion input.

1. Introduction

In anti-seismic safety evaluation of arch dam, the accurate indication of the impact of so-called "radiation damping" i.e. the dissipation of dynamic seismic energy toward infinite foundation as well as the definition of its corresponding reasonable seismic motion input mechanism are important preconditions for ensuring the correctness of the evaluation result [1]. In dynamic analysis of

[1] This work is supported by the Postdoctoral Science Foundation (2013M540989), Independent Research Subject of State Key Laboratory of Simulation and Regulation of Water Cycle in River Basin (2015TS05).

finite element of arch dam, the artificial border conditions are usually set up at the foundation section of finite elements for simulating infinite foundation radiation damping, so as to ensure no reflection of scattered wave in passing through the artificial border inside the finite calculation area. On the basis of the artificial border model of viscoelasticity, according to the concept of border element with consistent equivalent viscoelasticity in the references [2,3], this article sets up a solid element of the same thickness on the border of the established finite element model in outward extending method along the boundary plane, which equivalently replaces the spring-damper imposed on border node and largely reduces the time of preprocessing. It studies the method of seismic motion input for the border element with consistent equivalent viscoelasticity, applies the artificial viscoelastic border and the border element with consistent equivalent viscoelasticity in earthquake response analysis of some high arch dam in China respectively, analyzes the dynamic response of dam in three-direction seismic load action and compares it with calculation results of traditional massless foundation model and studies the impact of infinite foundation radiation damping upon arch-dam earthquake response.

2. Seismic Motion Input

The rigidity and damping matrix of artificial border element with consistent viscoelasticity can be derived out of the spring-damping parameter of artificial viscoelastic border and then, the equivalent parameter of solid border element is obtained in virtue of the equivalent principle of element matrix [2,3]. According to the characteristics of artificial viscoelastic border, total wave field is divided into free wave field and scatter wave field. External source wave field is uniformly treated as free field. The energy in scattered wave field is absorbed by the equivalent viscoelastic border element, and free wave field can change into equivalent node load and impose on the border.

With consecutive displacement condition and mechanical equilibrium condition, the movement equation of any node b on artificial border can be defined as follows:

$$m_b \ddot{u}_{bi}^m(t) + C_b \dot{u}_{bi}^m(t) + K_b u_{bi}^m(t) = F_{bi}^f(t) + F_{bi}^s(t) \tag{1}$$

Where, K_b and C_b are artificial border parameters of the node b, $F_{bi}^f(t)$ and $F_{bi}^s(t)$ are the equivalent node loads that the free field and scattered field of simulated border impose on artificial border node. Among the rest, a stress imposing on artificial border node for simulating the scattered field is supplied by viscoelastic border, instead of additional load imposed on the border node. In simulating the free field of the border, the load to be imposed on viscoelastic border node comprises two parts: one is the force required for overcoming the rigidity and damping of artificial border element, and the other is the stress field of free field the border at artificial border. Detailed formula is as follows [4]:

$$F_{bi}^{f}(t) = K_{bi}u_{bi}^{f}(t) + C_{bi}\dot{u}_{bi}^{f}(t) + \sigma_{bi}^{f}(t)A \tag{2}$$

Where, $F_{bi}^{f}(t)$ is the load to be imposed on the border node b along the direction i in free wave field conditions; K_{bi} and C_{bi} are artificial border parameters of the border node b along the direction i respectively; $u_{bi}^{f}(t)$ is free field of former consecutive medium border node b along the direction i; A is the influenced area of the border node b in artificial border plane; $\sigma_{bi}^{f}(t)$ is the stress field generated by the fluctuation of the free field of the border and can be derived in Generalized Hooke Law.

3. Impact of Infinite Foundation Radiation Damping upon Arch-dam Earthquake Response

The dam is some concrete arch dam, of which the top elevation is 1867.5m and the dam peak is 130m. The elevations of regular water reservoir, dead water level and silt are 1866m, 1825m and 1796m respectively, and the buoyant unit weight of silt is 500kg/m^3. The dam features totally four transverse joints, of which dynamic touch non-linear effect in earthquake is simulated in constraint function method [5~7]. 1.5 times of dam height along the direction of upper and lower reaches, left and right banks and depth are taken for 3D finite element dispersion of the dam and its foundation as a whole, where the whole model is divided into 16788 units and 20734 nodes. The coordinates are taken as follows: X direction is across the river and points to the left bank; Y direction is along the river and points to the upper reach; Z is the vertical direction. The finite element grids of arch dam-foundation system and transverse joint position of the dam are in Figure 1 and 2 respectively.

The concrete material parameters of the dam are: elastic modulus $E = 18\text{GPa}$, dynamic elastic modulus higher than static elastic modulus by 30%. Poisson ratio $\mu = 0.167$, density $\rho = 2400\text{kg}/\text{m}^3$, linear swelling coefficient of dam concrete $\alpha = 1.0\times10^{-5}/{}^{o}C$, friction coefficient between transverse joints $f = 0.7$; material parameters of the rock in dam foundation are as follows: elastic modulus $E = 17.5\text{GPa}$, Poisson ratio $\mu = 0.23$, density $\rho = 2700\text{kg}/\text{m}^3$.

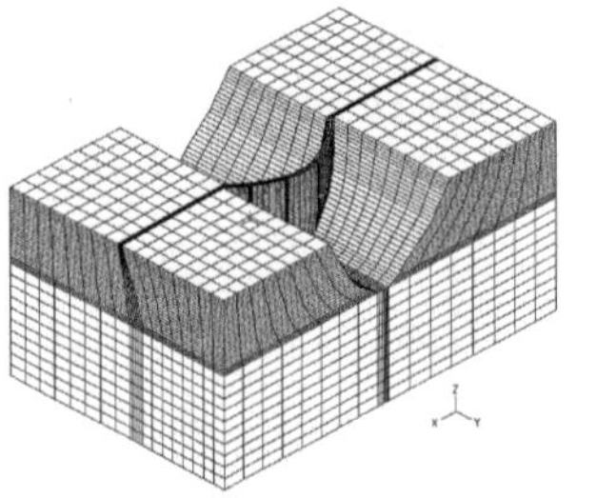

Fig. 1 Finite element grids of arch dam-foundation system.

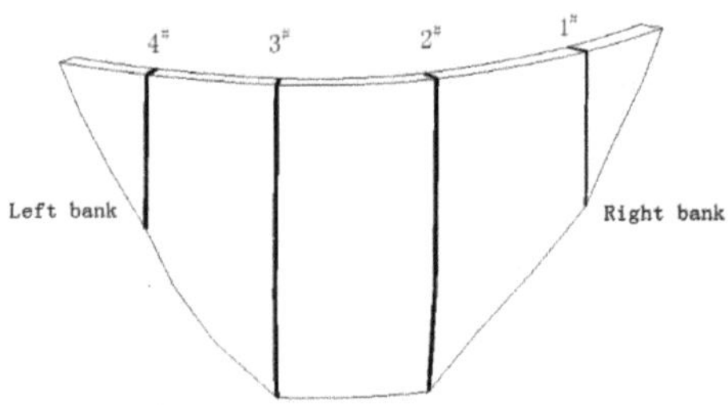

Fig. 2 Position of transverse joint of the dam.

A combination of load calculation is: regular water reservoir level + silt + dead weight of dam + designed temperature reduction + earthquake load. In this calculation, Rayleigh damping is used for defining the total damping matrix of the system i.e. $\xi = 0.05$. Dynamic water pressure is simulated in the modified Westergaard added mass formula.

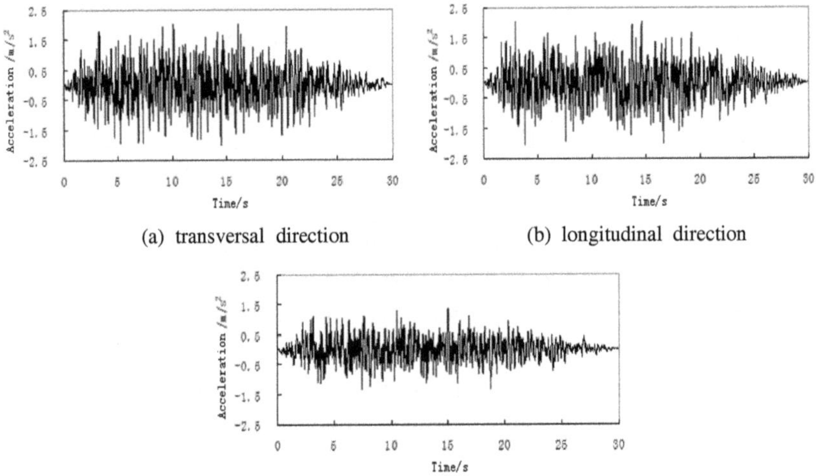

(a) transversal direction

(b) longitudinal direction

(c) vertical direction

Fig. 3 Acceleration time histories.

The horizontal peak acceleration of the bedrock with the transcendental probability P_{50}=10% of 50-year design benchmark period (equal to a recurrence period of about 500 years) is taken as the designed earthquake. Horizontal peak acceleration of the bedrock is 0.209g, and 2/3 of the horizontal acceleration is taken as the vertical peak acceleration i.e. 0.139g. 0.35s is taken as the characteristic site period, and the max value of reaction spectrum i.e. β_{max} =2.4. According to the design reaction spectrum in Design Criteria on Earthquake

Resistance of Hydraulic Constructions (DL5073—2000), artificial earthquake acceleration time-history at three directions on different phases are generated, with the acceleration time-history curves in Figure 3. The existence of transverse joint makes the calculation model become a non-linear system, and causes the malfunction of overlapping principle. Therefore, the static analysis on arch dam-foundation system is done firstly, on the basis of which a dynamic analysis is conducted for the whole system in implicit time-history analysis method. The time step in the calculation is 0.02s, with total duration of 30s.

Figures 4–6 presents the value charts including envelope value of main stress in upper reach and lower reach planes of the arch dam in traditional massless foundation, artificial viscoelastic border, border element with consistent equivalent viscoelasticity and other conditions respectively. It shows that a distribution rule of dam stress calculated for massless foundation model, artificial viscoelastic border and border element with consistent equivalent viscoelasticity is uniform by and large. Due to the opening and closing of transverse joint in earthquake, the tensile stress along arch direction in middle and upper part of dam plane on the upper reach is released, and the high tensile stress is mainly located in lower arch terminal of arch dam, the high tensile stress in dam plane in lower reach is mainly in middle and upper part of the dam plane; and the high tensile stress in dam plane in upper reach is mainly in middle and upper part of dam plane, and the tensile stress of dam plane in lower reach is mainly at arch terminals on both banks.

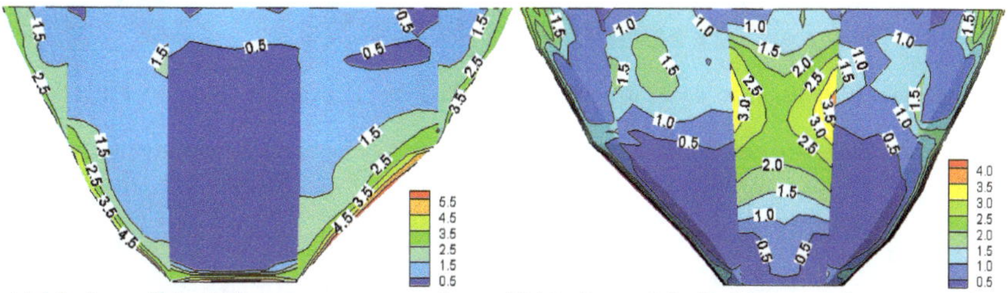

(a) Maximum Principal stress on upstream face (b) Maximum Principal stress on downstream face

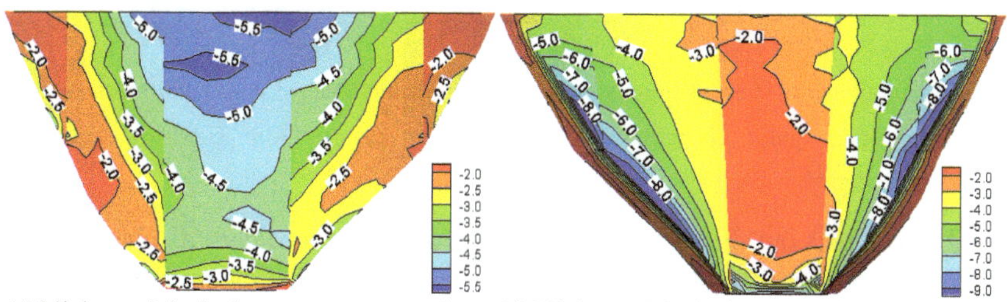

(c) Minimum Principal stress on upstream face (d) Minimum Principal stress on downstream face

Fig. 4 Envelope values of principal stresses (massless foundation, MPa).

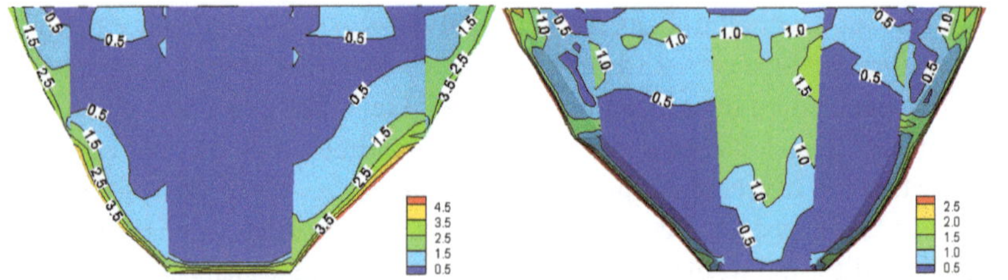

(a) Maximum Principal stress on upstream face (b) Maximum Principal stress on downstream face

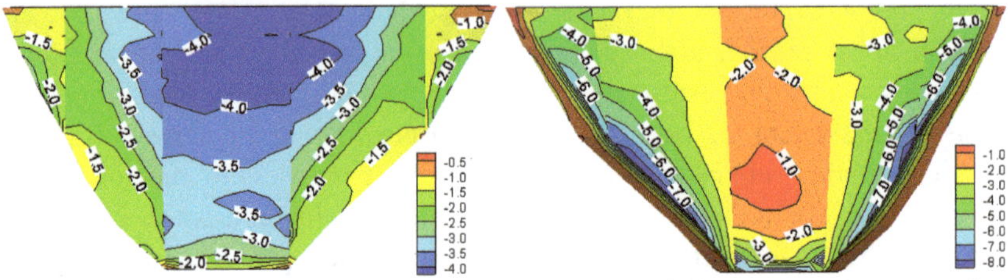

(c) Minimum Principal stress on upstream face (d) Minimum Principal stress on downstream face

Fig. 5 Envelope values of principal stresses (viscoelastic border, MPa).

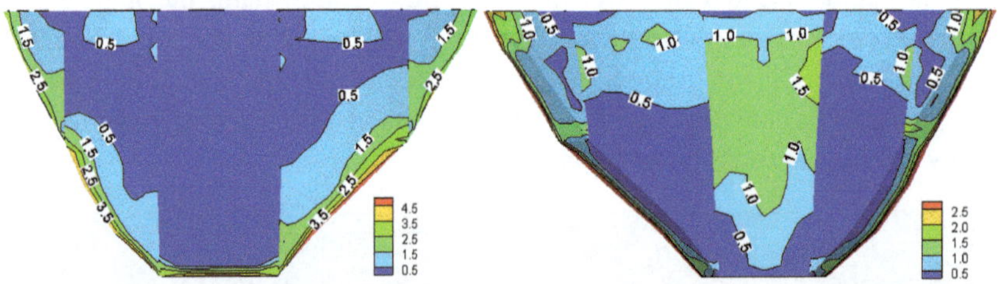

(a) Maximum Principal stress on upstream face (b) Maximum Principal stress on downstream face

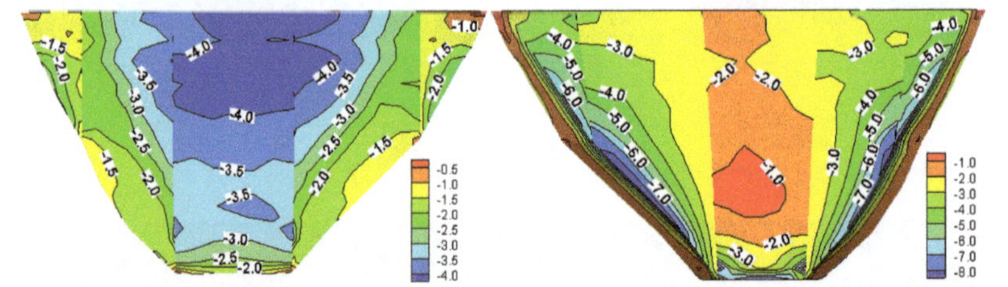

(c) Minimum Principal stress on upstream face (d) Minimum Principal stress on downstream face

Fig. 6 Envelope values of principal stresses (border element with consistent equivalent viscoelasticity, MPa).

Table 1 lists out the maximum values and positions of dam displacement at three directions in different border conditions. It shows that the maximum values of displacement of viscoelastic border and border element with consistent equivalent viscoelasticity at three directions are extremely close, and due to the fact that both have taken into account the long-distance foundation radiation damping, the maximum displacement responses of these two decline in comparison with massless foundation model, and the maximum displacement across and along the river declines by about 8% and 19% respectively, and the displacement along vertical direction declines by about 6%.

Table 1 Comparision of the maximum displacement results of the dam in different border conditions.

Border condition	Displacement along transversal direction(cm)	Displacement along longitudinal direction(cm)	Displacement along vertical direction (cm)
Massless foundation	2.00	-6.19	-2.16
Viscoelastic border	1.85	-5.02	-2.03
Consistent equivalent viscoelasticity border element	1.85	-5.03	-2.05

Table 2 lists out the maximum values and positions of the opening of transverse joint of the dam in different border conditions. It shows that the maximum opening value of massless foundation model occurs close to the top of 4# transverse joint of left arch terminal and is 14.30mm; and the opening values and distribution rule of transverse joints calculated for viscoelastic border and border element with consistent equivalent viscoelasticity are nearly uniform, of which the maximum opening values both occur on the top of 1# transverse joint close to the right arch terminal and are 6.66mm and 6.57mm respectively, and infinite foundation radiation damping obviously cuts off the maximum opening degree of the transverse joint of the dam by about 54%.

Table 2 Comparision of the maximum opening of transverse joints in different border conditions.

Border condition	1# transverse joint (mm)	2# transverse joint (mm)	3# transverse joint (mm)	4# transverse joint (mm)
Massless foundation	11.61	9.66	8.49	14.30
Viscoelastic border	6.66	3.28	2.80	4.48
Consistent equivalent viscoelasticity border	6.57	3.45	2.89	4.46

4. Conclusion

This article studies the border element with consistent equivalent viscoelasticity as well as the method and technology for wave input on this border. With some high arch dam in China as example, it applies artificial viscoelastic border and border element with consistent equivalent viscoelasticity in seismic response analysis of arch dam-foundation system of infinite foundation radiation damping respectively, analyzes dynamic response of the dam in three-direction earthquake load action, compares with calculation results of traditional massless foundation model and studies the impact of infinite foundation radiation damping upon arch-dam earthquake response. The calculation results reveal that infinite foundation radiation damping can obviously lower the seismic response of arch dam.

Acknowledgment

This research was financially supported by the Postdoctoral Science Foundation (2013M540989), Independent Research Subject of State Key Laboratory of Simulation and Regulation of Water Cycle in River Basin (2015TS05).

References

1. Chen Houqun. Discussion on seismic input mechanism at dam site [J]. Journal of Hydraulic Engineering, 2006, 37(12): 1417–1423.
2. Liu Jingbo, Gu Yin, Du Yixin. Fenves. Consistent viscous-spring artificial boundaries and viscous-spring boundary elements [J]. Chinese Journal of Geotechnical Engineering, 2006, 28(9): 1070-1075.
3. Gu Yin, Liu Jingbo, Du Yixin. 3D consistent viscous-spring artificial boundary and viscous-spring boundary element [J]. Engineering Mechanics, 2007, 24(12): 31–37.
4. Zhao Jianfeng, Du Xiuli, Han Qiang, Li Liyun. An approach to numerical simulation for external source wave motion, 2007, 24(4): 52–58. (in Chinese).
5. Bathe K J, Chaudhary A. A solution method for planar and axisymmetric contact problems [J]. Int. J. Num. Meth. in Eng., 1985, 21:65-88.
6. Eterovic A, Bathe K J. On the treatment of inequality constraints arising from contact conditions in finite element analysis [J]. Computers and Structures, 1991, 40(2): 203-209.
7. Bathe K J, Bouzinov P A. On the constraint function method for contact problems [J]. Computers and Structures, 1997, 64(5): 1069-1085.

Ecological Effect Evaluation Method of Permeable Slow -Traffic System

Man-liang Li[a,*], Xue-yan Zhou[b] and Yu-xiang Tian[c]
Chang'an University, Xi'an, Shannxi, China
E-mail: [a]gl01@cha.edu.cn, [b]xueyan0229@163.com and [c]561637264@qq.com

Most of concrete constructions built on urban ground surface are impermeable materials, which are very bad for urban ecosystem. This paper studied evaluation methods of permeable slow-traffic system though its drainage effect, noise reduction effect and thermal island effect reduction. The results show: as for drainage effect, permeability coefficient increase with asphalt mixture void ratio; non-fines concrete combined with graded gravel penetrates the most quickly, followed by graded gravel base and cement stabilized macadam combined with graded gravel. For noise reduction effect, the acoustical absorptivity of permeable concrete increase with the void ratio rising. And for thermal island effect reduction, temperature difference between surface and middle course of permeable pavement is much larger than that of other types of pavement structures, which illustrates that permeable pavement can alleviate thermal island effect positively. The results suggest that drainage effect, noise reduction effect and heat island effect reduction can be used to evaluate permeable slow-traffic system reasonably.

Keywords: Road engineering; permeable slow-traffic system; noise reduction effect; thermal island effect.

1. Introduction

In the modern urbanization construction, urban surface is covered by buildings and water-blocking materials gradually, thus produces "artificial desert" on ecology. Nowadays, urban infrastructure pavement consists of urban road, non-motorized vehicle lane, district and park are almost use waterproofing materials, and those pavements make up a large proportion of the city total area [1, 2]. The bound waterproof pavement destroyed urban surface ecological balance seriously [3, 5]. Furthermore, the bound waterproof pavement is adverse to mitigate city noise pollution. In addition, the "thermal island effect of city" would be increased by the interaction of bound waterproof pavement [4, 6].

* This work is supported by Central University fund project (2014G1211003).

Nowadays, numerous researches have been conducted about permeable pavement. For example, deliver permeability concrete pavement material, permeable base layer, and permeability road surfacing [5, 6]. Present permeable pavement is almost used in slow-traffic system that consists of lump slow trip mode such as pedestrians, bicycles and buses [4, 5]. The existing city permeable pavements increase permeable space and city air permeability, regulate urban climate and keep ecological balance effectively [3, 6]. However, permeable pavement researches almost focus on pavement material performance, little research results have been reported at structure, design and suitability of permeable slow - traffic system. Simultaneously, there is still no investigation at present about applying effect of permeable slow-traffic system. Accordingly, conduct deep research on permeable slow-traffic system can deepen and enlarge study areas of permeable pavement.

2. Drainage Performance Analysis of Permeable Slow-Traffic System

2.1. *Drainage effect analysis of pervious concrete pavement and permeable brick pavement*

This paper used laboratory test to analyze void ratio and hydraulic conductivity of permeable pavement. The results are shown in table1, where using TVR is the abbreviation of total void ratio, CVR is the abbreviation of continuous voids, HC is the abbreviation of hydraulic conductivity.

Table 1 Void ratio and hydraulic conductivity of permeable asphalt mixture.

item	SBS modified asphalt OGFC			TPS modified asphalt OGFC		
	gradation I	gradation II	gradation III	gradation I	gradation II	gradation III
TVR (%)	17.0	20.23	23.1	17.0	20.1	22.9
CVR (%)	12.8	16.2	19.8	12.8	16.2	19.8
HC (10-2cm/s)	2.37	3.08	3.33	2.31	3.02	3.25

In Table 1, with the increasing of void ratio and continuous voids, hydraulic conductivity grew gradually, proved that permeable asphalt mixture has good permeability. Compared with gradation I, hydraulic conductivity of SBS modified asphalt OGFC gradation II increased by 30.0% and gradation III increased by 40.5%; hydraulic conductivity of TPS modified asphalt OGFC gradation II increased by 30.7% and gradation III increased by 40.7% by the same token.

This paper used outdoor test study drainage property of graded gravel base, non-fines concrete combined with graded gravel and cement stabilized macadam combined with graded gravel. According to the test principle of "total rainfall-overflow volume" = "permeation volume", the three pavement relationships between penetration depth and time are shown in figure1.

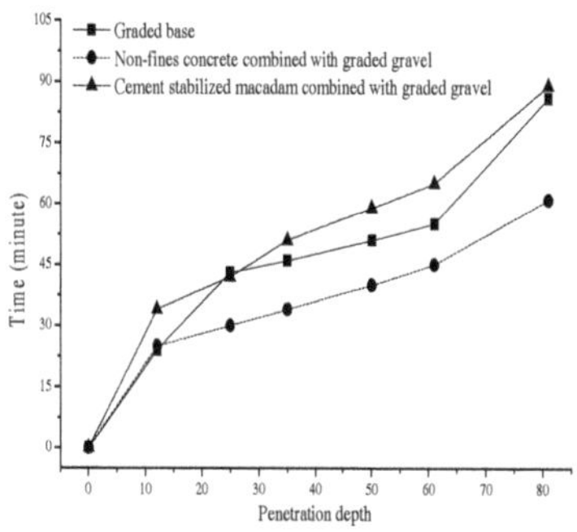

Fig.1 Relationships between penetration depth and time on drainage course.

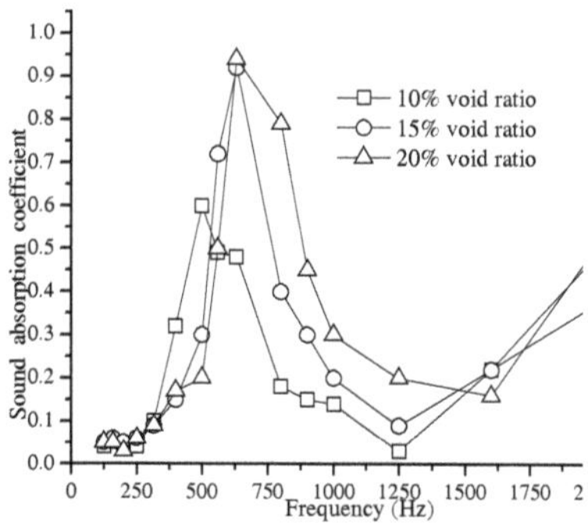

Fig. 2 Pervious concrete sound absorption coefficient curves with different void ratio.

According to Figure 1, The total penetration time of graded base, non-fines concrete combined with graded gravel and cement stabilized macadam combined with graded gravel was 1h 26min, 1h 1min and 1h 29min respectively. That showed that the penetration property of non-fines concrete combined with graded gravel is the best, followed by graded gravel base and cement stabilized macadam combined with graded gravel.

2.2. *Drainage effect analysis of permeable asphalt pavement*

Technical specification for permeable asphalt pavement (CJJ/T190) regulate permeable asphalt concrete void ratio is 18% to 25%. Technical specification for pervious concrete pavement (CJJ/T135-2009) regulate pervious concrete void ratio is 11% to 17%. Based on drainage effect analysis of permeable pavement, we combined trials and relevant provisions, used mixture void ratio to classify drainage effect of permeable pavement. In terms of permeable asphalt pavement, the void ratio of very good level was (23% 25%], good level was (20%, 23%] and fair level was [18%, 20%]; in terms of pervious concrete pavement, the void ratio of very good level was (15%, 17%], good level was (13%, 15%] and fair level was [11%, 13%].

3. Noise Attenuation Effect Analysis of Permeable Slow-Traffic System

3.1. *Noise attenuation effect analysis of permeable asphalt pavement*

As volume index, void ratio consists of connected void ratio and closed void ratio. The sound absorption coefficient mean and peak in different void ratio of OGFC-13 mixture are shown in Table 2, where using DVR is the abbreviation of design void ratio, AVR is the abbreviation of actual void ratio, CVR is the abbreviation of connected void ratio, SACM is the abbreviation of sound absorption coefficient mean, SACP is the abbreviation of sound absorption coefficient peak, PF is the abbreviation of peak frequency.

Table 2 Permeable pavement sound absorption coefficient in different void ratio.

DVR (%)	AVR (%)	CVR (%)	SACM	SACP	PF (Hz)
16	15.80	9.43	0.341	0.639	900
18	17.65	11.26	0.400	0.693	1000
20	19.56	13.01	0.402	0.669	1000
22	21.48	14.96	0.424	0.842	1000
24	23.32	17.89	0.428	0.826	900

In Table 2, the sound absorption coefficient peak and mean of permeable asphalt pavement grew with void ratio increasing in all. For example, compared with 16% void ratio, the permeable asphalt pavement with 18% void ratio increased by 17.3%; the permeable asphalt pavement with 24% void ratio increased by 25.5%.The peak frequency was focus on 900 to 1000 Hz.

This paper used OGFC-13 specimen as reference, tested OGFC-10 sound absorption coefficient with different void ratio and connected void ratio respectively, and then studied the influencing rule of asphalt mixture aggregate size for acoustical absorptivity. The results are shown in Table 3.

Table 3 Permeable pavement sound absorption coefficient in different particle size.

Gradation	DVR (%)	AVR (%)	CVR (%)	SACM	SACP	PF(Hz)
OGFC-13	20	19.56	16.2	0.402	0.669	1000
OGFC-10	20	20.63	14.5	0.330	0.495	500
	23	22.63	16.2	0.432	0.736	1800

From Table 3, for OGFC mixture with the same connected void ratio, the OGFC-10 mixture has larger acoustical absorptivity than OGFC-13 mixture. However, acoustical absorptivity of OGFC-10 reduced at the same void ratio. Based on above analysis, there was a closer relationship between acoustical absorptivity and OGFC mixture connected void ratio.

3.2. *Noise attenuation effect analysis of pervious concrete pavement*

The sound absorption coefficient of pervious concrete specimen with 10%, 15% and 20% void ratio were tested in this paper. The sound absorption coefficient curves are shown in Figure 2.

In Figure 2, sound absorption coefficient peak increased with void ratio increasing. Compared with 10% void ratio pervious concrete specimen, the specimen with 15% void ratio increased by 9.1%; compared with 15% void ratio, 20% void ratio specimen increased by 27%. Sound absorption coefficient peak occurred from 500Hz to 800Hz. Sound absorption coefficient appeared low ebb in 1250Hz or so, and then tended to grow along with frequency increasing.

3.3. *Noise attenuation effect classification of permeable slow-traffic system structure*

Based on above noise attenuation effect analysis, we used mixture void ratio to classify noise attenuation effect. That for permeable asphalt pavement, the void ratio of very good level was (20%, 25%], good level was (18%, 20%]; for pervious concrete pavement, the void ratio of very good level was (15%, 17%], good level was (11%, 15%].

4. Thermal Island Effect Analysis of Permeable Slow-Traffic System

4.1. *Analysis of thermal island effect reduction*

Urban thermal island effect was caused by urbanization, and it became more and more obvious with the rapid expand of city-size. Because permeable pavement could adjust air temperature and humidity, so it is benefit to mitigate urban thermal island phenomenon. Some researchers tested temperature of permeable pavement, SMA pavement surface and middle course. The results are shown in table4, where using SF is the abbreviation of surface temperature, MCT is the abbreviation of middle course temperature, TD is the abbreviation of temperature difference between surface and middle course, ATD is the abbreviation of average temperature difference.

Table 4 Temperature comparison of surface and middle course.

Pavement type	number	SF(°C)	MCT(°C)	TD(°C)	ATD(°C)
Permeable asphalt pavement	1	38.4	30.4	8.0	7.7
	2	38.2	30.8	7.4	
Pervious concrete pavement	3	38.4	32.2	6.2	6
	4	39.0	33.2	5.8	
Permeable brick pavement	5	39.4	31.9	7.5	7.5
SMA pavement	6	39.2	36.3	2.9	2.4
	7	39.0	36.6	2.4	
	8	38.0	36.0	2.0	

From Table 4, for permeable pavement, temperature difference between surface and middle course was higher than 6°C, while for SMA pavement, it was just 2.4°C, which showed that there has little accumulated heat in permeable pavement. Compared with SMA pavement, the average temperature difference between surface and middle course of permeable asphalt pavement increased by 3.2 times, pervious concrete pavement increased by 2.5 times and permeable brick pavement increased by 3.1 times, proved that permeable pavement was helpful to mitigate urban thermal island effect.

4.2. *Classification of thermal island effect reduction*

Based on above analysis about thermal island effect reduction, we used temperature difference between surface and middle course to evaluate and classify thermal island effect reduction of permeable pavement. The results are shown in Table 5, where the unit was °C.

Table 5 Classification standard of reducing thermal island effect.

Pavement type	very good	good	fair	poor	very poor
Permeable asphalt pavement	≥8	(6,8]	(4,6]	[2,4]	<2
Pervious concrete pavement	≥6.5	(5,6.5]	(3,5]	[2,3]	<2
Permeable brick pavement	≥7.5	(6,7]	(4,6]	[2,4]	<2

5. Summary

(1) In terms of drainage effect, permeability coefficient grew along with increasing of mixture void ratio and continuous void ratio; non-fines concrete combined with graded gravel penetrates the most quickly, followed by graded gravel base and cement stabilized macadam combined with graded gravel; proposed drainage effect classification standard of permeable slow-traffic system, that were "very good" , "good" and "fair".

(2) As for noise attenuation effect, sound absorption coefficient mean and peak grew along with void ratio increasing; at the same connected void ratio, sound absorption property of little particle size was better than large particle size, while at the same void ratio, the conclusion was opposite; proposed corresponding void ratio of noise attenuation effect classification standards of permeable pavement.

(3) For thermal island effect reduction, compared with SMA pavement temperature difference, permeable asphalt pavement increased by 3.2 times, pervious concrete pavement increased by 2.5 times; permeable brick pavement increased by 3.1 times. Proposed the classification standard of permeable pavement, that were "very good", "good", "fair", "poor" and "very poor".

References

1. C H Wang, J J Zhao, X H Wang, X Q Wang, S G Di. *Study on Compaction Characteristics of Solidified Mud with Different Proportion of Curing Agent, C. Advanced Materials Research,* Vols. 535-537 (2012), 1807-1810.
2. X H Wang, M M Yu, C H Wang. *Study on Cross Sectional Optimization System of Green Ecotype Urban Road,* C The 11th national urban road and traffic engineering academic conference (2011).
3. Y Q Wang, LY Sun, C J Sun. *Reasons in forming system and solutions of our country big city traffic problems,* J. Urban problem, (2007), 75-80.
4. Q S Song. *Study of urban green transportation system* D. Hua Zhong University and Technology, 2006.
5. W D Ding, M Liu, S P Du. *Transportation Means and Urban Green Traffic, J. of Wuhan Uni. of Sci. & Tech.* (Natural Science Edition), J. (2003) 50-53.
6. X G Yang, *Developing the public transportation, constructing an urban green traffic system,* J. China Mayors (2001).

The Hysteretic Behavior of Prefabricated Hollow Shear Wall*

Zhang Guowei†, Xiao Wei‡, Wu Kunlun, Zhan yuan and Li Chuanming
Civil Engineering, Beijing University of Civil Engineering and Architecture, Beijing, China
‡E-mail: Xiaowei@stu.bucea.edu.cn
www.bucea.edu.cn

Hollow shear wall generally applied to multi-story building and it can solve the problem of heavy self-weight with ordinary shear wall use in low-rise buildings. However, it is difficult to guarantee the quality of hollow shear wall at the site, so the paper presents prefabricated hollow shear wall. It has a lot of merits, such as small volume, easy to transport, convenient construction and so on. But study the seismic properties of prefabricated hollow shear wall is still very few, especially the seismic properties of post-cast strip. For the above reasons, the paper produced four specimens to simulate prefabricated hollow shear wall. Experimental results show that the prefabricated hollow shear wall has good seismic performance and the existence of post-cast strip and holes is not influenced structure seismic property. So it can be used in multi-story buildings.

Keywords: Prefabricated hollow shear wall; seismic properties; post-cast strip.

1. Introduction

The concept of "building industrialization" is becoming more and more important in modern buildings and it also gave birth to a lot of new technology, prefabricated shear wall is one of them. It is not only reduce the wetting operation and change "site construction" as a "factory construction ", but also greatly improve the construction speed and the comfort of the structure.

In this paper we are going to discuss a new type of shear wall is called prefabricated hollow shear wall based on the traditional technology. Traditional shear wall is mainly suitable for high-rise residences, but when it was used for multi-story buildings will cause an increase of weight and stiffness and lead to the buildings have strong reaction in the earthquake.[1] Prefabricated hollow shear wall overcomes these shortcomings and has the characteristics of factory

---

* This research is sponsored by BUCEA Urban Rural Construction and Management Industry Research Development Collabration Post Graduate Training Centre.
† Work partially supported by Young Talent Program (2014) Foundation.

production. So the quality of it can be guaranteed. In addition, due to the air sandwich in the wall its heat preservation and insulation are better than traditional shear wall.[2] Prefabricated hollow shear wall will have good application prospect in the multi-story buildings.

2. The Experiment

2.1. *Test method*

The paper is aimed to study seismic performance of reinforced concrete hollow shear wall. There are a lot of structural seismic experiment methods, mainly includes the pseudo static test, pseudo dynamic test and simulated earthquake shaking table experiment and so on.[3] This experiment is based on the pseudo static test which is a inelastic seismic response of the structure research method. In the process of the test applying low cycle loading to obtain the structure hysteresis curves. Finally establish restoring force model to research failure mode and ductility performance of the structure.

2.2. *Model making*

The ratio of model 1 high to thickness is 13 which is called general shear wall.[4] It is used to simulate the shear wall structure, frame - shear wall structure and shear wall in frame-core tube structure. General shear wall mainly used to assure lateral stiffness of the structure, providing basic seismic capability and dissipation of earthquake energy.

The ratio of model 2 high to thickness is 6.5 which is called short shear wall. It is gradually rise in recent years because it is helpful for building layout and can reduce self-weight. But because of short shear wall seismic performance is not better than general shear wall and has little experience in the application of earthquake zone, so more researches is needed.[5] The test consists of two models and each model making two shear wall. The wall size is shown in Table 1.

Table 1 Test specimen size.

Specimen number	Length	Width	Height	Diameter of the holes
HWV1	1100	200	2600	120
HW2	1100	200	2600	120
LWV3	1100	200	1300	120
LW4	1100	200	1300	120

Note: The unit of length, width, height and diameter is millimeter. The unit of load is KN and the value of rate of the holes is percentage. Zero means doesn't apply vertical load.

2.3. *Test loading device and the load system*

In order to prevent the occurrence of horizontal slide in the test via anchor screw through the reserved anchor hole to fix specimen on the ground. Setting steel beam to clamp specimen base in the horizontal direction. Two of the specimen need applying vertical load. Vertical load using hydraulic jack loaded before the experiment and remains constant during the testing process.

Horizontal load applied with hydraulic servo loading system. Before specimen yield is load control and after yield is displacement control. Then yield displacement of the specimen is defined as standard displacements and load to the specimen damage on the basis of integer multiple standard displacement. Specimen loading device is shown in Figure 1.

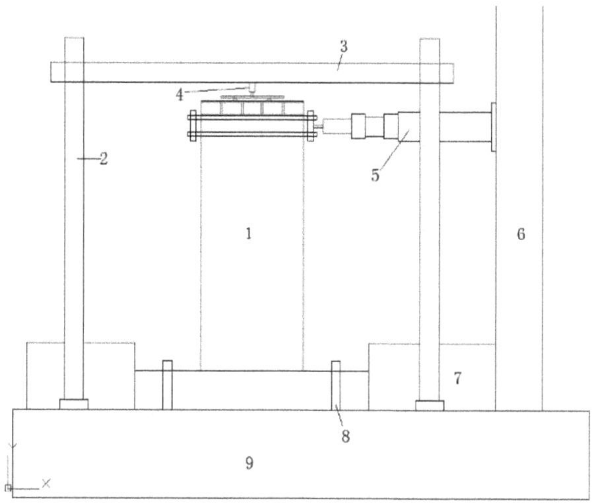

1 Specimen, 2 Portal frames, 3 Beam, 4 Vertical loading device, 5 Horizontal loading device, 6 Reaction wall, 7 pedestal, 8 earth anchor, 9 test platform.

Fig. 1 The loading device.

3. The Experimental Results and Analysis

3.1. *Hysteresis curve of load and displacement*

Loading a loop to get load - displacement curve is called hysteresis curve. According to the shape of the hysteresis curves to judge specimen failure characteristics. In general, the greater area of hysteresis curves, the stronger capacity of energy dissipation. The following list all specimen hysteresis curves.

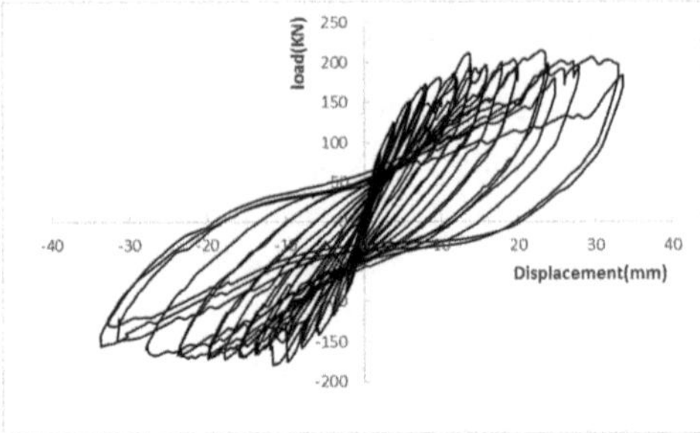

Fig. 2 Hysteresis curves of HWV1.

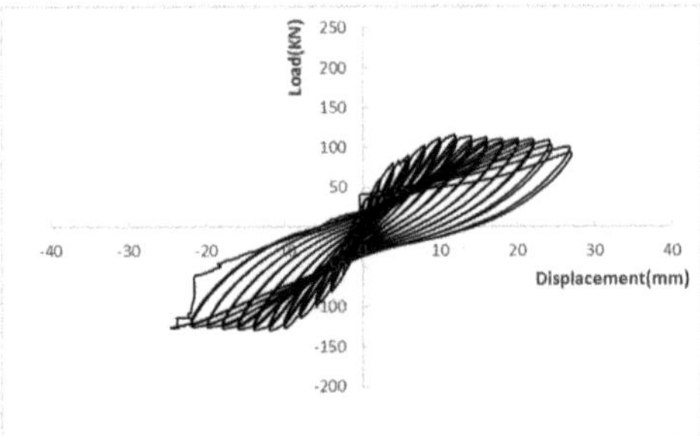

Fig. 3 Hysteresis curves of HW2.

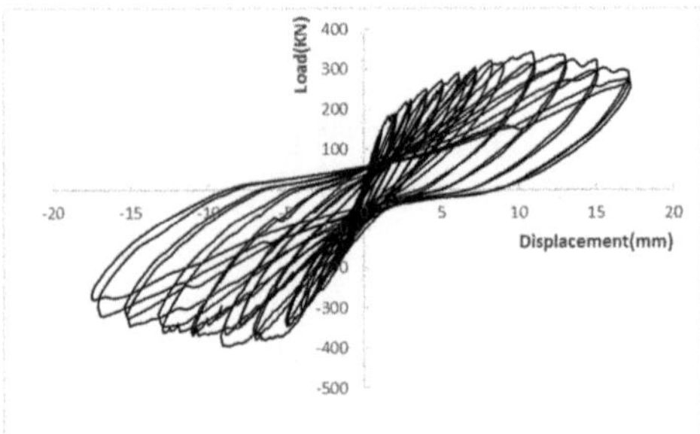

Fig. 4 Hysteresis curves of LWV3.

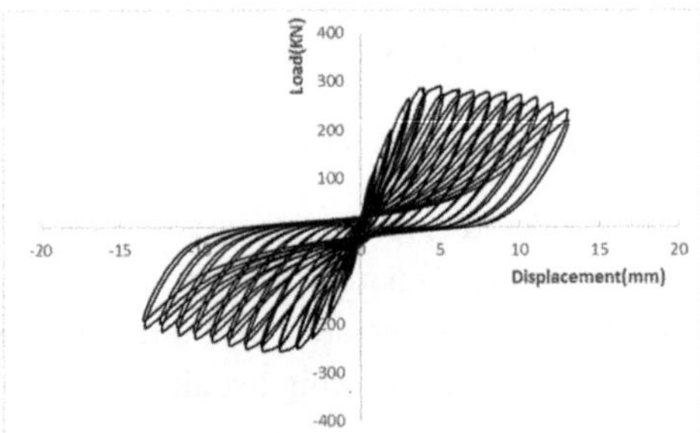

Fig. 5 Hysteresis curves of LW4.

3.1.1. *Hysteresis curves of load and displacement for HWV1*

Fig. 2 shows that the hysteresis curves are substantially linear in elastic phase. When the first cracks appeared (F = 123 KN) the area of the hysteresis curves began to increase slowly which indicate that the specimen began to energy dissipation. As it reaches the yield load (F = 178KN) the hysteresis curve starts to become arched, but pinching is not obvious which it is indicated that the specimen doesn't appear shear deformation and slip before yield. After the specimen yield the force increase slowly instead the displacement growing fast and the area of hysteresis curve significantly increase. All these indicate that the specimen has good energy dissipation capacity.[6] After that the slope of hysteresis curve begins to the decline rapidly which indicate stiffness degradation.

3.1.2. *Hysteresis curve of load and displacement for HW2*

As is shown in Figure 3 the load and displacement of specimen HW2 is much smaller than specimen HWV1 because of without vertical load and the property of specimen HWV1 and HW2 is essentially the same feature in elastic. When the first crack appeared (F = 60KN) the hysteresis curve presents arched and there is obvious pinching effect which is indicated slip influence and reflected the plastic deformation capacity of specimen HW2 is relatively strong. When it reaches the yield load (F = 92KN) hysteresis curve transit from the bow to the inverse S-shaped and it becomes full. All of the phenomena indicated that there is more slippage impact and the capacity of energy dissipation is very well.

3.1.3. *Hysteresis curve of load and displacement for LWV3*

As it is shown that hysteresis curve approximated a straight line when the specimen HWV1 in elastic in Figure 4. But when the specimen appeared cracks hysteresis curve begins to increase and present fusiform. It is shown that the specimen starts to dissipate energy and the strength of the specimen is gradually rising. As it approaches the yield load (F = 293KN) hysteresis curve present arched but pinching is not obvious which it is indicated that the specimen doesn't appear the influence of shear deformation and slip before yield. After yield hysteresis curve presents inverse S-shaped and its area began to increase rapidly due to slipping and crack developed. It proved that the specimen has a big slip and energy dissipation capacity. In addition, the slope of the hysteresis curve begins to decline significantly and the strength of the specimen increase slowly which are indicated stiffness degradation. When the load increases to the maximum load (F = 342 KN) displacement of the specimen is increasing rapidly and load of the specimen is declining slowly. We consider the load drops to 85% of maximum load as specimen destruction.

3.1.4. *Hysteresis curve of load and displacement for LW4*

Compare Figure 4 with Figure 5 we know that performance of specimen LWV3 and LW4 are basically the same in elastic. When it appeared cracks the hysteresis curves present arched with obvious pinching which is indicated shear deformation and slip. As the specimen yield (F = 252) pinching phenomenon is more pronounced due to the development of diagonal cracks and shear deformation. When the load increases to the maximum load (F = 290 KN) displacement of the specimen is increasing rapidly, load of the specimen is declining slowly and the area of the hysteresis curve starts to increase. All of this indicate specimen LW4 has excellent energy dissipation capacity. Finally hysteresis curve is Z-shaped and it is indicated that diagonal cracks have been fully developed and there is a lot of slip.

By comparing the hysteresis curves of the four specimens we know that the vertical load can improve crack load, yield load, maximum load and ultimate load and can reduce the slippage of the specimen.

3.2. *Skeleton curve*

Skeleton curves of each specimen are shown in Figure 6. Some conclusions could be drawn from the skeleton curve, such as yield load, yield displacement, deformation and so on. It can be seen from the skeleton curve that every specimen exhibited the similar properties in elastic. Displacement increases rapidly and load increases slowly after specimens yield. Displacement of the specimen increases along with the height of the wall.

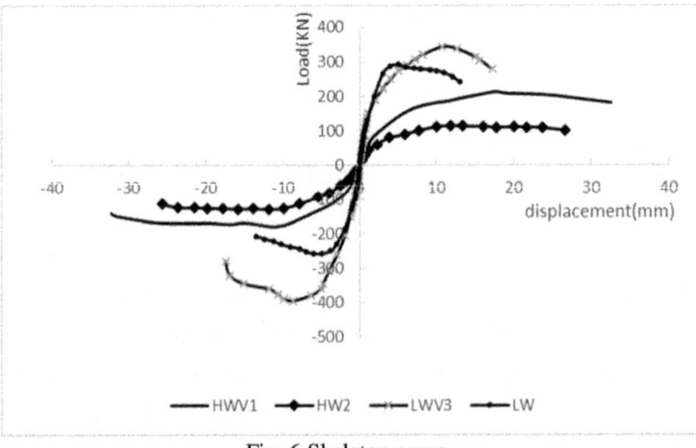

Fig. 6 Skeleton curve.

3.3. *Ductile properties*

Ductility reflects plastic deformation ability of structure or component before its load does not reduce significantly and it's important to evaluate seismic performance. We usually use ductility factor to determine the structure or component ductility and is shown in Table 2.

Table 2 Ductile properties of all specimens.

Specimen number	Yield load	Yield displacement	Maxim um load	displacement of corresponding to the maximum load	Ultimate displacement	Ductility factor
HWV1	178	9.16	213	17.54	32.38	3.53
HW2	92	6.42	116	11.72	26.69	4.16
LWV3	293	4.23	342	8.14	13.89	3.28
LW4	252	2.76	291	4.87	12.65	4.58

Note: Yield load and yield displacement are determined using the energy equivalent area method. The unit of yield load and maximum load is KN and the unit of displacement is mm.

It can be seen from Table 2 that the yield load of specimen HWV1 and LWV3 is greater than the corresponding specimen HW2 and LW4 due to axial load. Yield displacement and ultimate displacement are also bigger than the specimen without vertical load.

Specimen HWV1 and LWV3 ductility factors are less than specimen HW2 and LW4 which it is indicated that vertical load makes the ductile lower. A further explanation, due to the existence of vertical loads it delays formation of plastic hinges and cracks. So the capacity of rotation and energy dissipation is reduced and shorten the process of yield to destroy. All of this make yield and ultimate displacement ratio decrease.

3.4. *Energy dissipation capacity*

Energy dissipation capacity is measured by the area of load - displacement hysteresis curve which is shown in Figure 7. In this test uses energy dissipation coefficient to measure the energy dissipation capacity of each specimen and energy dissipation coefficient calculated as in Eq. (1).

$$\psi = \frac{S_{ABCD}}{S_{OEF}+S_{OGH}} \tag{1}$$

Where: S_{ABCD} is the area of envelope of hysteresis curve.

S_{OEF} and S_{OGH} are the area of triangle OEF and OGH.

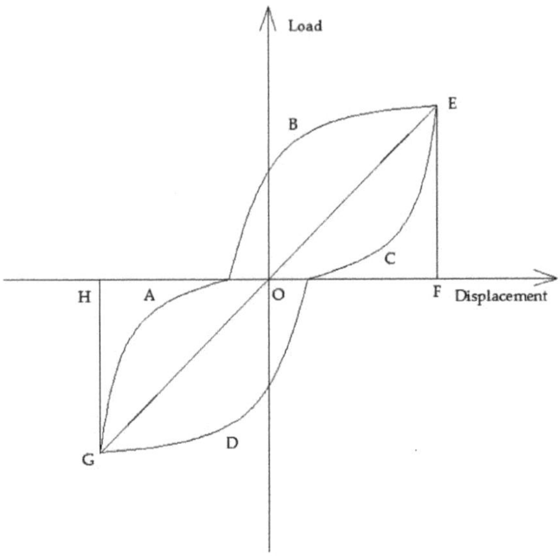

Fig. 7 Triangle OEF and ODH.

It can be seen that the energy dissipation of the four specimens is very well from Table 3. Post-cast strip and hollows don't weaken energy dissipation capacity of the specimen. If the wall has better ductility and more uniform cracks its capacity of energy dissipation will be much better.

Table 3 Energy dissipation coefficient of each specimens.

EDC	HWV1	HW2	LWV3	LW4
ψ	1.60	1.40	1.44	1.54

Note: EDC (Energy dissipation coefficient) is a dimensionless number.

3.5. *Stiffness analysis*

Stiffness is the ability to resist deformation under external loads of the structure and it is an important indicator to ensure the serviceability limit stat of the structure. The stiffness of the specimen is present by secant stiffness in pseudo static test. In other words it is the ratio of absolute value of the maximum and minimum loads and their corresponding absolute value of displacements in each circle. Stiffness is calculated as in Eq. (2).

$$K = \frac{|+F_i|+|-F_i|}{|+X_i|+|-X_i|} \tag{2}$$

Where: F_i is the maximum load in i-th time cycle.

X_i is the maximum load in i-th time cycle.

The stiffness degradation curves of each specimen is shown in Figure 8. As it can be seen from the stiffness degradation curves: The stiffness of specimen reduced with the increases of its height and the initial stiffness of the low wall is much bigger than the tall wall.

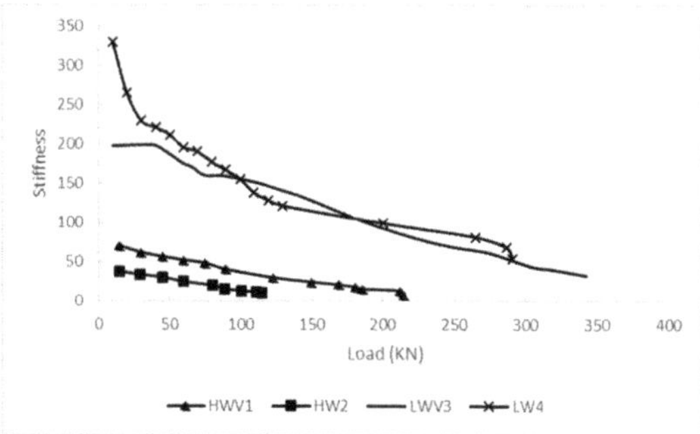

Fig. 8 Stiffness degradation curves.

Stiffness degradation curve of specimen HWV1 and HW2 substantially parallel and its stiffness degradation process is very slow and smooth. In addition stiffness mutation did not occur. On the other hand initial stiffness of the low wall is relatively higher which is indicated that the specimen is not easily deformed under external loads. Stiffness decreased relatively slow of specimen LWV3 because of the presence of vertical load, but the stiffness of the specimen LW4 has two significant turning point. At first stiffness decreased rapidly and after a while stiffness begins to fall gently due to cracks are appeared.

3.6. *The impact of depth-width ratio*

Failure characteristic and shear strength of wall are related to shear forces and moments of the failure plane and it is represented by shear span ratio generally. Define computational formula of generalized shear span ratio as $\lambda = \frac{M}{Vh_0}$. For shear walls it is calculated by calculate shear span ratio and it is also called depth-width ratio. It is calculated as in Eq. (3).

$$\lambda = \frac{a}{h_0} \tag{3}$$

Where: a means horizontal distance from the load point to the bottom of the specimen.

h_0 is the effective width of the specimen cross section.

As it is shown in table 4 the larger depth-width ratio, the lower shear strength and vertical load can increase shear strength of the specimen.

Table 4 Depth-width ration of specimen.

Specimen number	Ratio of height to width	Horizontal load	Shear strength
HWV1	2.4	213	0.068
HW2	2.4	115	0.037
LWV3	1.2	342	0.109
LW4	1.2	291	0.092

Note: The unit of horizontal load is KN. Shear strength is calculated by $\frac{V}{f_c b h_0}$.

4. Conclusions

Mechanical behaviors and failure modes of sheer wall are influenced by depth-width ratio. Depth-width ratio greater than 2 is bending shear failure and depth-width ratio between 1 and 2 is shear failure. Depth-width ratio is also has great impact on stiffness and the specimen with high depth-width ratio will has small initial stiffness. It is indicated that the specimen is easily deformed, but the stiffness degradation is relatively slow instead specimen with little depth-width ratio stiffness degradation is rapidly. In addition, the lower depth-width ratio, the greater shear strength. Vertical load has a great impact on the mechanical properties and ductility of shear walls. It can improve the crack load, yield load and ultimate load of sheer wall, but it will reduce the ductility of the specimen. As we can see that precast hollow concrete shear wall has good seismic performance from the hysteresis curve of the specimen. Because of the force increases slowly and the displacement grows fast so the area of hysteresis curve significantly increase, all of this indicated that precast hollow concrete shear wall has good ductile properties. Destructions of the wall mainly occur in the roots of the specimen and concrete exfoliated both in tensile and compressive direction in the end. It doesn't appear destructions of hollows and post-poured strips in the experiment which it is indicated that hollows and post-poured strips will not weaken shear seismic performance.

References

1. Qiongmei Wang, Gang Wang, Shufang Xu. "Seismic behaviors of hollow sheer wall analysis [J]." Sichuan Building Science, Oct. 2006, Vol. 32 No. 5: 156-160.
2. Tao Meng. "Seismic performance experimental and theoretical study on precast concrete hollow wall [D]." Beijing University of Technology, 2009.
3. JGJ101-96. "Specification of Testing Methods for Earthquake Resistant

Building [S]."
4. Xixi He, Linqing Huang. "Design of Tall Building Structures [M]." Wuhan University of Technology Press: 2007:112-119
5. Zhangfeng Zhu, Zhengxing Guo. "Test research on seismic performance of plane model of new precast concrete short-limbed sheer wall [J]." Journal of Harbing Institute of technology, Apr. 2012, Vol. 44 No. 4: 94-99.
6. Yongxin Ma, Shansuo Zheng. "Structure Testing and Inspection in Civil Engineering [M]." Higher Education Press: 2008: 69-83.

Pseudo-Dynamic Test Methods on Substructure Considering Variable Axial Force

Zhang Guowei[1], Zhan Yuan[2,*], Wu Kunlun[1], Xiao Wei[1] and Guo Yurong[3]
[1]*Civil Engineering, Beijing University of Civil Engineering and Architecture, Beijing, China*
[2]*Central China Real Estate Limited, Zhengzhou, Henan Province, China*
[3]*Civil Engineering, Hunan University, Changsha, Hunan Province, China*
[*]*Email: zhanyuan@stu.bucea.edu.cn*
www.bucea.edu.cn

During seismic action, frame columns are under reversed load. Unexpected damage of column elements may occur because of the continuous variation of axial force due to overturning moment caused by the earthquake and vertical seismic force which affect the stability of the whole structure. Therefore, the influence of the variable axial force should be considered in evaluating accurate characteristics of force and deformation of frame columns under cyclic loading. This paper presents an evaluation of hybrid simulation test method on substructure with columns under variable axial loads.

Keywords: Column; variable axial force; pseudo-dynamic test; hybrid simulation; substructure.

1. Introduction

As building technology develops, more and more high-rise, super tall building and long-span bridges appear. In these buildings, frame columns are the most important elements to bear the vertical load and the lateral force. The seismic performance is also affected greatly by frame columns. Much theoretical analysis and experimental study on seismic performance of different kinds of columns have been done in the past decades. A quasi-static test was conducted on concrete filled square steel tube (CFST) columns by Kyushu University in Japan in 1965. Hysteresis curve of the columns was gotten by combining test data and time-history analysis results. Sakino and Tomii [1] investigated the hysteretic behavior of 15 square CFST columns with quasi-static tests. Sakino et al. [2] studied seismic performance of 13 circular CFST columns by cyclic loading. Nakanishi et al. [3] carried out quasi-static tests on square CFST columns for ultimate load and ductility. Yokoyama [4] conducted cyclic tests of square CFST columns with reinforcement ring-steel beam joints. Reinforced concrete columns subjected different axial compression ratios were tested by Huang Xingsong et al. [5] to investigate the affection of axial force on columns during earthquake. Li Hongnan et al. [6] carried out cyclic loading tests with two orthogonal horizontal forces under constant axial compression to study strength and stiffness degradation of reinforced concrete columns under multidimensional load. Lv Xilin et al. [7] conducted tests on RC columns under constant axial force to investigate mechanical behaviors of RC columns. Many experimental studies on seismic behaviors of frame columns have been carried out, but most of the tests are mainly concerned with cyclic horizontal force under constant axial loading without considering the affections of variable axial compression on seismic performance of frame columns. It has been proved that mechanical behaviors and seismic performance of columns are greatly affected by variable axial forces. In this paper, pseudo-dynamic test methods on substructure were studied considering variation of axial force when applying axial load on column specimens during the test. Pseudo-dynamic test methods.

2. Development of Pseudo-Dynamic Test

Pseudo-dynamic test method means that computer analysis combines with actuator solving the structure dynamics equation. This method was first proposed by M. Hakuno in 1969 [8] which made seismic tests being able to simulate the effects of earthquakes acceleration. Since then, pseudo-dynamic test method is widely used for studying the seismic behavior of structures and their components. During pseudo-dynamic test, initial displacement of seismic response of structures is calculated firstly with dynamic equations. Then the initial displacement is applied to the tested substructure with actuator measuring the restoring force with sensors. Moreover, then with the restoring force and next step ground acceleration, the next-step target displacement is calculated. By this way, the response history curves of acceleration, speed, displacement with restoring force of structure or component elements are gained. The dynamic equation used during pseudo-dynamic test is given as,

$$Ma + Cv + Ku = P \tag{1}$$

Where M, C, K is mass matrix, damping matrix and stiffness matrix respectively; a, v, u is the acceleration vector, speed vector and displacement vector of the nodes respectively; P is the load vector.

2.1. *MDOF pseudo-dynamic test of substructure*

There are two types of pseudo-dynamic test methods. One is that applied load to the whole structure, the test results match the actual situation quite well.

However it cost much money on making test model and enlarges the equipment demand. The damage of the structure often occurs only in certain parts or local members. Other parts are still working well. So another test method is that applied load to the substructure that are easily destroyed or some members with complex nonlinear characteristics during earthquake. The other parts with elastic state could be simulated by computer. Combine the results of the load actuator and the computer to calculate the seismic response of the overall structure. This method is named pseudo-dynamic test methods of substructure or hybrid simulation test.

During an earthquake, the seismic oscillation is multidimensional. Damage investigation and analysis shows that the damage of the structure suffers the multidimensional seismic oscillation which is more serious than the destruction of the structure suffers the one-dimensional seismic action. The purpose of this paper to research the pseudo-dynamic test method of substructure loaded in the vertical and horizontal directions. The impact of the variable axial force on the seismic performance of frame columns can be simulated better in this new method.

Principle of variable axial force test method

2.2. *Multi-directional loading pseudo-dynamic test of substructure*

Currently, there are two main methods of the experimental study on variable axial force under horizontal cyclic loading, which are the coupled variable axial force and uncoupled variable axial force. The coupled variable axial force means that the axial force and the horizontal load (or the displacement) are applied simultaneously and reach their maximum or minimum value at the same time. Well, as for the other one, the specimens are still under the axial force and the horizontal load without considering the correlation of them. For both of the methods above, the impact of vertical seismic load on the frame column are not considered adequately. Thus, for the frame column, a single point can be applied in multiple directions by using methods of the substructure pseudo-dynamic test in order to simulate the axial force and displacement of frame column under the real seismic action.

For the substructure pseudo-dynamic test, we need consider the impact of both of the horizontal and vertical loads on loading controlled by force or displacement. In order to consider the change of the axial force in all time, there always are two methods. The first one is to combine the pseudo-dynamic test control software to apply a load and displacement on the substructure and the finite element software to calculate the load and displacement. For the other one, with using the feedback of reaction from the actuator after applying the initial displacement on the test substructure, we can calculate the next step displacement of experiment substructure by the structural dynamic equation to complete the horizontal loading circularly. Well, the variable axial force under seismic action has mainly based on the horizontal seismic action, gravity second-order effect and the vertical seismic action. However, when the earthquake occurred in the past, vertical seismic waves were not recorded completely. Due to technical limitations, we only consider the impact of horizontal seismic action on the variable axial force in this paper.

2.3. *Application of numerical integration method*

Numerical integration method is divided into implicit integration method and explicit integration method. The implicit integration method, which is stable unconditionally, is difficult to be uses in the pseudo-dynamic test., because calculating the displacement of the next step in the implicit integration method needs the next step restoring force which must be measured by the actuator. Therefore, the explicit numerical integration methods are always used in the most of Pseudo-dynamic tests. However, the explicit integration method needs a small schedule to get a stable algorithm. Finally, a new method, combined numerical integral method is found for pseudo-dynamic test of substructure.

2.4. *Explicit numerical integration method*

As solving the dynamic equation, the explicit numerical integration method only needs the information of the previous step. It mainly concludes central difference scheme, explicit Newmark scheme and modified Newmark scheme, etc. Central difference scheme is a typical explicit integration method. The velocity and the acceleration is assumed respectively as follows

$$v_i = \frac{d_{i+1} - d_{i-1}}{2\Delta t} \tag{2}$$

$$a_i = \frac{d_{i+1} - 2d_i + d_{i-1}}{\Delta t^2} \tag{3}$$

take v_i and a_i into equation (1), then the equation can be expressed as:

$$d_{i+1} = \left(M + \frac{\Delta t}{2}C\right)^{-1} \times \left[2Md_i + \left(\frac{\Delta t}{2}C - M\right)d_{i-1} - \Delta t^2\left(r_i + f_i\right)\right] \tag{4}$$

2.5. *Implicit numerical integration method*

Implicit numerical integration method needs the information provided not only in the previous step, but also in the current step to solve the dynamic equation. It mainly concludes Wilson-θ method, implicit Newmark-β method, and α method, and so forth. In the pseudo-dynamic test, α method is the most studied implicit method. It can be expressed by the equations

$$Ma+(1+\alpha)Cv_{i+1}-\alpha Cv_i+(1+\alpha)r_{i+1}-\alpha r_{i1}=(1+\alpha)-\alpha f_i \quad (5)$$

$$v_{i+1}=v_i+\Delta t(1-\gamma)a_i+\gamma a_{i+1} \quad (6)$$

$$d_{i+1}=d_i+\Delta tv_i+\Delta t^2\left[\left(\frac{1}{2}-\beta\right)a_i+\beta a_{i+1}\right]\gamma a_{i+1} \quad (7)$$

Where, the stability and damping characteristics are controlled by α, β, γ. When $\beta=\left.(1-\alpha)^2\right/4$, $\gamma=\frac{1}{2}-\alpha$, $-\frac{1}{3}\le\alpha\le 0$, this method is stable unconditionally.

2.6. *Combined numerical integration method*

Combined numerical integration method is mainly used in the pseudo-dynamic test of substructure. Well, the explicit numerical integration method is used in the experiment substructure and the implicit integration method is used in the calculate substructure. CDM-Newmark method is a more direct combined numerical integration method, which can be expressed as follows

$$\begin{bmatrix} M^E & 0 \\ 0 & M^I \end{bmatrix}\begin{Bmatrix} a^E \\ a^I \end{Bmatrix}+\begin{bmatrix} K^{EE} & K^{EI} \\ K^{IE} & K^{II} \end{bmatrix}\begin{Bmatrix} d^E \\ d^I \end{Bmatrix}=\begin{Bmatrix} F^E \\ F^I \end{Bmatrix} \quad (8)$$

Where E = explicit part, I = implicit part.

3. Loading Method of Variable Axial Force

3.1. *Load under different fixed axial force*

Current researches on the seismic performance of frame column are mainly concentrated on applying horizontal cycle load on frame column under different fixed axial force. With the study that focuses on the mechanical performance, failure mode and the capacity of energy dissipation under the different axial force, this method becomes the most common way to study the seismic performance of frame column. However the disadvantage of this method is that the axial force is always fixed during the change of horizontal force and displacement. It is different from the actual way and cannot reflect the actual failure mode of frame column.

3.2. *Loading method of coupling variable axial force*

Without considering the vertical seismic action, the change of the axial force of the frame column results from the overturning effect and $P-\Delta$ effect under the horizontal seismic action. The existing variable axial force experiments mostly focus on the coupling variable axial force, that is, the change of the axial force is regular. There are many different changing ways, for example that the change of axial force is directly proportional to transversal displacement at the top or the end of the column. Huang Xiang [9], though the hysteretic performance of 6 reinforced concrete column under variable axial force, has studied proportional change between axial force and displacement. However it is still different from the real one. During the earthquake, the axial force changes with the earthquake acceleration irregularly, which may leads to unexpected damages.

3.3. *Uncoupled variable axial load*

The methods above are all through horizontal reciprocating load experiments of frame column with settled axial force previously, which cannot simulate the actual situation. Yang Hong, Bai Shaoliang [10] studied the reinforced concrete columns under the variable axial force caused by horizontal earthquake, and analyze the factors leading to axial force changing and the relationship between axial force and moment of the column end. They propose that it is mostly corresponding to the actual situation when axial force changes proportional to the bending moment during the experiment. Wang Xunliu [11] made a comparison with uncoupled variable axial load and coupled variable axial load through reinforced concrete column test. It is believed that the coupling variable axial force may make the seismic performance decline on the direction of smaller axial force load, however the uncoupled variable axial force can cause the unstable phenomenon like "jump" of bearing capacity of the frame column. Due to the randomness of the uncoupled variable axial force, we should pay more attention to its effect on the column frame. Thus, under horizontal seismic action, this paper argues that the change of the axial force is mainly caused by lateral displacement of dead-load gravity center in the upper structure. That is, when the lateral movement of the column takes place, the upper dead-load gravity center and point of action will offset, which cause the axial force component changes. Firstly, through the numerical integration method above, the research can get test substructure horizontal displacement loading value d_{i+1} before every time step, then it is supposed to calculate the change of the axial force value by d_{i+1}. So circle reciprocating loading like that can realize the dynamic calculation of variable axial force. The calculation diagram is shown as Fig. 1.

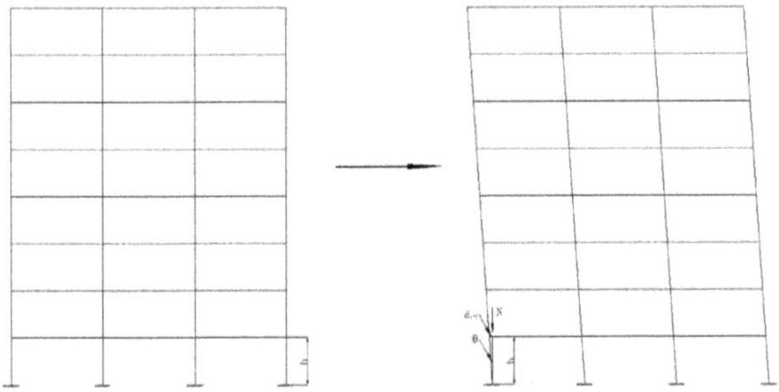

Fig. 1 Calculation diagram of variable axial force.

As shown above in Fig. 1. Assume the bottom layer is the experiment substructure. The vertical loads they born are mainly from the superstructure of the main. Represented by N. The next step horizontal displacement applied to the experiment substructure is represented by d_{i+1}. The height of the experiment substructure is represented by h. Then:

$$\sin\theta = {}^{d_{i+1}}\!/_{h} \tag{9}$$

When displacement of experiment substructure reach d_{i+1}, the axial force component along the rod can be expressed as:

$$N_{i+1} = N \cdot \cos\theta = N \cdot \sqrt{1-\left({}^{d_{i+1}}\!/_{h}\right)^2} \tag{10}$$

If there are n spans at the bottom of the test substructure. The bearing capacity of the side column can be calculated as:

$$\begin{aligned} N_{i+1} &= N \cdot \cos\theta + n \cdot N \cdot \sin\theta \\ &= N\left(\sqrt{1-\left({}^{d_{i+1}}\!/_{h}\right)^2} + n\left({}^{d_{i+1}}\!/_{h}\right)\right) \end{aligned} \tag{11}$$

The axial force in the every step can be calculated by the equation (11). Then apply the axial force to the experiment substructure. The flow chart of pseudo-dynamic test of substructure under variable axial force is shown as Fig. 2.

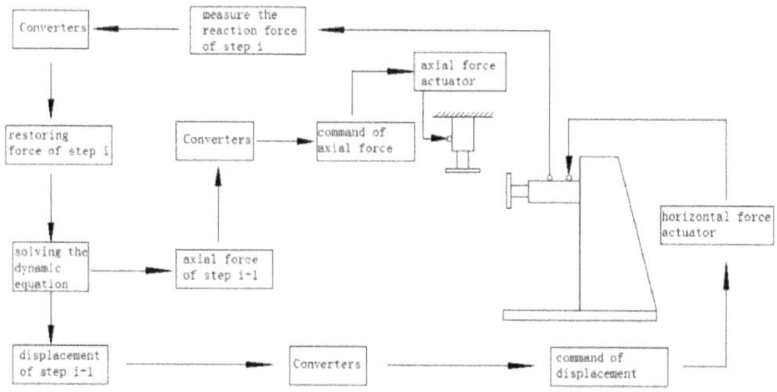

Fig. 2 Flow chart of pseudo-dynamic test of substructure under variable axial force.

3.4. *Load testing procedures combined with the finite element software*

The program of variable axial load test combined with finite element software calculated by iterative loop, the method of substructure pseudo-dynamic test above combined with dynamic loading can reflect the actual dynamic response of the structure under seismic action better. However workload of the development for the substructure pseudo-dynamic test procedures is heavier. Most of the existing pseudo dynamic test procedure is usually developed by experimenters themselves ignoring certain degrees of freedom to simplify structure model, whose ability of the numerical simulation is weaker than the professional finite element software relatively. For example, the overall structure is analyzed by using layer shear model in a substructure pseudo-dynamic test, which cannot simulate the component in the key parts which stress complicated comprehensively in the structure. Aiming at the defect, we can use better finite element software combined with pseudo-dynamic test control software to test any part of the structure, while the rest of the simulation can make full use of the function of the existing finite element software. S.P.S chneider et al. [12] based on the DRAIN - 2D structure analysis program developed a substructure pseudo-dynamic test program. Thus, we can choose complex loading components in the structure as the substructure test and the rest were simulated by computer. Feng Fan, Wang Qiang et al. [13] combined the finite element software ABAQUS with pseudo-dynamic control software OpenFresco to realize the complex components of substructure pseudo-dynamic test. On the basis of these studies, in order to realize accurate nonlinear calculation of concrete structure in the compute, we will combine nonlinear analysis software OpenSees with of control system NetSLab developed by Hunan university. By utilizing OpenSees with its strong ability of nonlinear computation, the study chose the frame column as test substructure. Besides, the rest of the structure would be computed by OpenSees with data dock transmission between the OpenSees and the NetSLab. In the end, substructure pseudo-dynamic test of concrete frame column can be realized.

4. Finite Element Simulation

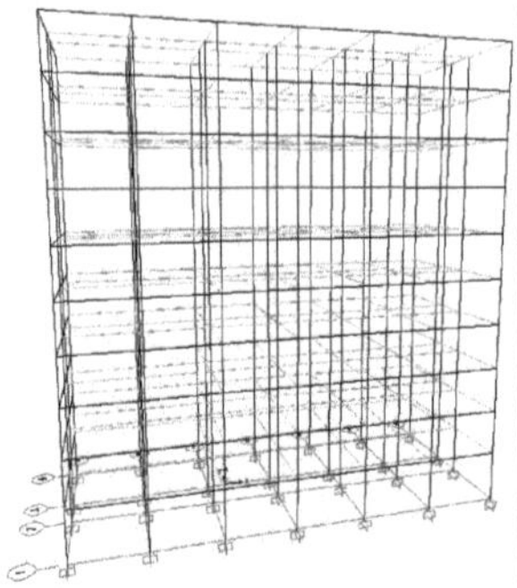

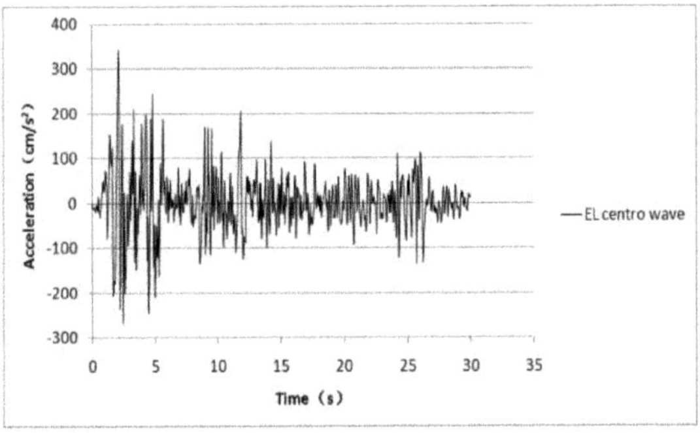

Fig. 3 Schematic of 10 layers CFST frame.

Fig. 4 Acceleration history of EL CENTRO.

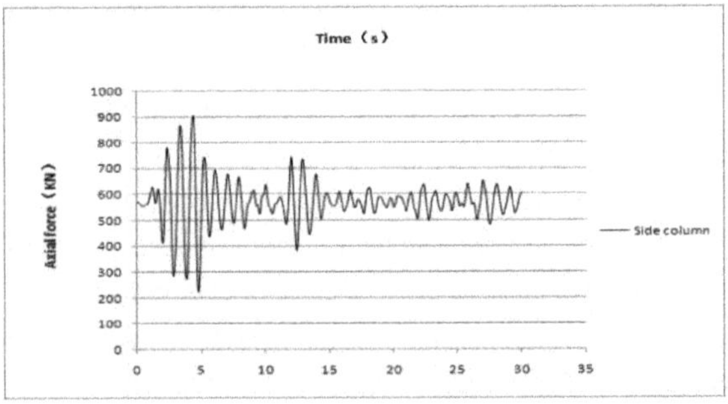

Fig. 5 Axial force history of side column.

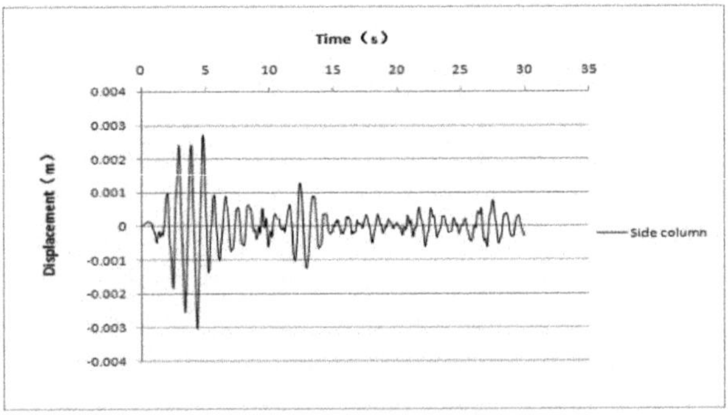

Fig. 6 Displacement history of side column.

A 10-story concrete filled steel tube frame model is made with FE software SAP2000, as shown in Fig.3. In order to simulate the axial force and displacement of the center column and side column of framework bottom layer under the seismic action, the following measures must be done. The axial force time history and displacement history of center column and slide column are shown as Figs. 5–8.

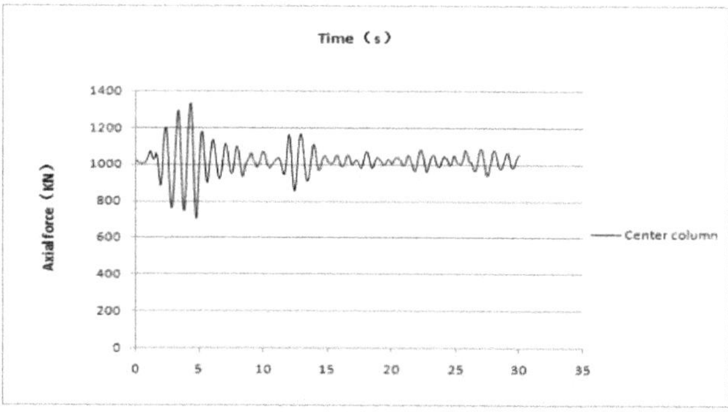

Fig. 7 Axial force history of center column.

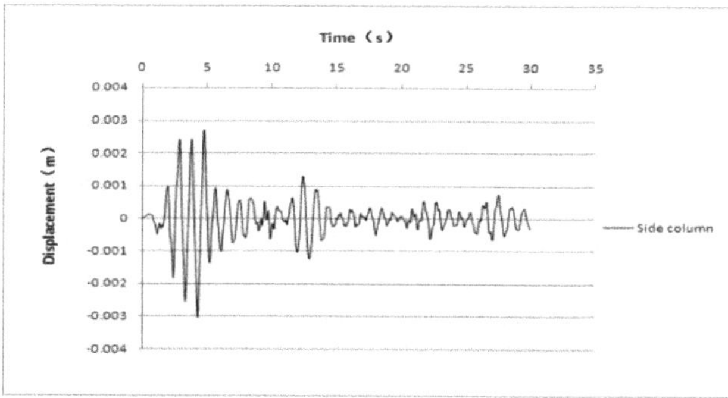

Fig. 8 Displacement history of center column.

It can be found from the above figures that the seismic acceleration will cause the horizontal lateral of frame columns under the horizontal seismic action. Then the axial force of frame columns will change as the horizontal lateral with the large amplitude of variation. Therefore, non-proportional changes in axial force have an important impact on the seismic performance of CFST. Axial compression ratio change caused by the variation axial force would result in more severe damage and destruction of the plastic hinge region. In the past research [14] on seismic behavior of CFST has been carried out in different axial compression ratio indicates that the flexural capacity of CFST would serious losses in the low axial compression ratio. Also the ductility of CFST would reduce in the higher axial compression ratio. Carrying capacity and stiffness of frame column degrade rapidly in the elastic-plastic phase result in the early destruction of frame columns. Therefore, influence of axial compression ratio on mechanical properties and seismic performance of CFST cannot be ignored. The result of simulation reflects the axial force of frame column change violently under horizontal seismic action.

5. Conclusions

With the theoretical analysis and simulation analysis of the behavior of frame structure under the horizontal seismic action, the change of the axial force of the frame column mainly results from the overturning effect and $P-\Delta$ effect only under the horizontal seismic action. And the amplitude of variation is obvious. However the variation of axial force can make the carrying capacity degrade rapidly and cause unexpected damage of frame columns. Thus this paper proposes a new test method of substructure under variable axial force. Such new method not only can compute the changes of axial force by the horizontal displacement but also can simulate more accurate dynamic response of frame column under seismic action.

References

1. Sakino K, Tomii M. Hysteretic behavior of concrete filled square steel tubular beam-columns failed inflexure [J]. Transactions of the Japan Concrete Engineering, ASCE, 1981, 3: 439-446.
2. Sakino K, Inai E, Nakahara H. Tests and analysis on elastic-plastic behavior of CFT beam-columns-U.S.-Japan cooperative earthquake research program [C]. Proceedings of the Fifth Pacific Structural Steel Conference, Seoul, Korea, 1998, 901-906.
3. Nakanishi K, Kitdaa T, Nakai H. Experimental study on ultimate strength and Ductility of concrete filled steel columns under strong earth quake [J]. Journal of Construction Steel Research, 1998, 51: 297–319.
4. Yokoyama Y, Morita K, kawamata Y. et al. Structural behavior of steel-beam to concrete – Filled square tube column connections reinforced with Inner ring stiffener [C]. Proceedings of the Third International Conference On steel-Concrete Composite Structures, 1991, 165-170.
5. Huang Xingsong, Study on behavior of reinforced concrete frame columns under low cyclic and pseudo-dynamic test of substructure. [D] Chongqing: Chongqing Architecture University, 1993.

6. Li Hongnan, Wang Qiang, Li Bing, Research on multidimensional quasi-static test of reinforced concrete frame columns. [J] Journal of Southeast University, 2002, 32(5): 728-732.
7. Lv Xilin, Lu Weidong. Experimental study on seismic performance of concrete filled square steel tube columns under the cyclic loading. [J] Journal of Building Structure, 2000, 21(2): 2-11.
8. Huang Liang. MDOF substructure pseudo dynamic testing and nonlinear seismic response analysis of frame-supported reinforced masonry shear wall. [D]Changsha, Hunan University, 2005.
9. Huang Xiang, Study on seismic performance of reinforced concrete columns under the rule variable axial force. [J] Fujian Architecture, 2003, 3: 46-48.
10. Yang Hong, Bai Shaoliang, A study on the loading method of varying axial force based on the elastic-plastic seismic response of structure. [J] World earthquake engineering. 2002, 18(2): 80-84.
11. Wang Xunliu, Lu Xinzheng, Ye Lieping, Analysis of earthquake-resistant behaviors for RC columns under variable axial loads. [J] Industrial Construction, 2007, 37(12): 71-75.
12. Wang Xiangying, Tian Shizhu, Zhang Hongtao, Song Kun, Hybrid testing method on substructure techniques for shaking table by position control of actuator. [J] World earthquake engineering, 2009, 6(25): 30-35.
13. Fen Fan, Wang Qiang, Wang Zhanfei, Research on Hybrid Simulation with Finite Element Software ABAQUS. [J] Structural Engineers, 2011, 1(27): 82-87.
14. Zhang Guowei. Research on Cumulative Seismic Damage of CFT Columns. [D] Changsha, Hunan University, 2009.

Study on Chloride Ion Penetration of Early Age Concrete Mixed Corrosion Inhibitor

Xiao Yi
School of Architectural and Surveying & Mapping Engineering, Jiangxi University of Science and Technology, Ganzhou, 341000, China
E-mail: 365711947@qq.com

Zhu Yunhui
Oujiang College, Wenzhou University, Wenzhou, 325035, China
E-mail: zhu-yunhui@163.com

Sun Fuxue
College of Architecture and Civil Engineering, Wenzhou University, Wenzhou, 325035, China
E-mail: sunfuxue@163.com

Li Han
School of Architectural and Mapping Engineering, Jiangxi University of Science and Technology, Ganzhou, 341000, China
E-mail: lihan1209@163.com

Chloride ions begin to erode concrete in early age. In this paper, the rule of diffusion coefficient and the development of effective porosity of early age concrete mixed corrosion inhibitor in different concentrations of salt solution are analyzed through coulomb electricity method and the effective porosity test. Results show that the chloride ion penetration resistance of early age concrete increase with increase of age, weaken with the increase of chloride ion concentration. Effective porosity decreases with the increase of age and the concentration of sodium chloride solution. Concrete mixed corrosion inhibitors can effectively reduce the coefficient of permeability, the early effect is better than the late.

Keywords: Early age concrete; corrosion environment; diffusion coefficient; corrosion inhibitor;

1. Introduction

As common material, concrete has suffered from a variety of corrosion of chlorine salt coming from environment, and chlorine salt erosion is studied by researchers [1-4] as one of the important factors that affect concrete durability deficiency. In literatures, most of authors developed the study by maintaining concrete to a certain age such as 7d or 28d, and then immersed concrete samples into salt solution for chloride ions to diffuse into concrete. This does not match the practical engineering, which is that concrete suffer the chlorine salt erosion from the early stage of the maintenance. In addition, engineers always improved durability performance of reinforced concrete by adding a certain amount of corrosion inhibitor into concrete, and few document reported influence of corrosion inhibitors to concrete. Therefore, early age concrete resistance to chloride ion penetration in chlorine salt corrosive environment under the action of corrosion inhibitor will be studied in this article.

2. Specimen Production and Experiment Scheme

Experimental material .Experiment use 42.5# ordinary Portland cement in Zhejiang province, which apparent density is 3150g/cm3, fineness is 350m2/kg, and the volume stability is qualified. Coarse aggregate: Granite stones for Wenzhou secondary macadam, particle size: 5~20mm, apparent density: 2650g/cm3. Fine aggregate: sand for Fujian fineness, modulus: 2.8. The moisture content: 3.7%. Mixing water: tap water. Slump: 180~220 mm, Corrosion Inhibitor: jus901 corrosion inhibitor produced in Beijing. The adding amount of corrosion inhibitor according to “Technical specification for application of corrosion inhibitor for steel bar” (JGJ/T 192-2009), in order to make the study and practical combination, the mixing proportion of concrete is Wenzhou OuFei sluice engineering, shown in table 1.

Table 1 Mix proportion of concrete.

corrosion inhibitoı (%)	Water cement ratio	Sand ratio (%)	Cement + sand + stone + water + corrosion inhibitor(Kg/m3)	Slump (mm)
5%	0.35	33%	500+569+1156+175+25	180-220
-	0.35	33%	500+569+1156+175	180-220

Experiment design: Concrete are mixed using mechanical mixer, after the completion of the concrete mechanical agitation, and poured into round PVC mold with size of 100mm×50mm to vibrate and erase. Specimens are numbered after forming, each group of 3 specimens, soaking in respectively of 0%, 3%, 5% and 8% sodium chloride solution to 3d, 7d, 14d, 28d.

Numbering rules: "Z + number": inhibitors + concentration. "N + number": sodium chloride solution+ concentration, "D + number": age + days

The chloride ion migration. Concrete chloride ion migration power test method is according to ASTMC 1202 standard measure. The instrument is the chloride ion diffusion coefficient of electric flux tester CABR - RCM6 made in academy of building materials of China, and the chloride ion migration is measured through the specimen power within 6h. According to the type (1) to calculate the permeability coefficient through the migration power [5], Test age: 3d, 7d, 14d and 28d.

$$\beta = 2.57765 + 0.00492Q \tag{1}$$

In type (1), β : the chloride ion diffusion coefficient($\times 10^{-12} m^2 / s$), Q : 6h total transfer capacity (C)

Effective porosity. Pore of concrete widely exists in the cement paste and aggregate and cement paste and aggregate interface, and can be divided into primary pores and secondary pores. Based on the analysis of pore fluids flow through porous media, only interconnected pores are meaningful. To introduce the concept of effective porosity, define it as a medium of interconnected pore volume and the ratio of the total volume of medium[6]:

$$n_e = (V_v)_e / V_b \tag{2}$$

In Type (2), $(V_v)_e$ is interconnected pores effectively.

After soaked to 3d, 7d, 14d and 28d of the concrete specimen, samples are weighted after dry the water on the surface of the specimen using wind drying oven, and the effective porosity is calculat by type (3).

$$\varepsilon_e = \frac{(m_l - m_0) \cdot p_c}{m_0 p_l} \tag{3}$$

In type (3) p_l : Density of water; p_c : Density of specimen after drying; m_l : Quality of the soaking specimens full of water. m_0 : Quality of the specimen after drying.

3. Results and Discussions

Penetration coefficient of chloride ions. The figure 1 (a) shows that chloride ion permeability coefficient was reduced in different degrees with the increase of immersion ages under the condition of the same concentration of sodium chloride. At the same time, coefficient of permeability decrease amplitude decreases with the increase of soaking concentration. A large number of experiments show that the main factors influencing the chloride ion diffusion coefficient of concrete are: water/cement ratio, curing age, admixture and the environment. The permeability coefficient of the specimens have larger decline from 3d to 14d, and 14d is a cut-off point. After 14d the permeability coefficient of decline slowed. The permeability coefficient increases with the increase of concentration of sodium chloride solution, and the permeability coefficient of concrete specimens is closer to changes in the concentration of 3% and 5% sodium chloride solution, However, the permeability coefficient of concrete in concentration of 8% sodium chloride solution both increased than before. Early concrete don't have the ability to resist chloride ion erosion. In order to improve life structure, corresponding measures should be taken to reduce the chloride ion in the early days of the concrete in engineering practice.

Effective Porosity. The figure 2 shows that the effective porosity of concrete decreases with the increase of age, and 7d as a cut-off point. The margin of the decrease of the effective porosity of concrete began to slow down in 7d. Results also show that the hydration of concrete internal cause pore size constantly decrease with the increase of age in the same concentration of sodium chloride solution. By the decrease of the effective porosity, the numbers of interconnected pores decrease faster than the speed of the reduction of the number of total porosity.

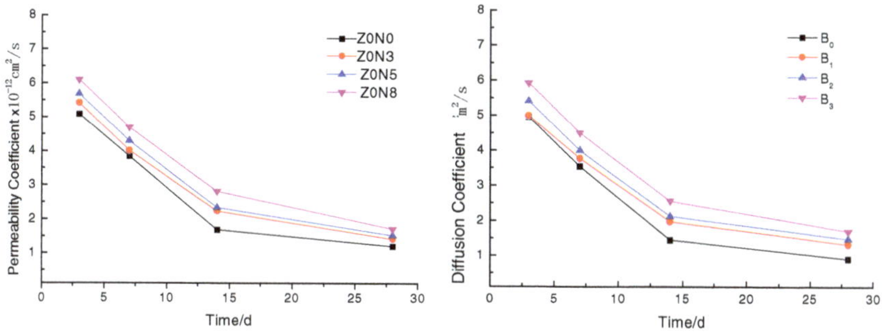

(a) (b)

Fig. 1 Permeability of chloride ion change with age.

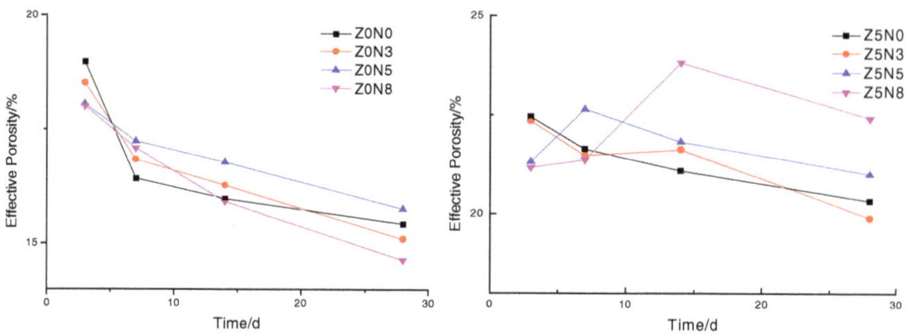

(c) (d)

Fig. 2 Effective porosity of concrete change with age.

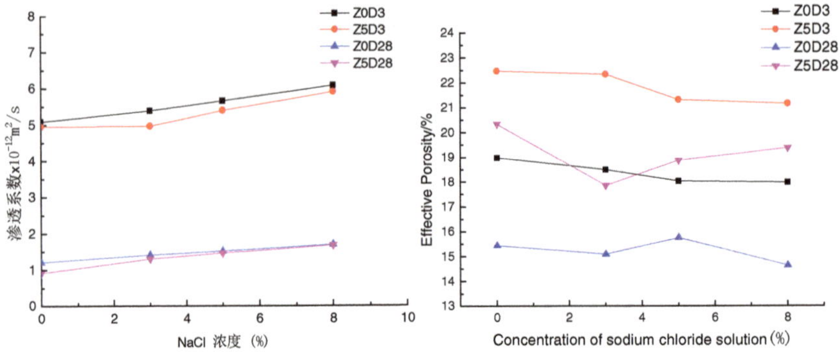

(d) (e)

Fig. 3 Permeability of chloride ion change with sodium chloride solution.

Corrosion Inhibitor: The figure 1(b) shows that the concrete which is mixed with a certain amount of inhibitor has similar rule to ordinary concrete along with age in total. Available by figure 3(e), by comparing the change of permeability coefficient in 3d and 28d, corrosion inhibitor can reduce the permeability coefficient of concrete to a certain extent. Concrete of 3d which mixed with corrosion inhibitor is more obvious than the 28d concrete. When the concentration of sodium chloride solution was 5%, the influence of 3d concrete is the most obvious. When concentration of sodium chloride solution was 0%, the influence of 28d concrete is the most obvious.

4. Conclusions

Here, we may draw the following conclusions.

(1) Early concrete don't have the ability to resist chloride ion erosion, and the permeability coefficient of concrete decreases with the increase of age. It can meet the requirements in the provisions of the durability of resistance to chloride ion penetration in 28d.

(2) Permeability coefficient decreases with the increasing of age in different concentrations of sodium chloride solution, and the permeability coefficient increases with the increase of concentration of sodium chloride solution under the same age.

(3) Concrete adding corrosion inhibitors can effectively reduce the coefficient of permeability, and the early effect is better than the late. With increase of the concrete effective porosity, the effective porosity firstly decreases and then increases with the increase of the concentration of sodium chloride solution, and early effect is better than late effect.

5. Acknowledgements

This work was financially supported by Natural Science Funding of Zhejiang Province (No. Y1101351) and the Science and Technology Planning Project of Zhejiang Province (No. 2013C33074). Authors wish to express great thank for financial support.

References

1. Odd E. Gjørv. Durability of Concrete Structures [J]. Arabian Journal for Science and Engineering.2011: 151-172
2. Abubaker, F; Lynsdale, C; Cripps, J. Laboratory study of the long-term durability of buried concrete exposed to Lower Lias Clay [J]. Construction & Building Materials.2014: 130-140
3. Zhu Jingsong, Ye Qing. Variation of Chloride-permeation Resistance of Concrete for Ocean Construction with Time at Early Ages [J]. Journal of Building Materiais.2006: 221-226
4. N. Holmes; R. O'Brien; P. A. M. Basheer. Engineering performance of a new siloxane-based corrosion inhibitor [J]. Materials and Structures. 2013: 1531-1543
5. FENG Nai-qian. Chlorine ion permeability and electrical conductance of high performance concrete[J].Concrete,2001: 1-7.
6. Wang Chenfei. Study on durability of Polypropylene Fiber Concrete in Chloride Environment[D]. Xian University of Architecture and Technology. 2012.

Research on Chloride Ion Diffusion Performance in Early Age Concrete under Dry-Wet Cycles

Li Han

School of Architectural and Mapping Engineering, Jiangxi University of Science and Technology, Ganzhou, 341000, China
E-mail: lihan1209@163.com

Zhu Yunhui*

Oujiang College, Wenzhou University, Wenzhou, 325035, China
E-mail: zhu-yunhui@163.com

Sun Fuxue

College of Architecture and Civil Engineering, Wenzhou University, Wenzhou, 325035, China
E-mail: sunfuxue@163.com

Xiao Yi

School of Architectural and Mapping Engineering, Jiangxi University of Science and Technology, Ganzhou, 341000, China
E-mail: 365711947@qq.com

In this paper, the chloride ion erosion resistance of early age concrete has been studied by chloride erosion experiment under dry-wet cycles including chloride ion concentration and chloride ion diffusion coefficient, through the analysis of chloride ion diffusion performance with different curing specimen. The experiment results show that the chloride ion concentrationand chloride ion diffusion coefficient increased significantly under dry-wet cycles, however, the chloride ion erosion resistance of concrete is greatly reduced, especially in the early age.

Keywords: Dry-wet cycles; early age concrete; chloride ion diffusion coefficient.

1. Introduction

In marine environment, the rust-eaten caused by ion eroding passive film is the main reason for the destruction of reinforced concrete, and the most important

* Corresponding author.

erosive ion is chloride ion. Because of that, concrete cover acting as the first defensive line plays an important role and how to improve resistance to chloride ion penetration becomes the main point of this paper.

At present, many domestic and abroad scholars have made research on this field. Considering time factor, Zhou Shengbin [1] and other people conclude that chloride diffusion coefficient reduces with prolongation of curing time. Through a lot of tests on different type of concrete, Tang [2] and the others found that the relationship between chloride diffusion coefficient and curing time is exponential function. However, the most of previous studies have focused on the long-term concrete erosion and didn't put enough energy on the erosion of early age concrete. Considering that, this paper is going to research into chloride ion diffusion performance in early age concrete under dry-wet cycles.

Reinforced concrete properties of Chinese rules and regulations [3] is based on the measured of 28d standard curing age. But, the construction of marine engineering concrete is general in site even under the seawater. Reinforced concrete eroded by the surroundings when it just formed, it hard to reach the curing condition of Chinese rules and regulations [3]. So, it is necessary to study the permeability of early age concrete when it just formed. In this paper. In this study, it has four kinds of curing conditions: standard curing in water, standard curing in seawater, dry-wet cycle curing in water and dry-wet cycle curing in seawater.

2. Experimental Program

2.1. *Materials*

Cement: Sheng Hua 325# ordinary Portland cement. Fine aggregate: river sand of Fujian province, continuous grading. Coarse aggregate: crushed stone, continuous grading, and size: 5~20mm. Mixing water: tap water.

2.2. *Mix proportions and experimental environment*

Table 1 Mix proportions.

NO.	W/C	Unit content (kg/m^3)			
		Cement (kg/m^3)	Fine aggregate (kg/m^3)	Coarse aggregate (kg/m^3) (kg/m^3)	Water (kg/m^3)
A	0.45	467	689	1034	210
B	0.40	425	596	1209	170
C	0.35	500	569	1156	175

Three kinds of different mix proportions were conducted in this study. The detailed mix proportions are showed in Table 1.

Solution concentration: 5% NaCl according to Zhejiang province marine environmental monitoring data. Temperature: constant temperature at 26℃. Humidity: relative humidity about 85%. Dry-wet cycle time: total 24h, 20h drying in constant temperature box and 4h wetting in solution of 5% NaCl.

2.3. *Preparation of specimens and measured items*

2.3.1. *Chloride ion concentration*

The size of specimens which is used for chloride ion concentration measurement is 100×100×100mm. The four faces were sealed by epoxy resin except the two opposites faces. Testing age was set to five levels: 3d, 7d, 14d, 21d and 28d. Specimens were put into different curing environments until they had reached the curing age. After that, specimens were put into drying oven to bake for about 6 hours in order to become measurable. Then their surface was milled by a concrete mill for 5 times and 2mm at a time. Totally, 10mm of the specimen's surface had been milled. In the end, chloride ion osmotic concentration of every stratum powders was measured by chloride ion rapid tester which was based on chloride ion selective electrode method.

2.3.2. *The chloride ion diffusion coefficient*

This experiment is conducted according to ASTM C1202. The size of specimens is Φ100× 50mm. Testing age was set to five levels: 3d, 7d, 14d, 21d and 28d. When the specimens were maintained to designated curing period, they were stay energized by 60V dc for 6 hours. The anode is 0.3mol/L NaOH, and the cathode is 3% NaCl. Feng Naiqian's study [5] has concluded the relationship between electric conduction quantity and chloride ion diffusion coefficient. The formula is given below:

$$D = 2.57765 + 0.00492 \times Q \tag{1}$$

D: chloride ion diffusion coefficient ($\times 10^{-9} cm^2/s$); Q: electric conduction quantity in 6h (coulomb).

Table 2 ASTMC1202 Quantity of electric charge and Chloride ion penetration performance.

Q(coulomb)	$D(\times 10^{-8} cm^2/s)$	Chloride ion penetration performance
>4000	>2.2258	High
2000~4000	1.2418~2.2258	Middle
1000~2000	0.7498~1.2418	Low
100~1000	0.3070~0.7498	Very low
<100	<0.3070	Negligible

3. Experimental Results

3.1. *Chloride ion concentration*

After the concrete specimens that were cured under different conditions had reached maintenance period, they were milled layer by layer to get each layer's chloride concentration. As illustrated in Fig. 1, Fig. 2, and Fig. 3:

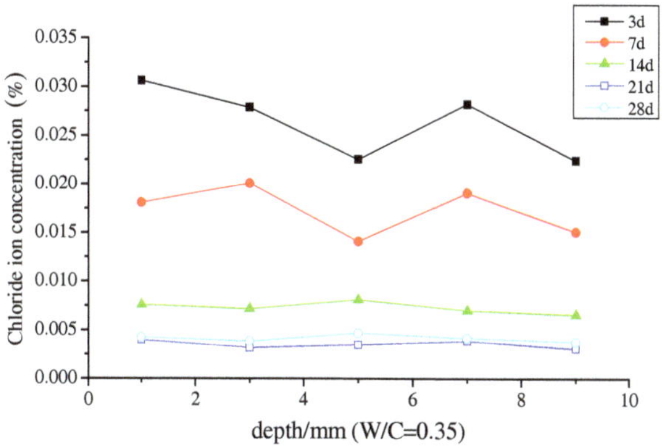

Fig.1. Standard curing in water

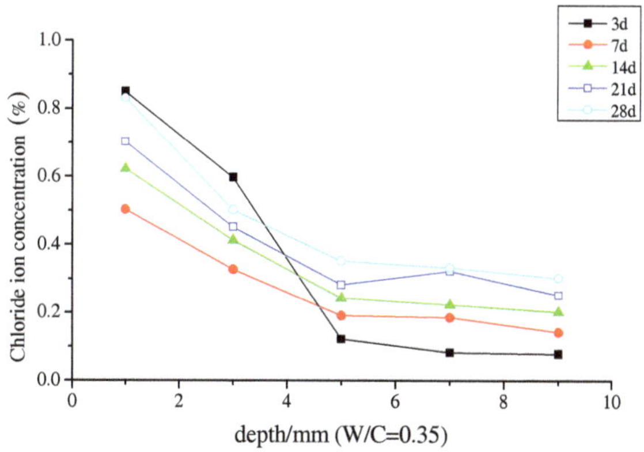

Fig.2. Standard curing in seawater

Fig. 1 shows that because the materials have residual chloride ion, there is micro-chloride in concrete raw materials which are cured in water. However, with the curing age increasing, the hydration reaction of cement become more sufficient and the measured chloride ion concentration will accordingly reduce. In Fig. 2, specimens are maintained in 5% NaCl solution until reaching to curing period, by observing, when the concrete is at early age, its chloride ion concentration changes greatly and the chloride ion concentration in the superficial layer is higher than it in the inside. It is because the absorption intensity is greater than the release intensity when the concrete is at early age, the chloride ion in marine environment could be quickly absorbed into concrete. With the ages increase, from the outside of concrete to the inside there will form a chloride ion concentration gradient. Accordingly, the absorption intensity of concrete will weaken and it turns into mainly depends on diffusion process. Fig.3 illustrates that under dry-wet cycles the chloride ion concentration of each layer has increased obviously and is twice that of curing in seawater, it is because dry-wet cycles have accelerated the absorption intensity and diffusion intensity of concrete.

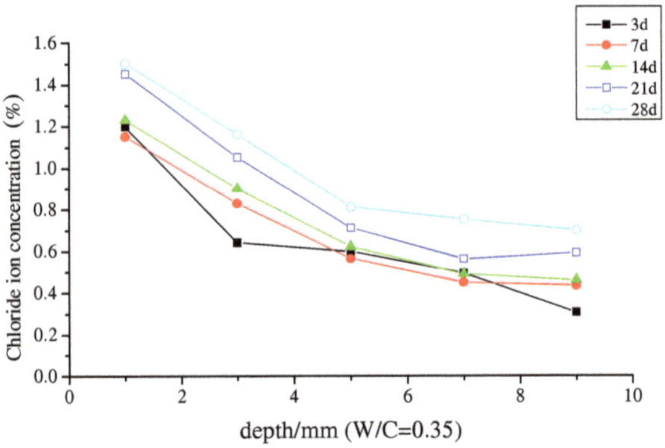

Fig.3. Dry-wet cycle curing in seawater

3.2. *Chloride ion diffusion coefficient*

The chloride diffusion coefficient of concrete under the same water-binder ratio and different curing conditions, as illustrated in Fig. 4, Fig. 5 and Fig. 6.

Dry-wet curing conditions observably influence the chloride diffusion coefficient of concrete, especially when the concrete specimen is cured in the 5% NaCl solution, the chloride diffusion coefficients of each period are much higher than the standard curing specimen. For example, when the w/b is 0.40, the chloride diffusion coefficient of concrete specimen 28d which is dry-wet cured in 5% NaCl solution is 1.42 times of the one which is cured under standard conditions. The reason is that, under drying conditions water in the NaCl solution will evaporate and the salinity of concrete surface porous solution will be higher, so that, when the specimen is immersed again there will be a chloride concentration difference between surface layer and internal part which will drive chloride ions to spread into concrete. However, except in early age the chloride diffusion coefficient of concrete specimen 28d doesn't have marked difference, it shows that dry-wet cycles will not influence the anti-chloride-permeability performances of concrete when it is cured in the water.

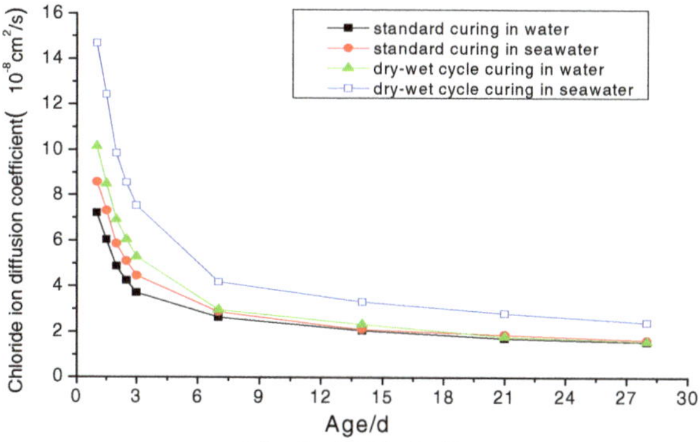

Fig.4. W/C=0.45

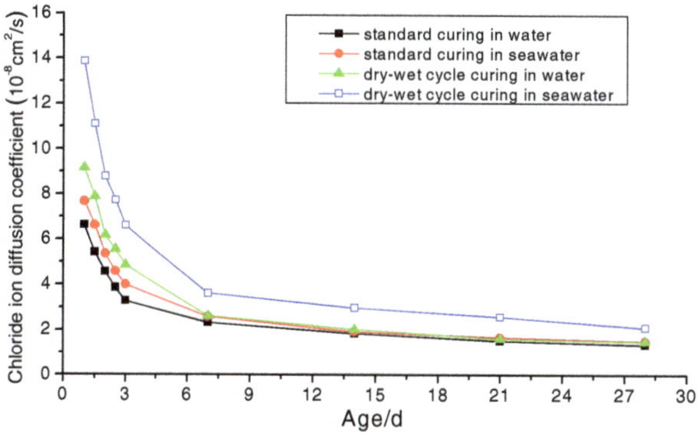

Fig.5. W/C=0.4

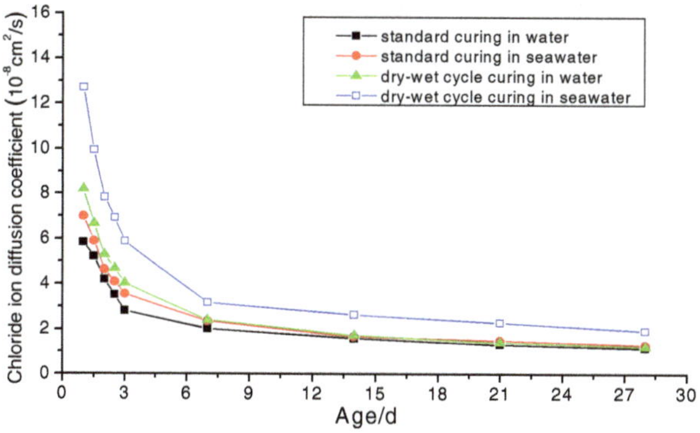

Fig.6. W/C=0.35

3.3. *The water-cement ratio*

In the same curing period, the chloride ion concentration of specimens greatly vary with different water-cement ratio. Fig. 4, Fig. 5, and Fig. 6. shows that the lower the water-cement ratio of concrete, the less the chloride diffusion coefficient. It concludes that low water-cement ratio could improve the chloride penetration resistance of concrete. This is because the water-cement ration of concrete is positive proportional to pore porosity. And the ion generally diffuse into concrete through porosity, so low porosity could cut down the number of ion's diffusion paths to make the concrete hard to be eroded. When the water-cement ratio drops to 0.4 from 0.45, the chloride diffusion coefficient of the specimen which is cured in water for about 28d accordingly down to $1.35\times10^{-8}cm^2/s$ from $1.57\times10^{-8}cm^2/s$, and when the water-cement ratio is 0.35, the chloride diffusion coefficient is $1.15\times10^{-8}cm^2/s$. These experimental data indicate that the water-cement ratio could significantly influence the chloride diffusion coefficient.

4. Conclusions

(1) Under the water curing conditions, the influence of dry-wet cycles on chloride resisting properties is small and pretty much the same with the standard curing in water; however, under the solution containing chloride ions conditions, as dry-wet cycles accelerate the erosion of chloride ion on concrete, chloride diffusion coefficient increases significantly and the resistance to chloride ion penetration of concrete decreases.

(2) When the curing time is longer, the chloride ion concentration will increase and chloride diffusion coefficient of concrete will decrease accordingly, and the range will stabilize as time past.

(3) Decreasing W/C could significantly improve the resistance to chloride ion penetration of concrete.

Acknowledgment

This work was financially supported by Natural Science Funding of Zhejiang Province (No. Y1101351), and Science and Technology Planning Project of Zhejiang Province (No. 2013C33074). Authors wish to express great thank for financial support.

References

1. Zhou Shengbin, Zhou Jian, Zhang Junzhi, Wang Jiandong. Experiment Study

on Relationship Between Chloride Diffusion in Concrete and Time. [J]. concrete, 2011, 04: 46-47.
2. Tang Lu-ping, Nilsson L O. Chloride Diffusivity in High Strength Concrete at Different Ages [J]. Nordic Concrete Research, 1992, 11(1): 162-170.
3. Ministry of Housing and Urban-Rural Development of the People's Republic of China. GB/T 50082—2009 Standard for test method of long-term performance and durability of ordinary concrete [S]. Beijing: China Building Book Shop, 2009.
4. Jin Wei-liang, Zhang Yi, Lu Zhenyong. Mechanism and Mathematic Modeling of Chloride Permeation in Concrete under Unsaturated State[J].Journal of the Chinese Ceramic Society, 2008, 10: 1362-1369.
5. Feng Nai-qian, Xing Feng. Chlorine Ion Permeability and Electrical Conductance of High Performance Concrete [J]. Concrete, 2001, 11: 3-7.
6. Chen Chun-lei, Shao Lin, Zheng Jian-jun. Diffusion Characteristics of Chloride Ions in Concrete under Cyclic Wetting-drying [J]. Concrete, 2009, 03:21-23.
7. Sun Fu-xue, Zhu Yun-hui, Chen Hai-ming. The Experimental Research for Chloride Ion Diffusion Function in High Strength Concrete [J]. Journal of China & Foreign Highway, 2009, 03:178-183.
8. Zhang Jun-zhi, Zhou Jian, Lu Lie. Influence of Exposure and Curing Time on Performance of Chlorine Ion Diffusion in Concrete [J]. Journal of Natural Disasters, 2011, 01:1-5.
9. Tae-Beom Min, In-Sung Cho, Won-Jun Park, Hyun-Kuk Choi, Han-Seung Lee. Experimental study on the development of compressive strength of early concrete age using calcium-based hardening accelerator and high early strength cement [J]. Construction and Building Materials, 2014, 04:208–214.

Study of Post-peak Stress-Strain curves of geo-materials based on Hoek-Brown Criterion

Hu Ai-yu
Architectural Institute, Nanjing Institute of Technology,
Nanjing 211167, China
942096120@qq.com

Hoek-Brown criterion is provided in FLAC3D software, but it is rarely applied. The main reasons is that the corresponding post -peak parameters are difficult to obtain. In the article aiming at Hoek-Brown criterion, evolution of different strength parameters and the corresponding stress-strain curves are studied by means of numerical analysis. Results show that the post-peak part of the stress-strain curve is much influenced by the evolution process of strength parameters and the confining pressure. The presented study may provide a heuristic method to determine the law of post-peak evolution of strength parameters of Hoek-Brown criterion.

Keywords: Hoek-Brown criterion; stress-strain curves; strength parameters.

If stress concentration in surrounding rock is more than the ultimate strength, deformation region will form a non elastic around. The mechanical behavior usually exhibited strain softening. V. Hajiabdolmajid gave a hard rock cohesion weakening friction reinforcement constitutive model for the constitutive model of CWFS based on Mohr-Colomb strength criterion[1]. In many cases, especially in the jointed rock mass, this criterion was not applicable .This criterion not only reflected the nonlinear failure characteristics, but also considered the rock strength, structure, stress state of rock and so on. Brown[2] adopted the principle to study analytical solution of the ideal elastic-plastic and elastic brittle plastic rock, Wang[3] improved it combining with the numerical method. The software FLAC3D is also including it, But on the whole was rarely applied. The major reasons is that it is difficult to obtain corresponding parameter of generalized criterion in the posterior segment[4]. Through numerical experiment, it was discussed on the media obeying the criterion that the corresponding stress-strain curve changed with different evolution process of strength parameters, and the influence on the curve of evolution process and the confining pressure was analyzed. It was also analyzed that the constitutive model of Hoek-Brown can not only describe hard and brittle material validly, but also can be adopted in brittle - ductile –plastic material such as soft rock. It provided some inspiration for the medium to determine the evolution of post peak strength parameters.

1. Strain softening model of Hoek-Brown

That compressive stress was positive was agreed on in this criterion, as:

$$\sigma_1 = \sigma_3 + \sigma_{ci}\left\{m_b \frac{\sigma_3}{\sigma_{ci}} + s\right\}^a \tag{1}$$

$$m_b = m_i \exp\left(\frac{GSI - 100}{28 - 14D}\right) \tag{2}$$

$$s = \exp\left(\frac{GSI - 100}{9 - 3D}\right) \tag{3}$$

$$a = \frac{1}{2} + \frac{1}{6}\left[\exp\left(\frac{-GSI}{15}\right) - \exp\left(\frac{-20}{3}\right)\right] \tag{4}$$

In the formula: σ_1 and σ_3—the maximum and minimum principal stress; σ_{ci}—the uniaxial compressive strength of rock. m_b, s and a can be obtained by type (2)(3)(4). Among them, m_i depended on the material constants of the rock properties; GSI was geological strength index; D was a parameter describing the influence degree on rock of the blasting damage or disturbance of stress relaxation, For the undisturbed rock mass, D=0; For serious disturbance of rock mass, D=1.

Hoek induced the elastic modulus and strength (represented by the uneasily compressive strength of rock) of rock mass after summing up a great deal of engineering properties of rock mass, also the integrity (represented by the rock mass quality classification index GSI), the relation between them was:

$$E_m = \sqrt{\frac{\sigma_{ci}}{100}} 10^{(\frac{GSI-10}{40})} \tag{5}$$

In this ideal model, parameters such as $\sigma_{ci,}$ m_b, s and a were mistaken as default constants, and this was not in line with the actual situation.

2. Evolution Law of Strength Parameters

At present, the finite difference software FLAC3D contains the above model, but it is rarely applied, and one of the main reasons is that it is difficult to obtain the corresponding parameters in the generalized Hoek-Brown criterion.

The criterion finally contained four parameters as σ_{ci}, m_i, D and GSI. Without considering the disturbance factor. They were reduced to 3. Changes in these parameters directly affected the stress-strain curve after the peak. Now, it is analyzed the several possible evolution law of rock parameters in failure process (body). And different indoor three axis simulation curve were gave with corresponding evolution law.

(1). Only GSI decreased (m_b, s decreased, a enlarged)

It was regarded as that m_b, s and a were the parameters in turn in elastic stage, and σ_{ci}, m_b, s_s, a_s, in plastic softening stage; and σ_{ci}, m_{br}, s_r, a_r, in plastic flow stage. From above, the change of parameters m_b, s and a, could be owned to the variation of GSI. According to its definition, softening rules could be assumed to be linear, as showed in Fig. 1.

In fig 1, GSI_0, GST_r, respectively, was the geological strength index of elastic and plastic flow phase. And $_e$, ε_r, respectively, was the strain variable of the two phases.

According to equation (2)-(4), strength parameters m_b, s decreased, and a enlarged.

(2) σ_{ci} and GSI both decreased

(3) σ_{ci}, m_i, s , GSI all decreased,

(4) only σ_{ci} decreased

(5) both m_i and GSI decreased

(6) only m_i, decreased

(7) m_i, enlarged (m_b, s enlarged), GSI decreased, σ_{ci} unchanged

(8) m_i, enlarged (m_b, s enlarged), GSI decreased, σ_{ci} unchanged, considering the confining pressure coefficient μ

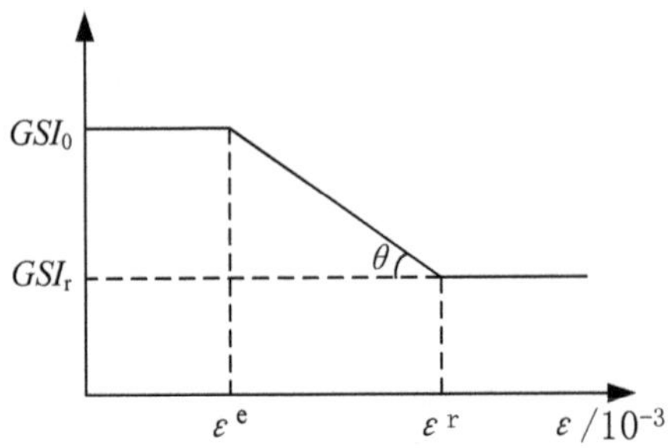

Fig. 1 Softening diagram of GSI.

In simulation of Jinping Baishan marble by the strength parameters m_b increasing, s decreasing, a increasing and σ_{ci} constant evolution, was used by Zhang Chunsheng.

(9) GSI decreased, m_i, decreased, confining pressure coefficient μ

3. Numerical test

The sample was 0.1m ×0.1m ×0.2m. Lateral confining pressure was applied, displacement was controlled in the vertical direction, and the top surface was applied non zero displacement, and the bottom surface was controlled, finally, one of the corners was constrained in the horizontal direction. Vertical displacement increased gradually. Numerical simulation only considered macro effect, without considering the rock by the localized loading process, similar to the three axle load test through indoor experiment to obtain rock strength parameters or the whole process curve. The deterioration of parameters were not happened at the same time, while combined in accordance with above ten cases, considering the confining pressure coefficient μ.

Table 1 Rock strength parameters.

feature description	σ_{ci} [MPa]	GSI	m_i	s	a
peak strength	140	100	9.0	1	0.5

4. Discussion about results of numerical experiments

These six figures were stress-strain curve individually considering deterioration of GSI only, deterioration of GSI and σ_{ci}, deterioration of m_i, σ_{ci}, GSI, deterioration of σ_{ci} , deterioration of GSI and m_i, deterioration of m_i and σ_{ci}, GSI decressed and m_i increased, GSI decreased, m_i increased, GSI decreased, m_i increased.

We can conclude that the variation of strength parameters after peak only affected the residual strength, but not the peak strength. Considering deterioration of σ_{ci} only, the residual strength was poorer than peak strength, and as σ_{ci} became smaller, it became smaller, with others unchanged. Comparison told us that the influence of *GSI* on residual strength was higher than σ_{ci}. With the decrease of GSI, also the residual strength reduced. The confining pressure was greater; the difference between the peak strength and residual strength was greater. This didn't match the stress strain of marble. We could see that the difference between the residual strength and the peak strength were smaller and smaller with the increasing of confining pressure. When confining pressure was 30MPa, the rock was an ideal plasticity. It can reflect the brittle ductility transformation characteristics of marble' stress strain curves, with confining pressure increased after its peak, but ductility length does not change.

5. Conclusion

Laboratory and field experiments show that geotechnical materials should stress - strain curve peak in the posterior region of the strain softening phenomenon with considerable universality.

Under external load, Strength of rock in the post peak stage was still able to bear external certain load. So the research of strength parameters evolution of rock in back peak has theoretical and practical significance on studying the bearing capacity of rock mass. In this paper, we study the evolution behavior of the rock strength parameters, and obtain the corresponding stress-strain curves of the Hoek-Brown strength criterion. In the broad sense, the parameters of Hoek-Brown strength criterion are more and more, and the final determination, GSI and the influence coefficient of confining pressure are studied. In this paper, 9 different combinations of 4 parameters were considered. Numerical simulation results showed that the evolution process of strength parameters had direct impact on the post peak stress - strain curves. Therefore, the mechanical properties of the rock and soil media must be reflected by the parameters of the strength parameters. The law of evolution were worthy of further study. The paper provided some inspiration for the medium obeying the rules of Hoek-Brown criterion to determine the evolution of post peak strength parameters.

Reference

1. Hajiabdolmajid V, Martin CD, Kaiser PK. Modelling brittle failure of rock [R]. Proceedings of the Fourth North American Rock Mechanics Symposium. Seattle. Washington. A.A. Balkema, Rotterdam, 2000.
2. Brown E T, Bray J W, Ladanyi B, et al. Ground response curves for rock tunnels [J]. Journal of Geotechnical Engineering, 1983, 109(1): 15-39.
3. Wang Y. Ground response of circular tunnel in poorly consolidated rock [J]. Journal of Geotechnical Engineering, 1996, 122(9): 703-708.
4. Zhang Chunsheng, Chen Xiangrong, Hou Jing, Chu Weijiang. Study of mechanical behavior of deep-buried marble at Jingping II hydropower [J]. Chinese Journal of Rock Mechanics and Engineering. 2009, 29 (10): 1999-2009.
5. Li Kong, Ge Xiurun, Li Chunguang. Method for three axial compression test to determine the rock softening parameters based on Hoek-Brown [J]. Chinese rural water and hydropower. 2011(8).

The Philosophy of Concrete Mix Design and Construction Technology Research under Hypothermia Environment

Xiao Chen[1,2,a], Zheng Li[2,b] and Xiongyi Liang[2,c]
[1] *Key Laboratory of Road Structure & Material Ministry of Transport, Beijing, China, 100088*
[2]*Wuhan University of Technology, Materials Science and Engineering, Wuhan, China, 430070*
Email: [a]chenxiao1981@whut.edu.cn, [b]13297064180@163.com and [c]1151270586@qq.com

Towards Tongtianhe Bridge located in high altitude alpine permafrost, the absence of the concrete mix data and other special circumstances, we do plenty of relevant research: concrete mix preliminary design, comparative study of the strength and frost resistance of putting two water reducer in concrete under standard conservation and outdoor conservation, and the pore structure of the incorporation of two water reducer paste are analyzed. The results shows that: the early strength type of polycarboxylic water reducer possesses good effect of low temperature, and it can better improve the internal pore structure of sample, increase frost resistance of concrete. In addition, under the special circumstances, we discuss the construction and maintenance technology of concrete in order to better serve the construction site.

Keywords: Concrete; mix strength; frost resistance; construction.

1. The Engineering General Situation

Tongtianhe Bridge is situated on the junction of Qumalaiand and Zhiduo county in Qinghai Yushu region, belongs to the provincial highway S308 line C contract section of highway engineering, full-bridge Pegs range: K212 + 146.900 ~ K213 + 303.100, a total length of 1156.2 m, span of 3 × 40m (approach bridge) + (53.5 + 6 × 100 + 53.5) m (main bridge) + two United 4 × 40m (approach bridge), the main bridge portion and the transition piers employ hollow thin-walled pier, 4 ~ 10 # main pier with highly for 82 ~ 88m, 5 # main pier (height-88m) is the highest across the board pier, known as "the first high pier in the senir-plateau" The bridge is located in Qinghai Province in southeastern Tongtianhe Canyon zone, belonging to the Tibetan plateau temperate semi-arid climate, altitude 4200m, major climatic characteristics: strong solar radiation, distinct wet and dry seasons, the temperature difference between the big day, the strong wind , the most cold -34.3 °C, the annual average temperature -3.3 °C [1].

In addition to the harsh environment in the region, the mechanical equipment of sand-stone factory is relatively backward, poor production of sand and gravel, and lack of concrete mix data under this environment, which not only causes inconvenience to the actual construction, but also brings a severe test to the quality of concrete materials and frost resistance of concrete structures. Therefore,it is necessary for optimizing the concrete mix design of bridge and to study its frost resistance and construction, maintenance technology, in order to accumulate experience and better service and actual construction.

2. Raw Materials and Test Methods

2.1. *Raw materials*

Using Qilian brand P•O 42.5 cement, of which the indicators meet the relevant standards. Water reducer: A common type of polycarboxylic water reducer called A and home-made polycarboxylic water reducer with the early strength called B. fine aggregate is from the Tongtianhe river sand, of which fineness modulus is 2.5. The lithology of coarse aggregate is limestone, of which size is 1 #: 5 ~ 10mm, 2 #: 10 ~ 25mm, flakiness: 13.4%.

2.2. *Test methods*

(1) Compressive Strength [2]: We make the slump of fresh concrete samples controllable from 160 mm to 180mm by adjusting the amount of water reducer. referring to "ordinary concrete mechanical test method standards" (GB / T5008-2002), forming 150mm × 150mm specimens are standard curing indoor and films the nature maintenance outdoor, testing its strength after conserving to the prescribed time limit.

(2) Frost Resistance [3]: Referring to "ordinary concrete long-term performance and durability test method standards" (GB/T50082-2009) antifreeze test - fast freezing method for testing when satisfying any of the three cases, the freeze-thaw cycles reach 300, the relative dynamic modulus of elasticity is reduced to 60% or less or the rate of weight loss reaches 5% or more, the test can be stopped.

(3) Pore Structure: Using the mercury analyzer (MIP) assays the pore structure of paste.

3. Experimental Research of Concrete Mix Design

3.1. *Impact of water-cement ratio and cementitious materials on concrete performance*

The impact of water-cement ratio and the amount of cementitious material on properties of concrete, the test results are shown in Table 1. Obviously, when we ensured that the workability of concrete was consistent: the compressive strength of the sample is rising trend with increasing amount of cementitious material. In the amount of cement 480 kg/m3 meet the prepared strength grade of C50 requirements of the main beam, and comparing the cement 440kg/m3 of the concrete strength, specimen used cement 480kg/m^3 strength improved 22.7%. When we used the amount of cementitious material 480kg/m^3, the amount of water reducer and compressive strength of sample trended down. Although water-cement ratio at 0.31, 0.33 can meet the strength requirements, both the intensity difference is not large, and when we used water-cement ratio of 0.31, the incorporation of water reducer was 2.20%. Taking into account the actual project economics, we use water-cement ratio of 0.33, water reducer of 2.00% [4].

Table 1 Impact of water-cement ratio and the amount of cementitious material on properties of concrete under standard condition curing.

Number	Cementitious material/ (kg/m^3)	W/C	Sand/ (kg/m^3)	1#Stuff /(kg/m^3)	2#Stuff /(kg/m^3)	H_2O/ (kg/m^3)	water reducer	collapsed slump /mm	compressive strength/ MPa
1-1	440	0.33				162.8	1.62%	175	51.2
1-2	460	0.33				170.2	1.80%	171	57.1
1-3	480	0.33				177.6	2.00%	180	62.8
1-4	500	0.33	627	223	894	185.0	2.30%	172	64.9
2-1	480	0.31				168.0	2.20%	187	64.1
2-2	480	0.33				177.6	2.00%	180	62.8
2-3	480	0.35				187.2	1.85%	176	58.2

3.2. *Effect of two kinds of water reducer and curing methods on concrete performance*

(1) Effect of two kinds of two kinds of water on the workability and mechanical properties of concrete

For the effect of the two water reducer on fresh concrete properties, the test results are presented on Table 2. Apparently, when using the water reducer B (dosage of 1.20%) can achieve the effect of water reducer A (dosage of 2.00%) , therefore the performance of water reducer B is better.

Table 2 Effects of two kinds of water reducer on concrete performance.

Types of water reducer	Cementitious material	W/C	Sand	5~10	10~25	H_2O	water reducer	collapsed slump/mm
A	480	0.33	627	223	894	177.6	2.00%	180
B	480	0.33				177.6	1.20%	174

The specimens formed were performed separately in the condition of a thin film of nature covering conservation and standard curing, which were tested the strength of 1d, 3d, 7d, 28d. The weather conditions seven days before the actual conservation was described in Table 3, and the strength test results were shown in Table 4. As we can see, under the same age period, the intensity of the concrete is: Standard Maintenance> Outdoor Maintenance, and after adding water reducer A and B, 28d standard curing strength compared to outdoor conservation increased separately 29.8%, 21.4%, and under the same curing conditions, after adding the water reducer B can better improve the strength of concrete. For the outdoor conservation and standards conservation, the 28d strength of concrete was increased 11.0% and 3.8% after joining the water reducer B.

Table 3 Actual weather conditions in the Project Department in September 2013.

Time period	9.10 Cloudy	9.11 Cloudy with sleet	9.12 Scouther	9.13 Sunny	9.14 Cloudy with sleet	9.15 Scouther	9.16 Sunny rain
Morn	2~4°C	1~2°C	0~2°C	0~3°C	-2~1°C	-2~0°C	1~3°C
Noon	10~12°C	9~11°C	5~7°C	7~8°C	4~6°C	2~3°C	5~7°C
Night	1~2°C	0~3°C	-1~0°C	0~2°C	-2~0°C	-1~1°C	0~2°C
Midnight	-5~0°C	-6~-2°C	-7~-3°C	-5~-1°C	-8~-4°C	-5~-2°C	-3~0°C

Table 4 Effects of two kinds of water reducer on the compressive strength of concrete.

Number	Curing system	Types of water reducer	1d	3d	7d	28d
A_1	Outdoor maintenance	A	4.2	24.2	35.1	48.4
B_1		B	12.2	32.7	44.3	53.7
A_0	Standard maintenance	A	21.9	39.7	47.9	62.8
B_0		B	26.7	47.1	56.5	65.2

In addition, compared the sample which added water reducing agent A with the sample which added water reducing agent B: outdoor conservation 1d, 3d, 7d and their compressive strength was increased separately by 190.5%, 35.1%, 26.2%, standard curing 1d, 3d, 7d and their compressive strength was increased by 21.9%, 18.6%, 17.9%, which showed the effect of improving the early strength of concrete outdoor significantly with low temperature curing specimens was better than under standard curing, therefore, the preparation of the reducing agent B has better low early strength effects, to some extent which can be better to shorten the template cycle, accelerate the construction schedule.

(2) Effect of two kinds of water reducer and curing methods on frost resistance of concrete

After curing specimen for 28d, testing its frost resistance, the results shown in Figure 1. Overall, the frost of curing specimens under the standard better than the specimen under outdoor conservation, after adding two kinds of water reducing agent A and B, the specimens under outdoor conservation whose antifreeze grade were F150, F200,the specimens under standard conservation whose antifreeze grade were F200, F225 [3,5]. It is easy to conclude that after adding water reducing agent B can better improve the frost resistance of concrete .

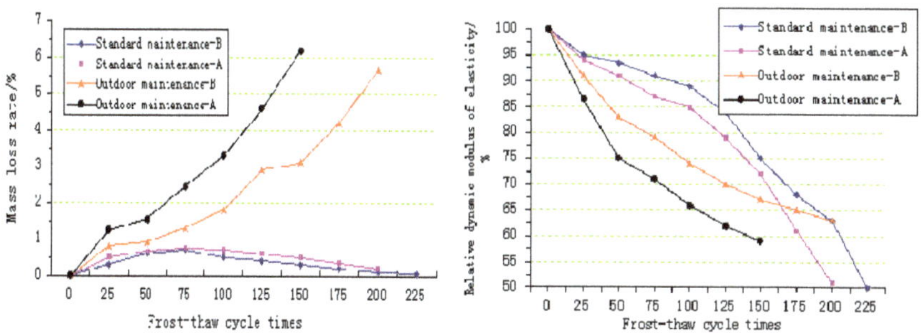

Fig. 1 Mass loss rate and the relative dynamic modulus of elasticity curves under the freeze-thaw cycles.

For the specimen's mass loss rate under the freeze-thaw cycles: Under the outdoor conservation, specimen's mass loss rate was on the rise with the increase in freeze-thaw cycles, after the freeze-thaw of specimen A1 cycled 150 times, the mass loss was 6.2%, after the freeze-thaw of specimen B1 cycled 200 times, the mass loss was 5.7%; under the standard conservation, the mass loss rate was reduced after showing an upward trend , which was due to changes in the mass of freeze-thaw test specimens which depends mainly on the quality of the test ablation amount and the amount of water absorption member, under the freeze-thaw cycle, the internal cracks and other defects in the sample is gradually increased, the water absorption increases, while the amount of water is greater than the exfoliation, the mass loss rate of the specimen is reduced.

For the specimen's dynamic elastic modulus under the freeze-thaw cycles: Under the outdoor conservation, specimen A1 and specimen B1's relative dynamic modulus of elasticity was reduced by a big margin in the pre-test, reduced the magnitude of slowing in the post-test, after the freeze-thaw of specimen A1 cycled 150 times, the relative dynamic elastic modulus was 58.9%, after the freeze-thaw of specimen B1 cycled 200 times , the relative dynamic elastic modulus was 62.2%; while under the standard conservation , specimen A0 and specimen B0's relative dynamic modulus of elasticity was reduced slowly in the pre-trial late but lower faster in the later period, compared to the strength of the data, it can be found that A1 and B1 belong to the low-intensity concrete, A0 and B0 belong to the high-strength concrete, it also shows that the freeze-thaw damage of high-strength concrete under standard conservation is suddenly , and ordinary concrete is not the same.

(3) paste pore structure analysis

Using two kinds of water reducer A and B prepared separately standard consistency of cement paste under the outdoor maintenance and standard maintenance. Then the samples conserved for 7d were tested its internal pore size, and the test results were shown in Table 5. Obviously, In both of the curing systems, water reducing agent B could better improve the internal pore structure paste, the porosity of paste with water reducing agent B decreased separately 4.6% and 2.2% in the condition of outdoor curing and standard curing. It could effectively reduce the amount of harmful holes that decreased separately 8.2% and 10.1% in the outdoor conservation and standard curing ,compared to adding water reducing agent A . To some extent, water reducing agent B can better improve the strength and frost resistance of concrete, which is in line with previous test results.

Table 5 The pore structure parameters of hardened cement paste of 7d in two curing systems.

Curing regime	Types of water reducer	Pore size parameters			
		Most probable pore size /nm	Average pore size /nm	porosity/ %	>200nm/ %
Outdoor curing	Water reducer A	21.29	37.50	16.0	32.6
	Water reducer B	18.60	20.35	11.4	24.4
Standard curing	Water reducer A	23.30	25.65	13.0	25.3
	Water reducer B	22.64	15.71	10.8	15.2

4. Construction and Maintenance Technology

(1) Control measures of the raw material's temperature

Construction in the winter, particularly when the temperature is below -5°C, water is mostly conducive to the heated material, usually when the temperature is above -15°C, the water should be heated to 60°C ~ 80°C, when the temperature is below -15°C,water can be heated to above 80 °C, but the cement is prohibited to contact directly with water whose temperature is above 80°C; coarse aggregates should be recovered by plastic sheeting or color of cloth, aiming at preventing rain and snow, if necessary, keeping them in the greenhouses; fine aggregates store in greenhouses or heating them by steam pipes or exhaust pipes which pass them into the internal , and cover them by plastic sheeting ,in order to prevent the rain and snow, and shall not contain frozen blocks, blocks of snow or ice, in addition, in order to better control the state of concrete, the moisture content should be measured regularly; besides, cement should not be heated.

Because antifreeze is directly related to results in antifreeze when concrete at the negative temperature environment and its effect on the strength of growth under the negative temperature environment, so the mixing amount should be strictly controlled, accurate measurement, assign designated persons to add. When faced with temperature changes larger, we should promptly notify technicians to mix and dosage adjusted according to temperature manual values and make records.

(2) Concrete Mixing

Before mixing, according to the external environment to do ready calculation and mixed thermal in order to determine the heating temperature of aggregate and water; when concrete is mixing, the hot water which is at 80°C may not be contact directly with the cement, it is good to prevent the phenomenon of cement quick-setting or false condensate, the correct order should be stirring: coarse aggregates, fine aggregates and hot water are premixed 30 ~ 60s, then add cement, additives, and the mixing time should be extended by 50% than normal temperature. Normal concrete slump generally controlled at 80mm ~ 100mm, pumping concrete slump can be controlled at 160mm ~ 180mm, excessive slump will cause the concrete segregation stratification, bleeding and other phenomena, it is not conducive to frost concrete, and cause the decline of hardened concrete's impermeability.

(3) Concrete transport

When construction in the winter, in addition to prevent the segregation of concrete, loss of excessive bleeding collapse, it should also prevent the loss of excessive heat during transport, and it should be combined with thermal calculation and the actual situation during transport, and take appropriate insulation measures, such as using cotton blankets banding. In addition, the temperature of the tank should also be concrete, pouring temperature, into the mold temperature should be monitored, when it is not met, it is necessary to take timely measures for the heating temperature of raw materials and the insulation measures during transport to adjust.

(4) Concrete pouring

For the pouring process in the cold regions , in addition to pay attention to the hierarchical placement (usually layered thickness of 20 ~ 30cm, not more than 50cm), it should also be strictly controlled pouring temperature (especially in rain and snow), when more than -15 °C,the temperature of bringing into the mold should not less than 6 °C ~ 8 °C, lower than -15 °C,the temperature of bringing into the mold should be raised to about 10 °C; concrete's vibrated should be uniform, vibrator should not a stay at a certain point for a long time,it may not appear excessive vibration or less vibration, leakage vibration; the part of the concrete which need to measure temperature, should also indwelling temperature thermocouple wire holes or buried.

(5) Concrete curing, temperature monitoring and split mold

Concrete curing is a especially critical link in the winter construction, in order to prevent the concrete hydration heat dissipation, conservation measures should be taken promptly after the completion of the concrete pouring: When the temperature is above -15 °C, we can use a layer of plastic sheeting and a layer of insulation cotton to prevent wind and keep temperature, while the temperature is below -15 °C, we should use one or two layers of plastic sheeting and two layers of insulation cotton to prevent wind and keep temperature, concrete structures for the windward side, edges protruding parts, easy to heat storage site should be strengthened insulation measures, and strengthen the monitoring of temperature. Temperature monitoring of concrete during the conservation: Before the frost of concrete reaches the critical strength, measured once every two hours, after reaching the antifreeze critical strength, measured once every six hours; If curing concrete by steam, the concrete should be controlled heating rate and the internal temperature and the maximum temperature should not exceed 40 °C. [6]

To ensure the sustainable development of concrete strength, after splitting mold, it is prohibited to directly exposed the concrete to the environment, the surface should be painted curing agent, and take the appropriate insulation, covered by moisture material, it can be removed after reaching the appropriate strength requirements.

5. Conclusion

(1) Based on the engineering of Tongtianhe Bridge, combined with the preliminary design lab mix, preferably cementitious material is 480kg/m^3, water-cement ratio is 0.33, the use of water reducing agent B, content is 1.2%.

(2) The strength of the sample under the nature conservation, frost

resistances are lower than the standard conservation: After adding A and B two kinds of water reducer, 28d standard conservation's strength is increased by 29.8% 21.4% when compared to outdoor conservation, under standard conservation, specimen antifreeze grade respectively are F200 and F225, outdoor conservation grade antifreeze specimen are F150 and F200.

(3) Water reducing agent B has good effect on early strength at low temperature, compared with adding A species of water reducing agent: Under outdoor conservation 1d, 3d, 7d, its compressive strength is increased by 190.5%, 35.1%, 26.2%, under standard conservation 1d, 3d, 7d, its compressive strength is increased by 21.9%, 18.6%, 17.9%, to a certain extent, it is able to better address local construction whose period is short and light construction problems.

(4) Water reducing agent B can better improve the internal pore structure of concrete, effectively reducing harmful number of holes, thereby improving the improvement of concrete frost resistance.

(5) Combined with the actual construction process of concrete, including raw material storage, concrete mixing, transportation, placement, maintenance, temperature monitoring and split mold are discussed.

Acknowledgments

This work was supported by the Opening Funding Supported by the Key Laboratory of Road Structure & Material Ministry of Transport, Beijing (KF201201) and the Fundamental Research Funds for the Central Universities (133237001).

References

1. Xiang Liu. *Study on the scour piles and reinforcement Tongtianhe bridge* [J]. Journal of Transportation Science and Technology of Qinghai, 2008-1.
2. Chen Kuen-suan, Shih Ming-hsiang. *Reliable evaluation method of quality control for compressive strength of concrete* [J]. Zhejiang University Science, 2005, 6(A) 8: 836-843.
3. Gao Song, Dai Li. *Study on frost resistance of concrete used in pavement of northeast China [J]. Applied Mechanics and Materials*, v 71-78, p 728-732, 2011, F.
4. Wang, Peng. *Study on the Synthesis and Properties of Polycarboxylate-type Water-reducer [J]. UMI Dissertations Publishing*, 2007. H461120.
5. Wagner, Dennis Jon. *Durability of concrete cured with antifreeze admixtures*

at temperatures below 0 degrees C [J]. UMI Dissertations Publishing, 1996. 1383616.

6. Evans, Christopher Michael. *The influence of fly ash and early-age curing temperature on the durability and strength of high performance concrete* [J]. UMI Dissertations Publishing, 1997. MQ28830.

The Seepage and Stability Evaluation of Daguangbao Landslide Dam

GUO Jian[a], SUN Jinkun[b] & WANG Jie[c]
School of Civil Engineering and Architecture, Panzhihua University, Panzhihua City, 617000, P.R. China
E-mail: [a]*pzh_gj@163.com*, [b]*66290838@qq.com*, [c]*542925605@qq.com*

The volume of Daguangbao landslide is very huge, whose accumulation has blocked the Huangdongzi valley, then produced two landslide dams. The water in upstream catchment leaks out from the deposit downstream along the original Huangdongzi valley. The seepage flow is greatly influenced by rainfall. The hydraulics method is applied to calculate the volume of seepage in five rainfall intensity; and it verifies that the seepage piping and soil flow are unlikely to happen; and then evaluates the stability of the debris flow area in downstream side. The conclusion is that part of the accumulation will in unstable state in torrential rain and earthquake condition.

Keywords: Daguangbao landslide; accumulation; seepage; piping; stability.

1. Introduction

Wenchuan earthquake on May 12, 2008 triggered the largest landslide in Asia--Daguangbao landslide, with a volume of 11.3×10^8 m^3 and an area of 7.8 km^2 [1~3]. The accumulation of the slides blocked Huangdongzi valley with the maximum thickness of 550m, which created two large landslide dams—Chuanlin landslide dam and Baiguolin landslide dam. It is found that there is water in them throughout the whole year and the water level rises dramatically at the rainy season when the seepage from the surface of accumulation rises with the increase of rainfall. Most of the seeping rainwater flows out from lower reach of Huangdongzi valley. Based on these features, the author of the present paper evaluates the seepage flow under different intensity of rainfalls and studies the effect of rainfall on the local stability of the Daguangbao accumulation.

2. The Basic Features of the Research Area

The research area is located in Gaochuan of Anxian Town, Mianyang, covering $30km^2$. Its altitude is from 1100m to 2950m with the difference of 1850m. According to the search need, this area is divided into three zones (Fig. 1): the catchment zone of the upper reach (Zone I), the landslide accumulation zone (Zone II), the catchment zone of the lower reach (Zone III). The following part introduces the characteristics of each zone.

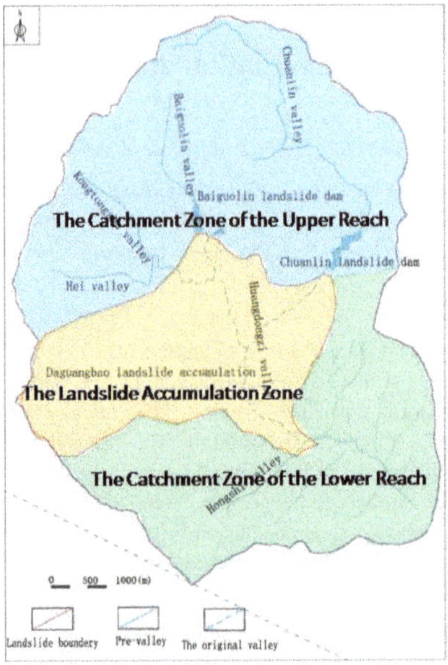

Fig. 1 The Zonation Map of Research Area.

(i) The Catchment Zone of the Upper Reach (Zone I)

Zone I is surrounded and sealed in by the watershed of the upper reach and one side of landslide accumulation. It covers an area of about 13.4 km^2. Within the zone are three tributaries—Hei valley, Baiguolin valley, and Chuanlin valley with the respective catchment areas of 3.4 km^2, 3.5 km^2 and 6.9 km^2.

Among the many landslide dams produced by the landslide, Chuanlin landslide dam and Baiguolin landslide dam are the largest, both of which never dries throughout the year. The water impounded is mainly supplied by rainfall and meltwater. Baiguolin landslide dam is 10～50m deep and Chuanlin landslide dam, 30～100m. The catchment seeps mainly downstream along the original valley to the lower reach.

(ii) The Landslide Accumulation Zone (Zone II)

The sliding mass of the Daguangbao landslide formed this accumulation zone with an area of about 7.8km^2 and a volume of 11.3×10^8 m^3. The displaced mass along the original Huangdongzi valley is deeper with a maximum thickness of 550m. The body of accumulation is made up mainly of chunks of rocks.

Around the middle of the accumulation distribute some solid rocks which have not yet disintegrated, and at the front part are small-sized debris.

(iii) The Catchment Zone of the Lower Reach (Zone III)

The flat area of this zone is about 9.2 km^2. Huangdouzi valley, which is fed by the eight tributaries within the zone, has large water flow at the rainy seasons and is very likely to trigger mud-soil flow.

3. Calculation of the Seepage in the Accumulation Zone

In the lower the reach of Daguangbao accumulation, there is water seeping out throughout the year, and the seepage varies with the change of seasons. Considering the amount of the seeping water is dependent on the rainfall, the seepage in different rainfall intensity has been evaluated. Five rainfall intensities in terms of Average Recurrence Interval are considered. They are P_1 (with 100 year recurrence interval), P_2 (with 50 year recurrence interval), P_5 (with 20 year recurrence interval), P_{10} (with 10 year recurrence interval and P_{20} (with 10 year recurrence interval), as is shown in Table 1.

Table 1 Rainfall intensity values.

Rainfall Intensity	P1	P2	P5	P10	P20
Cumulative Rainfall (mm)	634.5	459	306.1	261.9	162.3

The seepage flow of Daguangbao accumulation zone includes two parts: the seepage from upstream catchment along the original Huangdongzi valley and the rainfall seeping down the accumulation surface.

3.1 *The calculation of the seepage along the valley*

The accumulation of Daguangbao landslide blocked Huangdongzi valley and generated two large landslide dams. Most of the rainfall and meltwater upstream collect in these two dams and Hei valley. The collecting water seeps along the original Huangdongzi valley to the lower reach of the valley. Given the complication of the issue, a hydraulic method is employed to calculate the seepage. Based on Darcy's law and the Dupuit Assumption, the method further assumes that the body of accumulation is homogeneous, and the base of the valley as well as two sides of the accumulation body is impervious.

Considering the employment of the two assumptions will make the calculation result greater than real seepage, the present paper will later compare the theoretical calculation seepage with the real seepage and thus propose a loss coefficient λ so as to correct the calculation result.

3.1.1. *Model of seepage flow*

The model is developed by using the hydraulic method and "the method of fragment", which is widely used in analyzing seepage flow of earthen dam. Dupuit's formula of gradually varied seepage flow is applied to each section. And assuming the flow through each section is the equal, joint solution is done. The calculation model is as follows:

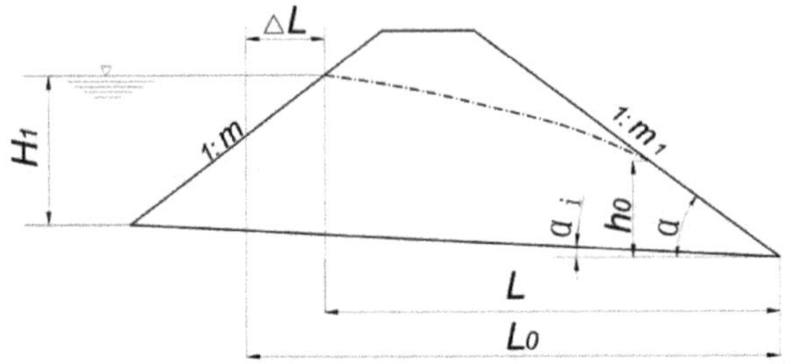

Fig. 2 The model of seepage flow.

The seepage flow of unit width q is evaluated through the following equation:

$$q = \frac{kH_1(H_1 + iL_0)}{L_0 + \sqrt{L_0^2 - H_1^2 \cot^2(\alpha - \alpha_i)}}. \quad (1)$$

where:

K—the permeability coefficient;

i—the gradient of dam foundation's impermeable layer, $i=\sin\alpha_i$;

αi— the angle between the horizontal plane and surface of dam foundation;

L—the horizontal distance from the intersection of upstream water surface and dam slope to the downstream dam toe;

α—the angle between the downstream dam slope and horizontal line;

$\triangle$L-- the alternative width, $H = (0.872P + 4.28)\times 10^{-2}$;

m-- the slope rate of upstream dam side;

L_0--the horizontal distance from the upstream vertical alternative plane to the downstream dam toe, $L_0=L+\triangle L$.

3.1.2. *The calculation of seepage flow along the valley*

As is shown by Fig. 1, the water in the catchment zone of the upper reach filtrates and flows from Hei valley, baiguolin valley and then to Huangdongzi valley. The section views of the seepage flow are shown in Fig. 3, Fig. 4 and Fig. 5.

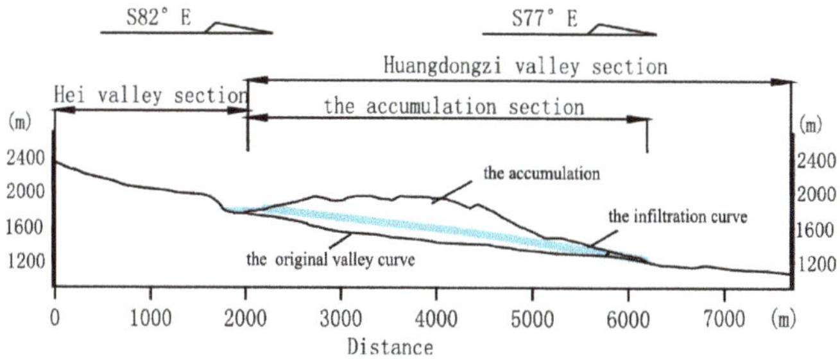

Fig. 3 The section view of seepage from Hei Valley to Huangdongzi Valley.

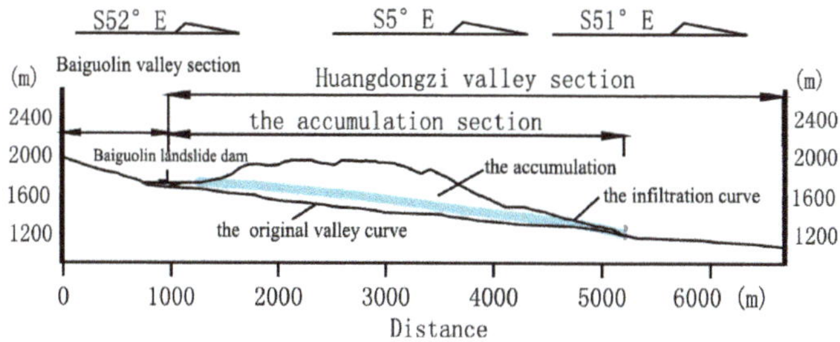

Fig. 4 The section view of seepage from Baiguolin Valley to Huangdongzi Valley.

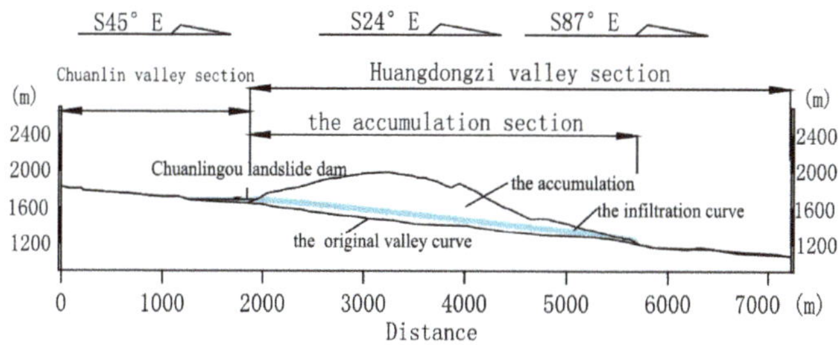

Fig. 5 The section view of seepage from Chuanlin Valley to Huangdongzi Valley.

Table 2 The physical parameters of seepage section view.

section view of seepage	k(m/h)	α_i(°)	i	α(°)	m	L (m)	$\triangle$L (m)	L_0 (m)
Hei valley-Huangdongzi valley	18	8	0.14	31	3.7	4021	261.18	4282
Baiguo valley-Huangdongzi valley	18	7	0.12	21	3.2	4077	233.18	4310
Chuanlin valley-Huangdongzi valley	18	7	0.12	14	1.9	3799	220.04	4019

The physical parameters for seepage calculation are presented in Table 2.

Substituting the variables in Eq. 1 with the above parameters, we get the seepage volume (per unit width) of different slope sections under different magnitude of rainfall. Meanwhile, using the same method, we arrive at the result that the theory seepage volume (per unit width) at the stable water level is 25.5 m^3/h. The onsite investigation shows that the real seepage volume is 19.6m^3/h. Hence the loss coefficient λ=0.77.

Substituting the variables in Expression (1) with the above parameters, we get the seepage volume (per unit width) of different slope sections under different magnitude of rainfall. Meanwhile, using the same method, we arrive at the result that the theory seepage volume (per unit width) at the stable water level is 25.5 m^3/h. The onsite investigation shows that the real seepage volume is 19.6m^3/h. Hence the loss coefficient λ=0.77.

Table 3 The volume of seepage along the valley.

	P1	P2	P5	P10	P20
Hei valley-Huangdongzi valley (m^3/h)	20.1	18.0	10.9	6.9	4.9
Baiguo valley-Huangdongzi valley (m^3/h)	22.7	19.1	15.5	10.2	8.5
Chuanlin valley-Huangdongzi valley (m^3/h)	46.0	36.1	31.3	24.7	21.9
Total volume(m^3/h)	88.8	73.2	57.6	41.7	35.3

3.2 *The analysis of seepage down from the accumulation surface*

3.2.1. *Seepage model down from the surface*

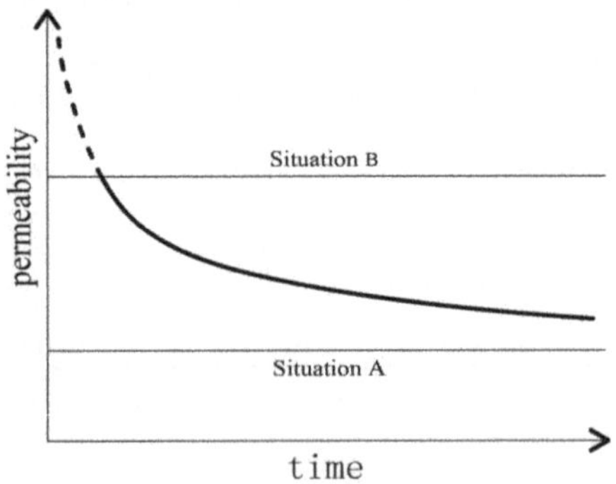

Fig. 6 Seepage model of rainfall from the accumulation surface.

Two situations should be considered in studying seepage down from the surface: First of all, permeability of the accumulation is always greater than rainfall intensity; secondly, due to the long duration and great intensity of rain, rainfall intensity is greater than the permeability of soil mass. These two situations are represented respectively by Situation A and Situation B (See Fig. 6).

In Situation A, all the rainfall infiltrates down the surface. In Situation B, at onset all the rainfall goes down the surface, but as it rains on and the saturation of soil increases, permeability decreases. Or the intensity of the rainfall is greater than the permeability of soil. Either the decrease of permeability or the greater intensity of rainfall will lead to the result that part of the rainfall can't pass through the soil and stays on the ground.

Made up mainly of bulk rocks, the accumulation of Dangguangbao landslide is of high permeability. And the onsite investigation has found that no water remains on the ground when it rains. Therefore, the study of the seepage of Daguangbao landslide needs to consider the Situation A only.

3.2.2. *The depth of infiltration*

Generally, infiltration depth of rainfall is ten time the amount of rainfall [6]. It can be estimated by using the following formula:

$$H = (0.872P + 4.28) \times 10^{-2}. \qquad (2)$$

In addition to the amount of rainfall, some other factors also influence the depth of infiltration, such as the duration of rain, the soil property and the intensity of rainfall. But the focus of the present study is on the volume of seepage flow, so only an initial estimate is needed.

According to Eq. 2, the rainfall infiltration depth in case of P_1 is about 5.6m, which has little impact on the hundred meter accumulation. So it is held that the seepage flow will neither infiltrate to the bottom of the valley nor seep out of the accumulation.

From the above analysis and calculation, it is concluded that the seepage flow of the lower reach is mainly from the seepage flow of the upper reach and the surface seepage of the accumulation can be neglected.

4. The Evaluation of Local Stability

After five years' deposit, the main body of accumulation of the Daguangbao landslide, which has undergone violent impact extrusion during the course of motion, is stable, but slides in some parts happens. The present study mainly focuses on the part of accumulation which poses threat to the safety of local people and their properties.

The present study, first of all, evaluates the possibility whether the seepage flow from the catchment of the upper reach will cause piping and soil flow at the accumulation, for in the case of the piping and soil flow at the accumulation, the water from the upstream catchment flows rapidly along the seepage passage and brings away the soil and stones, which will lead to the overall instability of the accumulation thus has very serious consequences.

Then the present research analyzes the stability of the flow area of debris at the lower reach of the accumulation. This flow area, formed by debris which is of smaller particle size, has lower permeability than the other part of the accumulation. Furthermore, the gradient of the area is steep (40°~55°) and under the erosion of rainfall, there formed many ditches of about 1-meter deep on the surface of the slope. In addition, the terrain shows that collapses have occurred in this area. Therefore, the instability of this area is likely to result in large amount of source materials being washed into the Huangdongzi valley. And a further rainstorm will induce mud-rock flow, posing severe threat to the residents in the lower reach.

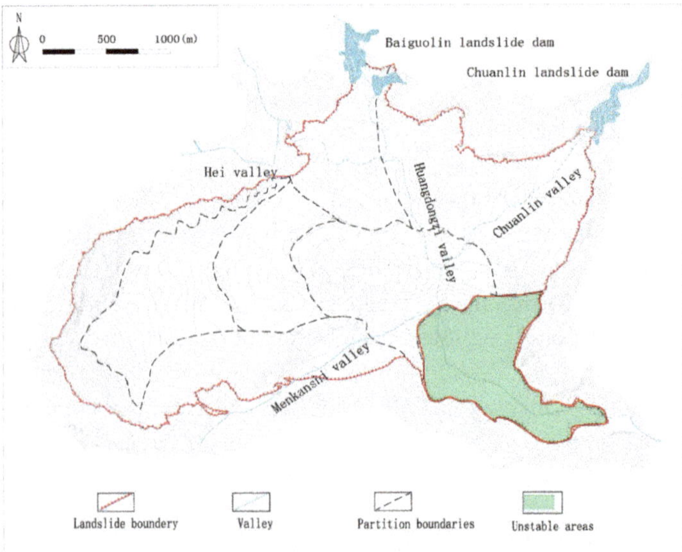

Fig. 7 The location plan of slope stability evaluation area.

4.1 *The judgment on seepage deformation*

The seepage deformation, including piping and soil flow, is determined mainly by the soil mass condition and the hydraulic condition.

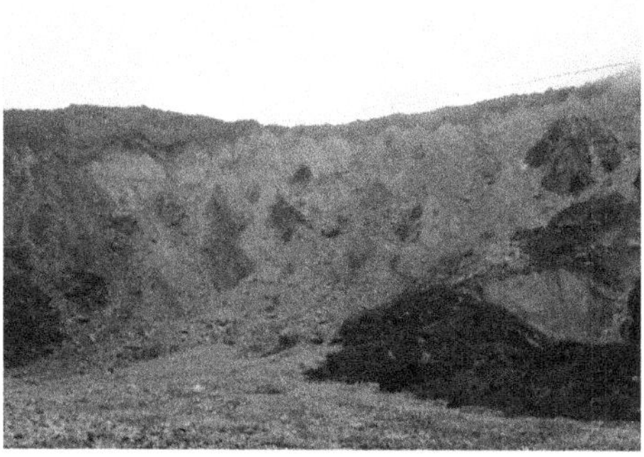

Fig. 8 Overall View of the Slope.

4.1.1. *The condition of soil mass*

Based on the principle that the volume of fine grains (filler grains) equals the void volume of coarse materials (framework grains), LIU Jie [7] has devised the following expression to calculate the content of fine grains:

$$P_z = \frac{\gamma_{d1} n_2}{(1-n_2)\gamma_{s2} + \gamma_{d1} n_2} \,. \tag{3}$$

where:

γ_{d1}—dry bulk density of fine grains

n_2—porosity of coarse grains in compact state

γ_{s2}—bulk density of soil grains of coarse materials.

Hence the criteria for judgment:

$$\begin{cases} P_Z > 35\% & \text{soil flow} \\ P_Z < 25\% & \text{piping} \\ 25\% < P_Z < 35\% & \text{soil flow and piping} \end{cases}$$

Through experiments in the labs and in the field, the calculation parameters for accumulation body of Daguangbao seepage flow area are: γ_{d1}=2200kg/m^3; n_2=30%; γ_{s2}=2500kg/m^3.

The result of calculation is P_Z=27.4%. Therefore, it can be inferred from the conditions of the accumulation body that both soil flow and piping can happen.

4.1.2. *The hydraulic condition*

The balance equation, devised by LIU Jie [7] based on deadweight, hydrostatic buoyancy and penetrating force which altogether work on the soil grains in the seepage field, is applied to calculate the critical hydraulic gradient for occurrence of piping:

$$I_{cn} = 2.2(G_s - 1)(1 - n)^2 \frac{d_5}{d_{20}} \tag{4}$$

In Eq. (4),

n—porosity;

Gs—soil mass proportion;

d_5 and d_{20}— the quality of the soil with smaller grain size is 5% and 20% respectively.

According to the experiments in the labs and in the field, the values of calculation parameters are:

n=28%; G_s=2.3; d_5=0.8mm; d_{20}=5mm.

From the calculation, the critical hydraulic gradient for occurrence of piping in the accumulation is 0.13. Therefore, it can be concluded that the piping will not happen.

4.2 *Stability evaluation of downstream debris flow area*

Through the long-term monitoring, it is found that local instability, in most of cases local collapses and rain erosion, occurs under the torrential rain. The app, Slide, is applied to search for the most risky slide face, and calculation is done to evaluate its stability. And the slope stability in the situations of normal condition, torrential rain and earthquake is studied. Fig. 9 shows the section view of the calculation and Table 4 demonstrates the calculation parameters.

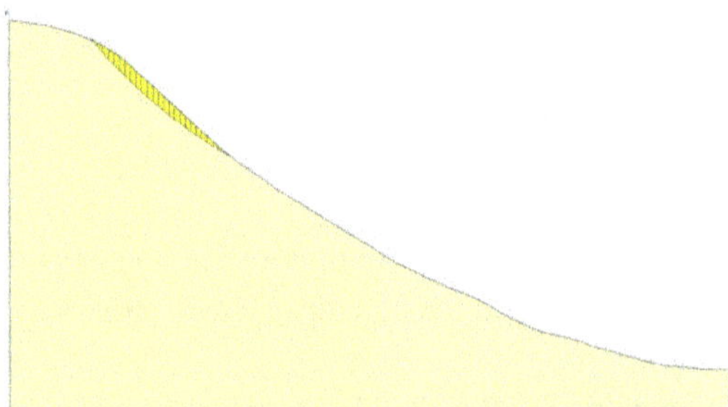

Fig. 9 The Section View of Slope Stability Calculation.

Given the seismic acceleration is 1.5g, the stability parameter values of the slope under three different conditions are presented in Table 5.

From the calculation results, it can be seen that the overall slide of the slope will not occur, but the upper part of the slope, which is in poor stability, tends to fail under the conditions of torrential rain and earthquakes.

Table 4 The physical and mechanical indexes of rock soil.

lithology	unit weight		shear stress in natural state		shear stress in saturated state	
	natural state	saturated state				
	KN/m3	KN/m3	C(kPa)	φ(°)	C(kPa)	φ(°)
blocky soil	21.70	22.20	28	35	20	30

Table 5 The landslide stability calculation results.

State	stability parameter	stability evaluation
normal	1.09	basically stable
torrential rain	0.97	unstable
earthquake	0.99	unstable

5. Conclusion

The bottom seepage flow of Daguangbao landslide accumulation comes mainly from the catchment of upper reach and it is subject to the influence of the rainfall intensity. As the accumulation body is generally stable, seepage flow will not cause piping or flow soil, but local collapses may occur. In the flow area of debris at the lower reach of the accumulation, overall sliding will not happen, but in torrential rain or earthquakes, local failures is likely to happen, and rainfall will wash the loose rocks into Huangdongzi valley, providing source materials for mud-rock flow.

6. References

1. HUANG Run-qiu, PEI Xiang-jun and LI Tian-bin, The Basic Characteristics and Formation Mechanism of Daguangbao Large-scale Landslide Triggered by Wenchuan Earthquake, *Journal of Engineering Geology,*16 (2008) 730-741.
2. HUANG Run-qiu, PEI Xiang-jun, ZHANG Wei-feng, et al. Further examination on Characteristics and Formation Mechanism of Daguangbao Landslide, *Journal of Engineering Geology*, 725-736, 17 (2009).
3. XU Qiang, PEI Xiang-jun, HUANG Run-qiu et al, *Large-scale landslides induced by the Wenchuan earthquake*, (Science Press, Beijing, 2009).
4. GU Wei-ci, *Design and Calculation of Earth Rockfill Dam*, (China Architecture and Building Press, Beijing, 2006).

5. LIU Xiang-yu, ZHANG Xi-tao, XIE Mo-wen, et al. GIS-based real-time assessment method of infiltration-stability of rainfall-induced landslide, *Chinese Journal of Geotechnical Engineering*, 34, 1627-1635(2012).
6. JIANG Xing-jiu, Study on the Calculation Method of Soil Retention after Rainfall Event, China Rural Water and Hydropower, 2, 44-46 (2006).
7. LIU Jie, *Seepage control of earth-Rock dams theoretical basis, engineering experiences and lessons*, (China Water Power Press, Beijing, 2006).

Experimental Study on Stress-Strain Relationship of Mud-Plaster Wall with Different Additives

Meng-Ting Tsai
Department of Architecture, National Taipei University of Technology,
1, Sec. 3, Zhongxiao E. Rd., Taipei 10608 Taiwan
E-mail: tsai@mail.ntust.edu.tw

Catur Prasetyo Hary
Department of Architecture, National Taiwan University of Science and Technology,
No. 43 Sec.4 Keelung Rd., Taipei 10607, Taiwan
E-mail: d10313801@mail.ntust.edu.tw

During 1999 Chi-Chi earthquake in Taiwan, numerous historical wooden buildings suffered serious damage. Most of these historical wooden buildings are important cultural property in Taiwan, and their damages are related to the mud-plaster wall. For investigating the structural behavior of the mud-plaster wall, and establishing the fundamental knowledge for seismic assessment, in this study, the most important element, mud, in the mud-plaster wall is tested with different additive, under compressive load, in order to observe the properties of these specimens. The obtained failure mechanism is discussed, and the followings results are concluded.

(1) Specimen with cement added will have best initial elastic modulus E.

(2) Specimen with hemp fiber added allows higher plasticity displacement.

(3) Specimen with clay added will not help increase the strength.

Keywords: Mud-plaster wall; initial elastic modulus; stress-strain relationship, additives.

1. Introduction

According to the past earthquake investigation, it is found that the damage of historical wooden buildings in Taiwan, as shown in Fig. 1(a), is closely related to the seismic resistance ability of mud- plaster walls. In order to improve the seismic resistance of these historical wooden buildings, the structural behavior of mud-plaster wall have to be completely understood by researchers and designers. The seismic resistance behavior can be illustrated and shown in Fig. 1(b). Mud-plaster wall rotates under seismic load, resulting in two coupling compressive load in the upper and lower mud-plaster wall. Due to the behavior that have been observed [1], a fundamental knowledge and properties of the most important element in the mud-plaster wall – mud that can properly evaluated and applied into the simulation of these walls is required and essential. In this study, the material properties of mud with different additives are generated from test under compressive load, in order to observe the stress-strain relationship of these mud specimens.

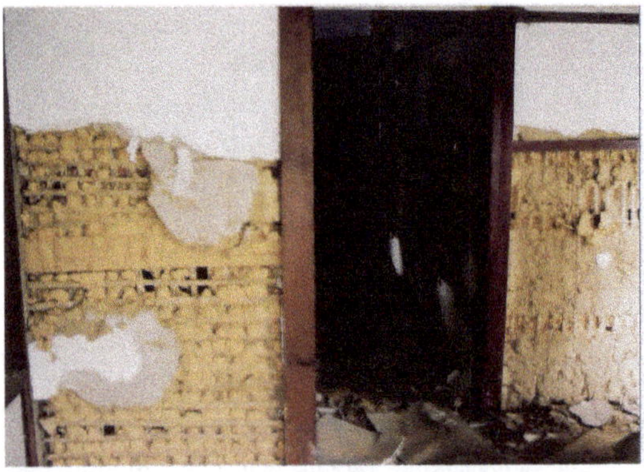

(a) Typical mud-plaster wall in taiwan.

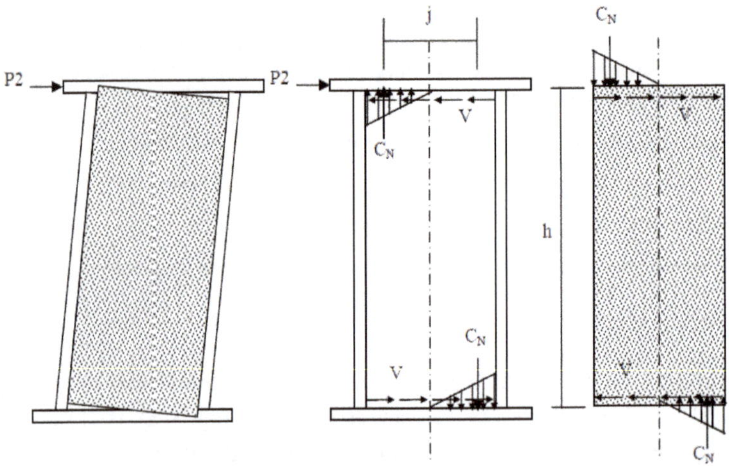

(b) Behavior of mud-plaster wall under seismic load

Fig. 1 Typical bamboo-mud-wall and its seismic resistance mechanism.

2. Test Specimens

The test of mud specimens with the different additives is to determine the basic properties. In this study, all the specimens are prefabricated into the mud cubic with size 5x5x5cm, as shown in Fig. 2(b). The mix proportions of mud and additives are fixed and described in Table 1, and the amount of water and straw added follow the experience of senior technician.

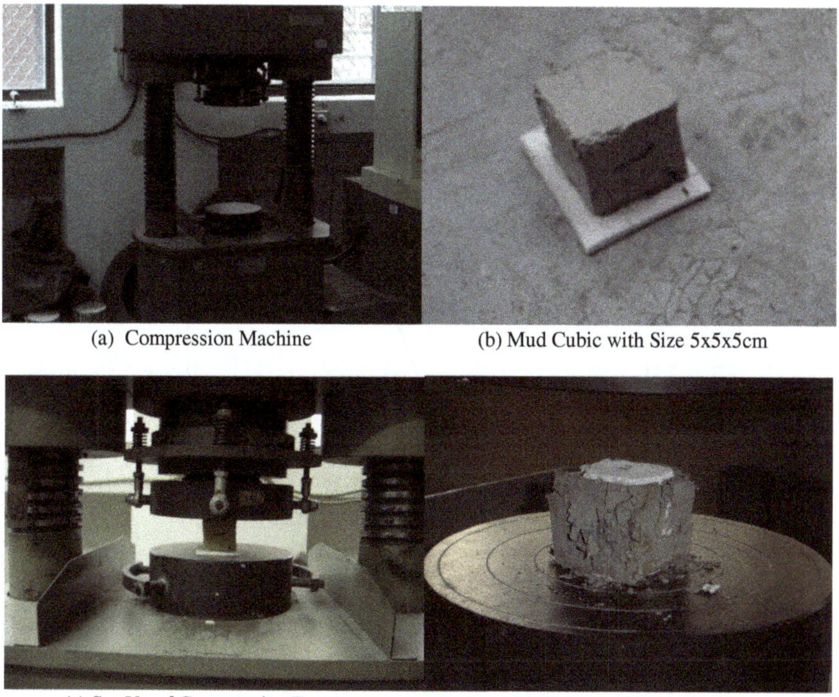

(a) Compression Machine (b) Mud Cubic with Size 5x5x5cm

(c) Set-Up of Compressive Test (d) Failure After Testing

Fig. 2 Setting-up of test and failure.

Table 1 Mix proportions of mud with different additives.

Specimen	Standard Mud	Additive		
	Clay:Straw:Husk	Hemp fiber	Clay	Cement
M0		–	–	–
MA		0.38	–	–
MB	130 : 1 : 5	–	18	–
MC		–	–	20

The mud used in this study is taken from Da-Su County (near Kaoshiung). Normally, the mud that has been used for the construction of mud-plaster wall is mixed with short rice straw and rice husk, and this kind of mixture is the prototype, called specimen Mo. The specimen MA is Mo with hemp fiber added, and the specimens MB and MC have clay and cement added respectively.

The upper and lower face of the specimen is cover by gypsum to make sure the face contacting with the machine is horizontally smooth, as shown in Fig. 2(b). And the test is taken place under a compression machine shown in n Fig. 2(a). It is noticed that, each specimens will have 1~2% shrinkage due to the mud properties, dry of the water inside the mud cubic. Hence, it is important to measure the compression area for each specimen again before test.

3. Test Results

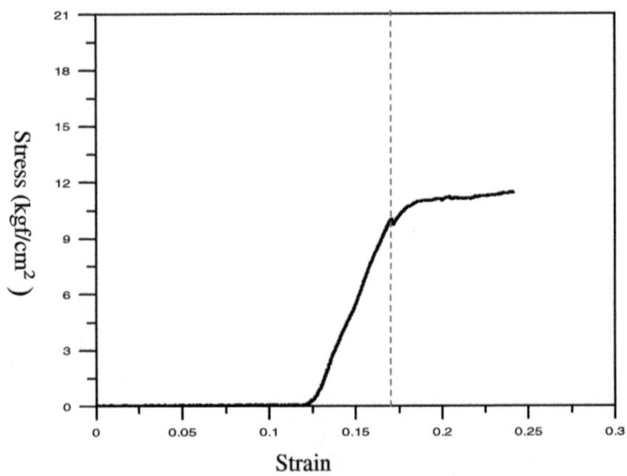

(a) Specimen M0 (pure mud)

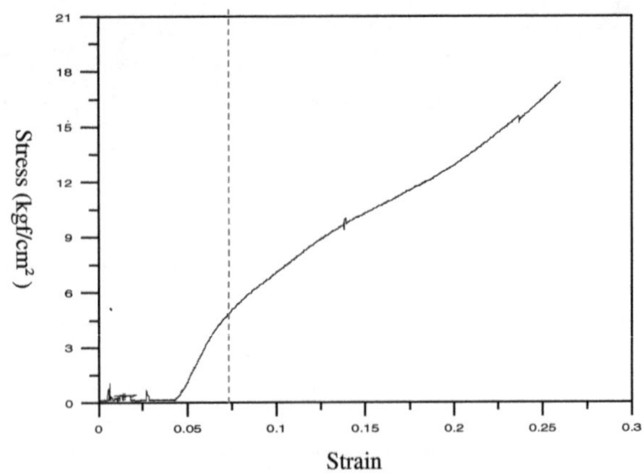

(b) Specimen MA (mud with Hemp fiber)

The testing result show that the mud with cement added will have best initial elastic modulus E(σ/ε), as illustrated in Fig 3(d). The initial elastic modulus E of pure mud specimens and mud with hemp fiber added are close. Mud with clay added is with the lowest initial elastic modulus E among all the specimens.

As for the failure performance of each cubic specimen, it is important to notice that, although specimen Mc has the highest elastic modulus E among all the specimens, the properties of the specimen Mc becomes brittle due to the effect of cement added. Therefore, once the crack happens, the elastic modulus E drops abruptly, as shown in Fig 3(d). Contrasting with specimen Mc, specimen MA (mud with hemp fiber added) is ductile, as shown in Fig 3(b). In the other word, specimens with hemp fiber added will have higher energy absorption ability.

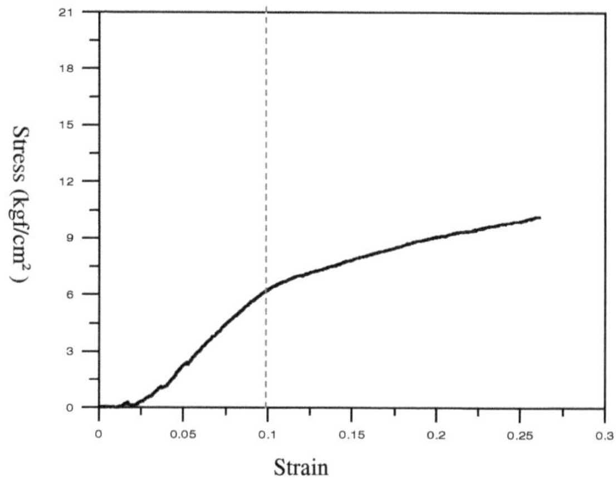

(c) Specimen MB (mud with clay)

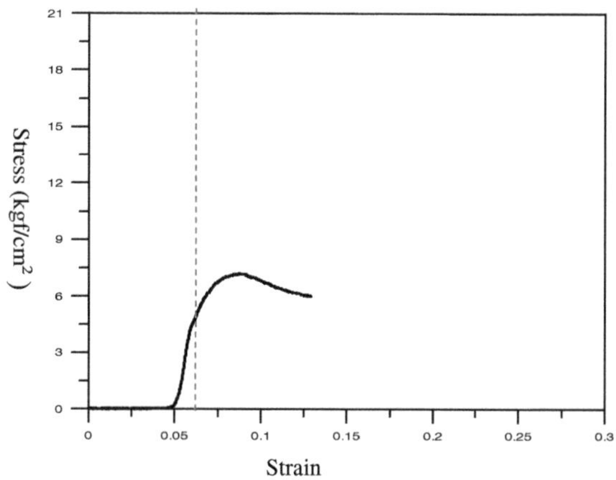

(d) Specimen MA (mud with cement)

Fig. 3 Stress-strain relationship of each testing specimen.

4. Summary

In this study, it is found that the mud with different additive used for historical wooden buildings, the stress-strain relationship changes visibly. In addition to load resistance increased, such as specimen Mc, the energy absorption of other specimen such as MA will be improved. As for the failure behavior of each specimen with different additives, the specimen with hemp fiber added makes the amount of crack reduced, however, the increasing of compressive load resistance ability is not observed.

The mud with cement added may increase the load resistance ability, however, it becomes brittle. Based upon the tests, the elastic modulus E and stress-strain relationship (Fig. 4) which has been obtained in this study can be used for establishing equivalent bracing model, which makes the simulation of mud-plaster wall under horizontally cyclic load become possible.

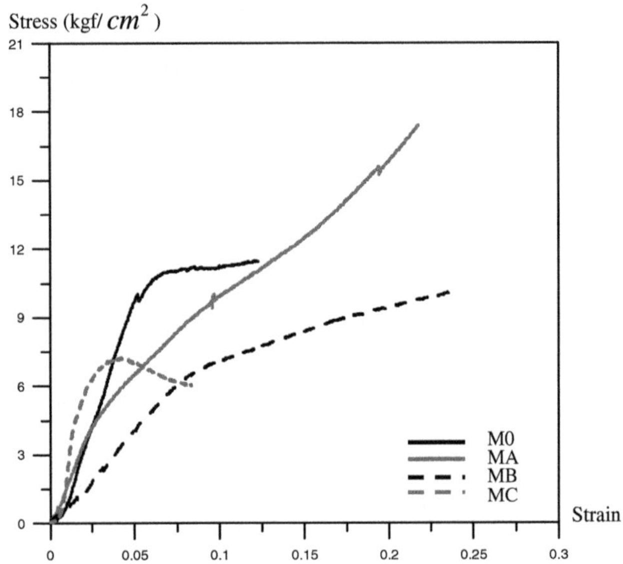

Fig. 4 Comparison of σ-ε curves with different mud additives.

References

1. Chia-Chi Chen, Ja-Shian Chang, Meng-Ting Tsai, Structural Behaviors of Japanese style Bamboo-Mud-Walls under Horizontal Cyclic Loading. *Journal of Architecture*, No. 62, pp. 91~116, Taiwan (2007).
2. Chen Chia-Chi, Chang Ja-Shian, Tsai Meng-Ting, Structure and Seismic Strengthening of Wall for Wooden Building During the Japanese-

Colonization (1) -The Tested and Analytical Study on Shear Capacity of the Clay Walls. *National Science Council NSC92-2625-Z-165-001* (2004).

3. Masato Nakao, Yutaka Yamazaki, Experimental Study of the Earthquake Resistance Performance of Mud-Plastered Walls. *13th World Conference on Earthquake Engineering*, Canada, Vancouver (2004).
4. Meng-Ting Tsai, Experimental Study and Equivalent Bracing Simulation for the Bamboo Mud-Wall of Japanese Wooden Buildings. *Master Thesis*, National Cheng-Kung University (2006).
5. Chen Chia-Chi, Tsai Meng-Ting, Chang Ja-Shian, Shih Chung-Hsien, Experiment Study of the Bamboo-mud-wall Used In Taiwanese Historic Building. *Proceedings of First European Conference on Earthquake Engineering and Seismology*, Geneva, Switzerland (2006).

Influence of SBS Inhibitor on Basic Performance of Modified Asphalt

Yanshuang Zhang,
Traffic Construction Engineering Quality Supervision Station of Tongliao City, Inner-Mongolia, 028000, China
Email: 253122797@qq.com

Wan Yu*
State Key Laboratory of Silicate Materials for Architectures, Wuhan University of Technology, Wuhan, 430070, China
Email: yuwan0523@163.com

The rheological properties and the components analyzing of styrene butadiene styrene (SBS) inhibitor modified asphalt was investigated by dynamic shear rheology (DSR) and four composition analyzer, respectively. Compared with the compositions and fundamental properties of asphalts, the results show that the addition of SBS inhibitor to asphalt results in reducing of the penetration and ductility and enhancement of the softening point. The complex shear modulus reduces slightly while the phase angle increases when the inhibitors are added. Meanwhile, the components of saturates and aromatics change slightly. With the increase of SBS inhibitor, the content of resin decreased and the content of asphaltene increased.

Keywords: Inhibitor; styrene butadiene styrene (SBS); physical properties.

1. Introduction

There are volatile organic compounds (VOCs) emission to the atmosphere from road asphalt [1-3]. In general, asphalt is a kind of viscoelastic materials and widely used in road paving, waterproofing, roadway maintenance and micro-surfacing material [4-6]. The softening point of asphalt was selected to evaluate the thermal stability of asphalt as an index, but the asphalt aging degree was characterized by the change of the softening point before and after aging [7-8]. Styrene butadiene styrene (SBS) inhibitor plays an important role in VOCs emission and absorption of asphalt and makes the components of asphalt change. Meanwhile, this changes will lead to the physical performance reduce and there is a big difference with the base asphalt [3,9-10].

* Corresponding author.

The basic properties of different compositions modified asphalt were investigated such as penetration, softening point, and ductility. And the rheological properties and chemical components of modified asphalt before and after aging were analyzed.

2. Materials and Methods

2.1. *Materials*

Asphalt with 90# penetration grade (dmm), Ring and Ball temperature of 47.3°C, which was measured according to ASTM D36-76, was used. SBS was produced by Changsha Power Chemical Technology Co, LTD.

2.2. *Methods*

Approximately 450g of asphalt PJ90 was first heated to 135°C with a thermoelectric heater. 3wt%, 4wt%, and 5wt% SBS inhibitor were added and then stirred for 1 hour with speed of 800 rpm. At the end, a high shear mixer was employed for another 1.5 hour with speed of 4000 rpm. Four types of asphalt binders were prepared.

3. Results and Discussions

3.1. *Basic performance of asphalt*

Their compositions and fundamental properties of modified asphalts were shown in Table 1.

Table 1 Compositions and fundamental properties of asphalt.

Compositions	Penetration 25°C, [0.1mm]	Ductility 10°C, [cm]	Softening point, [°C]
PJ 90	82.1	128.5	47.3
PJ 90+3%SBS	69.5	56.7	54.0
PJ 90+4%SBS	67.7	59.2	59.8
PJ 90+5%SBS	65.3	62.7	602

In Table 1, with the increase of SBS inhibitors, the penetration and ductility of inhibitor modified asphalt decreased, whereas the softening point increased gradually. The decrease of the penetration of asphalt shows that the addition of SBS inhibitor improves the consistence of asphalt. The addition of SBS inhibitor makes the ductility of asphalt declined largely and the reduction rate is almost 100%. It shows that the SBS inhibitor can reduce the low-temperature ductility and there is a certain negative impact on the low temperature properties of asphalt. However, with the addition contents of SBS inhibitor increasing, the softening point has raised. The softening point will reach to 60.2°C and increase by 12.7°C, when the addition contents reached to 5%. This suggests that the addition of SBS can significantly improve the high temperature performance of asphalt.

3.2. *Complex shear modulus (G*)*

The addition of SBS makes the complex shear modulus of PJ90 asphalt in the scanning scope (0-80 °C), with the increase of temperature, the complex shear modulus tend to downward trend, and the PJ90 plural trend are similar to the influence of shear modulus, complex shear modulus curve basically coincide with each other, as the Fig. 1. It shows that SBS inhibitor modified asphalt has a good high temperature property.

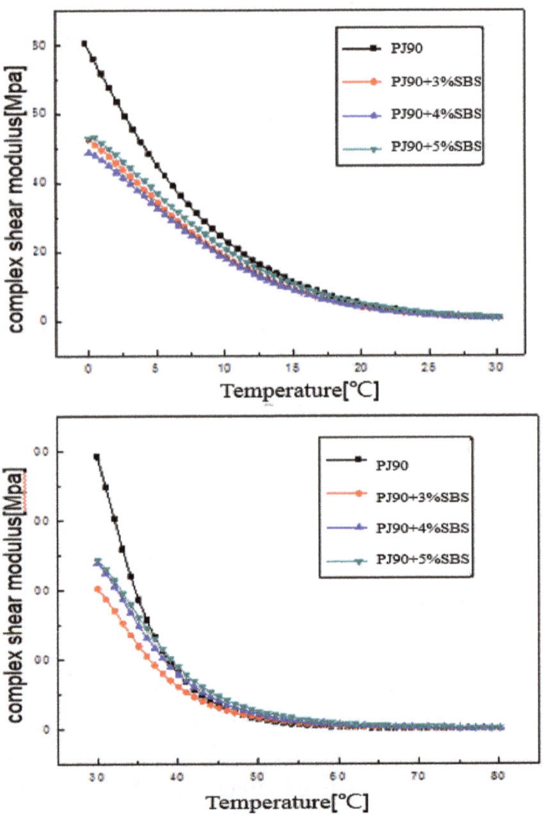

Fig. 1 Complex shear modulus of SBS inhibitors to modified asphalt.

3.3. *Phase angle (δ)*

With the increase of temperature, the sample of phase angle increases gradually, the elastic characteristics of asphalt is abate, and the cohesive characteristics of asphalt is reinforced with addition of different proportion SBS inhibitors. As show in Fig. 2(a), the phase angle of asphalt in the test range (0-30°C) increased, and the increase of degree will decrease with the increase of scanning temperature. It indicated that SBS inhibitor modified asphalt has a better low temperature property than base asphalt and the more the inhibitor, the better the low temperature rheological properties are.

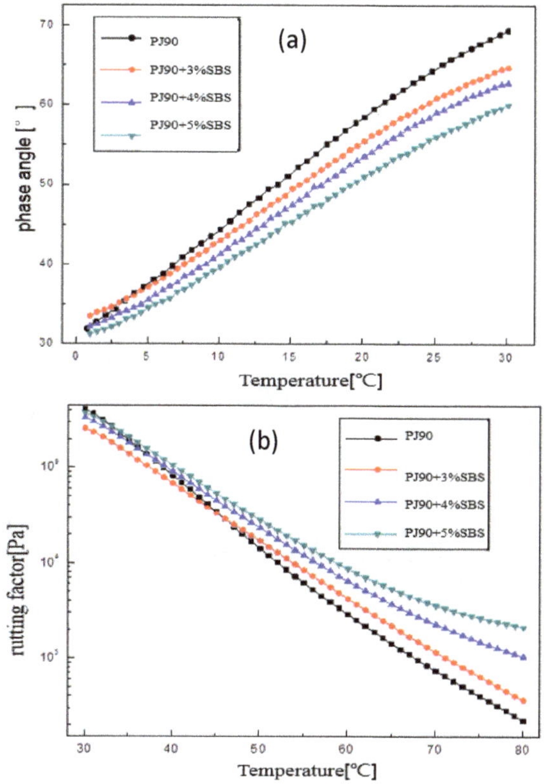

Fig. 2 (a) Phase angle and (b) rutting factors of SBS inhibitors to modified asphalt.

3.4. *Rutting factor (G*/sinδ)*

SHRP recommended that rutting factor (G*/sinδ) was equal to 1kPa to evaluate the highest temperature of asphalt designs [11]. The rutting factor is the evaluation index to resist the high temperature of asphalt, the greater the rutting factor, the greater the resistance of high temperature is. As the Fig. 2(b), the rutting factor of SBS inhibitors of modified asphalt decrease with the increase of temperature. The difference is more and more bigger between the rutting factor of modified asphalt and base asphalt, that may be associated with the network structure of SBS.

3.5. *Four component analysis*

Four components analysis was measured by thin layer chromatography detection (TLC-FID) method using four components analyzer and get the signal diagram. The qualitative location is the retention time: saturate Rt<0.2min, aromatics 0.2min<Rt<0.32min, resin Rt>0.32min, as the Fig. 3. According to the order of the exhibition, it is obviously that appears four peak from left to right and it may be saturates, aromatics, resins and asphaltenes. The content of these four components can be calculated by calculating the area of the peak.

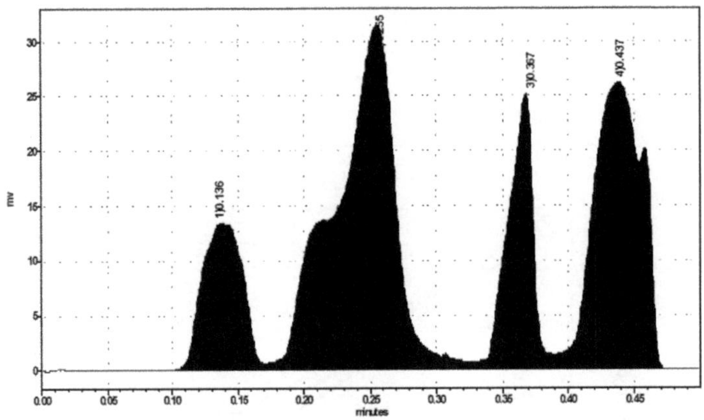

Fig. 3 The chromatogram of four components analysis.

Table 2 Four components of asphalt.

inhibitor	wt%	saturate	aromatics	resins	asphaltenes
SBS	0	5.7813	64.9223	20.6933	8.60320
	3	6.2915	64.6474	18.4318	10.6293
	4	6.2819	64.2830	18.5990	10.8362
	5	7.3423	64.0842	18.0539	10.5196

Compared with the four component, the asphaltene reduces slightly and play a role in lubrication and flexible of asphalt. The more the content, the more flexible the asphalt is. On the contrary, the litter the content, the harder the asphalt is. At the same time, the content of asphaltene increased with the addition contents of SBS inhibitor increasing. The physical properties of SBS inhibitor modified asphalt decreased such as penetration and ductility, while the softening point increased.

4. Summary

Compared with the four component, the asphaltene reduces slightly and play a role in lubrication and flexible of asphalt. The more the content, the more flexible the asphalt is. On the contrary, the litter the content, the harder the asphalt is. Meanwhile, with the increase of asphaltene and SBS inhibitor, the penetration and ductility decreased, while the softening point increased.

Acknowledgments

The authors acknowledge the financial supported by the National Key Scientific Apparatus Development Program from the Ministry of Science and Technology of China (No. 2013YQ160501), National Basic Research Program of China (973 Program No. 2014CB932104) and National Project of Scientific and Technical Supporting Programs funded by Ministry of Science & Technology of China (No. 2011BAE28B03).

References

1. Boczkaj, A. Przyjazny, M. Kaminski, Characteristics of volatile organic compounds emission profiles from hot road bitumens, Chemosphere. 107 (2014) 23-30.
2. B. Tang, U. Isacsson, Chemical characterization of oil-based asphalt release agents and their emissions, Fuel, 85 (2006) 1232-1241.
3. P.Q. Cui, S.P. Wu, Y. Xiao, and H.H. Zhang, Study on the deteriorations of bituminous binder resulted from volatile organic compounds emissions, Construction and Building Materials. 68 (2014) 644-649.
4. X.X. Zhou, G.F. Zhang, R.M. Liu, and L. Zheng, Molecular simulations of anti-aging mechanisms on nano-LDHs modified asphalt. Key Engineering Materials. 599 (2014) 198-202.
5. J.Q. Zhu, B. Birgisson, N. Kringos, Polymer modification of bitumen: advances and challenges, European polymer journal. (2014) 1-41.

6. S. P. Wu, J. Han, L. Pang, M. Yu, and T. Wang, Rheological properties for aged bitumen containing ultraviolet light resistant materials, Construction and Building Materials. 2012, 33, 133-138.
7. J. Wei, Z. Liu, Y. Zhang, Rheological properties of amorphous poly alpha olefin (APAO) modified asphalt binders, Construction and Building Materials. 48 (2013) 533-539.
8. A. Perez-Lepe, F.J. Martinez-Boza, C. Gallegos, Influence of the processing conditions on the rheological behavior of polymer-modified bitumen, Fuel. 82 (2003) 1339-1348.
9. X.M. Huang, S.P. Wu, Y.L. Wang, Asphalt and asphalt mixture. Southeast university press, Nanjing, 2002.
10. H. Fu, L. Xie, D. Dou, Storage stability and compatibility of asphalt binder modified by SBS graft copolymer, Construction and Building Materials. 21 (2007) 1528-1533.
11. D.A. Anderson, D.W. Christensen, H.U. Bahia, Binder characterization and evaluation volume 3: physical characterization, SHRP-A-369, Strategic Highway Research Program. Washington, DC 1994.

CHAPTER 6

Material Science and Engineering

The Surface Modification of Tourmaline Powder with Allyl Glycidyl Ether and Characterization

Yingmo Hu
Beijing Key Laboratory of Materials Utilization of Nonmetallic Minerals and Solid Wastes, National Laboratory of Mineral Materials, School of Materials Science and Technology, China University of Geosciences, Beijing, 100083
E-mail: huyingmo@cugb.edu.cn
www. cugb.edu.cn

In order to prepare polymerizable organic tourmaline, allyl glycidyl ether (AGE) modified tourmaline powder had been investigated in details by focusing on the experimental parameters of turbidity and subsidence time in liquid paraffin. The experimental results indicated that the organic modified tourmaline have a good dispersity in organic solvent when the weight ratios of AGE to tourmaline was 0.8, weight ratios of the solvent to tourmaline was 4.0, reacted at 140°C for 6h. And the structure of organic modified tourmaline was also characterized by means of IR, XRD and SEM.

Keywords: Tourmaline; Polymerizable tourmaline; Modified tourmaline.

1. Introduction

Tourmaline have been widely applied in the field of environmental protection [1], health care [2,3], medicine [4,5] and building materials [6] and so on for its special performances of far infrared radiation [7], releasing negative ion [8] and weak galvanic current [9] et al. Tourmaline was regarded as novel material of 21 century that could improve environment and beneficial to health [10]. However tourmaline powders are difficult to combine with polymer firmly for its great distinguishing surface properties from polymers, and its applications have been largely restricted [11,12]. If the double bond-containing organic group could introduced into the surface of tourmaline by means of the surface modification of tourmaline to prepare polymerizable organic tourmaline, and then polymerize to get tourmaline-containing functional polymer that have the special performances of far infrared radiation and releasing negative ion, it would have significance on people's health care, developments of novel products and high-worth integrative utilization of functional mineral resource.

In this work, the modified condition of tourmaline powders with allyl glycidyl ether as modifier were studied by focusing on the experimental parameters of turbidity and subsidence time in liquid paraffin, and the modified tourmaline's structures were characterized.

2. Materials and Methods

2.1. *Materials and instruments*

Tourmaline powder with the diameter of d_{50} 1.75 μm and d_{97} 5.23 μm (purity: 98%) was purchased from Yanxin Mineral Co. Ltd., Hebei, China; allyl glycidyl ether (CP grade)was obtained from Baishun Chemical Co. Ltd., Beijing; N, N-dimethylformamide (DMF, AR grade) was purchased from West Long Chemical Co. Ltd; liquid paraffin was purchased from Tianjin Fuchen Chemical Reagent Factory.

The testing devices were including PerkinElmer Spectrum 100 Fourier transform infrared spectroscopy (Shanghai Co.), Rigaku D / max-rA 12kw X-ray diffraction (Japan), SEM images were observed by Hitachi Model S-450 scanning electron microscope, and SGZ-2-type nephelometer (Shanghai Yue Feng Instrument)

2.2. *Allyl glycidyl ether modified tourmaline*

In a 100 ml three-necks flask, 5g super fine tourmaline powder and a certain amount of allyl glycidyl ether in 50 ml anhydrous DMF were added and stirred at 120°C for 6 hours. The samples were separated by centrifugation of mixtures, then washed three times with ethanol and acetone respectively, and finally dried and grinded to be characterized.

2.3. *Turbidity measurements*

In a 100 ml beaker, 1.0 g modified tourmaline powder was added into 80 ml liquid paraffin, the solution was kept for 12 hours statically after 5 minute sufficient mixing, the turbidity of the upper liquid was measured by SGZ-2-type nephelometer.

2.4. *Subsidence time measurements*

2.0g modified tourmaline and 30mL liquid paraffin was added into 100mL beaker, stirred adequately 15min. Then take 10mL into graduated cylinder and let's to stand, and check the time that the upper clear liquid settle to 5mL. The longer of subsidence time, the better of modified effect of tourmaline.

3. Results and Discussion

3.1. *The optimization of reaction conditions*

The modified effect of tourmaline powder with allyl glycidyl ether under various conditions were studied by focusing on the experimental parameters of turbidity and subsidence time in liquid paraffin.

3.1.1. *The effect of reaction time*

The effect of reaction time on modified tourmaline with allyl glycidyl ether was shown in Figure 1. It was concluded that the turbidity and subsidence time of modified tourmaline in liquid paraffin changed with reaction time as the similar trend, and reach the maximum value at 6 hours. Therefore, 6 hours was selected as the optimized reaction time.

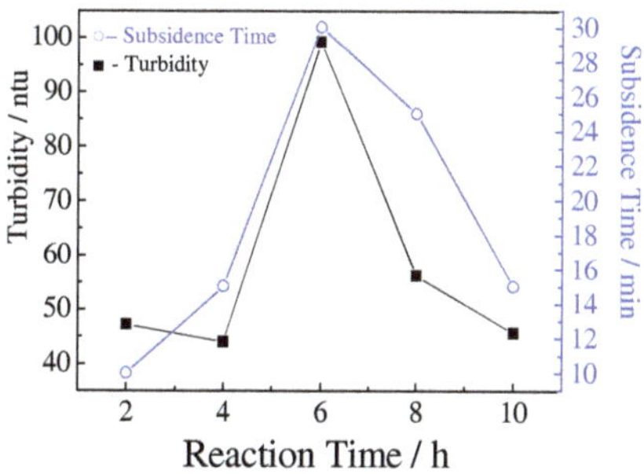

Fig. 1 The effect of reaction time on modified tourmaline.

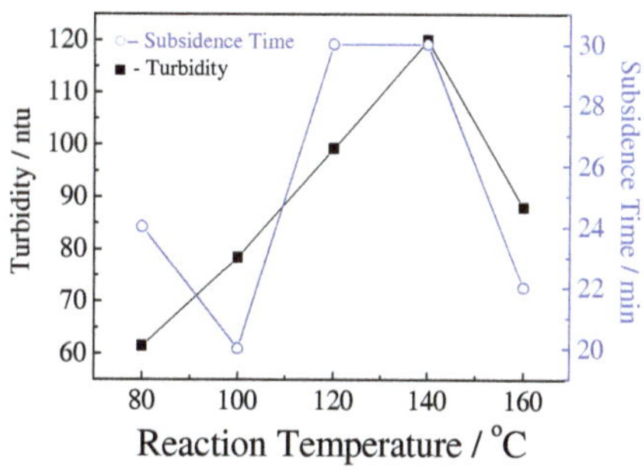

Fig. 2 The effect of reaction temperature on modified tourmaline.

3.1.2. *The effect of reaction temperature*

The effect of reaction temperature is shown in Figure 2. Figure 2 shows that the turbidity of modified tourmaline in liquid paraffin increased firstly and then fall down with the temperature continuous raising, with the maximum value at 140°C, the 140°C was selected as the optimized reaction temperature. And the subsidence time of modified tourmaline in liquid paraffin were the best at the period of 120 ~ 140°C, which had a good hydrophobic property.

3.1.3. *The effect of weight ratios of AGE to tourmaline*

The effect of weight ratios of AGE to tourmaline was shown in Figure 3. Figure 3 reveales that the turbidity and subsidence time of modified tourmaline in liquid paraffin had the same trend with increasing of the weight ratios of AGE to tourmaline, and both had the maximum value when the weight ratio of AGE to tourmaline was 0.8. presenting an excellent hydrophobic property.

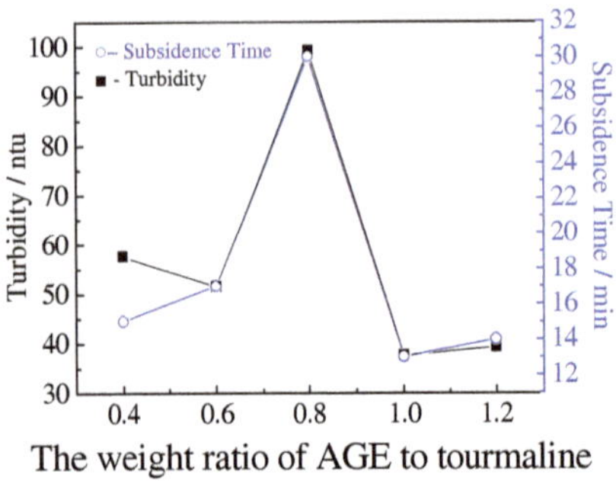

Fig. 3 The effect of weight ratios of AGE to tourmaline on modified tourmaline.

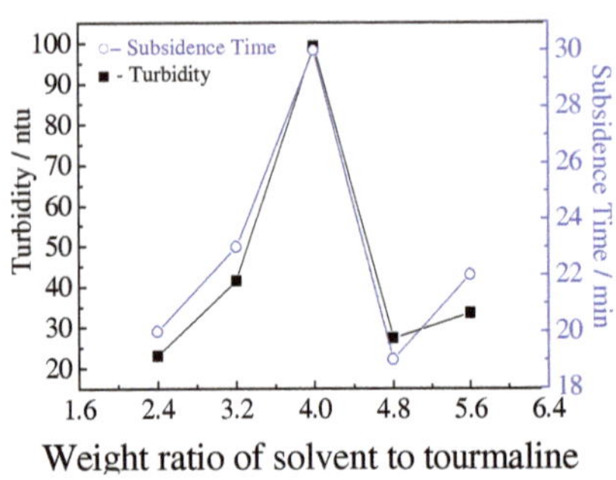

Fig. 4 The effect of the weight ratios of the solvent to tourmaline tourmaline.

3.1.4. *The effect of the weight ratios of the ore slurry*

The effects of the weight ratios of the solvent to tourmaline on the modification of tourmaline were shown in Figure 4. The curves indicate that both the turbidity and subsidence time of modified tourmaline in liquid paraffin increased sharply with increasing of the weight ratios of the solvent to tourmaline at beginning, and fell down with the continuous increasing of the weight ratios of the solvent to tourmaline. The optimum weight ratio of the solvent to tourmaline was selected to be 4.0.

3.2. *The characterization of modified tourmaline*

3.2.1. *IR Spectra Analysis*

The infrared spectra of unmodified and modified tourmaline with AGE were shown in Figure 5. In Figure 7a, unmodified tourmaline[13] have absorption bands at 3558 cm^{-1} (–OH group), 1272 cm^{-1} (B-O group) and 975 cm^{-1} (Si-O group). By comparison with Figure 7a, the IR spectrum of modified tourmaline (Figure 7c) shows that absorption bands of methyl (2963 cm^{-1}), methylene (2861 cm^{-1}), double bond (1629 cm^{-1}) of allyl have appeared. Besides those, the absorption shape of tourmaline almost unchange clearly but all wavelengths shift corresponding to unmodified tourmaline owing to the electronic effect of allyl glycidyl group. This indicats that allyl glycidyl chain has been introduced in the surface of tourmaline to get polymerizable organic modified tourmaline.

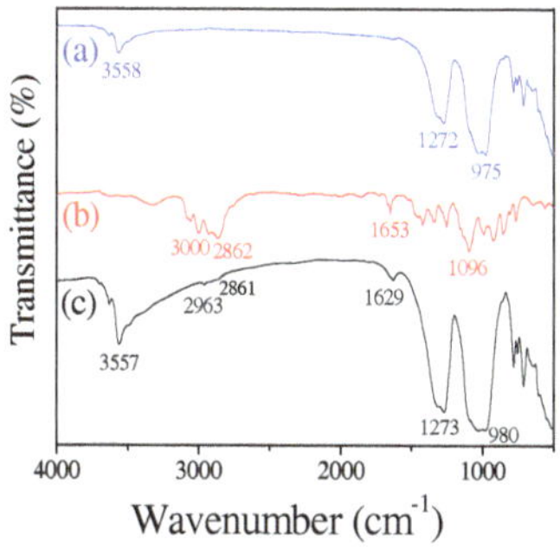

Fig. 5 The IR spectra of (a) unmodified tourmaline, (b) AGE, (c) modified tourmaline.

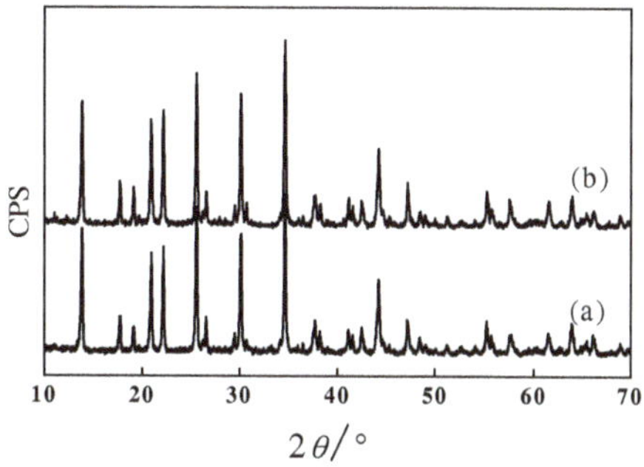

Fig. 6 The XRD spectra of (a) unmodified tourmaline and (b) modified tourmaline.

3.2.2. *XRD pattens*

XRD spectra of unmodified and modified tourmaline are shown in Figure 6. The major peaks of unmodified tourmaline (Figure 6a) are observed at 2θ of 13.8°, 21.0°, 22.0°, 25.5°, 26.7°, 30.3°, 34.7°, 44.3°, 47.1°, 55.3°, 57.7°, 61.5°, 63.9°, while the major peaks of modified tourmaline locate at the same 2θ and no other phases are detected. The two nearly identical spectra indicate that the modifications of tourmaline do not alter tourmaline's crystal structure.

3.2.3. *SEM images*

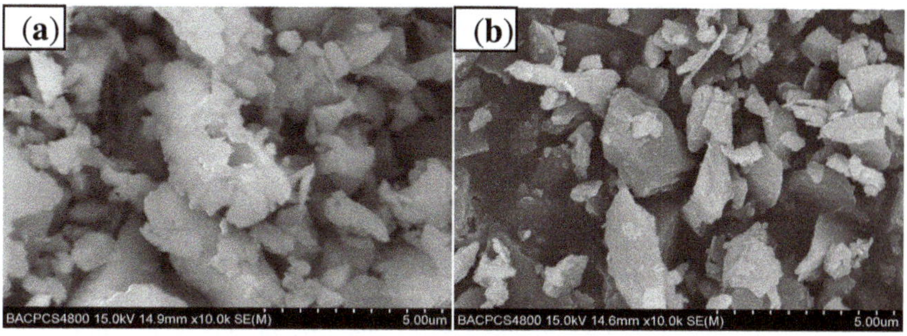

Fig. 7 SEM images of unmodified (a) and modified (b) tourmaline.

Figure 7 shows the SEM images of unmodified and modified tourmaline. Some conglomeration in unmodified tourmaline particles is apparent (Figure 7a), and no agglomerates were observed in modified tourmaline particles (Figure 7b). These results are attributable to the strong polar surfaces of the tourmaline particles before modification facilitated the easy conglomeration of the particles.

And the surface polarity of the tourmaline decreased after the organic modification, the surface energy was depressed, therefore the dispersivity of the tourmaline particles was improved.

4. Summary

The surface modification of tourmaline with allyl glycidyl ether was investigated, and optimized the modified conditions with parameters of the turbidity and subsidence time of modified tourmaline in liquid paraffin. The experimental results showed that the organic modified tourmaline with allyl glycidyl ether have a good dispersity in organic solvent when the weight ratios of AGE to tourmaline was 0.8, weight ratios of the solvent to tourmaline was 4.0, reacted at 140°C for 6h. The IR spectra revealed that allyl glycidyl chain has been introduced in the surface of tourmaline to get polymerizable organic modified tourmaline, and the modified tourmaline kept the same crystal structures as the unmodified one, but the hydrophobic property of tourmaline's surface was improved clearly. The investigation of tourmaline-containing functional polymer is also under way.

Acknowledgments

This work is supported by the National Natural Science Foundation of China (No. 51372233).

References

1. D. L. Guerra, S. P. Oliveira, E. M. Silva, A. C. Batista, Adsorption of uranyl on beryl and tourmaline, kinetics and thermodynamic investigation. *Int. J. Min. Proc.* **102–103**, 25 (2012).
2. C. P. Wang, L. Yu, Z. Y. Zhang, B. L. Wang, H. W. Sun, Tourmaline combined with Phanerochaete chrysosporium to remediate agricultural soil contaminated with PAHs and OCPs, *J. Hazard. Mat.* **264**, 439 (2014).
3. R. Z. Orlowski, Novel Agents for Multiple Myeloma to Overcome Resistance in Phase III Clinical Trials, *Seminars in Oncology*, **40**(5), 634 (2013).
4. Y. Zheng, Y. Liu, A.Q. Wang, Fast removal of ammonium ion using a hydrogel optimized with response surface methodology, *Chem. Eng. J.* **171**(3), 1201 (2011).
5. P. P. Gostner, M. Bonelli, P. Pernter, A. Graefen, A. Zink, New radiological approach for analysis and identification of foreign objects in ancient and historic mummies, *J. Arch. Sci.* **40**(2), 1003 (2013).

6. G. K. Zhang, X. Qin, Efficient photocatalytic degradation of gaseous formaldehyde by the TiO_2/tourmaline composites. *Mat. Res. Bull.* **48**(10), 3743 (2013).
7. C. C. Zhao, L. B. Liao, Z. G. Xia, X. N. Sun, Temperature-dependent Raman and infrared spectroscopy study on iron–magnesium tourmalines with different Fe content Original Research Article, *Vib. Spectr.* **62**, 28 (2012).
8. K. Jiang, T. H. Sun, L. N. Sun, H. B. Li, Adsorption characteristics of copper, lead, zinc and cadmium ions by tourmaline. *J. Envir. Sci.* **18**(6), 1221(2006).
9. W. B. Aleksandra, N. N. Lucyna, A Raman microspectroscopic study of organic inclusions in "watermelon" tourmaline from the Paprok mine (Nuristan, Afghanistan). *Vibr. Spectr.* **57**(2), 248 (2011).
10. G. D. Harald, The "chessboard" classification scheme of mineral deposits: Mineralogy and geology from aluminum to zirconium. *Earth Sci. Rev.* **100**(1–4), 1(2010).
11. Y. M. Hu, J. Bian, X. Yang, Q.L. Wang, Studies on Lauroyl Chloride Modified Tourmaline Powder. *Adv. Mat. Res.* **287-290**, 245 (2011).
12. Y. M. Hu, X. Yang, The surface organic modification of tourmaline powder by span-60 and its composite, *Appl. Surf. Sci.* **258**(19), 7540 (2012).
13. P. S. R. Prasad, D. S. Sarma, Study of structural disorder in natural tourmaline by infrared spectroscopy, *Gond. Res.* **8**(2), 265 (2005).

Conductive Polyaniline/Cellulose Nanocrystals Composite for Ammonia Gas Detection

Qian Wu[a], *Yun–Feng Qin*[b], *Long Chen*[c] *and Zong–Yi Qin*[d]

State Key Laboratory for Modification of Chemical Fibers and Polymer Materials, and College of Material Science and Engineering, Donghua University, Shanghai, 201620, China
E-mail: [a]310224877@qq.com, [b]qinyunfeng2010@sina.com, [c]happyjack@dhu.edu.cn, [d]phqin@dhu.edu.cn
www.dhu.edu.cn

Cellulose nanocrystals were extracted from cellulose raw material through hydrothermal process, and then polyaniline layer was coated on the surface of cellulose nanocrystals via in-situ chemical oxidative polymerization of aniline monomers. The resulting nanocomposite was investigated by scanning electron microscopy, Fourier transform infrared spectrometry, thermal gravimetric analysis, and gas sensing measurement. The results show the nanocomposite with good core-shell structure exhibited high thermal stability. For ammonia gas detection, high sensitivity, relative fast response, short recovery time, and good reproducibility can be achieved for the nanocomposite.

Keywords: Polyaniline; cellulose nanocrystals; nanocomposite; gas sensing; ammonia.

1. Introduction

Nanoconductive polymers have caused a great interest because of their low size and terrific electrical conductivities. Among those polymers, polyaniline is considered as the most promising conductive polymer owing to its unique properties such as acid/base doping/depoing chemistry, strong chemical stability, cheap and easy preparation and so on.[1,2] However the application range of polyaniline is limited due to its worse mechanical properties and easy to agglomeration. Recently, cellulose nanocrystals have been demonstrated to make up a promising new class of renewable nanomaterials as a support for conducting polymers due to their unique properties including nano-dimensions, high strength and light weight.[3,4] In this work, ultrathin polyaniline layer was coated on the surface of cellulose nanocrystals through in-situ chemical oxidative polymerization of aniline monomers, and its possible application as a gas sensing materials should be evaluated.

2. Experimental

2.1. *Materials*

Aniline monomers ($C_6H_5NH_2$) with a molar mass of 93 g/mol and a density of 1.02 g/cm^3 were purchased from Pinghu Reagent Co. Ltd. Ammonium peroxydisulfate (APS), hydrochloric acid (HCl) were obtained from Guoyao Group Chemical Reagent Co. Ltd., and used as received without any further purification.

2.2. *Preparation*

The cellulose nanocrytals were firstly extracted from cellulosic raw materials through hydrochloric acid hydrolysis under hydrothermal condition. The obtained product was washed with de-ionized water several times until it has a pH level of 7. Then the nanocomposite was prepared by chemical oxidation polymerization of aniline in the presence of the cellulose nanocrystals mentioned above. Firstly, cellulose nanocrystals were dispersed into 100 ml 1 M solution of HCl, and then 1 M HCl solution of aniline monomers were added into the above suspension under ultrasonic treatment for 30 min in an ice bath. When 1 M HCl solution containing the APS was added dropwise, the polymerization reaction of polyaniline carried out. After about 6 h, the resulting products were filtered, washed with deionized water several times, and then dried under vacuum at 60°C for 48 h. For comparison we also prepared pure polyaniline in the same way.

2.3. *Characterization*

The morphologies of nanocomposite were observed on HITACHI S-4800 field emission scanning electron microscopy (FE-SEM). The chemical structures were characterized on a Nicolet NEXUS 670 FTIR spectrometer with a resolution of 4 cm^{-1} over 32 scans. The thermal properties were characterized on a NETZSCH TG 209 F1 thermogravimetric analyzer at a heating rate of 20°C min^{-1} under nitrogen stream with a flow rate of 20 mL min^{-1}. The gas sensing properties were evaluated by monitoring the variation in the resistance as a function of time for different ammonia concentrations by using a digital multimeter (Agilent 34401A).

3. Results and Discussion

Morphology 3.1. Figure 1 gives the morphologies of celloluse nanocrystals and the resulting nanocomposite. The rod-like morphologies of celloluse nanocrystals could be observed, and its average diameter and length were about 20-30 nm and 200-250 nm, respectively. Due to polyaniline layer was uniformly coated to the surface of celloluse nanocrystals, the nanocomposite exhibited similar rod-like morphology but larger diameter. The results show that the nanocomposite had a good core-shell structure.

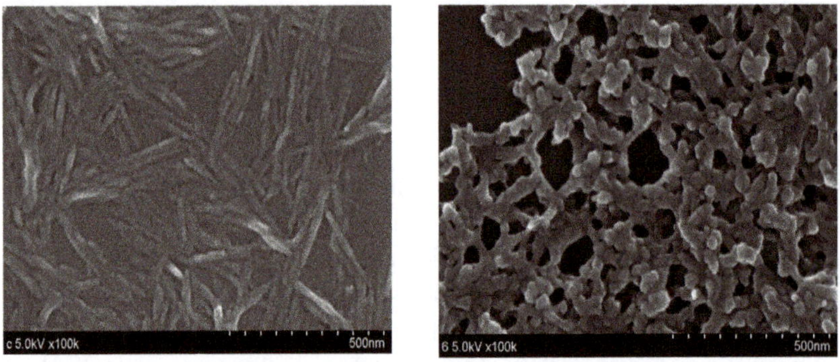

Fig. 1 SEM images for celloluse nanocrystals (left) and the resulting nanocomposite (right).

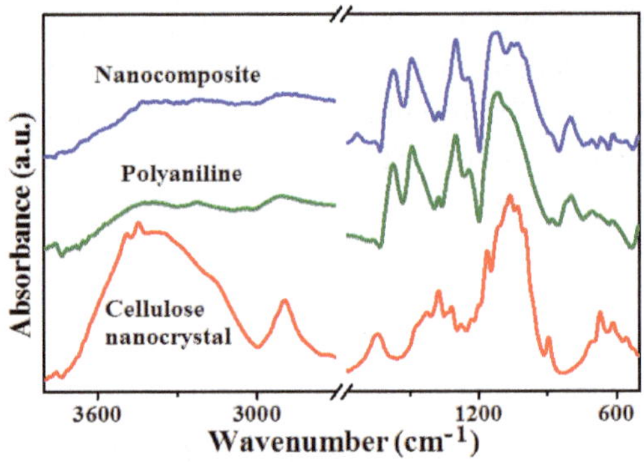

Fig. 2 FT–IR spectra of cellulose nanocrystals, pure polyaniline and the resulting nanocomposite.

Chemical structure 3.2. Figure 2 shows FT-IR specta of pure polyaniline, celloluse nanocrystals and the resulting nanocomposite. All the characteristic peaks of celloluse appeared in the FT-IR spectra. The bands at 1061, 2890, and 3406 cm^{-1} could be assigned to -C-O-C- stretching vibration, and the stretching vibration of aliphatic -CH_2 and -OH, respectively, and the bands at 1126, 1297, 1490, and 1568 cm^{-1} attributed to in-plane band vibration of C-H on the 1, 4-

desubtituted ring, C-N stretching vibration mode of the N-Ph-N unit, and C=C stretching vibration of benzenoid and quinoid rings, respectively. [5] These characteristic peaks of celloluse in the specta of the nanocomposite became weak due to the coverage of polyaniline layer. All the expected peaks of PANI, e.g., N-H-hydrogen bonding, C-N stretching, C-H-bonding, aromatic ring, benzenoid and quinoid ring deformations also appeared in the infrared spectrum of the nanoocomposite, however, some shifting in position is observed, which might be due to the interaction between cellulose nanocrystals with polyaniline.

Thermal stability 3.3. Figure 3 displays the TGA curves for cellulose nanocrystals, pure polyaniline and the resulting nanocomposite. For cellulose nanocrystals, three main degradation processes took place with the increase of the temperature. The initial stage of weight loss appearing before 100°C could be ascribed to the volatilization of H_2O, the second process which occurred near 285°C to 380°C was due to the remove of the molecular fragment such as -OH and $-CH_2-OH$, and the third process would be attributed to the decomposition of cellulose chains. For polyaniline, the weight loss below 120°C was attributed to volatilization of water absorbed by the polymer in the form of moisture. With the increasing of the temperature, weight losses observed for polyanilines in this temperature range have been attributed to evolution of the dopant and/or smaller chain oligomers. For temperatures higher than ~365°C, a significant weight loss takes place for both polyanilines, which could be attributed to thermal decomposition of the main molecular chain of the polymer. It can be clear found that the addition of cellulose nanocrystals improved greatly the thermal stability of polyaniline.

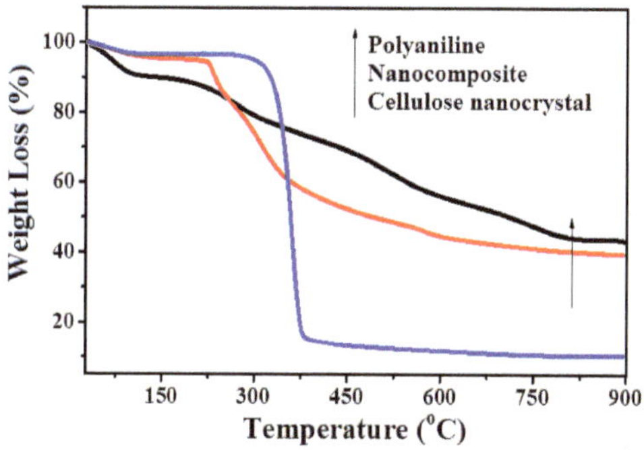

Fig. 3 TGA curves of cellulose nanocrystals, pure polyaniline and the resulting nanocomposite.

Sensing property 3.4. The response curves of the nanocomposite for the repeated exposure and removal of ammonia vapor with various concentrations were recorded at room temperature as shown in Fig. 4. The sensitivity can be represented by the relative resistance change (R/R_0), in which R_0 and R are the resistance for the nanocomposite before and after exposure to the ammonia vapor, respectively. It can be observed in Fig. 4 that when the composite fibers exposed to ammonia vapor, a rapid increase in the $\Delta R/R_0$ was found, which could be mainly contributed to the deprotonation of polyaniline. It is clear that a rapid response occurred when the nanocomposite exposed to ammonia vapor, and reached a maximum value within less than 10 s, and the recovery time varied slightly for less than 100 ppm ammonia vapor. Moreover, low detection limit of 10 ppm for composite fiber can be achieved. The high sensitivity of polyaniline coated cellulose nanocrystals may be attributed to the high surface area of the nanocrystals, which provided more active sites for the adsorption of ammonia molecules.

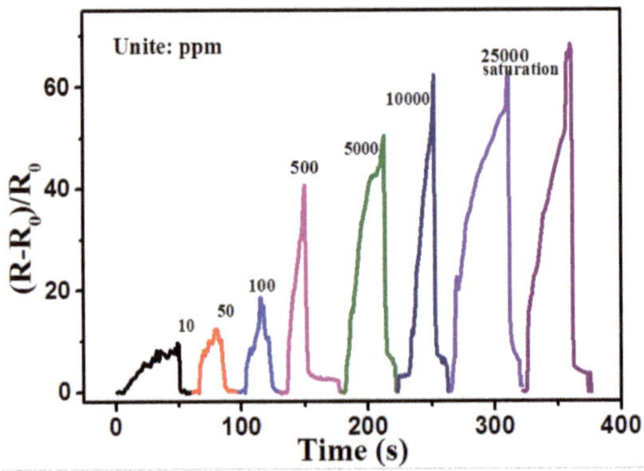

Fig. 4 Response curves as a function of time for cellulose nanocrystals, pure polyaniline and the resulting nanocomposite with various ammonia gas concentrations.

4. Summary

A simple and effective method to fabricate gas sensing nanocomposite based on polyaniline coated cellulose nanocrystals for ammonia detection has been demonstrated. The nanocomposite was prepared by in situ chemical oxidation polymerization of aniline in the presence of rod-like cellulose nanocomposite. The nanocomposite with good core-shell structure and high thermal stability were found to be highly responsive to gaseous ammonia over a wide concentration range, indicating a great potential in gas sensing applications.

Acknowledgments

Financial support from the Fundamental Research Funds for the Central Universities (2232013A3–02) is gratefully acknowledged.

References

1. T. Merian and N. Redon, Z. Zujovic, et al. Ultra sensitive ammonia sensors based on microwave synthesized nanofibrillar polyanilines, Sens. Actuators B **203**, 626 (2014).
2. A.L. Kukla, Y. M. Shirshov, S. A. Piletsky, et al. Ammonia sensors based on sensitive polyaniline films, Sens. Actuators B **37**, 135 (1996).
3. H. Peng, G. F. Ma, W. M. Ying, et al. In situ synthesis of polyaniline/sodium carboxymethyl cellulose nanorods for high-performance redox supercapacitors, J. Power Sources **211**, 40 (2012).
4. Y. C. Xie, Z. Y. Qin, J. Li, Preparation and characterization of conductive polypyrrole-nanocellulose crystal composite materials, J. Textile Research 34, 15 (2013).
5. J. Liu. Y. Lin, L. Liang, et al. Templateless assembly of molecularly aligned conductive polymer nanowires: A new approach for oriented nanostructures, Chem. –Eur. J. 9, 604 (2003).

The Catalytic Wet Air Oxidation of Phenol with Fe_2O_3 Nanoparticles

Duo Heng Cui, Yue Wan and Xu Chun Song†
Department of Chemistry, Fujian Normal University,
Fuzhou, P. R. China
†E-mail: songxuchunfj@163.com
www.fjnu.edu.cn

The Fe_2O_3 nanoparticles have been prepared by the co-precipitation and followed by calcination process. The as-prepared Fe_2O_3 nanoparticles were characterized by scanning electron microscopy (SEM), transmission electron microscopy (TEM), energy-dispersive X-ray analysis (EDS), and X-ray diffraction (XRD). Catalytic wet air oxidation of phenol with molecular oxygen using the Fe_2O_3 nanoparticles catalyst at different temperatures has been studied. The results showed that the catalytic activity of the Fe_2O_3 nanoparticles for phenol degradation can be increased with increasing the temperature, and the degradation of phenol catalyzed by the Fe_2O_3 nanoparticles fits the first-order kinetics.

Keywords: Fe_2O_3; catalytic wet air oxidation; phenol.

1. Introduction

The presence of organic compounds in the industrial wastewater has become a great concern due to toxicity to all living organism and their resistance to natural degradation. With the ever-increasing interest in environmentally friendly processes, catalysis is attracting considerable interests due to its potential in solving global environmental [1, 2]. Phenol is very harmful to organisms because it may cause health effects on the digestive system, heart, eye, lung, liver, skin and others. Therefore, people have been taking action to treat wastewaters containing phenol before entering the water stream. The catalytic wet air oxidation is a option to treat wastewaters containing phenol. The Co_3O_4 nanocubes was synthesized by a hydrothermal route, and tested for degradation of phenol in aqueous solution [3]. And the results show that Co_3O_4 nanocubes has the highest catalytic activity. Catalytic wet air oxidation of phenol with molecular oxygen using Co-doped Fe_3O_4 nanoparticles catalyst at mild operating conditions (308.15-353.15K) has been studied, and cobalt ions doping can improve the catalytic activity of Fe_3O_4 nanoparticles in phenol degradation [4]. The Fe/activated carbon catalyst exhibits the high catalytic performance for the catalytic decomposition of phenol in aqueous solution [5]. The catalytic activity towards the catalytic degradation of phenol over Co_3O_4 nanorods was studied under continuous bubbling of air through the liquid phase [6]. To the best of our knowledge, the investigation on the catalytic wet air oxidation of phenol by Fe_2O_3 nanoparticles has never been reported before. In this work, we report the catalytic wet air oxidation of phenol with oxygen using the Fe_2O_3 nanoparticles. The catalytic performance of the Fe_2O_3 nanoparticles for the phenol degradation in aqueous solution was investigated.

2. Experimental Section

2.1. *Synthesis of the Fe_2O_3 nanoparticles*

The Fe_2O_3 nanoparticles were synthesized via the co-precipitation and followed by calcination process. Experimental details were as follows: 4.56g of $FeSO_4 \cdot 7H_2O$ and 4.44g of $FeCl_3 \cdot 6H_2O$ were dissolved in 60 ml of 0.01M HCl to form a transparent solution. Then the mixture was added to 80 ml of NH_4OH (3M) with the reaction mixture vigorously stirred at 80°C for 3h. After the reaction was completed, the precipitate was filtered, washed several times with distilled water and anhydrous ethanol, and dried in an oven at 50°C for 24h. The as-prepared products was further calcined at 550°C for 4h.

2.2. *Characterization*

The morphologies of the as-prepared products were characterized using a Hitachi S-4700 field emission scanning electron microscope (SEM, scanning voltages 15 kV) and Tecnai G2 F30 transmission electron microscopy (TEM, accelerating voltage 200 kV). The composition of the products was investigated by energy dispersive X-ray detector (EDS, Thermo Noran VANTAG-ESI). The phase structure of the obtained products were analyzed with a Thermo ARL SCINTAG X'TRA diffractometer using Cu Kα radiation (λ= 0.154056 nm), and recorded with 2θ ranging from 20–80°C.

2.3. *Catalytic experiments*

The catalytic wet air oxidation of phenol was carried out in a 50 mL reactor containing 100mg/l of phenol solution. Then 0.05 g of the Fe_2O_3 nanoparticles were placed in reactor. The reactor was attached to a stand and dipped in a water bath with a temperature controller, and air was continuously bubbled during the reaction. The catalytic experiments were carried out at 308.15K, 323.15K, 338.15K and 353.15K, respectively. At given reaction time intervals, analytical samples were drawn from the suspension and subsequently centrifuged to remove the Fe_2O_3 catalysts. The concentration of phenol was analyzed by measuring the absorptions at wavelength 270 nm using a UV759S UV-Vis spectrophotometer.

3. Results and Discussion

The morphology and the particle size of the Fe_2O_3 nanoparticles were investigated by SEM and TEM. Fig. 1a shows a representative SEM image of the Fe_2O_3 samples, clearly indicating that the prepared Fe_2O_3 products are nanoparticles with crystallite size of 80-120 nm. Fig. 1b shows TEM image of the Fe_2O_3 nanoparticles. The TEM image of the Fe_2O_3 nanoparticles further confirms that as-prepared products consist of nanoparticles. The detailed structure of the Fe_2O_3 nanoparticles were further investigated by HRTEM (inset of Fig. 1b). It can be seen that clear lattice fringes have easily manifested the high crystallinity of the samples. The fringe spacing of the samples is about 0.368nm, which correspond to the (012) atomic spacings.

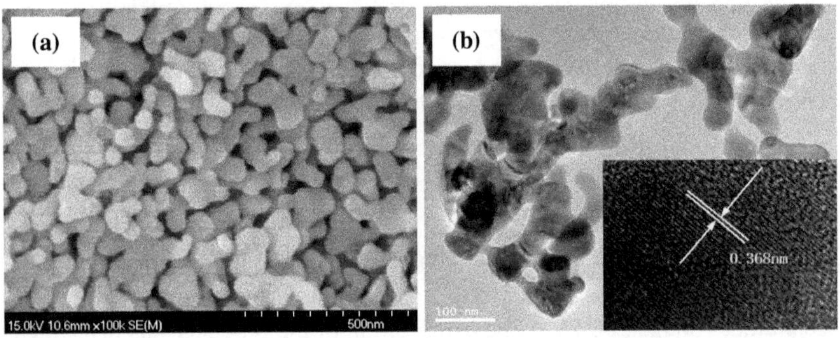

Fig. 1 SEM(a) and TEM (b) images of the Fe_2O_3 nanoparticles.

Energy dispersive spectrometry (EDS) analysis was used to determine the element composition of the Fe_2O_3 nanoparticles and the results were shown in Fig. 2. The obvious signals for Fe and O elements were observed, and the resulsts from EDS confirm that the molar ratio of Fe/O existed in the Fe_2O_3 nanoparticles is 2/3. This result would be reasonable to believe that the the final products is Fe_2O_3. No other elements can be detected in Fig. 2, indicating the high purity of the Fe_2O_3 nanoparticles.

The phase structure of the Fe_2O_3 nanoparticles were analyzed by powder X-ray diffraction. Fig. 3 shows the XRD patterns of the as-obtained products at 550°C. It can be seen that all of the peaks of the XRD pattern can be indexed to α-Fe_2O_3 (JCPDS Card No. 39-1346). The XRD patterns indicate that Fe_2O_3

nanoparticles were obtained at 550°C under calcination. No characteristic peaks of other impurity phases have been detected, indicating that the final product is of high purity.

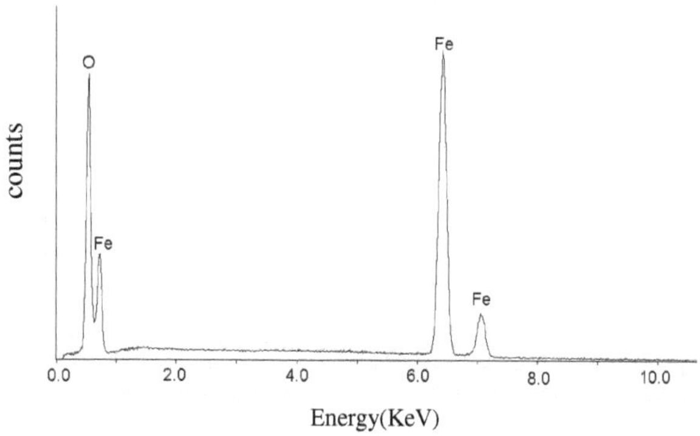

Fig. 2 EDS spectrum of the Fe_2O_3 nanoparticles.

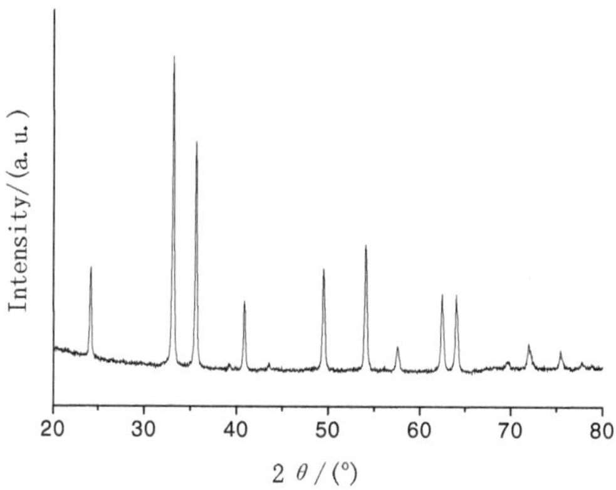

Fig. 3 XRD pattern of the Fe_2O_3 nanoparticles.

The catalytic activity of the Fe_2O_3 nanoparticles on the oxidation of phenols has been studied in the presence of air as oxidant. Fig. 4 shows the catalytic efficiency of the as-obtained sample for phenol degradation at different temperatures. It can be seen that percentage of phenol degradation is 21.8, 25.2, 40.9, and 83.7% within 12h over the Fe_2O_3 nanoparticles at 308.15K, 323.15K, 338.15K and 353.15K, respectively. The catalytic activity of the Fe_2O_3 nanoparticles for phenol degradation can be increased with the temperature increased. The degradation of phenol can be catalyzed by the Fe_2O_3 nanoparticles fits the first-order kinetics and the catalytic reaction can be described by:

$$\ln\left(\frac{C}{C_0}\right) = -kt \tag{1}$$

Where C_0 is the initial concentration, C is the concentration of phenol during the degradation time, k is the apparent rate constant and t is the degradation time. As can be seen from Fig. 5, k is found to be 0.01656, 0.02151, 0.03788 and 0.13086 h^{-1} (the correlation coefficient of linear fitting R = 0.9206, 0.9839, 0.9916 and 0.9578) for the Fe_2O_3 nanoparticles at 308.15K, 323.15K, 338.15K and 353.15K, respectively.

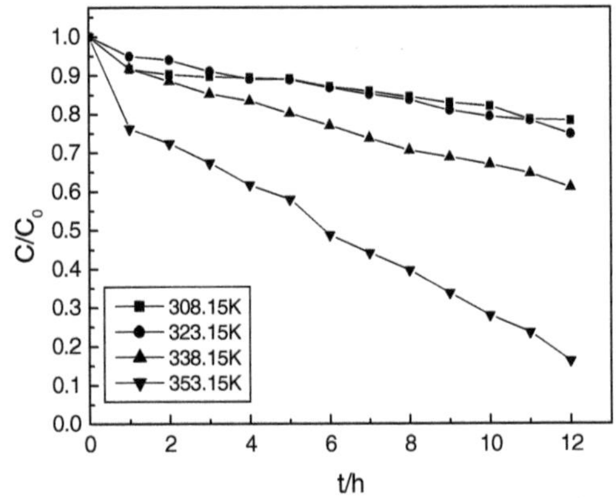

Fig. 4 Degradation rate of phenol at different temperatures.

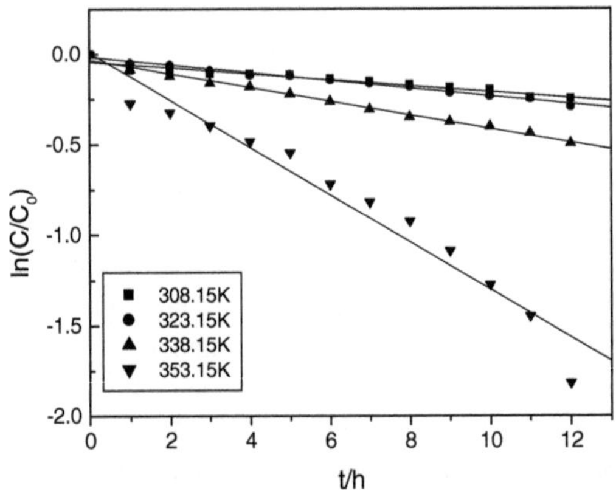

Fig. 5 First-order plots for the catalytic degradation of phenol by the Fe_2O_3 nanoparticles.

4. Conclusions

In summary, the nano-Fe_2O_3 catalysts have been successfully synthesis. The results show that the prepared Fe_2O_3 products are nanoparticles with crystallite size of 80-120 nm. The Fe_2O_3 nanoparticles are a kind of novel environmental friendly material to be used for degradation of phenol. The Fe_2O_3 nanoparticles showed the high catalytic performance for the catalytic degradation of the aqueous phenol. The reaction of the degradation of phenol by the Fe_2O_3 nanoparticles fits the first-order kinetics model. The present work suggests that the Fe_2O_3 nanoparticles is a promising catalyst for environmental remediation.

References

1. Y. Hardjono, H. Sun, H. Tian, C. E. Buckley and S. Wang, Synthesis of Co oxide doped carbon aerogel catalyst and catalytic performance in heterogeneous oxidation of phenol in water, *Chem. Eng. J.* **174**, 376 (2011).
2. W. T. Li, W. Z. Huang, H. Zhou, H. Y. Yin, Y. F. Zheng and X. C. Song, Synthesis and photoactivity enhancement of Ba doped Bi_2WO_6 photocatalyst, *Mater. Res. Bull.* **64**, 432 (2015).
3. X. C. Song, Z. A. Yang, Y. F. Zheng and H. Y. Yin, Catalytic degradation of phenol by Co_3O_4 nanocubes, *Current Nanosci.* **9**, 128 (2013).
4. X. C. Song, Y. F. Zheng and H. Y. Yin, Catalytic wet air oxidation of phenol over Co-doped Fe_3O_4 nanoparticles, *J. Nanopart. Res.* 15, 1856 (2013).
5. A. Quintanilla, J. A. Casas, A. F. Mohedano and J. J. Rodriguez, Reaction pathway of the catalytic wet air oxidation of phenol with a Fe/activated carbon catalyst, *App. Catal. B* 67, 206 (2006).
6. T. L. Lai, Y. L. Lai, C. C. Lee, Y. Y. Shu and C. B. Wang, Microwave-assisted rapid fabrication of Co_3O_4 nanorods and application to the degradation of phenol, *Catal. Today* 131, 105 (2008).

Co-Effect of Oxygen and Spontaneous Polarization on Resistance Variation in Y-Mn co-doped $BaTiO_3$ Ceramics Through Heat Treatment

Fangzhou Zhao† and Quanxi Cao

School of Advanced Materials and Nanotechnology, Xidian University, Xi'an, Shaanxi, China

†E-mail: 422980526@qq.com

In low oxygen partial pressure atmosphere, resistance variation of Y-Mn co-doped barium titanate ($BaTiO_3$) through 500℃ ~ 700℃ heat treatment which could be a convenient method to reduce resistance of sintered elements, was investigated. Co-effect of oxygen and spontaneous polarization during this process was discussed qualitatively to explain the different quantity variation of room temperature resistance and maximum resistance in resistance-temperature (R-T) characteristic profiles.

Keywords: $BaTiO_3$; oxygen; spontaneous polarization; heat treatment.

1. Introduction

Barium titanate ($BaTiO_3$) based positive temperature coefficient resistance (PTCR) is widely used in electronics industry, systematic research on interactions between oxygen concentration and resistance of the elements has been conducted these decades [1, 2, 3]. Degradation of the PTC behavior caused by oxygen loss in reduced ambient has been demonstrated by authors. Simultaneously origination of PTC effect has been confirmed from the grain boundary and the importance of spontaneous polarization (P_s) is recognized gradually [4, 5, 6, 7, 8, 9].

Due to the complexity of grain boundary the elements are sensitive to composition and process conditions. Hence it is difficult to obtain a quantitative model of interaction between Ps and various defects. Nevertheless through certain heat treatment we could achieve a qualitative model consisting of oxygen loss and spontaneous polarization regions.

We investigated the variety of resistance of Y-Mn co-doped $BaTiO_3$ through 500°C ~ 700°C heat treatment in low oxygen partial pressure atmosphere. Elements exhibited weaker PTC effect and the maximum resistance (R_{max}) had a significantly larger decrease than room temperature resistance (R_{25}).

Concerning treatment temperature, except oxygen concentration, factors which could affect element resistance changed little contrast to sintering temperature (1350°C). We believe the resistance variation is mainly caused by oxygen loss. Hence we could discuss a model of nearly one parameter (oxygen concentration) for convenience. In this contribution, the influence of oxygen was discussed with respect to P_s.

The less decrease in R_{25} revealed that a large proportion of losing oxygen in heat treatment was compensated by P_s before the treatment. Simultaneously huge decrease in R_{max} showed that overall oxygen loss mainly contributed the barrier height of untreated elements in elevated temperature. By proposing qualitatively model, we consider the oxygen loss region is closer to grain boundary core than spontaneous polarization region, outside which the oxygen loss resulted in ΔR_{25}. Based on discussion of boundary structure in $BaTiO_3$ PTCR, we analyzed the relationship between P_s and oxygen loss through heat treatment and the reasonability of our model.

2. Experiment

2.1. *Resistance reduction*

Sintered at 1300°C in air atmosphere, Y-Mn co-doped $BaTiO_3$ PTCR were prepared through conventional solid method. We labeled the elements as 1# and 2# (20 specimens each group, coated aluminum as electrodes) whose average R_{25} were around 1KΩ and 5KΩ, respectively.

Appropriate amount $MgCO_3$, $ZnCO_3$, NH_4HCO_3, $(CH_3COO)_2Ca$, $SrTiO(C_2O_4)\cdot 4H_2O$ and powders of carbon, iron, zinc and aluminum (mol% of 0.30, 0.30, 0.30, 2.99, 0.60, 50.75, 14.93, 14.93 and 14.90, respectively) were mixed as resistance reduction reagent to create low oxygen partial pressure atmosphere. 1# and 2# elements were separately placed in two covered ceramic crucibles with mass ratio to the reagent of 3:1. The crucibles were heated to 500°C~700°C for 60min~180min in a muffle furnace.

Resistance-temperature (R-T) characteristic were measured by ZWX-B PTCR R-T characteristic automatic measurement system (Huazhong University of Science and Technology, China) and the representative results of one specimen in each group were showed in Fig. 1.

To the two specimens, decrease of R_{max} was much larger than that of R_{25}. Comparative data were showed in Tab 1. Other specimens in two groups had similar situation.

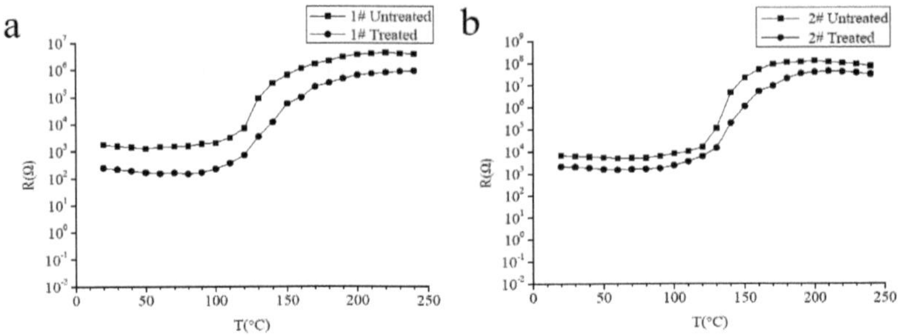

Fig. 1 Representative R-T characteristic: (a) Group 1; (b) Group 2.

Table 1 Resistance variation of specimens through heat treatment.

Group	Untreated		Treated			
	R_{25} [KΩ]	R_{max} [MΩ]	R_{25} [KΩ]	R_{max} [MΩ]	ΔR_{25} [KΩ]	ΔR_{max} [MΩ]
1#	1.674	4.27	0.234	0.91	1.44	3.36
2#	6.459	123	2.042	42.7	4.507	80.3

2.2. *Resistance restoration*

To eliminate the effect of stress relief in grain boundaries [10], the two treated groups were placed in empty crucibles without resistance reduction reagent and undergone the same process in the muffle furnace as before. Their R_{25} restored to the state before the heat treatment.

3. Mechanism Analysis

After heat treatment, ΔR_{25} was dramatically less than ΔR_{max}, which can't be explained just considering the oxygen consumption. To discuss why the same amount of consumed oxygen resulted in different variation of R_{25} and R_{max}, phase transition around Curie temperature (T_c) and grain boundary structure should be taken into account.

3.1. *Model of heat treatment effect in grain boundaries*

According to Heywang's model [11], in grain boundaries of donor-doped $BaTiO_3$ ceramic, dopants and defects formed approximate two-dimensional acceptor interface. The interface constituted Shottky barrier on grain surface and formed high resistance layer in elevated temperature.

Adsorbed oxygen in grain boundary makes great contribution to element resistance [1]. Usually, oxygen diffusion along grain boundary is more active than grain interior [12, 13] especially in temperature range of our experiment.

Oxygen concentration change should be primarily responsible for ΔR_{25} and ΔR_{max} contrast to other factors (stress relief, other defects diffusion, etc) in grain boundary. For simplicity, one model in single boundary with respect of P_s is proposed in Fig. 2.

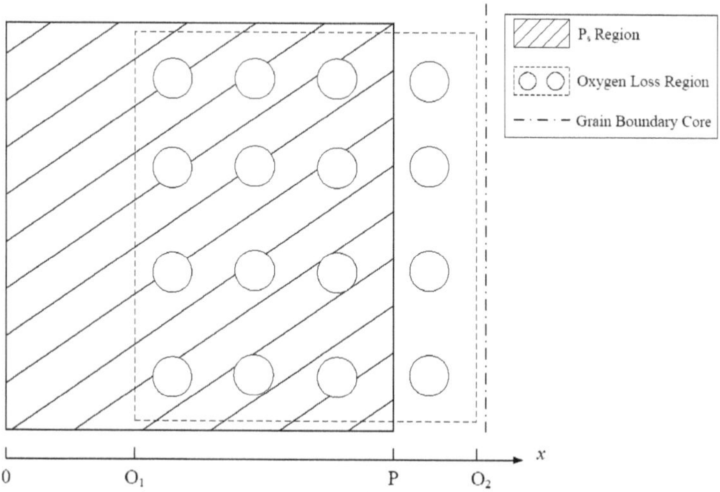

Fig. 2 Single grain boundary model with respect of P_s and oxygen loss. X axis and points is for comparison with Fig. 3.

As previously described, when P_s existed, compensated regions in grain boundaries were main conductive paths [14]. Combined with our experiments, decrease of R_{25} revealed that boundary barrier consisted by oxygen was not completely compensated.

Referred to calculation of Chao Fang and Liangyan Chen [15] which revealed acceptors had a higher concentration near grain boundary core, we consider oxygen loss region (O_1 to O_2) is closer to boundary core than Ps region (0 to P) in Fig. 2. In this model, we assume acceptor state oxygen was completely compensated in overlap area (O_1 to P) of oxygen loss region and P_s region at room temperature. Outside P_s region (P to O_2), oxygen loss in heat treatment is the origin of ΔR_{25}. And the huge ΔR_{max} could represent the resistance value from losing oxygen in grain boundaries when $T > T_c$.

For further explanation, in Fig. 3 we define oxygen concentration in grain boundary as a function of x (using the same x axis as Fig. 2). Thus ΔR_{25} and ΔR_{max} can be treated in appropriate integral form. Since elements contain various boundaries, relationship between ΔR and oxygen concentration can be described as follows.

$$\Delta R_{25} \propto \int_{P}^{O_2} \left[C_0(x) - C_1(x) \right] \mathrm{d}x. \quad (1)$$

$$\Delta R_{max} \propto \int_{O_1}^{O_2} \left[C_0(x) - C_1(x) \right] \mathrm{d}x. \quad (2)$$

Thus we can explain the difference of ΔR_{25} and ΔR_{max} qualitatively and the reasonability of our model could be illustrated furthermore.

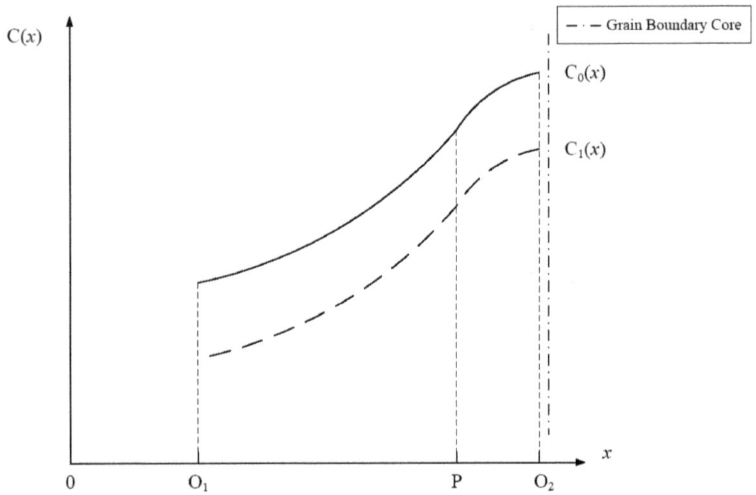

Fig. 3. Variation of oxygen concentration through heat treatment. $C_0(x)$ and $C_1(x)$ are oxygen concentration profiles before and after heat treatment respectively.

3.2. *Reasonability of the model*

The PTC effect originates in the grain boundary only and behaves differently in each boundary [5]. Makoto Kuwabara, Ken-ichiro Morimo and Tatsuya Matsunaga [7] investigated R-T characteristics of strictly single-grain boundaries in semiconducting barium titanate ceramic bars. The R-T characteristics can be classified into three types: (1) normal type PTCR characteristics, (2) saw-tooth type PTCR characteristics and (3) flat type PTCR characteristics. Thus, distribution of the first two kind boundaries actually dominates the R-T characteristics of elements.

Effect of grain boundaries microstructure on R-T characteristics has been confirmed [16]. Grain orientation is the primary factor impacting resistance behavior of single grain boundary. Relative experimental evidence on bi-crystals indicated that the high-coherent grain boundaries, e.g., low angle and coincidence site lattice boundaries (Σ3, Σ5, and Σ9 grain boundaries) showed low or even no PTC-effect, while the incoherent or random large angle grain boundaries were electrically active [16, 17, 18].

Conclusion above is important to our experiment because adsorbed oxygen is difficult to generate in coherent boundaries [19]. Thus we can focus on the situation in ordinary boundaries with low coherence which should mainly affect resistance variation through heat treatment. In these boundaries, P_s component vertical to the boundary is less than that in coherent boundaries. The region edge affected by polarization is further from the boundary core. Thus compensation of absorbed oxygen is weaker than the situation in coherent boundaries. Our model above showed this in a qualitative manner.

Stress relief and grain orientation are important factors affecting element resistance. Concerning with these, we firstly confirmed that the resistance decrease was not caused by stress relief because that kind of decrease is irreversible. Secondly grain orientation is dominated in early stage of sinter process in element manufacture [20] and it is fixed in later high temperature process. Temperature of our treatment couldn't provide appropriate dynamic for grain reorientation.

In conclusion, we believed our treatment nearly just changed one parameter (oxygen concentration around grain boundary region) and could give a qualitative explain to experiment phenomenon.

3.3. *Compensation mode of spontaneous polarization*

Since grain orientation didn't change through treatment, distribution of P_s intensity also remained unchanged. Based on resistance variation of heat treatment, compensation mode of P_s isn't just subtracting a constant resistance from R_{max}. P_s can decrease elements resistance in proportion to R_{max}. Hence we can treat compensation of P_s as a proportional one.

According to our model, width of spontaneous polarization region is in proportion to that of grain boundary. This ratio remained constant during the heat treatment. We consider the proportional property of microstructure may result in proportional compensation of P_s.

4. Conclusions

According to experiment conditions and analysis, conclusions can be made as follows.

1. In oxygen loss during the heat treatment, the part which couldn't be completely compensated by P_s below T_c formed ΔR_{25}. Total oxygen loss in grain

boundaries formed ΔR_{max}. Resistance of elements is determined by P_s and oxygen concentration in boundaries.

2. P_s compensated the grain boundary barrier in proportion to R_{max}. We believe this originated from width of P_s region is in proportion to that of grain boundary.

If R-T character and profile of oxygen concentration versus position in a single grain boundary can be obtained exactly before and after heat treatment, it is possible to acquire the compensation range of P_s.

3. Our experiment provided a convenient method to treat sintered elements for resistance control. In actual production, it is possible to reduce element resistance more effectively. Elements with resistance exceeding customers' requirement could be treated to obtain access to market again.

References

1. G. H. Jonker, Halogen treatment of barium titanate semiconductors, *Mater. Res. Bull* **2**, 401 (1967).
2. M. Kuwabara, Determination of the potential barrier height in barium titanate ceramics, *Solid-State Electron* **27**, 929 (1984).
3. F. D. Morrison, A. M. Coats, D. C. Sinclair and A. R. West, Charge compensation mechanism in la-doped $BaTiO_3$, *J. Electroceram* **6**, 219 (2001).
4. G. H. Jonker, Some aspects of semiconducting barium titanate, *Solid-State Electron* **7**, 895 (1964).
5. H. Nemoto and I. Oda, Direct examination of PTC action of single grain boundaries in semiconducting $BaTiO_3$ ceramics, *J. Am. Ceram. Soc* **63**, 398 (1980).
6. B. Huybrechts, K. Ishizaki and M. Takata, Experimental evaluation of the acceptor-states compensation in positive-temperature-coefficient-type barium titanate, *J. Am. Ceram. Soc* **75**, 772 (1992).
7. M. Kuwabara, K. Morimo and T. Matsunaga, Single-grain boundaries in PTC resistors, *J. Am. Ceram. Soc* **79**, 997 (1996).
8. J.H. Hou, Z.L. Zhang, W. Preis, W. Sitte and G. Dehm, Electrical properties and structure of grain boundaries in n-conducting $BaTiO_3$ ceramics, *J. Eur. Ceram. Soc* **31**, 763 (2011).
9. J.L. Liu, S.P. Gong, L. Quan, B.B. Chen and D.X. Zhou, Reoxidnation effects of Ba excessive barium titanate ceramics for laminated positive temperature coefficient thermistors, *J. Am. Ceram. Soc* **95**, 1640 (2012).

10. G.S. Liu and R. D. Roseman, Secondary thermal treatment effect on PTCR $BaTiO_3$, *J. Mater. Sci. Lett* **18**, 1875 (1999).
11. W. Heywang, Bariumtitanat als sperrschichthalbleiter, *Solid-State Electron* **3**, 51 (1961).
12. A. Hasegawa, S. Fujitsu, K. Koumoto and H. Yanagida, The enhanced penetration of oxygen along the grain boundary in semiconducting barium titanate, *Jpn. J. Appl. Phys* **30**, 1252 (1991).
13. W. Preis and W. Sitte, Modeling of fast diffusion along grain boundaries in oxide ceramics, *Solid State Ion* **179**, 765 (2008).
14. S. B. Desu and D. A. Payne, Interfacial segregation in perovskites I Theory, *J. Am. Ceram. Soc* **73**, 3391 (1990).
15. C. Fang and L.Y. Chen, The PTCR effect induced by grain boundary segregation in acceptor, *Advanced Materials Research* **750-752**, 1003 (2013).
16. K. Hayashi, T. Yamamoto and T. Sakuma, Grain orientation dependence of the PTCR effect in niobium-doped barium titanate, *J. Am. Ceram. Soc* **79**, 3669 (1996).
17. K. Hayashi, T. Yamamoto, Y. Ikuhara and T. Sakuma, Formation of potential barrier related to grain-boundary character in semiconducting barium titanate, *J. Am. Ceram. Soc* **83**, 2684 (2000).
18. S. Y. Choi, J. P. Buban, M. Nishi, H. Kageyama, N. Shibata, T. Yamamoto, S. J. L. Kang and Y. Ikuhara, Dislocation structure of low-angle boundaries in Nb-doped $SrTiO_3$ bicrystals, *J. Mater. Sci* **41**, 2621 (2006).
19. H. Ogawa, M. Demura, T. Yamamoto and T. Sakuma, Estimation of PTCR effect in single grain boundary of Nb-doped $BaTiO_3$, *J. Mater. Sci. Lett* **14**, 537 (1995).
20. J. Seaton and C. Leach, Evolution of low sigma grain boundaries in PTC thermistors during sintering, *J. Eur. Ceram. Soc* **25**, 3055 (2005).

Research on the Powder TiH_2-45Al-4Sn by Mechanical Alloying*

Zhou Huimin[a], Chen Hua[b] and Zou Yang[c]
School of Material Science and Engineering, Changchun University of Technology, Changchun, China
Email: [a]1182822159@qq.com, [b]chenhua@mail.ccut.edu.cn, [c]413821193@qq.com

Mechanical alloying (MA) as a powder metallurgy method is often used to prepare materials with ultrafine grain and special structure difficultly obtained in conventional ways. In this paper, the $TiH_2$45Al4Sn (at. %) composite powder was mechanically milled by high energy ball milling. The crystalline grain size, morphology and phase characteristic of milled powder with different milling time were investigated by XRD, SEM and TEM. The results show that with the milling time increasing, the powder particles are refined rapidly in the initial stage and then gradually become stable. The new phase Ti_2Sn_3 is formed by mechanical alloying (MA) of TiH_2, Al, Sn powders during milling which resulted particles refinement to very small size. The homogeneous and dense Ti_2Al and Ti_2Sn_3 intermetallic compounds are obtained after vacuum hot pressing sintering, which microstructure is composed of equal axial Ti_2Al as matrix and fine Ti_2Sn_3 particles. Because of the addition of Sn, Ti-Al intermetallic compounds formation is inhibited during MA and sintering. However, Sn contributes to the formation of Ti_2Al phase which which is difficult to be obtained with the conventional method of casting and forging.

Keywords: TiH_2, Al, Sn; powder; mechanical alloying.

1. Introduction

Mechanical alloying is a feasible method for preparing fine and homogeneous alloy powder, which can not only increase the structure uniformity of the sintering sample but also improve its strength and ductility [1-6]. Moreover, Some intermetallic compounds difficultly obtained by conventional way can be got by this method [7-10]. This paper studies the mixed powder particle and phase change characteristic in the high-energy ball milling process as well as the combination reaction of Ti-Sn and Ti-Al to lay the foundation for the application of this alloy.

* This work is supported by No.51371038 of the National Natural Science Foundation.

2. Experimental

TiH_2 and Sn powder (average particle size above 50μm, purity>99%) and Al powder (average particle size above 74μm, purity>99.5%) were used as experimentally raw materials to fabricate alloy powder. The powder with chemical composition of TiH_2-45Al-4Sn (at.%) was milled by three dimensional high-energy pendular ball mill. The optimized milling parameters are as follows: Powder was firstly mixed for 30 minutes at the speed of 330r/min then milled to 40h at the speed of 400r/min. In the process of ball milling, sufficient cooling was needed after successive 5h milling to prevent powder from overheating and take some powder out. The ratio of grinding ball to mixed powder was 10:1, and the grinding ball made of GCr15 has two different diameters of 10mm and 15mm respectively. Alcohol was added as a control agent at room temperature. Structural transformation of the powder during high energy ball milling was observed by X-ray diffraction (XRD), electron microscopy (TEM) and scanning electron microscope (SEM).

3. Results and Discussion

3.1. *The morphology and phase characteristic of milled powder*

The mixed powder collided with the grinding ball and tank inside wall and was extruded by them, which made powder particles deform, crush and refine. In the initial stage, the powder particles were refined quickly, and then wouldn't be changed and tend to be stable. However, welding and aggregation occurred later in the high energy ball milling.

The morphology and microstructure of original powders are illustrated in Fig. 1(a)-(c). It shows that TiH_2 powder particles are in irregular shapes, Al particles emerge in spherical shapes and Sn particles are mainly oval-shaped. The difference of the morphology of original powders is caused by different preparation processes. Elemental powder underwent obvious refinement after high energy ball milling. The microstructure and morphology of the milled powders evolved for different milling time in the case of high energy ball milling (550r/min) are illustrated in Fig. 2. The particle size of the mixed powder decreased quickly in the first 10h but the particle size distribution is nonuniform with the visible TiH_2 particles in irregular shape (Fig. 2(a)). Al and Sn powders were easily bonded to the powder particles TiH_2 in the process of milling because of their low hardness. After milling for 20 h, TiH_2 powder particles were changed from irregular shape to circular shape and there are small particles of Al and Sn distributing on the surface of TiH_2 particles with a size of 30μm(Fig. 2(b)).

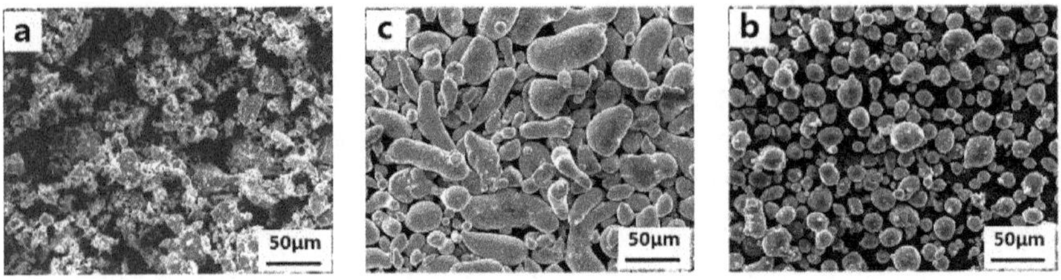

Fig. 1 SEM micrographs of the original powders of (a) TiH2; (b) Al; (c) Sn.

As shown in Fig. 2(c)-(d), particles became smaller and more homogeneous with further milling. However, the surface energy of milled powder enhanced after refinement and appeared aggregation because of mutual adsorption of powders, subsequently forming even larger particles. Furthermore, cold welding and combination between powder particles were found owing to the continuing collisions with high energy The result is also verified by TEM and XRD shown in Fig. 3.

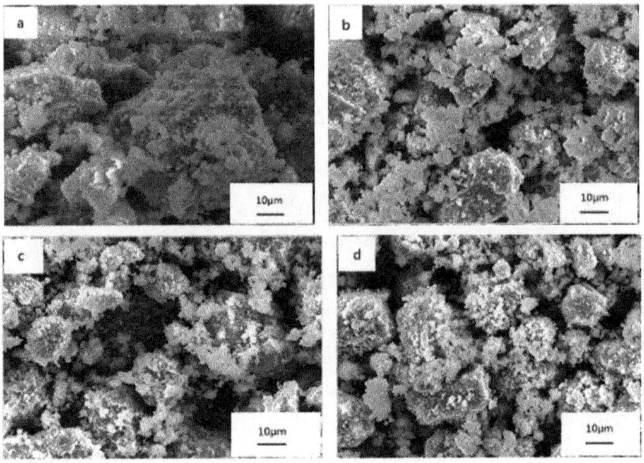

Fig. 2 SEM micrographs of TiH2-45Al-4Sn powders mechanically milled for (a)10h; (b)20h; (c)30h ; (d)40h.

The TEM morphology and electron diffraction photographs of powders mechanically milled for 20h, 35h and 40h are showed in Fig. 3. That is layer structure inserted by some smaller particles with a size of a few nanometers (Fig. 3(a)-(b)). Formation of this "sandwich" structure is the result of fracture and continuing welding under successive collision of high speed and forceful pressure high energy. Through the transmission diffraction spot analysis, the phase marked by the arrow in Fig. 3(a) and (b) is Ti_2Sn_3. Ti and Sn were synthesized because of the gradual refinement of powder with high interfacial energy and the increasing of the rate of diffusion between atoms of powder.

Consequently the new phase was generated easily under the low-temperature condition when the powder particles were refined to a certain extent. The intermetallic compounds between Ti and Al wouldn't be found during the ball milling, which demonstrates that chemical affinity between Ti and Sn is larger.

The TEM morphology and regional diffraction spots of powders milled for 40h are showed in Fig. 3(c). As the milling time increases, the particle diameter of the powder constantly decreased but appeared agglomeration. The powder sheet is thin within the diffraction region and the intermittent polycrystalline ring showed the phase is $TiH_{1.94}$, illustrating TiH_2 decomposition occurs during milling and the ball milling process is advantageous to H to escape.

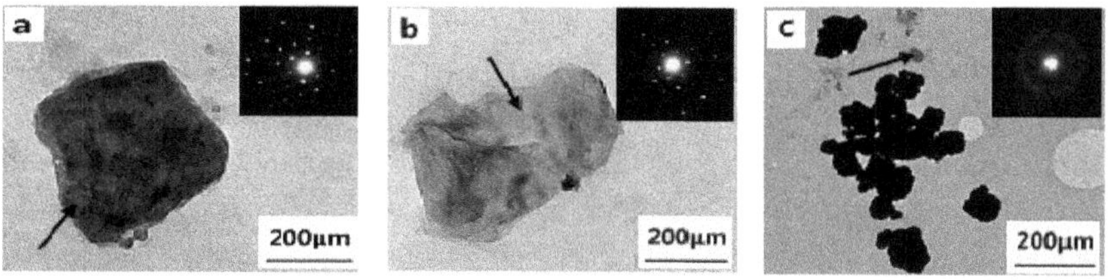

Fig. 3 The TEM morphology and electron diffraction photographs of TiH2-45Al-4Sn powders mechanically milled for (a) 20h; (b)35h; (c)40h.

The X-ray diffraction patterns of Ti-Al-Sn composite powders milled for different milling time are shown in Fig. 4. It is noted that the peaks of three kinds of elemental powder are obvious in the early stage. Subsequently the peak broadening is observed with the milling time increasing. Sn element powder gradually disappeared when milled for 20h. Formation of Ti_2Sn_3 phase also coincides with the analysis of TEM of the powder milled for 20h. The peak of Al exists all the time and gradually broadens, indicating Al powder underwent refinement in the milling process for 40 h. In the mean time, with the milling time increasing, the peak of TiH_2 broadens obviously and H element escapes from the TiH_x continuingly.

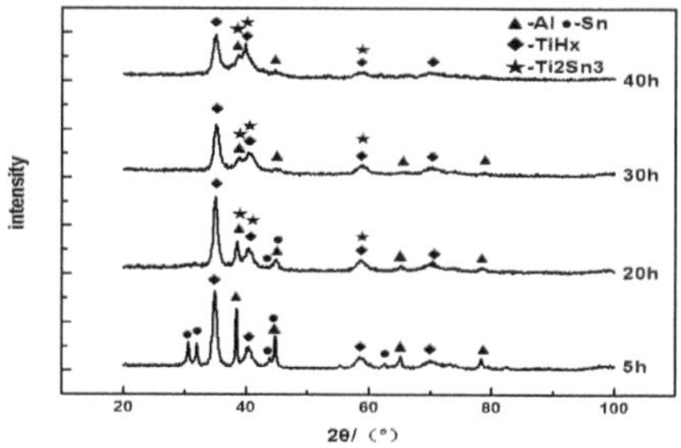

Fig. 4 The X-ray diffraction patterns of Ti-Al-Sn composite powders milled for different milling time.

3.2. *Sintered Organization*

The SEM micrograph and X-ray diffraction of Vacuum sintering microstructure of the powder milled for 40h are showed in Fig. 5. The sintered structure is very homogeneous and dense (Fig. 5(a)). It can be concluded that the structure consist of Ti_2Al and Ti_2Sn_3 intermetallic compounds. The microstructure is composed of equal axial Ti_2Al as matrix and fine Ti_2Sn_3 particles. As is shown above, Ti_2Sn_3 phase had been formed during the milling process so its grain size is very small, only a few nanometers.

When the fine powder including TiH_x phase sintering, it decomposed firstly with H all escaping, then Ti and Al combined rapidly to form Ti_2Al phase whose structure is fine with the small grain size about 2-5 μ m.

Compared with TiH_2-45Al, Ti_2Sn_3 and Ti_2Al were formed with Sn addition (Fig. 5(b)) and the sintered TiH_2-45Al generated Ti_3Al and TiAl phases. Obviously, formation of compound phase between Ti and Al is inhibited with Sn addition, subsequently gaining the Ti_2Al phase difficultly obtained with the method of casting and forging.

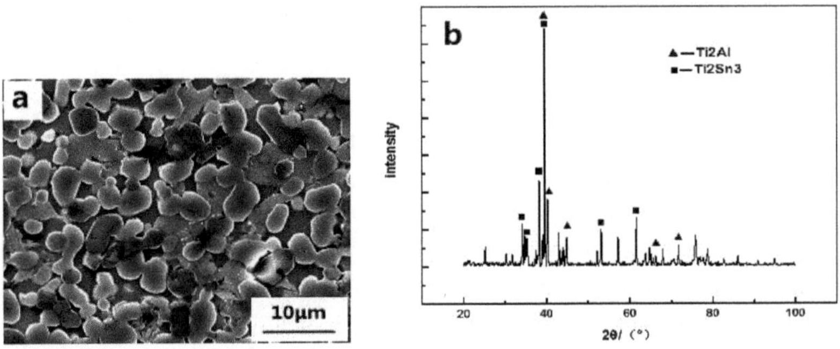

Fig. 5 The SEM micrograph (a) and X-ray diffraction (b) of Vacuum sintering microstructure with milled powder for 40h.

4. Conclusions

1) As the milling time increases, the particle size of the TiH_2-45Al-4Sn mixed powder gradually stabilizes form the initial rapid refinement. Ti and Sn powders are synthesized to generate Ti_2Sn_3 phase during the ball milling process. Theoretically different valence compounds can be formed with Ti and Al, but only Ti_2Al phase appears in the experiment, which indicates that chemical affinity between Ti and Sn is larger.

2) The more homogeneous and dense structure can be obtained under vacuum hot pressing condition. The microstructure is composed of equal axial

Ti_2Al as matrix and fine Ti_2Sn_3 particles. Ti_2Sn_3 phase can be formed during the milling process, so its grain size is very small.

3) Because of the addition of Sn, Ti-Al intermetallic compounds formation is inhibited during MA and sintering. However, Sn contributes to the formation of Ti_2Al phase which is difficult to be obtained with the conventional method of casting and forging.

Acknowledgments

The authors would like to thank the National Natural Science Fund (No. 51371038) for providing financial support.

References

1. Forouzanmelu N, Karlmzadeh F, Enayati M H. Study on solid-state of nanocrystalline TiAl synthesized by mechanical alloying [J]. Journal of Alloys and Compounds, 2009, 471(1/2): 93-97.
2. Couret A, Molenat G, Galy J, Thomas M. Microstructures and mechanical properties of TiAl alloys consolidated by spark plasma sintering [J]. Intermetallics, 2008, 16(9): 1134-1141.
3. Bhattacharya P, Bellon P, Averback R S, Hales S J. Nanocrystalline TiAl powders synthesized by high-energy ball milling: Effects of milling parameters on yield and contamination [J]. Journal of Alloys and Compounds, 2004, 368(1/2): 187-196.
4. Moon K II, Lee K S.A study of the microstructure of nanocrystalline Al-Ti alloys synthesized by ball milling in a hydrogen atmosphere and hot extrusion [J]. Journal of Alloys and Compounds,1999, 291(1/2): 312-321.
5. Li Z W, Gao W, Zhang D L, Cai Z H. High temperature oxidation behaviour of a TiAl-Al2O3 intermetallic matrix composite [J]. Corrosion Science, 2004, 46(8): 1997-2007.
6. Wu Y, Hwang S K. Microstructural refinement and improvement of mechanical properties and oxidation resistance in EPM TiAl-based intermetallics with yttrium addition [J]. Acta Material, 2002, 50(6): 1479-1493.
7. Wang G X, Dahms M. TiAl-based alloys prepared by elemental powder metallurgy [J]. Powder Metallurgy International, 1992, 24(4): 219.
8. Moll John H, McTiernan Brian J. PM TiAl alloys: the sky's the limit [J]. MPR, 2000, 18: 18.

9. Kumaran S, Chantaiah B, Sriniwasa Rao T. Effect of niobium and aluminum additions in TiAl prealloyed powders during high-energy ball milling [J]. Material Chemistry and Physics, 2008, 108 (1): 97-101.
10. Xiao shulong, Tianjing, Xu lijuan and so on, Such as the two-step plasma sintering fine grain milling and discharge TiAl alloys [J]. Metal Materials and Engineering, 2011, 40 (5): 880-884.

Effect of Co Addition on Martensitic Transformation, Mechanical And Magnetic Properties of Polycrystalline $Ga_{42.5}Mn_{29}Ni_{28.5}$ High Temperature Ferromagnetic Shape Memory Alloys*

Rong Xin[2], Shuo Yang[2] and GuiFu Dong [1,†]
[1]*College of mechanics, Dalian University, Dalian 116622, China*
[2]*Department of physics, Dalian University, Dalian 116622, China*
[†]*E-mail: dgfu0451@sina.com*

The $Ga_{42.5}Mn_{29}Ni_{28.5-x}Co_x$ (x=0,1) samples showed higher martensitic transformation temperature of 816℃ and 470℃. The decrease of transformation temperature maybe is due to substitution of Ni by Co which has a smaller ion diameter and lower valence electrons. Additionally, Co doping can significantly enhance Curie temperature and saturation magnetization of $Ga_{42.5}Mn_{29}Ni_{28.5}$ alloy. Also, the highest Curie temperature of 255°C is obtained in $Ga_{42.5}Mn_{29}Ni_{27.5}Co_1$ alloy, this is about higher 200°C than that of the $Ga_{42.5}Mn_{29}Ni_{28.5}$ alloy. In addition, the compressive strength and compressive strain are obviously enhanced by the addition of 1 at.% Co. It can be seen that the fracture surface of $Ga_{42.5}Mn_{29}Ni_{28.5}$ and $Ga_{42.5}Mn_{29}Ni_{27.5}Co_1$ alloy exhibit typical brittle characteristics with an intergranular pattern.

Keywords: $Ga_{42.5}Mn_{29}Ni_{28.5-x}Co_x$; martensitic transformation; curie temperature; mechanical properties.

1. Introduction

Several previous investigations show that the non-stoichiometric Ni_2MnGa alloys exhibit great potentials as high-temperature shape memory alloys (HTSMAs) [1–3]. However, it has been revealed that introducing a ductile γ phase into the martensite matrix of NiMnGa alloys by fourth elements addition, such as Co, Cu, Fe [4-6], or substitution of Ni for Ga [7,8], also substantially affects phase transformation and mechanical behavior of Ni-Mn-Ga alloy to improve their work ability and ductility. However, it is found that the effect of γ phase is two sided [4,6,8]. On the one hand, the presence of ductile γ phase can hinder the movement of dislocation and the propagation of the cracks thereby enhances the ductility of the alloy. On the other hand, since γ phase does not participate in the reversible martensitic transformation and seriously hinders the

* This work is supported by etc, etc.
† Work partially supported by grant 2-4570.5 of the Swiss National Science Foundation.

reorientation of martensitic variants in two-phase NiMnGa-based alloys, it will deteriorate the shape memory effect (SME) of the alloy. There is a pressing need to develop HTSMAs with single-phase. Therefore, practical application of high-temperature shape memory NiMnGa alloy is limited due to its second phase existed and low T_{C}.

Recently, S.R. Barman reported that a new ferromagnetic shape memory alloy Ga_2MnNi with the T_M and T_C are 780 K and 330 K [9]. However, the lower T_C and high brittleness of Ga_2MnNi alloy greatly limits their practical application. Therefore, it is important to further investigate for Ga_2MnNi alloy. The purpose of our study was to investigate for the first time the effect of Co addition on the microstructure, Curie temperature, saturation magnetization and transformation behavior of polycrystalline $Ga_{42.5}Mn_{29}Ni_{28.5}$ alloy. It was found that the Curie temperature, saturation magnetization of $Ga_{42.5}Mn_{29}Ni_{28.5}$ alloy could be remarkably increased by substituting 1 at.% Co for Ni, Also, the highest Curie temperature of 255℃ is obtained in $Ga_{42.5}Mn_{29}Ni_{27.5}Co_1$ alloy, this is about 200℃ higher than that of the $Ga_{42.5}Mn_{29}Ni_{28.5}$ alloy. In addition, the compressive strength and compressive strain are obviously enhanced by the addition of 1 at.% Co. At the same time, it can be seen that the fracture surface of $Ga_{42.5}Mn_{29}Ni_{28.5}$ and $Ga_{42.5}Mn_{29}Ni_{27.5}Co_1$ alloy exhibit typical brittle characteristics with an intergranular pattern. In this work, we main purpose is to identify the martensitic transformation behavior, mechanical and magnetic properties and microstructure changes in the $Ga_{42.5}Mn_{29}Ni_{28.5-x}Co_x$ (x=0,1) alloys.

2. Experimental

The veritable composition of alloy $Ga_{42.5}Mn_{29}Ni_{28.5-x}Co_x$ was prepared by non-consumable arc-melting in an argon atmosphere using 99.97 mol% electrolytic Ni plate, 99.5 mol% electrolytic Mn plate, 99.99 mol% Ga and 99.99 mol% Co. The obtained ingot was sealed into a quartz tube with a vacuum of 10^{-4} Torr and annealed firstly at 600℃ for 48 h, then 400℃ for 24 h, followed by quenching into the ice-water to achieve high chemical order. The martensitic transformation characteristics was monitored by Differential Scanning Calorimetry (PE Diamond DSC) and Thermo-gravimetric analysis (TGA) in temperature range of -200~1000℃ with a heating and cooling rate of 20 K/min. The microstructure and composition of experimental alloys were examined by using an Mx2600FE Scanning Electron Microscope (SEM) equipped with a microanalysis system. X-ray diffraction (XRD) measurements were performed as a means of crystal structure determination using a Rigaku D/max-rB with Cu

Kα radiation. The Curie temperatures of alloys were measured by DC susceptibility. Saturation magnetization measurements were taken using physical property measurement system (Quantum Design) in an applied field up to 5 T. Finally, compression tests at ambient temperature were conducted using an Instron-1186 Model machine which maintained a strain rate of 0.1 mm min-1, by applying compressive stress along casting direction.

3. Results and Discussion

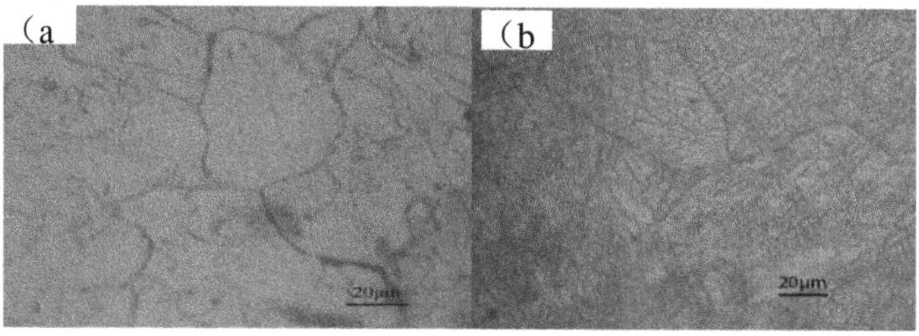

Fig. 1 The SEM image of the $Ga_{42.5}Mn_{29}Ni_{28.5-x}Co_x$ (x=0,1) alloys, (a) $Ga_{42.5}Mn_{29}Ni_{28.5}$; (b) $Ga_{42.5}Mn_{29}Ni_{27.5}Co_1$.

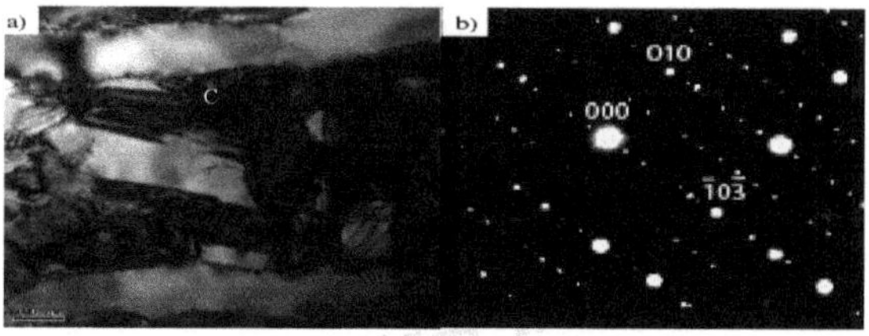

Fig. 2 TEM bright-field images and the corresponding EDPs in $Ga_{42.5}Mn_{29}Ni_{27.5}Co_1$ alloy. (a) bright-field image, (b) EDP from area C in (a).

Fig. 1 illustrates the secondary electron image of $Ga_{42.5}Mn_{29}Ni_{28.5-x}Co_x$ (x=0,1) alloys. The $Ga_{42.5}Mn_{29}Ni_{28.5}$ sample has typical morphology of parent phase, as shown in the Fig. 1(a). Typical unitary martensitic phase morphology is observed at room temperature in the $Ga_{42.5}Mn_{29}Ni_{27.5}Co_1$ annealed specimen, as shown in the Fig. 1(b). As shown in Fig. 1(b), straight plate twinned martensitic variant are clearly observed at room temperature. The TEM images in Fig. 2(a) and the corresponding EDP in Fig. 2(b) show that the large-plate-like martensite variants in the alloy. The martensitic lath of $Ga_{42.5}Mn_{29}Ni_{27.5}Co_1$ alloy exhibitions each other perpendicular, as shown in the Fig. 2(a). Nevertheless, the electron diffraction pattern shows that $Ga_{42.5}Mn_{29}Ni_{27.5}Co_1$ alloy is 7M martensite with monocline structure, namely, between the two main spots there are six weak diffraction spots. However, it is worth noting that the alloy with anamorphic martensitic lath, it is suggest that there are a lot of stress field in alloy, thereby resulting in the metamorphosed martensite.

The XRD patterns for the annealed $Ga_{42.5}Mn_{29}Ni_{28.5-x}Co_x$ (x=0,1) samples were collected at RT. Fig. 3 shows the RT XRD patterns of annealed samples. According to the XRD results, the $L2_1$ crystal Structures of $Ga_{42.5}Mn_{29}Ni_{28.5}$ sample can be indexed the austenite peaks appear with lattice parameters $a = b =$ 0.5930 nm and $c =$ 0.5684 nm in the Fig. 3(a). The $Ga_{42.5}Mn_{29}Ni_{27.5}Co_1$ sample exhibits some pattern of reflections can be indexed within a monoclinic martensite structure with lattice parameters $a =$ 0.4367 nm, b =2.9538 nm, $c =$ 0.5552 nm and β =90.60, as shown in the Fig. 3(b). This result agrees with that of SEM.

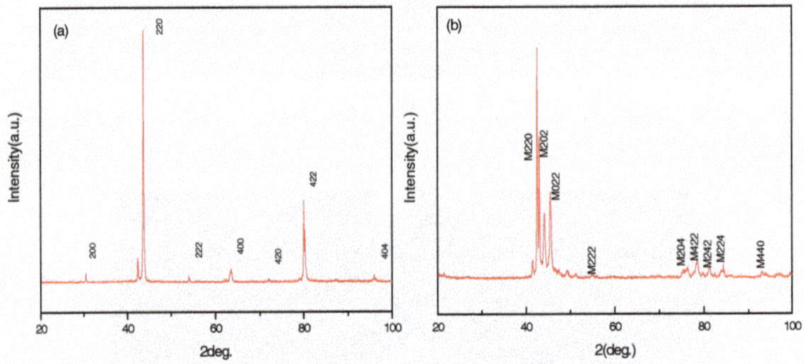

Fig. 3 XRD patterns of the $Ga_{42.5}Mn_{29}Ni_{28.5-x}Co_x$ alloys , (a) $Ga_{42.5}Mn_{29}Ni_{28.5}$; (b) $Ga_{42.5}Mn_{29}Ni_{27.5}Co_1$.

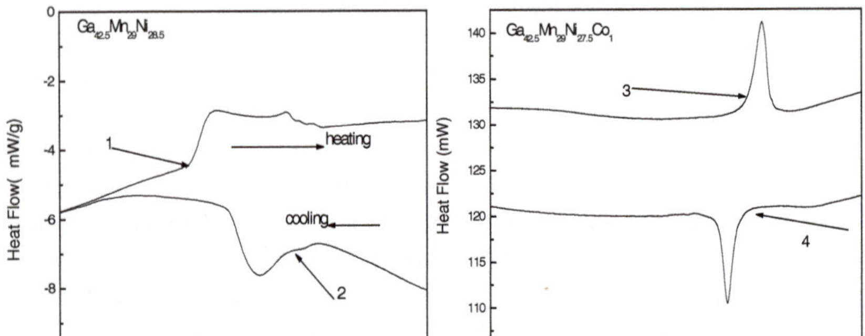

Fig. 4 DSC curves of the $Ga_{42.5}Mn_{29}Ni_{28.5-x}Co_x$ (x=0,1) alloys.

Fig. 4 presents the DSC curve of the $Ga_{42.5}Mn_{29}Ni_{28.5-x}Co_x$ (x=0,1) alloys, which shows that a one-step thermoelastic martensitic transformation occurs upon cooling and heating. The forward martensitic transformation starts (M_s) around 865.5 ℃ and finishes (M_f) at 785.1 ℃, while the reverse transformation starts (A_s) and finishes (A_f) at 741.4℃ and 890.4℃, respectively. $Ga_{42.5}Mn_{29}Ni_{27.5}Co_1$ compared to the $Ga_{42.5}Mn_{29}Ni_{28.5}$ sample, martensitic transformation and reverse transformation temperature for $Ga_{42.5}Mn_{29}Ni_{27.5}Co_1$ samples decreases above room temperature by substituting 1 at.% Co for Ni. Data for annealed $Ga_{42.5}Mn_{29}Ni_{27.5}Co_1$ sample is not available from this study since the characteristic temperatures are too low to be detected by the test equipment.

It is generally believed that the change of the electronic concentration (*e*/*a*), the atom size factor and the precipitated phase will significantly affect the martensitic transformation temperature of Ni–Mn–Ga alloys [10]. The number of valence electrons is 10 for Ni, 7 for Mn, 3 for Ga, and 9 for Co, respectively. The valence electron concentrations of $Ga_{42.5}Mn_{29}Ni_{28.5-x}Co_x$ (x=0,1) alloys negative from 6.155 to 6.145 with the addition of Co content. For the $Ga_{42.5}Mn_{29}Ni_{27.5}Co_1$ alloy, it is obvious that decrease of its martensitic transformation temperatures is consistent with the decrease of *e*/*a*. Therefore, the approachcan also be applied to case of quaternary $Ga_{42.5}Mn_{29}Ni_{28.5-x}Co_x$ (x=0,1) alloys with a proper composition range. In addition, the decrease of transformation temperature may be due to substitution of Ni by Co which has a smaller ion diameter and lower valence electrons. In this regard, the modified alloy composition caused by substituting 1 at.% Co for Ni is still considered to be the main contributor to the change in transformation temperature. Therefore, the decrease of the transformation temperature is mainly due to alters the composition of the alloy and the electronic concentration (*e*/*a*).

Fig. 5(a), (b) show the temperature dependencies of low-field Dc magnetic susceptibility of the $Ga_{42.5}Mn_{29}Ni_{28.5-x}Co_x$ (x=0,1) alloys during heating. It is found that there is characteristically abrupt change in such susceptibility curves for both specimens, corresponding to the magnetic transition. In addition, it can be obviously seen that for the $Ga_{42.5}Mn_{29}Ni_{28.5}$ alloy, the Curie temperature is 55°C, and that $Ga_{42.5}Mn_{29}Ni_{27.5}Co_1$ specimen is 255°C. Therefore, it can be seen from Fig. 5 that Co addition has an affect on Curie temperature. As is well known, the chemical composition of material significantly affects the Curie temperatures of Heusler-type Ni–Mn–Ga ferromagnetic shape memory alloy. Thus it is reasonable to believe that the content of Ni in the alloy is changed by substituting Co for Ni, and results in the variation of the composition of the alloy, and further investigation is still needed. Therefore, our experimental data is sufficient to make an unambiguous conclusion about the mechanism responsible for change of T_c by substituting 1 at.% Co for Ni.

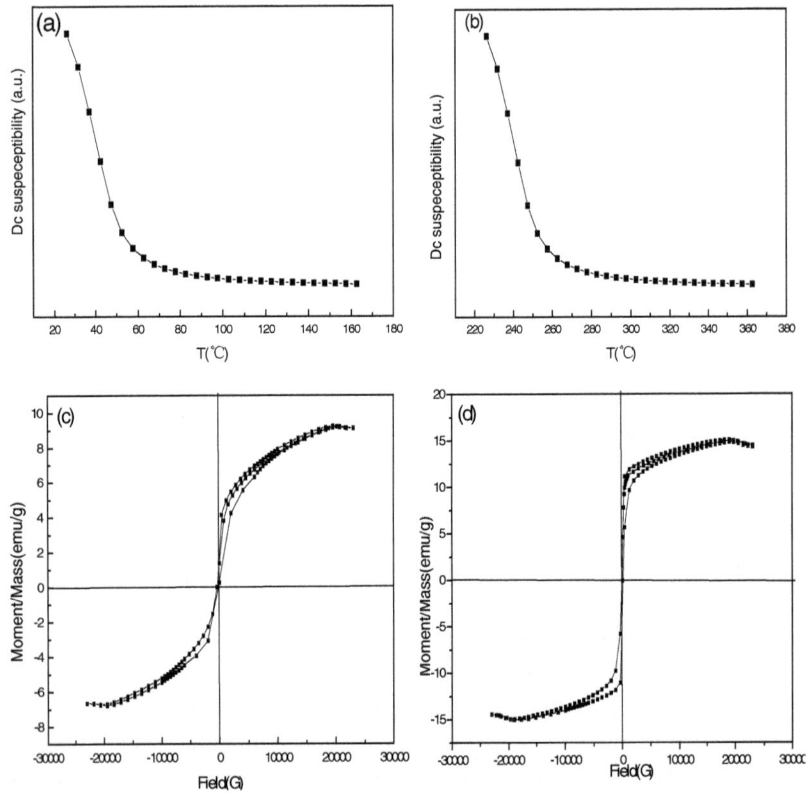

Fig. 5 The Curie temperature dependence and magnetisation curves for $Ga_{42.5}Mn_{29}Ni_{28.5-x}Co_x$(x=0,1) alloys, (a) $Ga_{42.5}Mn_{29}Ni_{28.5}$; (b) $Ga_{42.5}Mn_{29}Ni_{27.5}Co_1$; (c) $Ga_{42.5}Mn_{29}Ni_{28.5}$; (d) $Ga_{42.5}Mn_{29}Ni_{27.5}Co_1$.

Fig. 5(c), (d) is measured the magnetization curve of $Ga_{42.5}Mn_{29}Ni_{28.5-x}Co_x$ (x=0,1) alloys at room temperature. It is clear that, all alloys reached saturation magnetization in fields up to 2 T. Magnetization curve of $Ga_{42.5}Mn_{29}Ni_{28.5}$ specimen measured at room temperature is shown in Fig. 5(c). The magnetization curve should be noted that the curve exhibits deflection at about -0.15 kOe and 0.25 kOe, as well as some hysteresis. These deflection points were observed in magnetization curves for the martensite phase and parent phase. A possible explanation of this deflection points may be that the alloy is composed of the regions with different magnetocrystalline anisotropy. Other possible reason is the existence of several martensitic twin variants with different orientations with respect to the field direction. For the case of 10M martensite easy and hard axisof magnetization are $[001]_{10M}$ and $[100]_{10M}$, respectively.

In order to investigate the effect of Co doping on the mechanical properties, compression tests were carried out at room temperature. All the samples were compressed to fracture. Fig. 6 shows the compressive stress–strain curves of solution-treated $Ga_{42.5}Mn_{29}Ni_{28.5\text{-}x}Co_x$ (x=0,1) alloys at room temperature. It can be seen that the compressive strength and compressive strain of Ga–Mn–Ni alloy are obviously enhanced by the addition of Co. The higher compressive strength and compressive strain are obtained for $Ga_{42.5}Mn_{29}Ni_{27.5}Co_1$ alloy, which is about 53 MPa and 2.5% higher than that of the $Ga_{42.5}Mn_{29}Ni_{28.5}$ alloy.

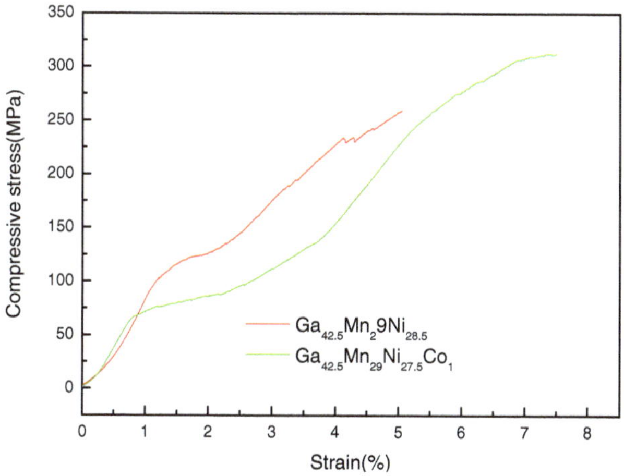

Fig. 6 RT compressive stress–strain curves of $Ga_{42.5}Mn_{29}Ni_{28.5\text{-}x}Co_x$ (x=0,1) alloys.

To clarify the fracture mechanism and investigate the nucleation and propagation of cracks in $Ga_{42.5}Mn_{29}Ni_{28.5}$ and $Ga_{42.5}Mn_{29}Ni_{27.5}Co_1$ alloys, the SEM observations of the fracture surfaces were performed, as shown in Fig. 7. It can be seen that the fracture surface of $Ga_{42.5}Mn_{29}Ni_{28.5}$ alloy exhibit typical brittle characteristics with an intergranular pattern, and this intergranular pattern becomes weaker. The fracture surfaces of $Ga_{42.5}Mn_{29}Ni_{27.5}Co_1$ alloy exhibits characteristics of brittle fracture, as evidenced have also been observed, as shown in Fig. 7(b). The mechanism of the brittle improvement is partly provided by the Co-alloying due to strengthen intergranular and intracrystalline in $Ga_{42.5}Mn_{29}Ni_{27.5}Co_1$ alloy. In addition, when deformed, the microcracks generated and propagated along the intergranular boundaries. At the same time, the effects will certainly increase the energy for the crack propagation, thus giving the increase of ductility.

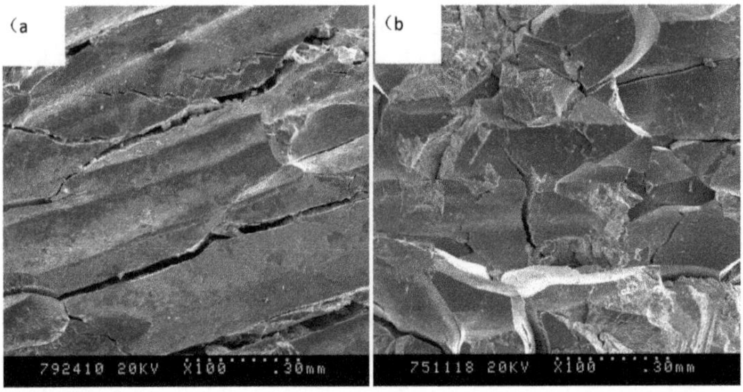

Fig. 7 SEM observations of the fracture surface of $Ga_{42.5}Mn_{29}Ni_{28.5-x}Co_x$ alloys after compression tests. (a) $Ga_{42.5}Mn_{29}Ni_{28.5}$; (b) $Ga_{42.5}Mn_{29}Ni_{27.5}Co_1$.

4. Conclusions

The $Ga_{42.5}Mn_{29}Ni_{28.5}$ sample has typical morphology of parent phase at room temperature; moreover, typical unitary martensitic phase morphology with monocline structure is observed at room temperature in $Ga_{42.5}Mn_{29}Ni_{27.5}Co_1$ specimen. The $Ga_{42.5}Mn_{29}Ni_{28.5}$ and $Ga_{42.5}Mn_{29}Ni_{27.5}Co_1$ samples showed a larger martensitic transformation temperature of 816℃ and 470℃. Additionally, Co doping can significantly enhance Curie temperature and saturation magnetization. The highest Curie temperature of 255℃ is obtained in $Ga_{42.5}Mn_{29}Ni_{27.5}Co_1$ alloy. The compressive strength and compressive strain are obviously enhanced by the addition of 1 at.% Co.

Acknowledgments

This study is supported by Postdoctoral Science Foundation of China (Grant No. 20100481218), Supported by Program for Liaoning Excellent Talents in University (LJQ2013131) and Young Doctor Startup Foundation of Dalian University, Natural Science Foundation of Dalian (No. 2013J21DW001).

References

1. V.A. Chernenko, E. Cesari, V.V. Kokorin, I.N. Vitenko. Scripta Metall Mater. 33 (1995), 1239.
2. Y. Li, Y. Xin, C.B. Jiang, H.B. Xu. Scripta Mater. 51 (2004), 849.
3. X. Jin, M. Marioni, D. Bono, S.M. Allen, R.C. O'Handley. J. Appl. Phys. 91 (2002), 8222.

4. Y.Q. Ma, L.H. Xu, Y. Li, C.B. Jiang, H.B. Xu, Y.K. Lee, Z. Metallkd. 96 (2005) 843.
5. Y.Q. Ma, S.Y. Yang, W.J. Jin, X.J. Liu, J. Alloy. Compd. 471 (2009) 570.
6. Y.Q. Ma, S.Y. Yang, Y. Liu, X.J. Liu, Acta Mater. 57 (2009) 3232.
7. Y.Q. Ma, C.B. Jiang, Y. Li, H.B. Xu, C.P. Wang, X.J. Liu, Acta Mater. 55 (2007) 1533.
8. Y. Xin, Y. Li, L. Chai, H.B. Xu, Scr. Mater. 57 (2007) 599.
9. S. R. Barman, Aparna Chakrabarti, Sanjay Singh, S. Banik, S. Bhardwaj, P. L. Paulose, B. A. Chalke, A. K. Panda, A. Mitra, A. M. Awasthi. Physical Review B. 78 (2008):146.
10. G.F. Dong, W. Cai, Z.Y. Gao. J. Alloy. Compd. 465 (2008) 173.

Effect of High Temperature Deformation and Tempering on the Microstructure and Properties of Nb Microalloyed Steels

Jian Chen[a], Yufei Li[b], Yongqiao Zhao[c] and Henghua Zhang[d]
School of Materials Science and Engineering, Shanghai University, Shanghai 200072, China
Email: [a]523517317@qq.com,[b]846178860@qq.com, [c]951064498@qq.com,[d]hhzhang@shu.edu.cn

Microstructure and properties in the tempering process of high temperature deformed Nb microalloyed Steels F40 had been studied by resistance heating and die casting machine. Results showed that in the process of resistance heating, temperature in central section of samples was higher than that in the edge. Fully austenitization was obtained when samples were heated to 1250°C. In the tempering process, the resistivity firstly decreased and then increased. Microhardness had the similar trend as resistivity except it decreased finally, which contributed to changes of microstructure and precipitated phases in the tempering process.

Keywords: Resistance heating; high temperature deformation; resistivity; microhardness.

1. Introduction

Nb microalloyed steels have been studied and used widely, such as in oil, automobile and other machinery industry [1]. Researchers have done a lot on the evolution process of precipitate in Nb microalloyed steels. A previous study [2-3] showed that before the formation of precipitates, it experienced the formation of clusters. Clusters played a very important role in the nucleation of the precipitates. Some works had also been done on the mechanism of the formation of clusters by 3DAP [4-5].

High temperature deformation of microalloyed steels was often investigated by using the Gleeble-3500 thermomechanical simulator, however, the resistivities and tensile properties of steels couldn't be analyzed as the limitation of sizes, so the method of heated by resistance heating [6-7] and deformed by die casting machine was used to study high temperature deformation. Resistance resistivity analysis is an effective method to study the precipitate of metals [8]. Solution temperature of microalloy elements was determined by measuring changes of resistivity when samples were heated to different temperatures [9].

The evolution of precipitate was also generally analyzed by measuring different resistivity for different aging times [10]. Microstructure and properties of high temperature deformed and tempered samples was studied by microhardness testers, optical microscopy and resistance instruments in this paper.

2. Experimental Materials and Procedures

2.1 *Materials and procedures*

Nb microalloyed Steel F40 plate (C: 0.06%, Si: 0.20%, Mn: 1.53%, Cr: 0.13%, Nb: 0.040%, Ti: 0.013%, Cu: 0.19%) with 3 mm in thickness was employed for this experiment. Resistance heating was used to heat samples by clamping with a pair of electrodes. The size of sample was 160×15×3mm. Temperatures in the process of resistance heating were analyzed by measuring at various locations. Schematic diagram of resistance heating were presented in Figure 1. High temperature deformation was carried out in horizontal die casting machine. The process was showed as Table 1.

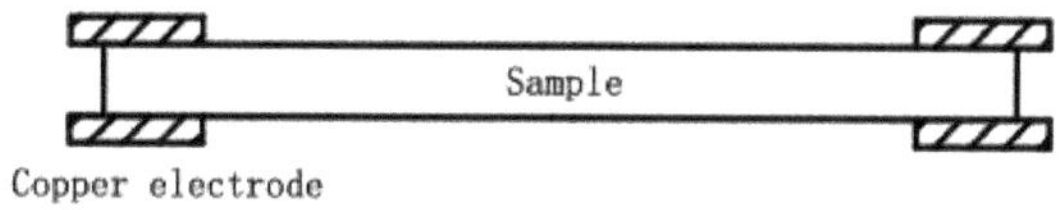

Fig. 1 Schematic diagram of resistance heating.

Table 1 Process parameters of the high temperature deformation.

Experimental Number	Austenitizing Temperature/ °C	Deformation Temperature/ °C	Deformation Amount	Cooling Mode
1	1250	1250	2%	Metal mold Cooling
2	1250	1250	9%	Metal mold Cooling
3	1250	1250	16%	Metal mold Cooling
4	950	950	9%	Metal mold Cooling

Temperature was measured with thermocouples welded on samples, deformation amount was controlled by gaskets with different thicknesses. Each deformed sample was cut into five blocks with size of 45×2.5×2.5mm. The blocks were tempered at 700°C for 0min, 5min, 15min, 30min, 60min, respectively. Microstructure analysis of as quenched and as tempered was studied. Alcohol solution containing 10% of nitric acid was used to reveal microstructure of samples. Microstructure was observed by optical microscopy. Evolution of age precipitated phases was analyzed by measuring microhardness and resistivity of samples.

3. Experimental Results and Discussions

3.1. *Distribution of temperatures in the process of resistance heating*

A new heating method was used in this experiment. Distribution of temperatures was also illustrated in Figure 2. It was shown from Figure 2 that temperature in the central section of samples was homogeneous. If the temperature of homogeneous section was controlled about 1250°C and length of whole heating section was 130mm, the length of homogeneous section was about 90mm, which can meet the requirement for high temperature deformation.

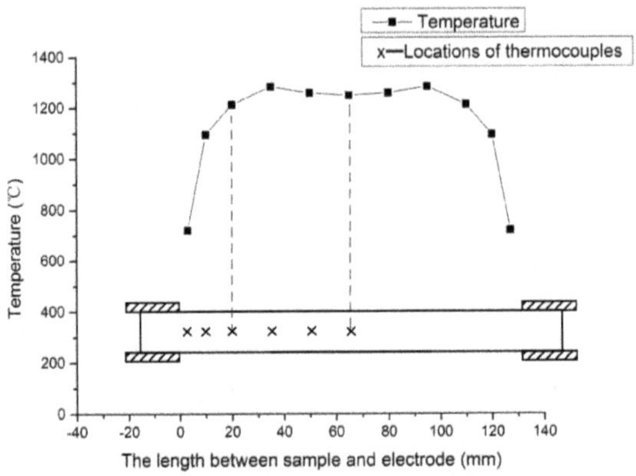

Fig. 2 Size of samples and locations of thermocouples and temperature distribution of resistance heating samples.

3.2. *Microstructure of microalloyed Steels F40 after high temperature deformation and die quenching*

Microstructure of F40 steels after high temperature deformation and die quenching was presented in Figure 3. Where a, b, c, d represented microstructure under different austenitizing temperatures and deformation amounts, respectively.

Results showed that when samples were heated to 1250°C without holding and then high temperature deformed and die quenched immediately to room temperature, they had completely transformed to lath martensite. From the microstructure of Figure 3(d), results showed when the sample was only heated to 950°C, it had incompletely austenitized, ferrite could also be seen in the microstructure. It indicated when the sample was resistance heated to the critical transition temperature, pearlite and ferrite changed into austenite in a short time, but the Fully austenitization needed more time.

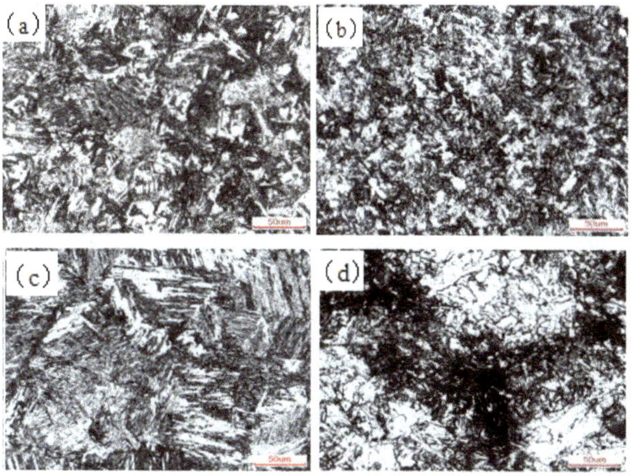

Fig. 3 Microstructure of samples after high temperature deformation and die quenching (a) 1250°C+ 2% (b) 1250°C+9% (c) 1250°C+16% (d) 950°C+9%. (austenitizing temperatures + deformation amounts).

3.3. *Microstructure and properties of as tempered samples*

Microhardness and resistivities evolution in the tempered samples were presented in Figure 4.

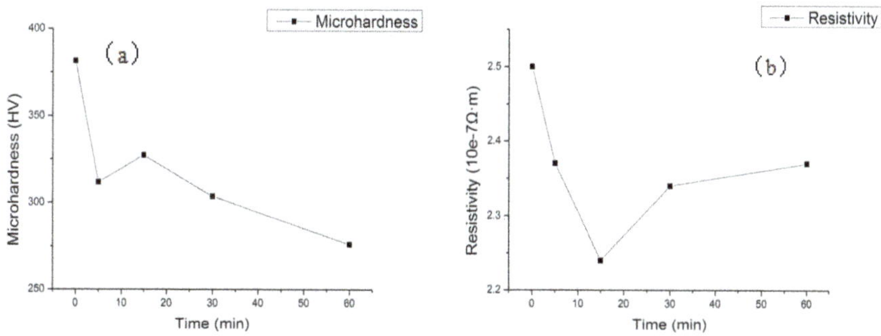

Fig. 4 Evolution of (a) Microhardness and (b) Resistivity during tempering in the tempered samples 3.

Microhardness of samples after high temperature deformation and die quenching was high as there was lath martensite in the microstructure. In the tempering process, martensite was decomposed into high temperature tempering martensite, so microhardness decreased. With the prolongation of tempering time, microhardness firstly increased and then decreased. In early tempering stage, precipitation strengthening played a very major role as fine carbides increased, microhardness was the highest when tempering for about 15 minutes. In the further tempering stage, microhardness decreased as carbides coarsened.

Before tempering, the resistivity of samples was 2.49*10e-7Ω·m.In the tempering process, C, Nb atoms continuously agglomerated and precipitated in the form of NbC precipitates, which made the content of solute atoms in matrix significantly decreased and the resistivity decreased. On the other hand, NbC precipitates caused the resistivity to increase slightly. Considering effects of two aspects, the resistivity of samples decreased in early tempering stage. When aging for 15min-20min, the precipitation of NbC had finished, the resistivity of samples was the lowest. As the carbides grew up, orientation relations between carbides and matrix changed from full coherent lattice to semi-coherent lattice which caused distortion and lead the resistivity to increase.

4. Summary

1. In the process of resistance heating, temperature distribution of samples showed high in the central section and low in the edge, when the length of whole heating sample was 130mm, the length of homogeneous section was about 90mm, which can meet the requirement of high temperature deformation.

2. When samples were heated to 1250°C without holding and then high temperature deformed and die quenched immediately to room temperature, they had completely transformed to lath martensite. However, if the sample was only heated to 950°C, it had incompetely austenitized and some ferrite still existed.

3. In the tempering process, the resistivity of samples decreased in early tempering stage and then increased, while microhardness increased slightly when tempered for about 15 min and then decreased. The resistivity of samples was the lowest while the microhardness was the highest when tempering for about 15 min.

Acknowledgments

The research work described in this paper was supported by the top disciplines in Metallurgical Engineering of Shanghai University.

References

1. Qi Junjie, Huang Yunhua, Zhang Yue. Micro alloyed steel [M]. Beijing: Metallurgical Industry Press, 1988.
2. Murayama M, Hono K. Role of Ag and Mg on precipitation of T1 phase in an Al-Cu-Li-Mg-Ag alloy [J]. Scripta Materialia, 2001, 44(4): 701-706.
3. Cerezo A, Hirosawa S, Rozdilsky I, et. al. Combined atomic-scale

modelling and experimental studies of nucleation in the solid state [J]. Philosophical Transactions of the Royal Society, 2003, (361): 463-477.
4. Wilde J, Cerezo A and Smith GDW. Three-dimensional atomic-scale mapping of a cottrell atmosphere around a dislocation in iron [J]. ScriptaMater. 2000, 43: 39-48.
5. Wu Jing, Zhang Heng-hua, ZHU Song-he. Investigation on nucleation process of precipitation in the microalloyed steel by three-dimensional atom Probe [J] Shanghai Metals, 2009, 31(3): 36-38.
6. Wu, Jing, Zhang, Heng-hua. Formation and growth rules of participate in niobium micro-alloyed steel [J]. Heat Treatment of Metals, 2011, 36(4): 4-7.
7. T. Maeno, K. Mori, K. Adachi Gas forming of ultra-high strength steel hollow part using air filled into sealed tube and resistance heating [M]. Journal of Materials Processing Technology 214 (2014): 97-105.
8. The National Machinery, Industry, Commission. Testing technology of metal physics [M]. Beijing: Machinery Industry Press, 1988, 35-40.
9. He Yizhu, He Lieyun, Zhang, Hui, Li Xiang, Chu Juefei. Method for detecting Nb (C, N) dissolving temperature of low-carbon microalloy steel by resistivity [P]. China: CN101929967 B, 2012. 6.6.
10. T. Mori K, Maeno T, Fukui Y, 2011. Spline forming of ultra-high strength gear drum using resistance heating of side wall of cup. CIRP Ann.: Manuf. Technoloy. 60(1): 299-302.

Preparation of Affinity Polymer Beads for Separating Sugary Proteins and Its Application

Manhua Liu[†], Xuluan Lin and Zhihua Li
Department of Biotechnology, Jinan University, Guangzhou, China
[†]291282744@qq.com

Renqiang Li
Department of Biotechnology, Jinan University, Guangzhou, China
trqli@jnu.edu.cn (corresponding anthor)

The Sepharose CL-6B column was made to separate ricinus communis agglutinin (RCA) from the crude extract of castor beans. RCA were immobilized on activated Sepharose 4B to prepare the affinity polymer beads, which was used to capture the proteins in rabbit plasma by affinity chromatography. Results showed that two polypeptides with molecular mass about 120 and 97 KDa were captured by these affinity polymer beads. The captured polypeptides were demonstrated to contain the carbohydrate. The affinity polymer beads for separating sugary proteins from biological samples were successfully prepared.

Keywords: Sepharose CL-6B; immobilized RCA affinity polymer beads; captured proteins by RCA; sugary proteins.

1. Introduction

There are many proteins in the plasma, including many glycoproteins [1], which have many important functions. Also, there is a lot of existance of biological samples containing sugary proteins. So far, to separate or purify the glycoproteins from biological samples is still difficult or complex. Obviously, the study offered a quick, effective biomaterial for the separation or purification of those glycoproteins from the biological samples is favor of a specific study of biochemistry of proteins.

Because the ricinus communis agglutinin (RCA) has high affinity and particular specificity for glycoconjugates containing terminal β-D-galactoside bond [2, 3, 4] this lectin could be selected as the ligands to capture those glycoproteins in plasma by affinity chromatography. So the aim of this study was to probe or establish an available material for quickly and effectively separating those associated glycoproteins in plasma by making an immobilized

RCA polymer beads based on the mechanism of affinity chromatography. For preparation of these affinity polymer beads, Sepharose CL-6B was used to separate RCA from castor seeds due to these gel carriers contain a large amount of β-galactoside bond originally [5]. Then an immobilized RCA affinity polymer beads was made and was applied to separate the associated proteins in the plasma.

2. Materials and Method

2.1. *Materials*

New Zealand white rabbits from Jinan University Experimental Animal Center, of which the plasma and red blood cells were prepared. The castor bean was from local market. Sepharose CL-6B and Sepharose 4B were from Amersham. BCA kit, epichlorohydrin, 1, 4-dioxane and all other chemicals used in SDS-PAGE or for buffers used in the column chromatography were of analytical or chemical grade and were purchased from Guangzhou Chemical Co. Ltd. (Guangzhou, China).

2.2. *Extraction and purification of the RCA*

The preparation of RCA crude extract was carried out according to the method of Niecolson[6]. The castor beans were bled in phosphate buffer (0.01mol/L, pH 7.2, containing 0.15mol/L NaCl). The sample after blender was centrifugated at 10000 rpm for 30 min at 4°C, supernatant was obtained, which was salted out with 60% saturation of ammonium sulfate, the precipitate was dissolved in a small amount of phosphate buffer, and then dialyzed against the same buffer.

The Sepharose CL-6B affinity chromatography column was prepared to purify the RCA from the crude extract. 12 mL of RCA crude extract was applied to the column of Sepharose CL-6B washed fully with equilibrium solution phosphate buffer at a flow rate of 0.3 mL per min. After being washed fully with equilibrium solution, eluting solution was applied to elute the column. A number of fractions at penetration peak and eluting peak at O.D.280 were collected respectively and were concentrated by vacuum cold drying apparatus, and dialyzed against deionized water before mixing with 1% SDS-mercaptoethanol solution as the SDS-PAGE sample. Gel concentration used in SDS-PAGE was 12%.

2.3. *Preparation of immobilized RCA affinity polymer beads*

After the Sepharose 4B beads were washed using 1mol/L NaCl and deionized water respectively at Buchner's funnel, 10 grams of these polymer beads were mixed with 6.5 mL 2mol/L NaOH, 1.5 mL epichlorohydrin and 15 mL 56% 1, 4-dioxane, shaken for 2 h at 40℃ for the activation of Sepharose 4B, and then were saturated in 0.1mol/L, pH 9.5 Na_2CO_3-$NaHCO_3$ buffer after being washed at funnel by using deionized water. The activated Sepharose 4B beads were mixed with 10 mL of RCA dissolved in the 0.1mol/L, pH 9.5 Na_2CO_3-$NaHCO_3$ buffer, shaken at 40℃ for about 24 h and washed at funnel using deionized water to collect the RCA that were not attached to the polymer beads. BCA kit was used to measure the RCA before and after mixed with the polymer beads. The immobilized RCA affinity polymer beads were made.

2.4. *Application of the immobilized RCA affinity polymer beads*

The immobilized RCA affinity polymer beads were used to establish a column with enough washed using equilibrium solution Tris-HCl buffer, then 10 mL of rabbit plasma diluted ten-folds were loaded to the column at a flow rate of 0.3 mL per min. After being washed fully with equilibrium solution, eluting solution was applied to elute the column. The same performance was done on the control column. The chromatography process was under real-time monitored and a number of fractions at penetration peak and eluting peak at O.D.280 were collected respectively, also freeze dried and detected by SDS-PAGE.

3. Results and Discussion

3.1. *Extraction and purification of RCA*

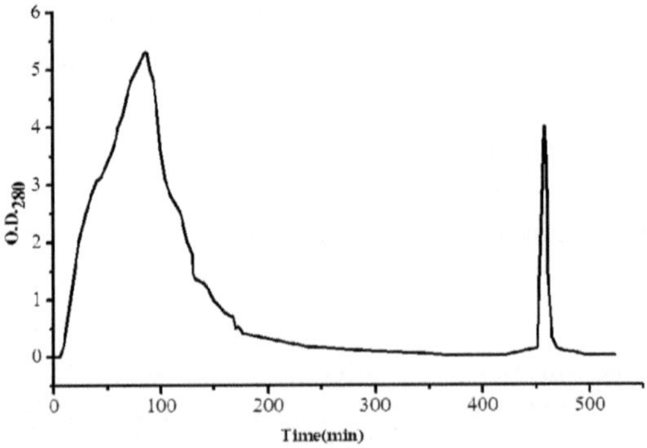

Fig. 1 Chromatography process of RCA crude extract on the Sepharose CL-6B column.

Big peak refers to those proteins haven't bound to the Sepharose CL-6B column, the second peak to the proteins captured by the column. The equilibrium solution was phosphate buffer (0.01mol/L, pH7.2, containing 0.15mol/L NaCl), and eluting solution was equilibrium solution containing 0.20mol/L of galactose.

The chromatography process of RCA crude extract from Sepharose CL-6B column was shown in Fig. 1. SDS-PAGE analysis of those proteins captured or uncaptured by β-galactoside bond in the Sepharose CL-6B column was shown in Fig. 2. The chromatography process of RCA by the Sepharose CL-6B column was very effective, not only in large numbers but also the pure RCA were obtained, which was reflected on SDS-PAGE pattern. RCA is a tetramer composed of two A-type and two B-type chains with about 130 KDa molecular mass[7, 8], of which the subunits are almost the same in 30-35 KDa. Further examination of agglutination of red blood cells (data not shown) demonstrated that the RCA sample possessed the activity, which explained too that the RCA had been obtained.

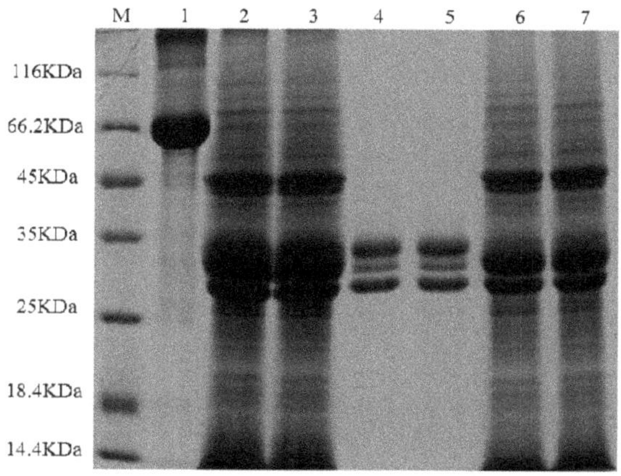

Fig. 2 SDS-PAGE pattern of RCA from the Sepharose CL-6B column.
M: protein markers. Lane 1: bovine serum albumin (BSA) Lane 2 and 3: RCA crude extract. Lane 4 and 5: elution peak of the column. Lane 6 and 7: penetration peak of the column.

3.2. *Application of the immobilized RCA affinity polymer beads*

BCA kit was used to calculate the RCA proteins fixed with Sepharose 4B beads. More than 1.73 mg RCA proteins were fixed by 1g wet Sepharose 4B beads. The chromatography process of rabbit plasma through the immobilized RCA affinity polymer beads was shown in Fig. 3. Some proteins were captured by these beads and their SDS-PAGE analysis was shown in Fig. 4. In control column, not any elution peak was appeared (date not shown).

Although the captured proteins in rabbit plasma by RCA were not so much (the second peak in Fig. 3), two kinds of polypeptides captured by the RCA were appeared with molecular mass about 120 and 97 KDa (Lane 2 in Fig. 4), respectively. In order to further verify the captured proteins, the UV absorption spectra of mixture of RCA and the captured proteins in vitro was examined (date not shown). Captured proteins and RCA showed their protein absorption character at near 280 nm respectively, but after they were mixed together, this character of absorption spectrum was almost disappeared, which explained that RCA could react with the captured proteins, it was RCA that pull-down those proteins. For understanding if the carbohydrate was attached to the captured proteins, the colorimetric phenol-sulfuric acid method [9] was used to examine the samples. Results of O.D.490 of the control, RCA, captured proteins and their mixture were 0, 0.141, 0.195 and 0.310, respectively, which explained that the carbohydrate were attached to both RCA and captured proteins, the latter may be the glycoprotein.

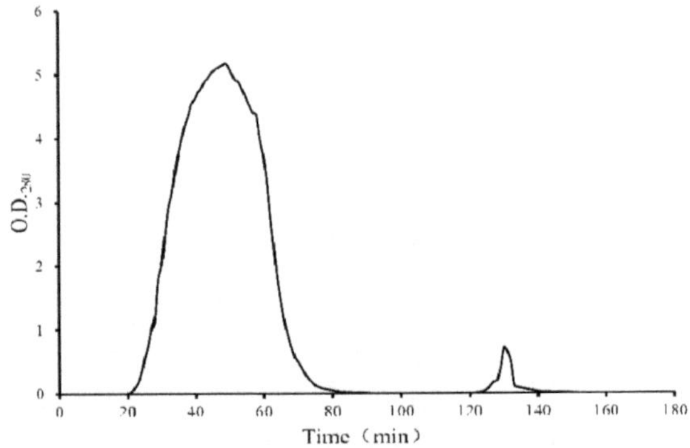

Fig. 3 Elution profile of RCA-binding protein on proteins immobilized RCA affinity polymer beads. Big peak refers to those proteins haven't bound to RCA, the second peak to the proteins captured by RCA. The equilibrium solution was 0.02mol/L, pH 7.4, Tris-HCl buffer, eluting solution was 0.02mol/L pH 4, NaAc-HAc buffer containing 0.15mol/L NaCl.

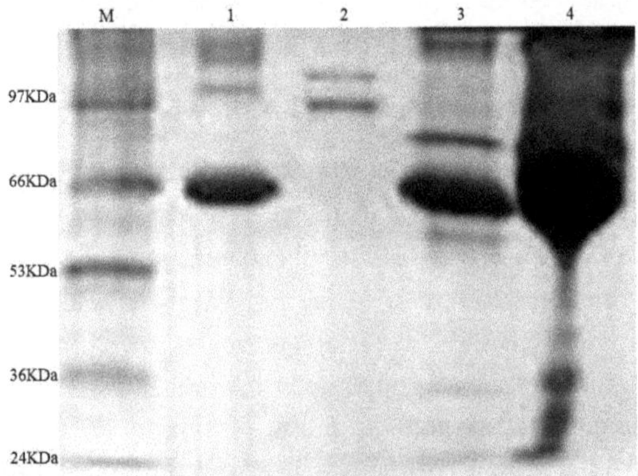

Fig. 4 SDS-PAGE pattern of rabbit plasma from immobilized RCA affinity polymer beads.
M: protein markers. Lane 1: bovine serum albumin (BSA) Lane 2: elution peak of RCA-Sepharose 4B column. Lane 3: penetration peak of the column. Lane 4: rabbit plasma.

4. Conclusions

An affinity chromatography of Sepharose CL-6B column was used to separate RCA, which was used to prepare the affinity polymer beads for separating sugary proteins. The application of these polymer beads demonstrated that the immobilized RCA affinity polymer beads could offer a quick, effective medium for the separation of sugary proteins from biological samples.

References

1. H.G. Schwick, H. Haupt. Purified human plasma proteins of unknown function. *Jap. J. Med. Sci. Biol.* **34**, 5 (1981).
2. Y. Wang, G. Yu, Z. Han, et al. Specificities of Ricinus communis agglutinin 120 interaction with sulfated galactose. *FEBS Letters.* **585** (2011).
3. J. Wu, A. Herp, A. Wu. Defining carbohydrate specificity of Ricinus communis agglutinin as Gal beta 1-->4GlcNAc (II)> Gal beta 1-->3GlcNAc (I)>Gal alpha 1-->3Gal (B)> Gal beta1-->3GalNAc (T). *Molecular Immunology.* **30** (1993).
4. A.Wu, J. Wu, T. Singh, et al. Recognition factors of Ricinus communis agglutinin 1 (RCA (1)). *Molecular Immunology.* **43**(2006).
5. S.G. De-Simone, C. C. Netto, E. P. Silva Jr. Simple affinity chromatographic procedure to purify beta-galactoside binding lectins. *J. Chromatogr B* **838**, 2 (2006).
6. G. L. Nicolson, J. Blaustein. The interaction of Ricinus communis agglutinin with normal and tumor cell surfaces. *Biochim Biophys Acta* **266**, 2(1972).
7. I. E. Liener. The lectins: *Properties, Functions, and Applications in Biology and Medicine,* (Academic Press, San Diego, CA, and London. 1986).
8. E. Rutenber, J.D. Robertus. Structure of ricin B-chain at 2.5 A resolution. *Proteins* **10**, 3 (1991).
9. S. K. Saha, C. F. Brewer. Determination of the concentrations of oligosaccharides, complex type carbohydrates, and glycoproteins using the phenol-sulfuric acid method. *Carbohydr. Res.* **254** (1994).

The Effect of Nano-Silica Sol in Different Concentrations on Mechanical Properties of Zirconia Ceramics*

Zheng Ruibin[a], Wang Siqian[b], Lin Tingting[c], Fan Jiangyuan[d], Dai Panpan[e] and Ma Jianfeng [f†]

School & Hospital of Stomatology, Wenzhou Medical University,
Wenzhou, 325027, China

Email: [a]robinsion.hunter@gmail.com,[b]wsq982004@163.com,[c]siyuemu@163.com [d]fanjfany@126.com, [e]dppdaisy@163.com, [f]dentistmacn@aliyun.com

The objective of this study was to examine the impacts on mechanical properties of zirconia ceramics after surface modification with different concentrations of nano-silica sol by sol-gel process. 40 zirconia ceramic blocks were randomly divided into 4 groups: Group A (control group): no surface treatment; Group B, C and D were respectively treated with 20%, 30%, 40% nano-silica sol via sol-gel process. The Vickers hardness, fracture toughness, flexural strength and microstructure of all samples were measured. The microstructure of cross-section of the ceramics was observed under scanning electron microscopy (SEM). There were no significantly differences on Vickers hardness, fracture toughness and flexural strength ($P>0.05$).The interlocking layer thickness of Group C was greater than that of Group B and Group D.30% nano-silica sol might be the optimal concentration used in the further clinical practice.

Keywords: Nano-silica sol; Zirconia; Sol-gel processing.

1. Introduction

The demand for aesthetics resulted in an increasing use of all-ceramic restorations in dental clinical practice [1]. In recent years, new high performance ceramics such as zirconia ceramics, which possess outstanding aesthetic appearance, biocompatibility, superior mechanical properties, high flexural strength and fracture toughness, are commonly used in restorative dentistry for copings and frameworks of fixed restorations [2]. However, the physical and bonding properties of zirconia ceramics are not completely satisfactory. To achieve long-term stability of bonding, the surface modification of zirconia ceramics is needed. Since zirconia ceramics do not contain a silica phase, the required silica phase for the chemical reaction to form a siloxane network that

* This work is supported by National Natural Science Foundation of China (grant no. 81271186) and New-Shoot Talented Man Plan Project of Zhejiang province (grant no. 2014R413063).

† Corresponding author.

strengthens the adhesion stress should be introduced firstly with the sol gel technology [3, 4].

Sol–gel technology is a simple, rapid and convenient way to prepare coatings at low temperatures. A thin layer with fine pores can be achieved by deposition onto a ceramic tube and the requirements for sol-gel process are a crack free, uniform coating and a good adhesion between the coating and the ceramic. It is worth mentioning that the inherent advantages of this technology are not only its low cost, but also the distinctive capability of homogenizing the prepared synthesis in a molecular level. Besides, the adhesion of the coating on the substrate is strong because of its chemical bonding. Wang Yu etc. utilized different concentration of silica (20 wt%, 30 wt% and 40 wt%) to modify the zirconia surface through sol-gel technology, the results showed 30% silica sol gained the highest bond strength between zirconia ceramics and resin composite after silica coating followed with silane coupling agent [5]. However, to update, no attempts have been yet made to investigate the impacts on mechanical properties of zirconia ceramics after surface modification with silicon sol through sol-gel process. In all, this study aims to investigate the effects of different concentration of silica sol modifying the zirconia ceramics through sol-gel process on Vickers hardness, fracture toughness, flexural strength and microstructure of zirconia, and lay foundation for clinical usage of silane coupling agent treatment before bonding.

2. Materials and Methods

2.1. *Preparation of specimens*

Forty presintered zirconia ceramic blocks (Upcera, Shenzhen, China) with a dimension of 38mm×10mm×2.5mm were fabricated by SC-20G CNC lathes (Shanghai Sigma Machine Co., Ltd.) and then they were completely sintered at the Kavo Everest CAD/CAM system. After that, all the ceramic blocks were ultrasonically cleaned in distilled water in KQ-600KDE CNC ultrasonic cleaner (Kunshan Ultrasonic Instrument Co., Ltd.) for 30 min and dried in DHG-9030A electro-thermostatic blast oven (Shanghai Precision Experimental Equipment Co.).

2.2. *Surface treatment with silica sol*

The prepared forty ceramic blocks were randomly divided into four groups (n=10) according to the following conditioning methods: Group A (control group): no treatment; Group B, C and D blocks were coated with 20%, 30% and

40% nano-silica sol by a spin coater (KW-4A,CHETMAT TECHNOLOGY INC, China) with its rotation speed 3000rpm and kept for 30sec respectively; Afterwards, specimens were placed in DZF-6020 vacuum chamber (Shanghai hengyi Scientific Instrument Co., Ltd.) to complete the transition of the gel drying process at room temperature (20°C) for 24h. After surface treatments, the specimens were placed in MIHM-VOGT muffle furnace (Mihm-Vogt, Germany) to be heated with temperature raising at the rate of 1°C/min till 400°C and kept for 30 min, finally all samples were put at room temperature to be tested for further study.

2.3. *The Vickers hardness (HV) and fracture toughness (Ft) test*

The HV and Ft of the specimens were tested by Wilson-Wolpert Tukon 2100B Vickers hardness tester (British Instron Company) with the loading 98N for 15 sec. The HV values could be showed by the computer with the method of sampling 5 times on the different positions of the specimens. After that, a diamond-shaped indentation was introduced to the surface of each specimen with indentation method, and the Ft values were calculated by the following equation:

$$K1C=P\ (b\pi)\text{-}3/2(tg\beta)\text{-}1 \tag{1}$$

P: the loading of fracture, β=68°, b: the crack length of specimens, mm.

2.4. *Three- point bending strength test*

Three-point bending strength of green parts and sintered parts were tested on an NDN-100 versatile mechanical test machine (KQL Testing Instruments Co., Ltd., China) with a span of 20 mm and a crosshead speed of 0.5 mm /min. Diameter of the indenter in the instrument was 4 mm. Force values sensor with 2000 N was used.

$$\sigma = \frac{3P\times L}{2b\times h^2} \tag{2}$$

P: the loading of fracture, L: span, b: the specimen's width, h: the specimen's thickness.

2.5. *Scanning electron microscope*

The fracture surfaces of different groups were observed under a JSM-6700F field-emission SEM (JEOL Ltd., Japan). In order to compare the interlocking layer thickness of zirconia and silica among the treated groups, the interlocking layer was measured at three different points in each SEM image; while five SEM images were taken for each sample.

2.6. *Statistical analysis*

The results were analyzed by factorial ANOVA and Fisher's least significant difference (LSD) t test (a = 0.05, SPSS 20.0).

3. Results and Discussion

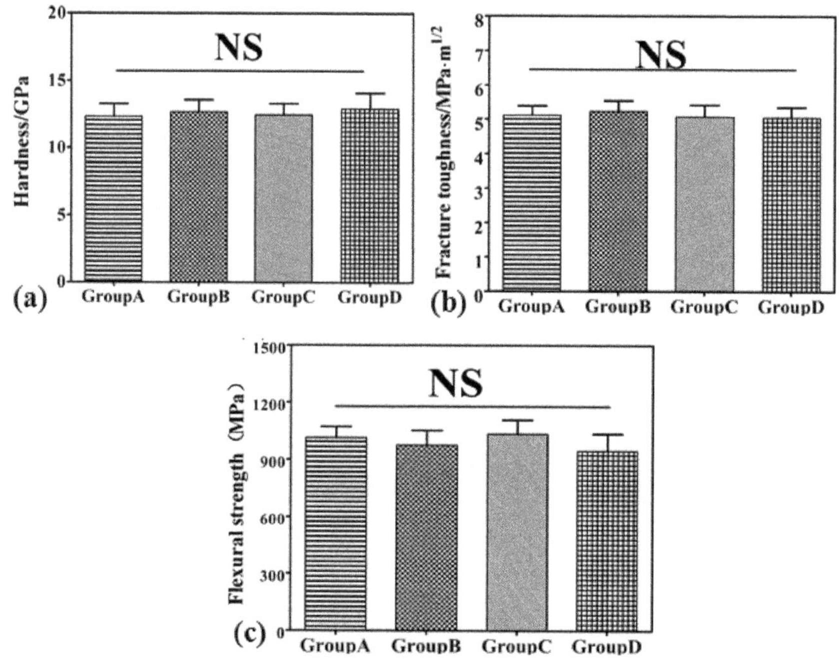

Fig. 1 Comparison of Vickers hardness (a) fracture toughness (b) and flexural strength (c) in different groups.

A growing body of evidence demonstrates that Sol-gel technology exhibits excellent properties to enhance the bonding strength between zirconia ceramics and resin composite. However, few reports have been conducted to evaluate whether this technology will have some impacts on the intrinsic mechanical properties of zirconia ceramics, meanwhile, the effect of concentration of silica sol has not been reported either. The Vickers hardness, fracture toughness and flexural strength of different groups are shown in Fig. 1. As demonstrated in Fig. 1, there were no significantly differences on Vickers hardness, fracture toughness and flexural strength of zirconia ceramics treated with 20%, 30% and 40% nano-silica through sol-gel technology. It indicated that so gel with different concentration of nano-silica exerted no deleterious effect on the mechanical properties of ceramics. The bending strength of four groups, using this same sol gel technology, were much higher than 300 Mpa, which fully met the required strength for making all ceramic crown and bridges in clinical practice [6]. This result further demonstrates that the addition of silica by sol-gel technology has promising property in its clinical work.

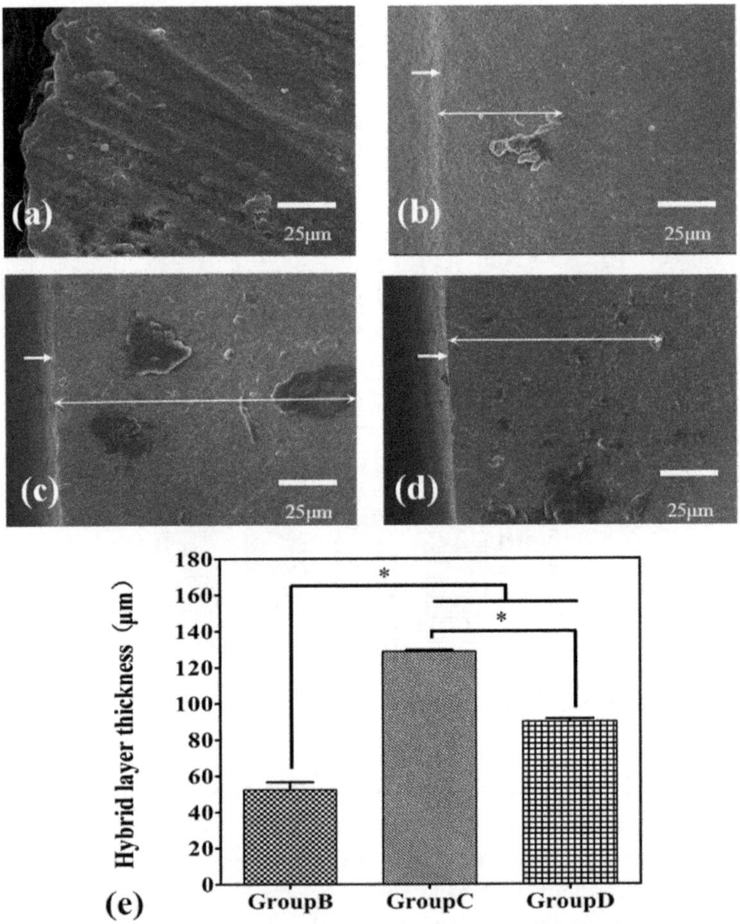

Fig. 2-(a-d) SEM photograph of cross-section of the specimen in different groups (magnification 1000×).: (a), Group A; (b), Group B; (c), Group C; (d), Group D; short arrow indicated surface of sample, two-way arrow indicated infiltration depth of gel. (e) Comparison of infiltration depth in interlocking layer of zirconia and silica of the treated group. * $p<0.05$.

The morphologies of cross-section of the sintered zirconia specimens of four groups are observed in Fig. 2. Fig. 2e. illustrates that the silica membrane is continuous and the hybrid layer thickness of zirconia and silica varied along with different concentration. According to measuring data, it was observed that the hybrid layer thickness of Group C (128.72±0.95μm) was greater than that of Group B (52.40±4.16μm) and Group D (89.96±1.47μm). There was also significant difference between Group B and D. The reason for this result may be related with characteristic of gel and also concentration effects. To some degree, the hybrid layer thickness increased along with increasing concentration of gel. That's why the hybrid layer thickness of 30% group is greater than that of 20% group. However, the high concentration of gel would enhance the agglomeration of nanoparticles, which might prevent the further infiltration in 40% Group. In comparison, Group C with 30% concentration silica sol exhibited better performance in regarding to hybrid layer thickness.

In a word, the present study presents that different concentration of silica sol did not have any negative effects upon mechanical properties of zirconia ceramics. Sol-gel technology is a low temperature method, suitable for preparation of ceramic membranes with pores in the nanometer range, which could create roughening and interlocking surfaces between the ceramics and the silica [7]. Meanwhile, the heating of silane on the surface of ceramics can eliminate water, alcohol and byproducts of the reaction and help to complete the condensation reaction of silane silica promoting the formation of siloxane [8]. In addition, previous studies have reported that silica coating on zirconia ceramics by sol-gel technique improved bonding to the zirconia surface [9]. Hence, zirconia crowns and bridges can be bonded after immediate pretreatment of Silane-coupling agents, which would enhance the bonding strength of zirconia ceramic restoration with resin binder in the clinical work.

4. Conclusion

(1) The addition of silica by sol-gel process did not affect mechanical properties of zirconia ceramics remarkably.
(2) The technology route of 30% nano-silica sol modifying the surface of sintered zirconia ceramics is realistic and feasible, laying the foundation for clinical silane coupling agent treatment before adhesion in the future.

Acknowledgments

This work is supported by National Natural Science Foundation of China (grant no. 81271186) and New-Shoot Talented Man Plan Project of Zhejiang province (grant no. 2014R413063).

References

1. A. Raut, P.L. Rao, T. Ravindranath, Zirconium for esthetic rehabilitation: an overview, Indian J Dent Res. 22 (2011) 140-143.
2. S. Nakamura, K. Yoshida, K. Kamada, M. Atsuta, Bonding between resin luting cement and glass infiltrated alumina-reinforced ceramics with silane coupling agent, J Oral Rehabil. 31 (2004) 785-789.
3. M. Kern, S.M. Wegner, Bonding to zirconia ceramic: adhesion methods and their durability, Dent Mater. 14 (1998) 64-71.
4. P. Derand, T. Derand, Bond strength of luting cements to zirconium oxide ceramics, Int J Prosthodont. 13 (2000) 131-135.
5. Wang Yu, Xie Haifeng, Zhang Feimin, Effects of surface modification with different concentration silica sol on bond strength of dental zirconia ceramic. J Pract Stomatol. 24 (2008) 518-521.
6. J.W. McLean, Evolution of dental ceramics in the twentieth century, J Prosthet Dent. 85 (2001) 61-66.
7. M. Eriksson, L.C. Klein, E. Liden, K. Lindqvist, Preparation of nanoporous silica-zirconia layers by in situ sol-gel method, Mater Sci Tech-Lond. 22 (2006) 611-614.
8. C. Shen, W.S. Oh, J.R. Williams, Effect of post-silanization drying on the bond strength of composite to ceramic, J Prosthet Dent. 91 (2004) 453-458.
9. C. Chen, G. Chen, H. Xie, W. Dai, F. Zhang, Nanosilica coating for bonding improvements to zirconia, Int J Nanomedicine. 8 (2013) 4053-4062.

Photodegradation of Rhodamine B Using Fe_3O_4@SiO_2@BiOBr Magnetic Photocatalyst

Qian Wen Cao, Yue Wan and Xu Chun Song†
Department of Chemistry, Fujian Normal University, Fuzhou, P.R. China
†E-mail: songxuchunfj@163.com
www.fjnu.edu.cn

A novel kind of magnetically photocatalyst Fe_3O_4@SiO_2@BiOBr was synthesized by hydrothermal method. Fe_3O_4 nanoparticles were firstly synthesized, and then got coated by SiO_2. The as-prepared product was coated by BiOBr finally. The character of Fe_3O_4@SiO_2@BiOBr was fully analyzed by transmission electron microscopy (TEM), scanning electron microscopy (SEM), X-ray diffraction (XRD), and reflectance spectroscopy (DRS). The as-prepared Fe_3O_4@SiO_2@BiOBr show good photocatalytic performance in degradation of rhodamine B under visible light irradiation. In addition, Fe_3O_4 performs good magnet, which plays an important role in Fe_3O_4@SiO_2@BiOBr samples, moreover, its nontoxicity, easy and cheap to get also give it many priority.

Keywords: Fe_3O_4; BiOBr; photocatalytic; rhodamine B.

1. Introduction

In the modern times, the environmental pollution is getting serious, as a result, green ways to deal with pollutant attract more and more attention, while the promoting magnetic separation technology comes into our eyes [1]. The semiconductor photocatalysis has attracted increasing attention due to their potential applications in water treatmen [2]. The synthesis of magnetic photocatalyst has been worked by Rao et al. using wet chemical method [3]. At the same time, bismuth oxyhalides is reported to be a promoting photocatalyst under visible light or UV irradiation, while BiOBr is special because its reaction to visible light [4]. Because of properties above, in our study, we prepared Fe_3O_4@SiO_2@BiOBr magnetic photocatalyst, in which Fe_3O_4 showed suitable magnet and silica as a linker connecting Fe_3O_4 and BiOBr.

2. Experimental Section

2.1. *Synthesis of Fe_3O_4@SiO_2 nanoparticles*

4.44 g $FeCl_3\cdot 6H_2O$ along with 4.56 g $FeSO_4\cdot 7H_2O$ were dissolved in 60 ml 0.01

M HCl solution and then added to the 80 ml 3 M $NH_3 \cdot H_2O$ solution dropwise under violent stirring. Kept the mixture at 80°C for 3h under continuous stirring and then separated it with an external magnet. Rinsed the obtained Fe_3O_4 nanoparticles with distilled water and absolute ethanol for three times respectively, and then got dried at 60°C for 6h. 0.4 g as-prepared Fe_3O_4 nanoparticles were dispersed ultrasonically in a mixture of 80 ml absolute ethanol and 20 ml distilled water, followed by continual addition of 1 ml concentrated $NH_3 \cdot H_2O$ solution and 1.6 ml TEOS. After vigorous stirring at room temperature for 6 h, the mixture was separated by an external magnetic field, rinsed with distilled water and absolute ethanol for several times and then dried at 60°C for 6 h.

2.2. *Synthesis of Fe_3O_4@SiO_2@BiOBr*

The Fe_3O_4@SiO_2@BiOBr composite were synthesized through a solvothermal process. First of all, 4 mmol $Bi(NO_3)_3 \cdot 5H_2O$ were dissolved in 30 ml EG, then added 0.12g Fe_3O_4@SiO_2 nanoparticles under violent stirring for 30 min. Subsequently, 4 mmol KBr dissolved in 10 ml EG were added dropwise to the above mixture under vigorous stirring for another 30 min to form a suspension precursor. Finally, the precursor was transferred into a 50 ml Telfon-sealed autoclave and kept at 180°C for 12h. After the solvothermal process, the as-synthesized photocatalyst was left to cool to room temperature naturally and separated by an external magnetic field, followed by rinsing with distilled water and absolute ethanol for several times, and drying at 60°C for 6 h.

2.3. *Characterization*

The morphology of the photocatalyst was characterized by scanning electron microscopy (SEM, Hitachi S-4700, 25 kV). The composition of the product was analyzed using energy dispersive X-ray detector (EDS, Thermo Noran VANTAG-ESI). The X-ray diffraction (XRD, Thermo ARL SCINTAG X'TRA with Cu Kα irradiation, λ= 0.154056 nm) was used to analyze the crystallinity. The UV-Vis diffuse reflectance spectrum (DRS, Lambda 850 UV-Vis spectrometer) was recorded in the spectral range of 200–800 nm and $BaSO_4$ was used as the reflectance standard.

2.4. *Photocatalytic experiment*

The photocatalytic performance of the photocatalysts was evaluated by the degradation of RhB under UV and visible light irradiation using a 300 W Xe lamp system. Before the photocatalytic activity test, 100 mg photocatalyst and

200 ml 10^{-5} M RhB solution were placed in dark and stirred for 30 min to reach an absorption-desorption equilibrium. Subsequently, in a certain interval of time, a certain volume of reacting solution was sampled and centrifuged at 10000 r/min for 5 min to ensure all the photocatalysts were separated. The concentration of RhB solution was analyzed at the maximum absorption wavelength 553nm with a UV759S UV-Vis spectrophotometer.

3. Results and discussion

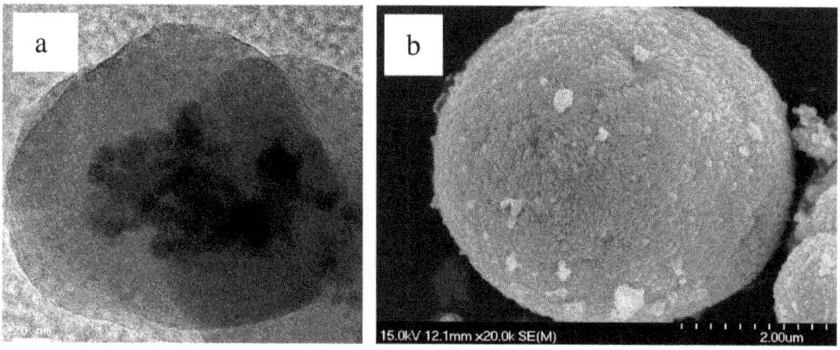

Fig. 1 TEM (a) image of Fe_3O_4@SiO_2 and SEM (b) image of the Fe_3O_4@SiO_2@BiOBr.

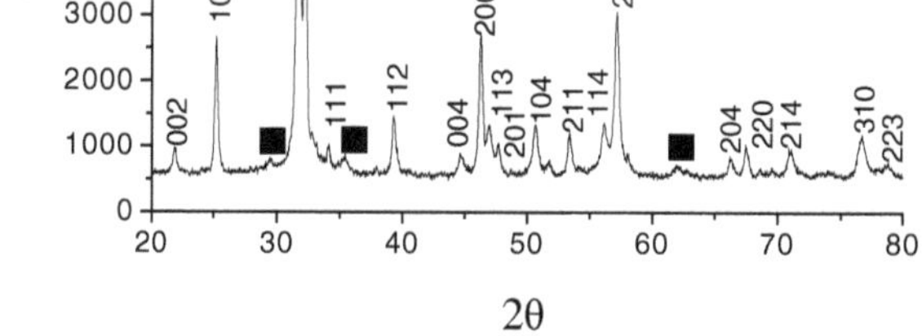

Fig. 2 XRD patterns of the Fe_3O_4@SiO_2@BiOBr.

As shown in Fig. 1a and Fig. 1b, they describe as-prepared particles Fe_3O_4@SiO_2 and Fe_3O_4@SiO_2@BiOBr. It is clear that Fe_3O_4 is well coated by SiO_2 from TEM. Besides, the SEM describes that the Fe_3O_4@SiO_2@BiOB shows spheres and the sample is composed of a large quantity of nanoplates and the nanoplates were combined and assembled into spheres.

The phase and structure of the products were examined by powder X-ray diffraction (XRD). As Figure 2 shows, the crystal planes (101), (102), (110), (112), (200), (104), (211) and (212) performs good agreement with the standard card of tetragonal BiOBr (JCPDS card no. 73-2061). And the existence of Fe_3O_4 is proved from the marked diffraction peaks showed above.

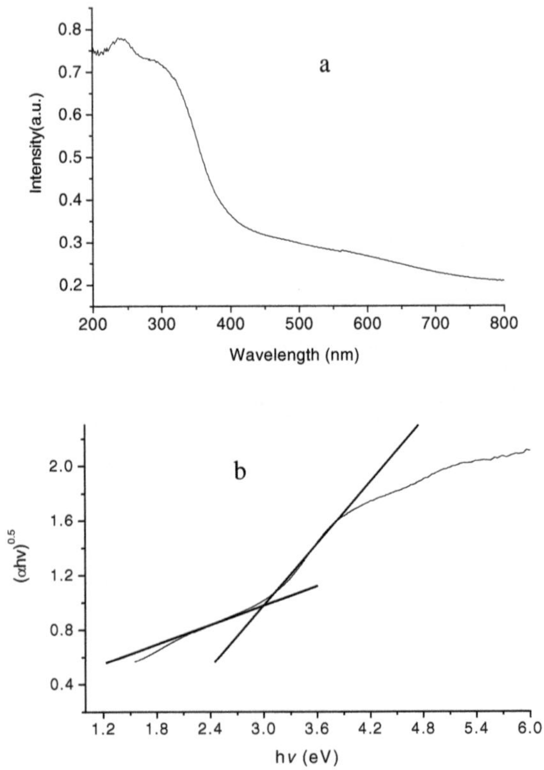

Fig. 3 (a) UV–vis diffuses reflectance spectra and (b) plots of the $(\alpha hv)^{1/2}$ versus hv of Fe_3O_4@SiO_2@BiOBr samples.

The UV–Vis diffuse reflectance spectra of the Fe_3O_4@SiO_2@BiOBr samples are displayed in Figure 3a. According to the spectrum, the Fe_3O_4@SiO_2@BiOBr samples mainly present the properties from the UV light region to visible light until about 450 nm. According to the fomular A(hv-Eg) n/2 = ahv and the picture above, where A, *a*, *v*, and *Eg* are the Planck constant, absorption coefficient, light frequency, and band gap, respectively. n is a coefficient determined by the type of transition considered, it is clear to be seen that the energy bandgap of the product samples is Eg = 3.0 eV (Figure 3b).

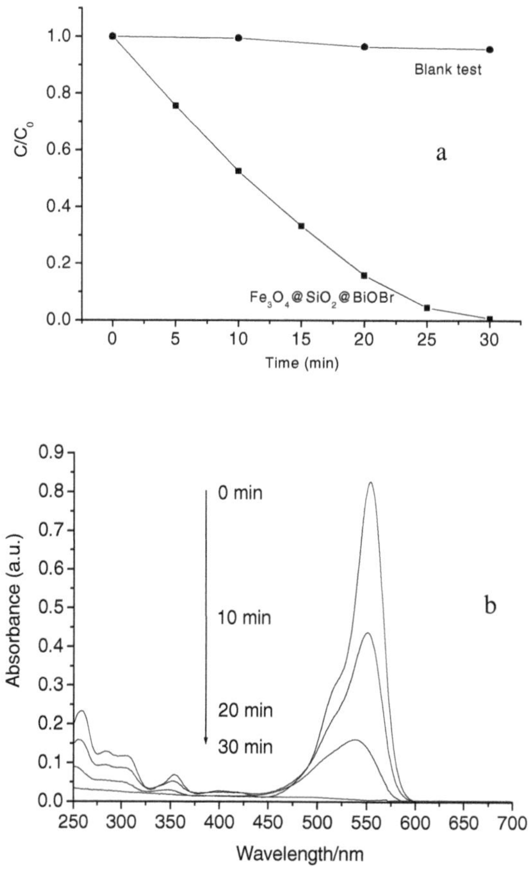

Fig. 4(a) The photocatalytic activity of the Fe_3O_4@SiO_2@BiOBr, (b) UV-vis spectral changes of the degredation of RhB dye by the Fe_3O_4@SiO_2@BiOBr.

It was by the decomposition of RhB aqueous solution that the photocatalytic performances of the Fe_3O_4@SiO_2@BiOBr were investigated under UV and visible-light irradiation at room temperature.The ratio of RhB concentration C and initial RhB concentration C_0 versus the photodegradation time was shown in Figure 4a. The blank test (no catalyst) exhibits that the amount and decomposition of RhB is negligible during the test period, while it is obvious that the RhB decomposes fast in 30 min with photocatalyst Fe_3O_4@SiO_2@BiOBr added. The photodegradation process was investigated by the major absorption band of RhB at 553 nm. From Figure 4b, it can be noticed that the intensity of the characteristic absorption peak of RhB decreases quickly as irradiation time goes by, and 99.85% of the RhB photodegradated in 30 min, with a shift of the maximum absorption peak to a lower wavelength. Besides, the catalyst is easy to be moved because of its magnetism.

4. Conclusions

We finished the photocatalyst Fe_3O_4@SiO_2@BiOBr successfully, and it exhibit high photocatalytic activity in degradation of RhB under UV and visible light irradiation. The information provided here suggests that the Fe_3O_4@SiO_2@BiOBr photocatalyst is a promising catalytic for water purification application and environmental remediation.

References

1. X. C. Song, Y. F. Zheng and H. Y. Yin, Catalytic wet air oxidation of phenol over Co-doped Fe_3O_4 nanoparticles, *J. Nanopart. Res.* **15**, 1856 (2013).
2. X. C. Song, W. T. Li, W. Z. Huang, H. Zhou, H. Y. Yin and Y. F. Zheng, Enhanced photocatalytic activity of cadmium-doped Bi2WO6 nanoparticles under simulated solar light, *J. Nanopart. Res.* 17, 134 (2015).
3. Y. R. Yao, W. Z. Huang, H. Zhou, X. Cui, Y. F. Zheng and X. C. Song, Synthesis of core–shell nanostructured magnetic photocatalyst Fe_3O_4@SiO_2@Ag_3PO_4 with excellent visible-light-responding photocatalytic activity, *J. Nanopart. Res.* 16, 2742 (2014).
4. Y. H. Feng, L. Li, J. W. Li, J. F. Wang and L. Liu, Synthesis of mesoporous BiOBr 3D microspheres and their photodecomposition for toluene, *J. Hazard. Mater.* **192**, 538 (2011).

Preparation and Characterization of Ordered Nano Multilayer of Synthesized Porphines-ZnTPP and TPETPP

Yong-Jian Chen[a] and Hai-Ning Cui[b]
Faculty of Electronic Information & Mechatronic Engineering, Zhao Qing University (526061), Jilin University (130012), P. R. China
†E-mail: [a]ok08@netease.com, [b]cuihaining2009@126.com
www.zqu.edu.cn

Rong Wang[c] and Shi-Quan Xi
Changchun Institute of Applied Chemistry, Chinese Academy of Sciences, Chang Chun 130022 P. R. China
E-mail: [c]Wangr@jlu.edu.cn

Synthetic porphyrins without long alkyi chains were used for forming monolayers and multilayers on substrates. The transmission electron micrographs (TEM), surface Pressure-area isotherms (Pi-A)isotherm, Spectral study and fluorescence lifetime measurement revealed the stable condensed films with measured molecular areas compatible with a vertical or tilted orientation of these molecules on the substrate, and the formation of aggregates as the main species in these films. The behavior for films of porphyrin mixed with stearic acid (SA) and arachidic acid (AA) was also studied.

Keywords: Porphine derivatives film; monomolecular layer; structural characterization.

1. Introduction

Porphyrins, as highly conjugated molecules, have been widely used as film materials because of their chemical stability and other various properties. Porphyrins constitute the functional unit of many proteins that are involved in catalytic and photo catalytic processes in biology. To study the interactions of macromolecules of porphyrins, the arrangement of these molecules in ordered solid state by Langmuir-Blodgett (LB) method presents a promising tool [1-3]. In this paper, the behavior of 5,10,15,20-tetrakis(4-phenyl)-21H, -23H-porphine Zn [ZnTPP] and 5,10,15,20-tetra-(p-theoxy carbonyl-benzene) porphine [TPETPP] monolayers at the air water interface was studied by Pressure-area isotherms (Pi-A) isotherm, TEM, Spectral and fluorescence lifetime study. The behavior for monolayers of porphyrin mixed with stearic acid (SA) and arachidic acid (AA) was also studied.

2. Experimental Details

Porphyrins were prepared according to the method reported in our previous paper [4]. Spectroscopic data and elemental analysis agreed with expectations. Chloroform and 1:1 dimethylsulphoxide (DMSO): chloroform was used as spreading solvents for synthetic and natural porphyrins respectively. In some cases blended films from individual porphyrins mixed with stearic acid (SA) and arachidic acid (AA)were deposited for spectral study. KSV-5000 Langmuir trough (Finland) with a Wilhelmy balance and domestic LB trough were employed for the surface pressure-area (Pi-A) isotherm measurements and the Langmuir-Blodgett (LB) films fabrication. The final replica of the sample film was then picked up on a copper grid for examination in a Hitachi H-500 electron microscope. The thicknesses of several films were determined by the folding method.

3. Results and Discussion

With a view to facilitate practical use and theoretical approached, one inevitably encounters three intractable problems in the monomolecular layer fabrication by using LB method, that are: 1. how to make a tighter arrangement of the molecule without the collapse of film happen; 2. how to make a looser arrangement of the molecule with a composed of domains of a certain size of the molecular area; 3. how to make a film with a good quality. Hence, Pi-A isotherm measurements and analysis become very important. Fig. 1 shows the Pi-A isotherms of ZnTPP and TPETPP monolayers at the air-water interface. The important data and properties of porphyrins ordered solid films from Pi-A isotherms are summed and shown in Table 1. It is seen from Fig. 1 and table 1 that the area per molecule in the films of synthetic porphyrins- ZnTPP is smaller than that of TPETPP, where the former differs from the latter in not possessing hydrophilic substituents. These polar groups with long chains would result in greater adhesion of the macro cycle face to the water and less cohesion between ring planes. The minimum area occupied by a porphyrin ring, lying flat, would be about 1.6 nm2 and the surface area of the edge is about 0.4 nm2. According to the area per molecule found in our study, we assume that the ZnTPP plane is oriented vertically onto the substrate and a tilted orientation for TPETPP is expected.

The porphyrin monolayers were transferred at 35 and 30 mNm-1 to substrates by a Z-deposition process for ZnTPP and TPETPP respectively. The morphology and thickness of the samples were observed by TEM operated at 30 kV and 100 kV respectively, and the picture for 3 layers of ZnTPP is given in

Fig. 2 as an example. The transmission electron micrographs show that the monolayers are composed of domains of a certain size. There is an approximate proportionality between the thickness of the films and the number of deposited monolayers; for example, the thickness of 3 layers of ZnTPP is 19, 14.7 nm. The measured average monolayer thickness of about 2.8, 4.8 nm is compatible with the rings orienting vertically on the substrate surface where an occupied area of the molecules would be expected to 0.6 nm2. Hence we assume that the films formed are ordered to some extent and the macrocycle plane of the ZnTPP is oriented vertically. TEM result is in accordance with the result of our work on polarized UV-vis spectra and above Pi-A result for both ZnTPP and TPETPP.

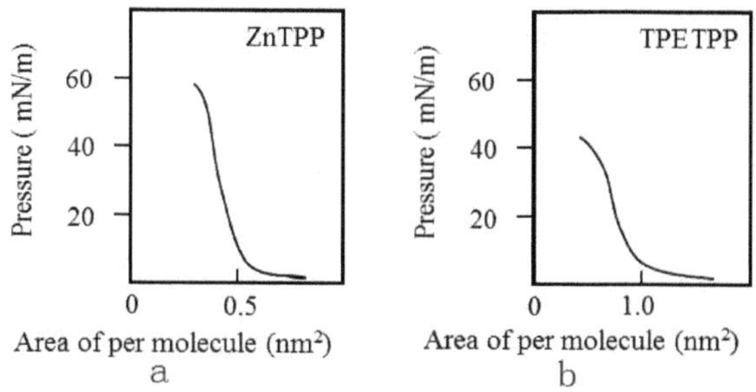

Fig. 1 Pressure-area isotherms of porphins: a. ZnTPP; b. TPETPP.

Table 1 Properties parameters of the -A isotherm about porphins layer on air-water interface.

Samples	Collapse Pressure mNm^{-1}	Transfer Pressure mNm^{-1}	The occupied area per molecule (nm^2) Under Zero Pressure	Under Collapse Pressure	Under Transfer Pressure
Zn TPP	55	35	0.58	0.31	0.37
TPETPP	41	30	1.13	0.78	0.81

As we know, fluorescence and fluorescence lifetime measurements are especially useful in the study of in ordered state systems, since both the absorption and fluorescence bands of included guest fluorophore are often overlapping with the bands of the free molecule, but the lifetimes are different in most cases. The study on fluorescence and fluorescence lifetime of porphyrins in ordered state - LB films was done. For example, the lifetime of ZnTPP in three monomolecular layers and in solution is 1.75 ns and 2.18 ns respectively. All spectra results tell us that the fluorescence lifetimes of porphyrins in ordered state films are noticeably shortened in comparison with those of solution samples. Mixed porphyrins ordered state enhances fluorescence by compartmentalizing and shielding the excited singlet species from quenching and non-radiative decay processes that occur in bulk solution, lengthening the lifetime of inclusion complex as compared to the free molecule. The short lifetime component is probably due to aggregated species in the film by analogy to similar phenomena in concentrated solution and in condensed films. In blended films dilution with SA or AA in a molar ratio up to 1:10 is not enough to reduce the probability of fluorescence quenching by aggregate formation. A small increasing tendency of lifetime shortening in multilayers could be due to non-radiative decay induced by coupling to the lattice modes.

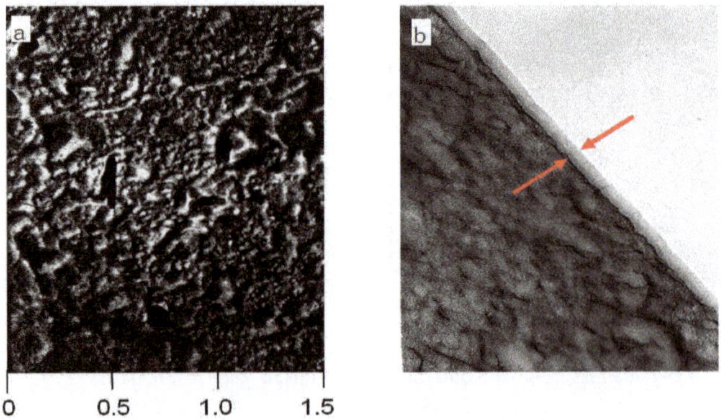

Fig. 2 TEM of 3 layers of ZnTPP films: a. The Surface morphology, scale-micrometer; b. The thickness of Multilayer: 19, 14.7nnm for arrow positions.

Acknowledgments

We acknowledge partial financial supports from Jointly Funded Project (No. 61179055) of Chinese Civil Aviation Authority and National Natural Science Foundation of China, Talent Grant (2013-ZQXY-05) of Educational Commission of Guangdong Province, China.

References

1. Michael G. Walter, Alexander B. Rudine, and Carl C. Wamser, J. Porphyrins Phthalocyanines 14, 759 (2010).
2. Lu-Lin Li and Eric Wei-Guang Diau, Porphyrin-sensitized solar cells, Chem. Soc. Rev., 2013, 42, 291-304.
3. S. Baker, M. C. Petty, G. G. Roberts and M.V. Twigg: Thin Solid Films, 1982, 99, 53.
4. Y.H. Yang and W.Y. Wang, Spectrosc. Spectral Anal. (China), 5(2) (1985) 16-21.

The Change on Aggregation of Column and Flake Structures of ZnO Films

Hai-Ning Cui[a] and Yong-Jian Chen[b]
Faculty of Electronic Information & Mechatronic Engineering, Zhao Qing University (526061), Jilin University (130012), P. R. China
E-mail: [a]cuihaining2009@126.com, [b]ok08@netease.com
www.zqu.edu.cn

B. Marí
Departament de Física Aplicada-IDF. Universitat Politècnica de València, Camí de Vera s/n, 46022 València, Spain

Since transparent conducting oxides can be as a buttom layer of complex film electrodes, electrodeposition technique may produce ZnO films depending on variety conditions and modified surface layers of substrates in electrochemical procedures. Here we invested the structure and morphologies of top ZnO layers by using modified surfaces of the substrate in the multilayer film-"ZnO-electrodeposition /ZnO(002)-sputtering /ITO/ glass".

Keywords: Electrodeposition; ZnO films; pentagonal flake structure; column structure; multilayer.

1. Introduction

Zinc oxide (ZnO) is one of the most promising materials for the fabrication of optoelectronic devices operating in the blue and ultraviolet (UV) region, owing to a direct wide band gap and a large exciton binding energy. It has been shown that ZnO thin films can be deposited electrochemically and that the films produced are of high structural quality [1]. ZnO layer made by electrodeposition method is for potential application of grade material and semiconductor junction devices. As we know, control of morphology and structures of oxides are of great importance for above applications and their implementation on technological devices. Zinc oxides had be obtained in different structures such as Pentagonal ZnO nanorods, hexagonal ZnO collunms, sheet nano-zinc oxide crystals with a hexagonal, pentagonal, rectangular or an irregular form etc. [2]. Different temperatures, solute and post-annealing for fabrication and characterations of ZnO films were systematically investigated by authors. In this paper, We will focus the structure of top layer ZnO, especially pentagonal flake structure, relation of morphologies and the surface of substrates.

2. Experimental Details

In the electrodeposition procedure of ZnO films a three electrode electrochemical cell is need. It contains a aqueous solution with 5 mM ZnCl2 and 100 mM KCl as supporting electrolyte and dissolved oxygen at 90 0C temperature [3]. The conducting substrate was set up as a working electrode and was located near the referential cathode at approximately 1cm. A potentio/galvanostat was used to keep a constant potential (-0.70 and -0.80 V) during the deposition. During the electrodeposition process four main growth variables- molarity ratios of solution, concentration of the solution, potential and modified surface of substrates have been controlled at a fixed time and temperature. The modified surface layer ZnO(002) of top of one substrate-ZnO(002)/ITO/ glass is made by reactive magnetron sputtering on ITO (indium tin oxide)/glass.

Scanning electron microscopy (SEM) images and quantitative elemental analysis were obtained by using a JSM 6300. The content ratio of elements in the film was obtained by means of Energy Dispersive X-ray Spectroscopy (EDX). For structural characterization it has been measured by an high-resolution X-ray diffraction (XRD) in the Θ-2Θ configuration with a copper anticathode (CuKα, 1.54 Å). Optical properties were monitored by transmittance using a Xe lamp and in association with a 500 mm Yvon–Jobin HR460 spectrophotometer using back-thinned CCD detector optimized for the UV–VIS range. Photoluminescences (PL) measurements were carried out at 6k-300k temperature using a He-Cd Laser as a light source at an excitation wavelength of 325 nm.

3. Results and Discussion

Generally electrochemical procedures permit the synthesis of ZnO films on different morphologies depending on the solute, concentrations of the solutions, temperature, PH value, and electrical potential, etc. Until now, these have been systematically investigated. In order to know that the variant morphologies of synthesised ZnO films depending on the surface of substrate, here the two kinds modified surfaces of substrates- thick ZnO(002)/ITO/glass and thin ZnO(002)/ITO/glass had been used in the electrochemical method.

Fig. 1 shows some SEM images of ZnO layers on thick ZnO(002)/ITO/glass substrates with a grow process in different deposition time from 100s to 1400 s.

The columnar structure, bundle of quasi column of ZnO predominantly normal to the substrate become dominant in different densities by adjusting the deposion condition with potential of –0.8 V (I:-0.3-1 mA) in Fig. 1(a) - (c).

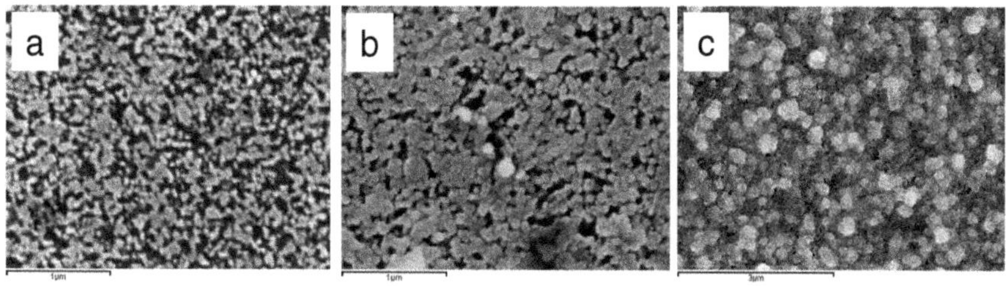

Fig. 1 SEM images of top ZnO film prepared by adjusting the potential and different deposition time on thick ZnO(002) /ITO/glass substrates. (a) –0.8 V, 100s, SEM: x40,0, scale: 1 micrometers; (b) –0.8 V, 500 s, SEM: x40,000, scale: 1 micrometers; (c) –0.8 V, 1400 s, SEM: x20,000; scale: 3 micrometers.

Fig. 2 shows two SEM images of ZnO layers on thin (50 nm) ZnO(002)/ITO/glass substrates with a grow process in different deposition time from 150s to 1400 s. The dominant flake structures with normal to the substrate (mark with #)and other angle appear eventually. There are a few of columnar structure, bundle of quasi column of ZnO (mark with *) by adjusting the deposion condition with potential of -0.7 V(I: -0.9-1.3 mA).

EDS analysis was selected in the photo of SEM. In its spectrum atomic percentage of O and Zn is 76.72% and 23.28% respectively. It indicates that there is larger intrinsic – Zinc vacancy (Vzn, Acceptors). The reason is (possibly) due to possibly the initial formation of an hydroxides in the solution, which would slowly dehydrates. In fact zinc hydroxide forms at room temperature by precipitation of Zn2+ by OH– addition [4], and it means and suggests that the film is Zn (OH)2 . This is why finally the zinc oxide film with Vzn forms and grows.

Generally it is realized that micro structure of ZnO film is of more functional and PL may gives much information about relation of the structure. There are various models being proposed to explain the complex PL band of ZnO materials. A strong PL emission peak at 370 nm is the intrinsic PL emission of ZnO crystallites due to the near band-edge emission (NBE). It had mostly been attributed to the radiative transition between electron (in conduction band) and hole (in valence band) recombination process, of course it corresponds to the bound exciton (BE). PL spectra of the ZnO thin films from the temperature of 6 k to 300 k were measured. Two broadening PL emissions at 350-440 nm and 471-770 nm, which belong to broader NBE and deep level emission (DLE) respectively, are observed.

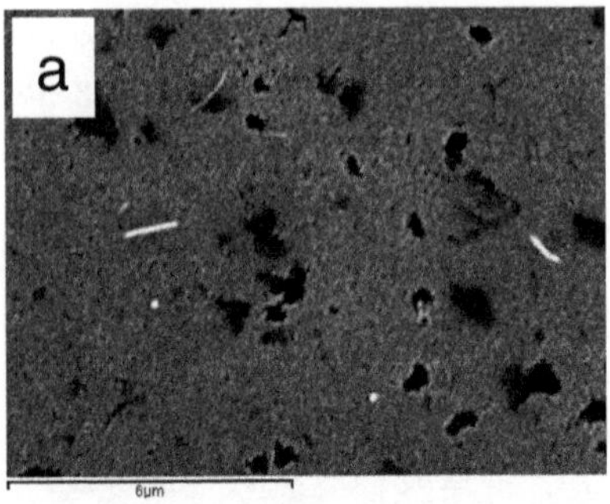

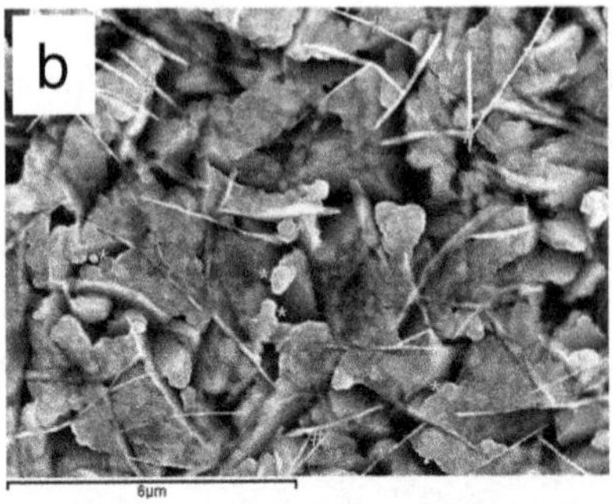

Fig. 2 SEM images of top ZnO film prepared by adjusting the potential and different deposition time on thin (50 nm) ZnO(002) /ITO/glass substrates. (a) –0.7 V, 150s, SEM: x,10,000, scale: 6 micrometers; (b) –0.7 V, 1400s, SEM: x,10,000; scale: 6 micrometers.

4. Conclusion

The ZnO on modified surfaces of substrates such as thick and thin ZnO(002) on ITO were prepared by the electrochemical method. We carried out the experiments by adjusting concentration of the solution, potential, substrate and deposition time. The combination of the effect of solution and potential on the growth of the film, the controlled aggregation structure of the column and flake top layer ZnO is obtained in the multilayer films-"ZnO-electrodeposition /ZnO(002)- sputtering /ITO/glass".

Acknowledgments

We acknowledge partial financial supports from Jointly Funded Project (No. 61179055) of Chinese Civil Aviation Authority and National Natural Science Foundation of China, Talent Grant (2013-ZQXY-05) of Educational Commission of Guangdong Province, China.

References

1. T. Pauporté, R. Cortès, M. Froment, B. Beaumont, D. Lincot, Chem. Mater. 14 (2002) 4702.
2. Zhifeng Liu, Zhengguo Jin, Jijun Qiu, Xiaoxin Liu, Weibing Wu and Wei Li, Preparation and characteristics of ordered porous ZnO films by a electrodeposition method using PS array templates, Semicond. Sci. Technol. 21 No 1 (January 2006) 60-66.
3. M. Tortosa, M. Mollar, B. Marí, Journal of Crystal Growth 304, 97 (2007) 97-102.
4. G. Deroubaix, P. Marcus, Surf. Interf. Anal.18 (1992) 39.

A Study of Duplex Melting Process with Blast and Medium Frequency Furnaces in the Production of Cast Iron*

Chen Xiang†, Zhou Wenwu and Li Yanxiang
School of Materials Science and Engineering, Tsinghua University
Beijing 100084, China
†*E-mail: xchen@tsinghua.edu.cn*

The differences of two melting process, which are conventional medium frequency furnace melting and duplex melting with blast and medium frequency furnaces have been investigated. It is shown that the short-cut duplex melting process resulted in higher undercooling of the iron melt, more undercooled graphite in the microstructure, higher tensile strength and hardness worsening the machinability depending on different conditions. Modification of composition, the carbon content in this study, and enhancing inoculation can eliminate the adverse influence of changing the melting process.

Keywords: Gray cast iron; melt iron quality; blast-induction duplex melting.

1. Introduction

In the conventional foundry, firstly, blast furnace liquid iron melt is poured to form pig iron and then heated again in the melting furnace such as cupola or induction furnaces. During the process, the latent heat of blast furnace iron melt is wasted in vain. Duplex melting process with blast and medium frequency furnaces has many advantages such as energy saving, high temperature, easy adjustment of composition, homogeneous ingredient, environment friendliness et al [1]. The duplex melting process will bring large magnitude of energy, economy and environment benefits and will be named short-cut melting process in the later context.

However, in cast iron especially for grey iron, the melt quality depends on the method in which it is obtained and the charge materials used [2]. Although there have already been some applications in practice [3-5], the shortcut melting process is limited to the production of high output volume common castings and there are a few studies on the influence of this process on the melt quality. To the best of the authors' knowledge, there has been no systematic investigation of

* This work is supported by National Science & Technology Major Project of China (No. 2012ZX04010-031).

the short-cut melting process with blast furnace and medium frequency furnace. In the present study, the influence of blast furnace liquid iron instead of pig iron, and the quantitative measurement and how to adjust the adverse effect has been researched quantitatively or qualitatively.

2. Experimental Procedure

This study has been executed for two stages. In the first stage, the data, including chemical compositions, thermal analysis curves and samples before and after inoculation, test bars et al, were collected as comparative standard with the conventional medium frequency furnace melting process, which is ongoing before the project is start. Then in the second stage, substituting liquid blast furnace iron for pig iron, the short-cut melting process trials were executed, with the same melting method and composition control target, and the real products were cast.

The charges have been prepared with pig iron or blast furnace iron melt, steel scrap, return, electrode graphite, ferro-silicon. The burdens for each product and each process are listed in Table 1. When the metal was totally molten and the temperature is higher than 1400℃, a sample was taken for chemical analysis by emission spectrometry and C-S analyzer. When needed, corrections were made just before the molten metal was superheated and hold for 10 minutes.

Before tapping and inoculation, a thermal analysis sample was poured. Inoculation was executed at the tapping spout. During operation, the dumpling of inoculant starts when the pouring ladle is filled 30% in weight and ends before the ladle is filled 80%. Just before the first ladle of iron melt was poured into the green sand mould, final chemical composition sample, thermal analysis heat and cylindrical test bar were poured.

Table 1 Experiment parameters for conventional and short-cut process.

	Steel scrap (Kg)	Return (Kg)	Pig iron (Kg)	Superheating temperature (℃)	Inoculant
Conventional	1650	2200	1650	1490-1510	FeSi0.4%BaSi0.1%
Short-cut	1500	1500	2000	1490-1510	FeSi0.4%BaSi0.1%

A self-developed quality measurement system for liquid metal [6] was used to record the thermal analysis curves before and after inoculation. Temperature was measured with a K-type thermocouple mounted in the thermal analysis sample cup of 30mm in diameter and 50mm in height. The acquiring speed of temperature is 5 readings per second. The thermal analysis operation consisted of sampling the iron with refractory spoon, getting ready and pouring into the cup rapidly when the oxide film is observed.

3. Results and discussion

3.1. *Results and discussion*

The resulting thermal analysis data was smoothed and the freezing zone, which from the start of solidification TL to the end of solidification TS, is intercepted automatically by the self-programmed software [7-9]. The final chemical analysis results are listed in Table 2 and the thermal analysis freezing zone curves collected for the conventional and short-cut melting process are shown in Fig. 1.

Table 2 Composition of the castings.

Element	Conventional & Short-cut	Short-cut after modification	σ
C	3.40	3.45	±0.05
Si	1.97	1.97	±0.05
Mn	0.69	0.69	±0.03
P	0.059	0.059	±0.009
S	0.060	0.060	±0.010
Cr	0.18	0.18	±0.04
Cu	0.46	0.46	±0.04
CE	4.01	4.06	±0.07

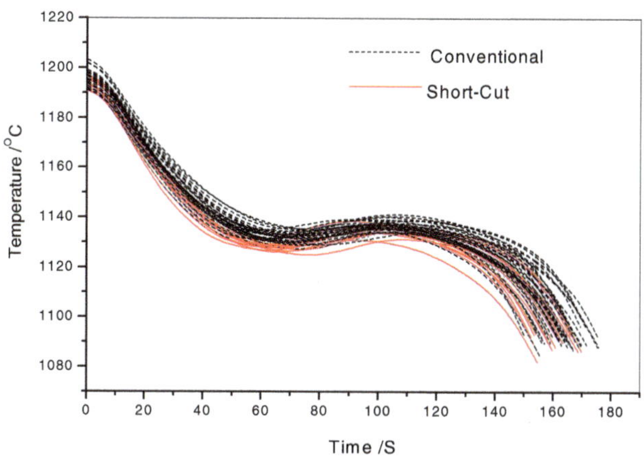

Fig. 1 Thermal analysis curves before inoculation for conventional and short-cut melting process.

It can be observed from Fig. 1 that, within the present set of experimental conditions, there is a trend of descending in the lowest eutectic temperature and shortening in the solidification time for short-cut melting process cast iron melt.

Therefore, it can be concluded that submitting blast furnace iron for pig iron will reduce the nucleation potential and aggravate the eutectic undercooling.

The test bars were machined to 20mm in diameter for tensile strength and hardness measurement, as well as metallographic examination. Fig. 2 shows the tensile strength and Brinell hardness obtained from the test bars for the trial furnaces. It can be calculated that the tensile strength increase about 4%, as well as the Brinell hardness increase about 9%.

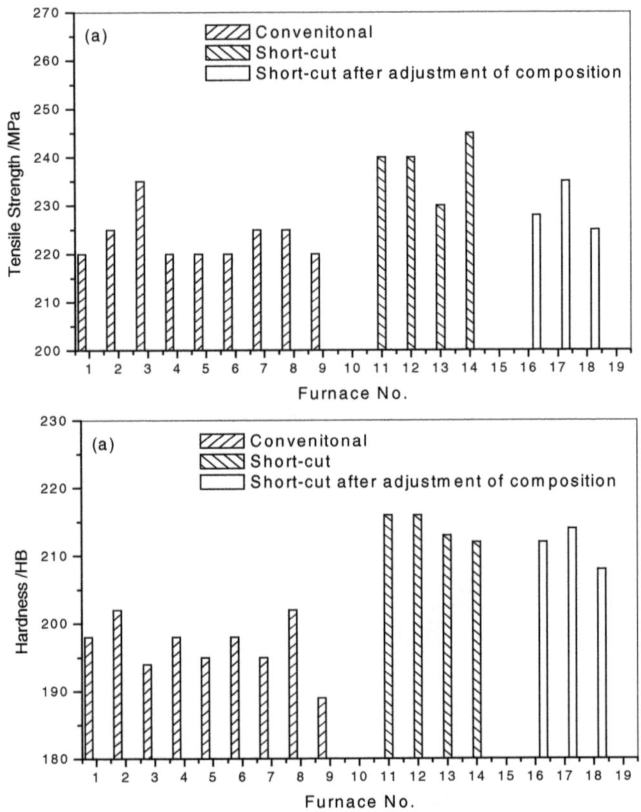

Fig. 2 Mechanical properties of test bars, a) Tensile strength, b) Brinell hardness.

The typical micrographs for two kinds of melting process in Fig. 3a and 3b illustrate the variation of graphite distribution in test bars. When the conventional melting process is used, the solidification structures are mainly randomly distributed A-type flake graphite, and the probability of undercooled graphite is little. While, with the short-cut process, the graphite structures are refined, but more undercooled graphites such as D or E-type graphite appear.

The microstructures can explain well the mechanical properties variation and the thermal analysis result.

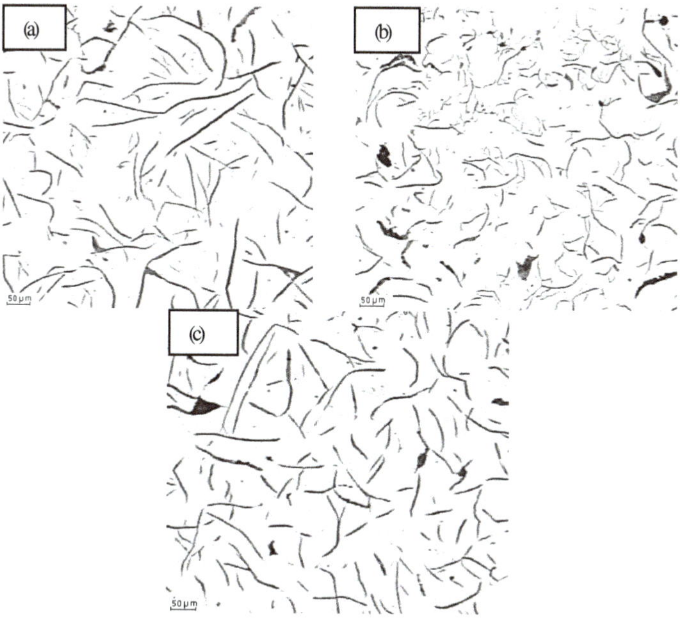

Fig. 3 Solidified structures of test bars for conventional and short-cut processes, a) conventional process, b) short-cut process, c) short-cut after modification of composition.

3.2. *Modifications in chemical composition*

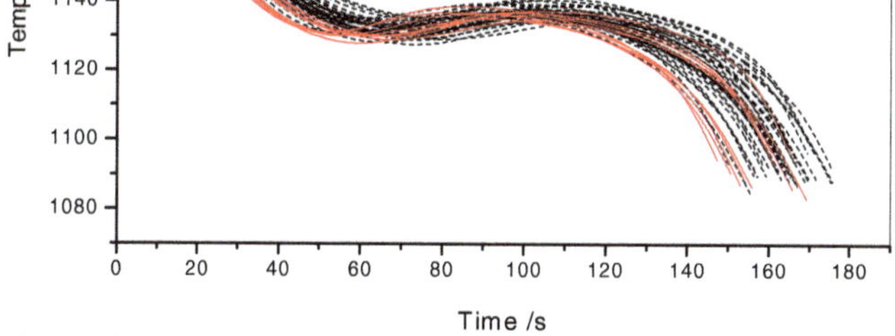

Fig. 4 Thermal analysis curves before inoculation for conventional and short-cut after modification of composition.

The increase of tensile strength is satisfying, however the problem originating in machining can be important when the increase of hardness is considerable. Therefore, it is necessary, for short-cut process, to make some adjustment so that the final result will be the same as the conventional process. In order to do this, the carbon content is increased about 0.05% (Table 2) keeping other elements unchanged and another 3 furnaces with short-cut process were executed. The relative results of thermal analysis, solidification microstructures and mechanical properties are given in Fig. 4, Fig. 3c and Fig. 2. It can be observed that, the eutectic nucleation ability is improved and the hardness decreased. According to the present results, it appears that, further increase of CE is needed to restore the mechanical properties as conventional process.

3.3. *Enhancing inoculation*

Inoculation is a most important method to control the melt quality in the foundry floor [10]. In order to eliminate the effect of submitting blast furnace for pig iron, enhancing inoculation from 0.1%BaSi to 0.35%BaSi is executed during this stage in stead of modification of chemical composition. Fig. 5 gives the inoculated thermal analysis curves collected before and after the measure is taken. It can be observed that, the nucleation ability is improved and even overrun the conventional ones. The mechanical properties collected are demonstrated in Fig. 6. It is calculated that tensile strength and hardness are both decreased to the level as conventional melting process.

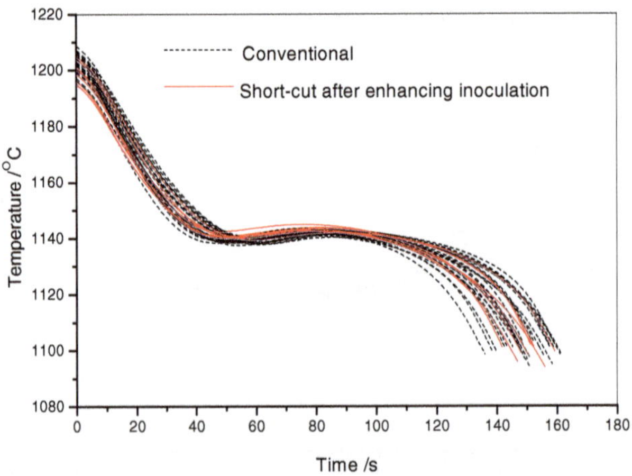

Fig. 5 Thermal analysis curves after inoculation for conventional and short-cut after enhancing inoculation.

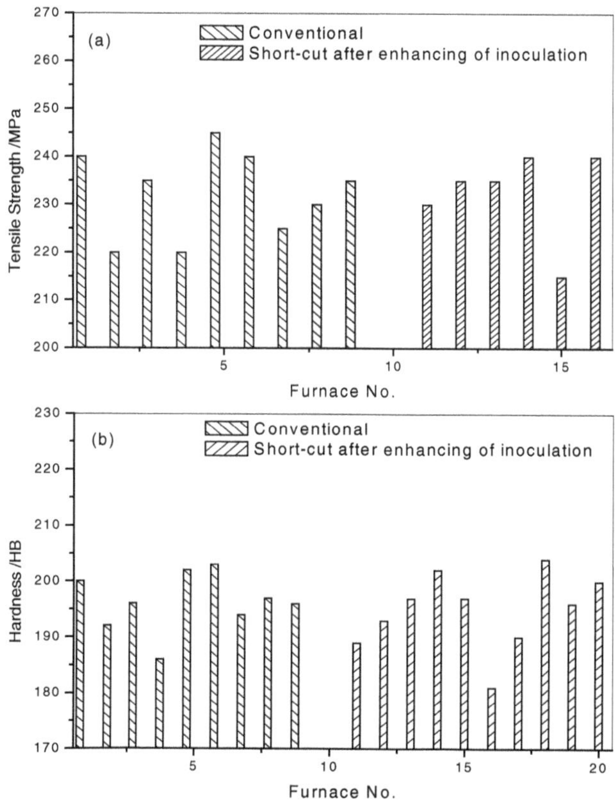

Fig. 6 Mechanical properties of test bars, a) Tensile strength, b) Brinell hardness.

3.4. *Discussion*

The results obtained from the two stages of experiments, are good exemplification of a hypothesis that the metal quality depends on the method in which it is obtained and the charge materials. The usage of blast furnace liquid iron in the production of casting has the potential of increasing the tensile strength and hardness to various extents depending on the charge and product. This phenomenon can be explained as follows.

On one hand, the number of heterogeneous nucleus may be smaller for short-cut iron melt. When the blast furnace liquid melt solidify to form pig iron, large quantity of bulk graphite, carbide and compound et al will come into being. After pig iron is melted again, these kinds of structures can be preserved to a certain extent because of dynamic reasons and exist in the form of unmelted crystalline graphite, clusters of carbon or Fe_3C, compound with high melting point et al. During later solidification, these micro structures can act as nucleus of primary and eutectic phase transformation. However, with the short-cut melting process, the favorable heredity of the pig iron as a component of the charge is absent. On the other hand, blast furnace liquid iron as part of the charge is hold in the medium frequency furnace with the state of high temperature over the melting point for enough time that the elements can disperse. Therefore, the distribution of element such as carbon and silicon may be more uniform in the micro scale for short-cut iron melt and less fluctuation of composition suppress nucleation and growth of graphite. At the same time, the good diffusivity of the added alloy makes low resistance of inoculation fading. Above analysis can be validated by the eutectic cell structures (Fig. 7) obtained from the thermal analysis sample before inoculation.

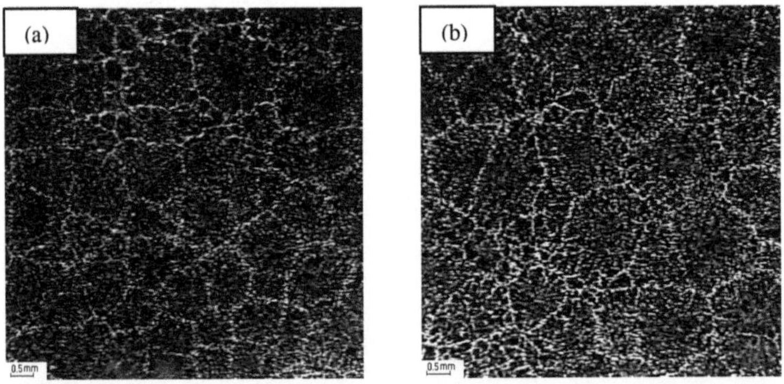

Fig. 7 Eutectic cells of solidified structures of conventional and short-cut processes, a) conventional, b) short-cut.

This study also shows that the adverse problems with the duplex short-cut melting process with blast and medium frequency furnaces can be resolved by modification of composition or enhancing inoculation. When the CE or inoculant is increased, the degree of activity of carbon in the iron melt is intensified, causing the precipitation of the graphite to start at higher temperature. Higher presence of graphite contributes to the decrease of hardness and better machinability.

4. Conclusions

Through the trial production on two products, the following conclusion can be made that the degree of undercooling increases when blast furnace liquid melt (with almost the same percentage with pig iron) is used instead of pig iron, remaining other parameter constant, accordingly, the microstructure deteriorate and the tensile strength and Brinell hardness increase dependently.

In the present study, two measures, which are modification of chemical composition and enhancing inoculation, were taken to eliminate the adverse influence of changing the melting process. It is validated that both the measures are effective.

References

1. X. J. Sun, Y. X. Li, X. Y. Wang, Analysis of cast iron production by duplex melting of blast and medium-frequency induction furnaces, *China Foundry Machinery Technol,* **2**, 1 (2005).
2. R. Sillén, R. Lisell, Optimization of Inoculation Practice by means of Thermal Analysis, http://www.novacast.se
3. V. A. Kurganov and V. V. Lesovoi, Casting ingot moulds from liquid blast-furnace instead of cupola iron in the general foundries of metallurgical works, *Steel in the USSR*, **5**, 546 (1975).
4. V. I. Sorokin, G. Y. Evseev and N. D. Kurochkina, Delivery and processing liquid blast furnace cast iron in machine-building works, *Liteinoe Proizvodstvo*, **4–5**, 14 (1995).
5. O. A. Pozhidaev and V. G. Grushevskij, Use of liquid blast furnace iron in iron foundries, *Liteinoe Proizvodstvo*, **4**, 8 (1998).
6. X. R. Xu, Intelligent Recognition of Thermal Analysis Cooling Curves and Evaluation of Melt Iron Quality, Master's thesis, Tsinghua University (2001).
7. Y. X. Li, X. R. Xu, Q. Wang and B. C. Liu, Evaluating Melt Iron Features by Computer Aided Recognition of Thermal Analysis Cooling Curves, *Inter. J. Cast Metals Research*, **16**, 42 (2003).
8. X. J. Sun, Y. X. Li, X. Chen, Identification and evaluation of modification level for compacted graphite cast iron, *J. Mater Process Technol*, **200**, 471 (2008).
9. X. Chen, H. Y. Geng, Y. X. Li, Study on the eutectic modification level of Al-7Si Alloy by computer aided recognition of thermal analysis cooling curves, *Mater Sci Eng, A* **419**, 283 (2006).
10. C. Q. Wang, *Inoculation Theory and Practice for Cast Iron*, 1st edn. (Tianjin University Press, Tianjing, 1991).

WPF-Based TFT-LCD Substrate Glass Measurement and Data Processing System

Guo Hua
Xi'an University of Technology
Xi'an Shaanxi, 710048, China
guohua@xaut.edu.cn

This paper presents a WPF – based TFT-LCD substrate glass measurement system, which utilizes the .NET's WPF technology to integrate the CNC control, data acquisition, Matlab data processing, SQL database and Office report forms in a complete special software system.

Keywords: Windows Presentation Foundation (WPF), TFT substrate glass, measurement.

1. Overview

With the development of electronic industry, the flat panel display products are showing a tremendous growth potential. As the upstream product of flat panel display industry chain, the demand of TFT-LCD ultra-thin glass substrate is particularly great. In the ultra thin glass substrate production line, the quality control is an essential link, the main measurement parameters are the glass thickness and warpage, which are also the main process parameters in the production process of ultra-thin glass substrate. The accurate measurement of ultra-thin glass substrate is an industrial problem, because it is large in area, extremely light and thin, and the measurement accuracy requirement is very high. The traditionalthin glass measurement uses the manual contact measurement method, featuring poor precision and low efficiency. This paper presents a special measuring instrument that utilizes a high- precision optical sensor and high- precision mechanical platform, combined with the software control, to make automatic measurement to the ultra-thin glass substrate.

This measurement system adopts the new WPF technology developed by the Microsoft Corporation to integrate the system control, data acquisition, data processing, database and reporting system and provide the users with a friendly interface of simple operation and convenient to use. The WPF (Windows Presentation Foundation) is one integral part of the NET Framework 3.0 launched by the USA Microsoft Corp, which is a development framework on the presentation layer based on the XML, NET Framework and vector drawing (vector graphic) technologies, regarded by the Microsoft as the next generation user interface technology to be widely used to the interface development in the next generation of Windows platform (Windows Vista). The WPF uses a new XAML (eXtensible Application Markup Language) language to develop interface, this shall well separate the interface development from the background logic to reduce the coupling degree, so that the user interface designer can have a better cooperation with the program developer to reduce the cost of maintenance and update. Based on the XAML and JavaScript, it can cross various platforms to integrate the CNC control, Matlab data processing and Excel reporting system into one body.

2. Measurement System

The main measurement parameters of TFT glass are of the glass thickness and warpage, these two parameters can directly affect the quality of glass and even the subsequent liquid crystal panel. The variation in the TFT glass thickness is particularly critical.

In the current production line in China, the glass thickness, including the average thickness and variation in the thickness in both the flow and non flow directions, is mostly measured by a digital micrometer to get the multipoint thickness value on the glass edge from the manual measurement, and manually work out the average thickness and the variation in thickness in the different directions. The shortcomings of this method are obvious, firstly, the difference of readings from different inspection personnel is larger, the measuring speed is slow, and it is difficult to get the thickness value of most part of glass. With the development of ultra-thin glass substrate towards the trend of new generation, the glass area is becoming larger and larger that it is more and more difficult for the thickness parameter of the edge part to reflect the thickness condition of the whole plate.

With the continuous development of modern science and technology, new measuring instruments and equipment with different principles instead of the micrometer in the glass thickness measurement field are studied, such as the ultrasonic thickness gauge, capacitance thickness gauge and various optical thickness gauges.

The prime advantage of the optical measurement method is of its non-contact nature, which can avoid the precision loss and probe damage problems, and can be used in some measuring sites where environment is relatively bad. The triangle method combined with the CCD detection technology is the most typical reflection type measurement method, it uses the reflected light beam from the top and bottom surfaces of glass under test to measure the glass thickness by the offset distance of the beam [1]. A improved method that uses the double laser sources symmetrically distributed on both sides of the normal line to reduce the measurement errors and improve the resolution by way of double light path compensation method [2]. It is also adopted the CCD-based displacement sensor to measure the displacement of top and bottom glass surfaces simultaneously to work out the glass thickness [3]. In addition, some researchers have proposed to use the circular interference fringe width of the glass to measure the glass thickness [4], as well as apply the low phase interference system to measure the glass thickness [5]. In recent years, some researchers have proposed an on-line glass thickness measurement method by application of laser heterodyne combined with the Doppler technique, to modulate the glass thickness information onto the phase difference and the frequency difference simultaneously, which is one of the main methods for accurate measurement of glass thickness. The conoscopic holography is a special engineering application of crystal optics in the polarized light interference process. The measurement system based on this method is a kind of common optical path measuring system, the advantages of this system are that the interference immunity is good, the operation is stable, efficient, and not affected by the surface properties of surface to be measured [6-8]. The Israel Scan Direct Company adopts has adopted the principle of conoscopic polarizer interference to have realized the high precision displacement measurement, the series sensor they developed for measuring distance, profile and thickness and measure the transparent surface with specula reflection, such as the glass, silicon wafer, wet coating, liquid surface and mirror surface [9]. The Germany Micro Epsilon Company adopts the spectral-confocal measurement principle, by using the special optical lens and through the catadioptric and spectral analysis of optical mechanism, to work out the changes in displacement from the reference surface to the target surface. This principle can also measure both the distance and displacement simultaneously. Of the sensor with measuring range to be 1mm, its initial measuring distance is 10mm, the measurement precision is 1.5μm, the working angle is ± 27°, the measuring speed is ranged from 100 Hz to 2000 Hz.

The spectral-confocal displacement sensor is developed based on in the confocal microscopy according the principle of spectral-confocal measurement. Its light source is not a single frequency laser, but the polychromatic light, after emitted, the polychromatic light shall go through the fiber coupler, after strict chromatic aberration correction through the lens system in the optical system, radiate the beam onto the surface to be measured to produce a spectral dispersion due to the action of color difference, forming a series of focus discrete in space. The monochromatic light focused on the object measured is reflected back to reach the sensor controller through optical fiber coupler, you can determine the frequency of the monochromatic light through the spectral analysis by spectrometer, as each frequency corresponds to a distance value, so the displacement can be reckoned by the frequency so detected. The distance values corresponding to the different spectra are calibrated before delivered at the factory, so that you can accurately measure out the distance from the optical probe to the surface of object to be measured, of course, the refraction coefficient of the object to be measured can be substituted into the distance value in the calibration process.

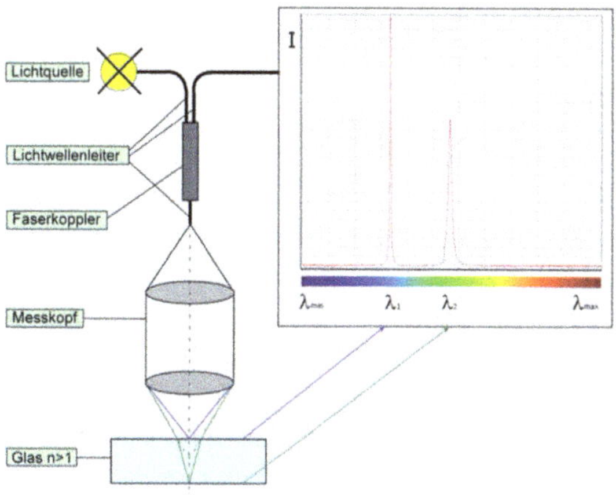

Fig. 1 Spectral-confocal measurement principle.

Based on the optical principle of such special structure design, the spectral-confocal sensor has a higher accuracy in the displacement and thickness measurement. It can also measure the transparent or translucent workpiece with thin coating, as the light of different frequencies is reflected from the contact surface of different materials, therefore we can analyze on the distribution of spectrum detected by spectrometer to determine the thickness of each material layer through detecting wavelength corresponding to each wave crest.

Through the comprehensive analysis and evaluation, the TFT substrate glass has adopted the spectral-confocal optical measurement sensor to have realized the non-contact, high precision and high speed measurement on the TFT glass thickness and warpage.

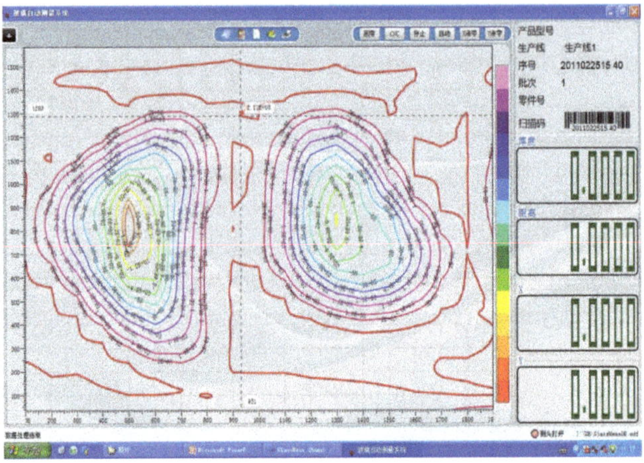

Fig. 2 Main interface of control system.

3. System Software Design

The whole software for the measurement system under this topic was developed by the VS2012 platform on the Windows platform. Of the language developed as the NET application, its grammar is concise, which adopts the object oriented design and carried out the error management by throwing and catching the exception object just like the Java. It can realize the expansibility control of instrument system and establish a beautiful, user friendly and powerful man-machine interface. At the same time it can be closely integrated with Web to provide the possibility for the establishment of measurement data analysis and processing LAN later.

The system software is composed of the following elements: the module for measurement path control, data processing and database management, the module for software interface design, the module for data processing by Matlab and measurement reporting module. The database management module is to store all the data measured in the SQL database for management and further processing. The software interface design module is used to design the interface appearance, using the WPF to conduct the interface rendering and design, and unified user interface UI. The Matlab is used for data processing, to call the Matlab engine through the .NET's platform invoke technology and data encapsulation technology, and hand over a lot of data processing, statistics and the error compensation workload to the Matlab software for execution, the results of such processing shall be sent back to software user terminal. This module can realize the error compensation of mechanical system, error compensation of geometric sense, error compensation of probe and environment compensation, at the same time it has still completed the basic operations of data statistics and measurement data processing work. The measurement data dynamic display and measurement chart module has realized the dynamic display of measuring position and result on the user terminal of software in the measuring process, as well as the display of measurement result icon on the software interface. The measurement reporting module shall generate the measurement report by calling the Office software.

4. WPF-Based Platform Invoke Technology

In the measurement system software design of this topic, as it is to use the Matlab, Excel and other mature software tools, at the same time, certain design of program is to be realized through the VC++ programming environment, therefore, the C# .Net-based platform invoke technology is particularly important.

As a mature and object oriented development language, the C++ has the extremely widespread application in the control field, both the control system and measuring sensor have provided the users with a set of C++ based development package, provided the application programming interface or a static library. You can not use the static library or the VC's .h headed files in the C#, in order to build a bridge in C# and VC, you need to add a new type into the C# solution, this new type can both contain the contents in the VC language you called and also can generate a dynamic link library, to be called by the C# main program. It shall generate a project in the solution of the C# program. This project can contain the VC static library and header files, when set up separately, it can generate a dynamic link library file that can be used by the C#.

In the measurement software under this topic, a lot of data are expected to be processed by the powerful Matlab software. It is recommended by the Matlab to use the COM (Component Object Model) to realize the interface between the Matlab and development environment. Matlab supports the transfer of the Matlab function needed into the generated components with its own COM Builder function. This method has the defect that the data types are incompatible, and some Matlab function can not be realized. Some scholars proposed to solve this problem by the .NET's platform invoke technology and data encapsulation technology [4-6]. When the C# .Net common language is used to run the platform invoke function of the library (CLR), it shall allow the managed code to call the unmanaged functions realized in the dynamic link library. In this case, the function of .NET's data encapsulation technology actually serves as an interacting channel between the managed interface and unmanaged interface.

5. Data Processing

In the measuring process of ultra-thin glass substrate, due to the vibration of mechanical platform, the changes in the power supply voltage of power network or the external electromagnetic or optical interference or other factors, there shall have noise appeared in the measurement data from the sensor, which can generate the errors for the parameter assessment. After a computer has obtained the original measurement data, it is necessary to conduct the related processing to the data to eliminate the errors, so as to make accurate evaluation on the parameters of glass substrate. This system adopts multiple data processing methods, uses the powerful data processing functions of Matlab to realize the measurement data processing and error evaluation. The sampling-data by this measurement system can be regarded as a discrete digital signal of equal time intervals. In theory, the measurement data should be a group of low frequency signal or more stable signal, as the high frequency interference can not be avoided in the industrial field so that the sampling data are mixed with some high frequency noise, which cannot be eliminated by way of preprocessing. In this paper the digital filter technology for digital signal processing is used to make further processing to the measurement data.

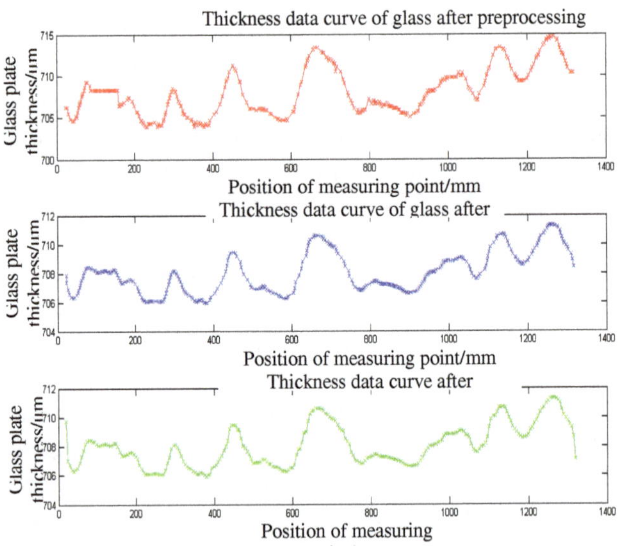

Fig. 3 Curve graph for the data processed by the filter interpolation.

As for the measurement data under this topic, in order to eliminate the noise signal mixed in the one dimensional measurement data, a digital low-pass filter can be added for the purpose of filtering. This method is realized by Matlab software. In order to represent the changes in measurement data before and after processing in a more clear manner, A group of measured data as an example to make the correlation analysis has been done. Figure 3 shows the changes in measurement data before and after processing

We first select a simple and ideal standard low-pass filter to make the low pass filter processing on the preprocessed data. The main codes are as follows:

```
Xs=fft(Y1);Y1 is the preprocessed dataindd2=40:346;
Xs(indd2)=zeros(size(indd2));
xd1=ifft(Xs);xd1=real(xd1);
plot(xd1);
disp(xd1);
```

After the noise in signal is suppressed by the digital filter, the spline interpolation algorithm shall be used to output a data point by the preset step length into the data after filtering for interpolation, using the spline function of Matlab toolbox. The graphs for the data after filter interpolation processing are shown in Figure 3.

It can be seen through the comparison of graphs that, after processed through the low pass filter, the thickness curve drawn by the discrete measuring points has become more smooth, this shows that the high frequency interference in discrete data has been eliminated.

The thickness measurement in both the flow and non flow directions

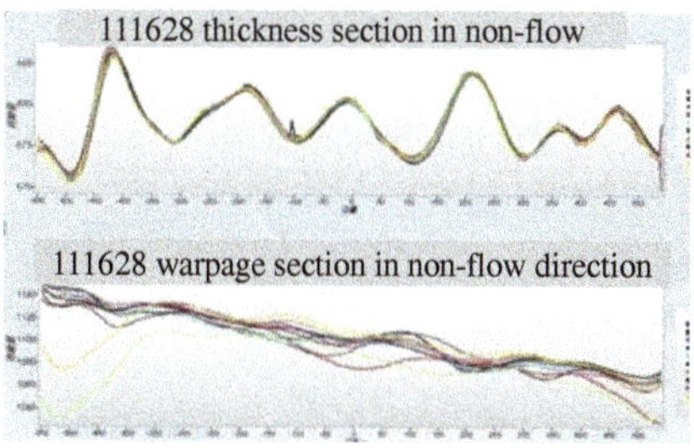

Fig. 4 Data reporting curve for the warpage of whole plate.

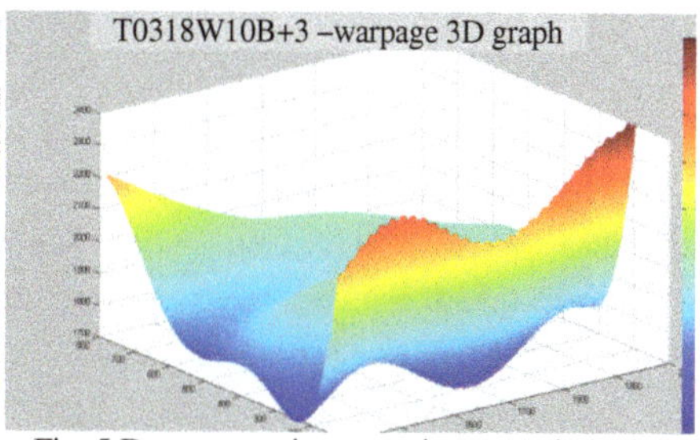

Fig. 5 Data processing reporting curve in both the flow and non-flow directions.

6. Conclusions

The WPF-based TFT substrate glass data acquisition and processing system introduced in this paper uses the WPF as the platform to integrate the control, data processing, report form and operation interface in one body in a organic manner, to have realized the TFT-LCD digital measurement system of ultra-thin glass substrate parameters, which is a new measurement scheme. This system has been successfully applied in practice. It is proved that the system framework, all the working modules, the system data communication and management are correct. It can be used in the similar systems. You can also use the TFT substrate measuring instrument as an intelligent data acquisition front end, to form a complete TFT glass digital measurement and quality control system together with other measuring instruments and equipment through the network.

References

1. Liu Lishuang, Zhang Yao, Lu Huiqing, et al. The CCD-based glass thickness online detection system [J]. Chinese Journal of Sensors and Actuators, 2006, 19(3): 652-654.
2. Wang Yutian, Yang Ni. The glass thickness measurement technology by double light path compensation method [J]. Chinese Journal of Sensors and Actuators, 2007, 20(6): 1428-1431.
3. Wang Wei, Wang Zhaoba. Study on the properties of CCD-based displacement sensor in the glass thickness measurement [J]. Instrument technique and sensor, 2006, 9: 44-45.
4. Kathrynj W, Richard R C, Gun Young-Lee. Quantitative in situ measurement of transfer film thickness by a Newton's rings method [J]. Article in Press, 2007, 10(4): 6-56.
5. Maru Yama H, Inoue S, Mitsu Yama T, et al. Low-coherence interferometer system for the simultaneous measurement of refractive index and thickness [J]. Appl Opt, 2001, 41(3): 1315-1322.
6. Li Yanchao, Zhang Liang, Yang Yanling, et al. The high-precision measurement of glass thickness by multi-beam laser heterodyne [J]. Chinese Physics, 2009, 58(08): 5478-5478.
7. Xie Wenjun, Lv Cen, Song Chen. Laser heterodyne Doppler second harmonic thickness measurement method [J]. Computer Measurement and Control, 2010, 18(8): 1721-1723.
8. Sirat Gabriel Y., Paz Freddy, Agronk Gregory, Wilner Kalman. Conoscopic holography SPIE of the International Society for Optical Engineering [J], USA, 2005, 5972: 021-026.
9. Scan Direct Ltd. NanoConoProbe Technic Parameter Sheet. Scan Direct Ltd.

Author Index

Lightning Source UK Ltd.
Milton Keynes UK
UKHW020730200220
359040UK00001B/1

9 789814 651004